MASTER TECHNIQUES IN ORTHOPAEDIC SURGERY

■

THE HAND

Second Edition

MASTER TECHNIQUES IN ORTHOPAEDIC SURGERY

■

Editor-in-Chief
Bernard F. Morrey, M.D.

Volume Editors

THE HAND
James Strickland, M.D.
Thomas Graham, M.D.

RECONSTRUCTIVE KNEE SURGERY
Douglas W. Jackson, M.D.

KNEE ARTHROPLASTY
Paul A. Lotke, M.D.
Jess H. Lonner, M.D.

THE HIP
Clement B. Sledge, M.D.

THE SPINE
David S. Bradford, M.D.
Thomas L. Zdeblick, M.D.

THE SHOULDER
Edward V. Craig, M.D.

THE WRIST
Richard H. Gelberman, M.D.

THE ELBOW
Bernard F. Morrey, M.D.

FRACTURES
Donald A. Wiss, M.D.

THE FOOT & ANKLE
Harold B. Kitaoka, M.D.

THE HAND

Second Edition

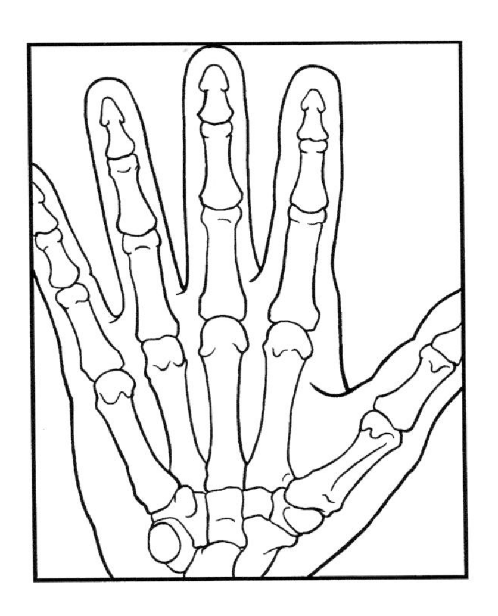

Editors

JAMES W. STRICKLAND, M.D.
Reconstructive Hand Surgeons of Indiana
Carmel, Indiana
Clinical Professor of Orthopaedic Surgery
Indiana University School of Medicine
Indianapolis, Indiana

THOMAS GRAHAM, M.D.
Chief
The Curtis National Hand Center
Vice-Chairman
Department of Orthopaedic Surgery
Decker Orthopaedic Institute
Union Memorial Hospital
Baltimore, Maryland

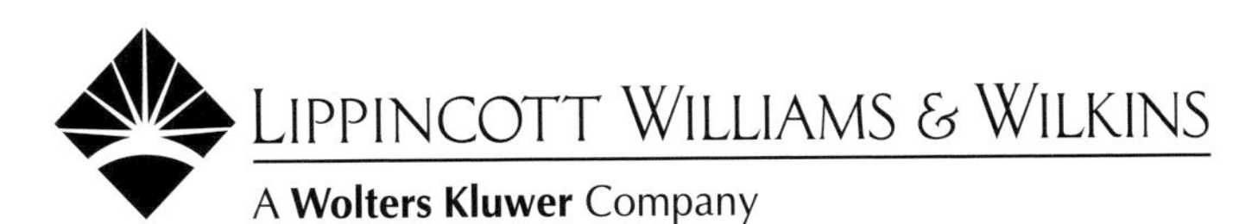
LIPPINCOTT WILLIAMS & WILKINS
A **Wolters Kluwer** Company
Philadelphia • Baltimore • New York • London
Buenos Aires • Hong Kong • Sydney • Tokyo

Acquisitions Editor: Robert Hurley
Developmental Editor: Stacey L. Sebring
Marketing Director: Sharon R. Zinner
Project Manager: Bridgett Dougherty
Manufacturing Manager: Ben Riviera
Production Services: Maryland Composition
Printer: Quebecor-Kingsport

530 Walnut Street
Philadelphia, Pennsylvania 19106 USA

351 West Camden Street
Baltimore, Maryland 21201-2436 USA

The publisher is not responsible (as a matter of product liability, negligence or otherwise) for an injury resulting from any material contained herein. This publication contains information relating to general principles of medical care which should not be constructed as specific instruction for individual patients. Manufacturer's product information should be reviewed for current information, including contraindications, dosages, and precautions.

Printed in the United States of America

Library of Congress Cataloging-in-Publication Data
The hand / editors, James W. Strickland, Thomas J. Graham.—2nd ed.
p. ; cm.—(Master techniques in orthopaedic surgery)
Includes bibliographical references and index.
ISBN 0-7817-4080-0
1. Hand—Surgery. I. Strickland, James W., 1936- II. Graham, Thomas J. III. Series: Master techniques in orthopaedic surgery (2nd ed.)
[DNLM: 1. Hand—surgery. 2. Hand Deformities—surgery. 3. Hand Injuries—surgery. WE 830 H23062 2005]
RD559.H3572 2005
617.5′75059—dc22

2004020877

The publishers have made every effort to trace copyright holders for borrowed material. If they have inadvertently overlooked any, they will be pleased to make the necessary arrangements at the first opportunity.

To purchase additional copies of this book, call our customer service department at (800) 638-3030 or fax orders to (301) 824-7390. For other book services, including chapter reprints and large quantity sales, ask for the Special Sales department.

For all other calls originating outside of the United States, please call (301) 714-2324.

Visit Lippincott Williams & Wilkins on the Internet: http://www.lww.com. Lippincott Williams & Wilkins customer service representatives are available from 8:30 am to 6:30 pm, EST, Monday through Friday, for telephone access.

10 9 8 7 6 5 4 3 2

I am honored to be a part of two winning teams.

Professionally—my partners, fellows and staff at the Curtis National Hand Center are the epitome of professionalism and collegiality. It is humbling to be a part of one of the greatest lineages in hand surgery and to be entrusted with the care of our patients and the training of those who will perpetuate our specialty.

Personally—my wife, CeCe, and my daughters, Margaret and Elizabeth, have made untold sacrifices without complaint or criticism. Ironically, my patients and students will never recognize the contributions they have made to many . . . but I do.

TJG

To my dad
James DeMotte Strickland
1909–1997
My hero, my inspiration, my best friend

JWS

■

TABLE OF CONTENTS

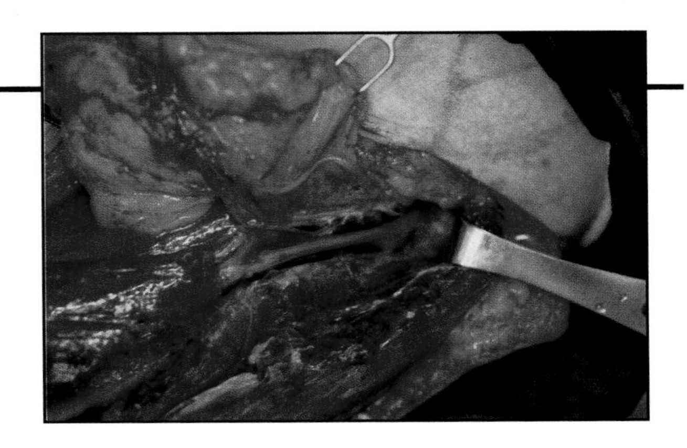

CONTRIBUTORS

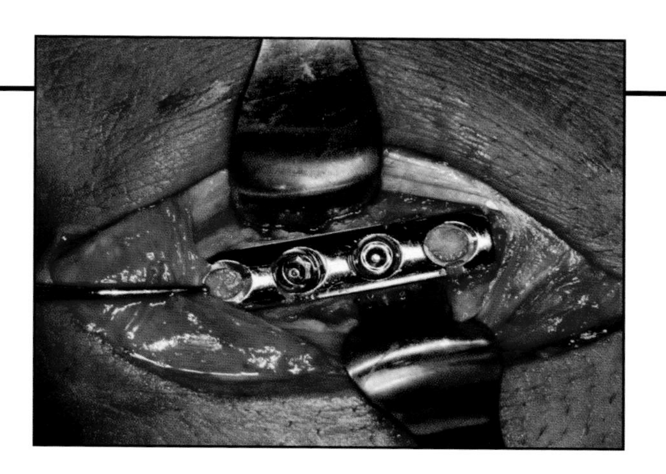

J. Robert Anderson, M.D.
Resident, Department of Orthopaedic Surgery, George Washington School of Medicine, Washington, DC

Donald S. Bae, M.D.
Instructor in Orthopaedic Surgery, Harvard Medical School, Boston, Massachusetts; Department of Orthopaedic Surgery, Children's Hospital Boston, Boston, Massachusetts

Richard W. Barth, M.D.
Assistant Clinical Professor, George Washington School of Medicine, Georgetown University School of Medicine, Washington, DC

Martin I. Boyer, M.D.
Department of Orthopaedic Surgery, Washington University School of Medicine, St. Louis, Missouri

John F. Dalton IV, M.D.
Department of Orthopaedic Surgery, Emory University, Atlanta, Georgia

Nickolaos A. Darlis, M.D., Ph.D.
Fellow, Upper Extremity Surgery, Department of Orthopaedic Surgery, Alleghany General Hospital, Pittsburgh, Pennsylvania

Konstantinos Ditsios, M.D.
Department of Orthopaedic Surgery, Washington University School of Medicine, St. Louis, Missouri

James R. Doyle, M.D.
Professor of Surgery Emeritus, Department of Orthopaedic Surgery, John A. Burns School of Medicine, University of Hawaii, Honolulu, Hawaii

Richard G. Eaton, M.D.
Clinical Professor, Department of Surgery, Columbia University, New York, New York; Chairman Emeritus, C. V. Starr Hand Service, St. Luke's-Roosevelt Hospital, New York, New York

Stuart J. Elkowitz, M.D.
Attending Hand Surgeon, Department of Orthopaedic Surgery, New York University Hospital for Joint Diseases, Northern Westchester Hospital, Putnam Hospital Center, New York, New York

Drew Engles, M.D.
Hand and Microvascular Surgeon, Summit Hand Center, The Crystal Clinic, Akron, Ohio

Donald C. Ferlic, M.D.
P/SL Professional Plaza West, Denver, Colorado

Alan E. Freeland, M.D.
Professor, Department of Orthopaedic Surgery and Rehabilitation, University of Mississippi Medical Center, Jackson, Mississippi

Steven Z. Glickel, M.D.
Associate Clinical Professor, Orthopaedic Surgery, Columbia University, New York, New York; Director, Hand Surgery, Orthopaedic Surgery, St. Luke's-Roosevelt Hospital, New York, New York

Thomas J. Graham, M.D.
Chief, The Curtis National Hand Center, Union Memorial Hospital, Baltimore, Maryland; Vice-Chairman, Department of Orthopaedic Surgery, Decker Orthopaedic Institute, Union Memorial Hospital, Baltimore, Maryland; Clinical Associate Professor, Departments of Orthopaedic and Plastic Surgery, Johns Hopkins University Hospital, Baltimore, Maryland

Todd M. Guyette, M.D.
The Curtis National Hand Center, Union Memorial Hospital, Baltimore, Maryland

Stephen M. Hankins, M.D.
Resident, Department of Orthopaedic Surgery, Drexel University, Philadelphia, Pennsylvania

Hill Hastings II, M.D.
Clinical Professor, Orthopaedic Surgery, Indiana University Medical Center, Indiana Hand Center, Indianapolis, Indiana; Attending Physician, Orthopaedic Surgery, St. Vincent's Hospital, Indianapolis, Indiana

Richard S. Idler, M.D.
Hand Surgery Associates of Indiana, Indianapolis, Indiana

Michelle A. James, M.D.
Associate Clinical Professor, Orthopaedic Surgery, University of California, Davis School of Medicine, Sacramento, California; Assistant Chief, Orthopaedic Surgery, Shriner's Hospital for Children, Northern California, Sacramento, California

Peter J. L. Jebson, M.D.
Chief and Associate Professor, Division of Elbow, Hand, and Microsurgery, Department of Orthopaedic Surgery, University of Michigan Medical Center, Ann Arbor, Michigan

Jesse B. Jupiter, M.D.
Hansjorg Wyss/AO Professor, Orthopaedic Surgery, Harvard Medical School, Boston, Massachusetts; Director, Orthopaedic Hand Surgery, Massachusetts General Hospital, Boston, Massachusetts

Brian M. Katt, M.D.
Deparment of Orthopaedic Surgery, University of Medicine and Dentistry of New Jersey, Robert Wood Johnson Medical School, New Brunswick, New Jersey

Joseph P. Leddy, M.D.
Professor and Chairman, Department of Orthopaedic Surgery, University of Medicine and Dentistry of New Jersey, Robert Wood Johnson Medical School, New Brunswick, New Jersey

Dean S. Louis, M.D.
Professor, Division of Elbow, Hand, and Microsurgery, Department of Orthopaedic Surgery, University of Michigan Medical Center, Ann Arbor, Michigan

Gary M. Lourie, M.D.
Assistant Clinical Professor, Department of Orthopaedics, Emory University School of Medicine, Atlanta, Georgia; Clinician, Hand Surgery, Department of Hand Surgery, Scottish-Rite Children's Medical Center, Atlanta, Georgia

Matthew M. Malerich, M.D.
Clinical Professor, Department of Orthopaedic Surgery, University of California, Irvine, Orange, California

Jennifer L. M. Manual, M.D.
Resident, Department of Orthopaedics, Brown University/Rhode Island Hospital, Providence, Rhode Island

Daniel J. Mastella, M.D.
Hand Surgery Fellow, Department of Orthopaedics, Thomas Jefferson University Hospital and The Philadelphia Hand Center, Philadelphia, Pennsylvania

John A. McAuliffe, M.D.
Hand Surgeon, Department Orthopaedic Surgery, Cleveland Clinic Florida, Weston, Florida

Michael A. McClinton, M.D.
Assistant Professor, Division of Plastic Surgery, Johns Hopkins Medical Institutions, Baltimore, Maryland; Attending Hand Surgeon, Curtis National Hand Center, Union Memorial Hospital, Baltimore, Maryland

Jorge L. Orbay, M.D.
Miami Hand Center, Miami, Florida

Kevin Plancher, M.D., M.S., F.A.C.S., F.A.A.O.S.
Attending in Orthopaedics, Singer Division, Beth Israel Medical Center, New York, New York; Associate Clinical Professor, Orthopaedics, Albert Einstein College of Medicine, Bronx, New York; Attending Surgeon in Orthopaedics, Stamford Hospital, Stamford, Connecticut; Orthopaedic and Sports Medicine PLLC, New York, New York

Keith B. Raskin, M.D.
Clinical Associate Professor, Department of Orthopaedic Surgery, New York University School of Medicine, New York, New York; Attending Physician, Department of Orthopaedic Surgery, New York University School of Medicine/Hospital for Joint Diseases, New York, New York

Lance A. Rettig, M.D.
Methodist Sports Medicine Center, Thomas A. Brady Clinic, Indianapolis, Indiana; Assistant Clinical Professor, Indiana University, Indianapolis, Indiana

Ioannis Sarris, M.D., Ph.D.
Fellow, Upper Extremity Surgery, Department of Orthopaedic Surgery, Alleghany General Hospital, Pittsburgh, Pennsylvania

Keith Alan Segalman, M.D.
Assistant Professor, Department of Orthopaedic Surgery, Johns Hopkins Hospital, Baltimore, Maryland; Curtis National Hand Center, Union Memorial Hospital, Baltimore, Maryland

John Gray Seiler III, M.D.
Clinical Associate Professor, Department of Orthopaedic Surgery, Emory University, Atlanta, Georgia; Georgia Hand and Microsurgery, Atlanta, Georgia

Steven S. Shin, M.D.
Chief Resident, Orthopaedic Surgery, New York University School of Medicine, New York, New York; Chief Resident, Orthopaedic Surgery, New York University Medical Center/Hospital for Joint Diseases, New York, New York

Dean G. Sotereanos, M.D.
Professor, Department of Orthopaedic Surgery, Drexel University, College of Medicine, Philadelphia, Pennsylvania; Vice-Chairman, Department of Orthopaedic, Surgery, Alleghany General Hospital, Pittsburgh, Pennsylvania

James W. Strickland, M.D.
Reconstructive Hand Surgeons of Indiana, Carmel, Indiana; Clinical Professor of Orthopaedic Surgery, Indiana University School of Medicine, Indianapolis, Indiana

John S. Taras, M.D.
Associate Professor, Department of Orthopaedic Surgery, Drexel University/Thomas Jefferson University, Philadelphia, Pennsylvania; Chief, Division Hand Surgery, Drexel University/Thomas Jefferson University, Philadelphia, Pennsylvania

Andrew L. Terrono, M.D.
Associate Clinical Professor, Department of Orthopaedics, Tufts University School of Medicine, Boston, Massachusetts; Chief, Hand Surgery, New England Baptist Bone and Joint Institute, Boston, Massachusetts

Matthew M. Tomaino, M.D., M.B.A.
Professor of Orthopaedics and Chief, Division of Hand, Shoulder, and Elbow Surgery, University of Rochester Medical Center, Rochester, New York

Joseph Upton, M.D.
Associate Professor, Division of Plastic Surgery, Harvard Medical School, Boston, Massachusetts; Surgeon, Division of Plastic Surgery, Department of Surgery, Children's Hospital, Beth Israel Deaconess Medical Center, Boston, Massachusetts

Peter M. Waters, M.D.
Associate Professor of Orthopaedic Surgery, Children's Hospital, Boston, Massachusetts

Arnold-Peter C. Weiss, M.D.
Professor, Department of Orthopaedic Surgery, Brown University, Providence, Rhode Island; Attending Hand Surgeon, Department of Orthopaedics, Rhode Island Hospital, Providence, Rhode Island

E. F. Shaw Wilgis, M.D.
Greater Chesapeake Specialists, Lutherville, Maryland

Robert Lee Wilson, M.D.
Pheonix Integrated Hand Surgery Fellowship, Pheonix, Arizona

Raymond A. Wittstadt, M.D., M.P.H.
Clinical Instructor, Part Time, Department of Orthopaedic Surgery, Johns Hopkins Hospital, Baltimore, Maryland; Attending Physician, Curtis National Hand Center Union Memorial Hospital, Baltimore, Maryland

ACKNOWLEDGMENTS

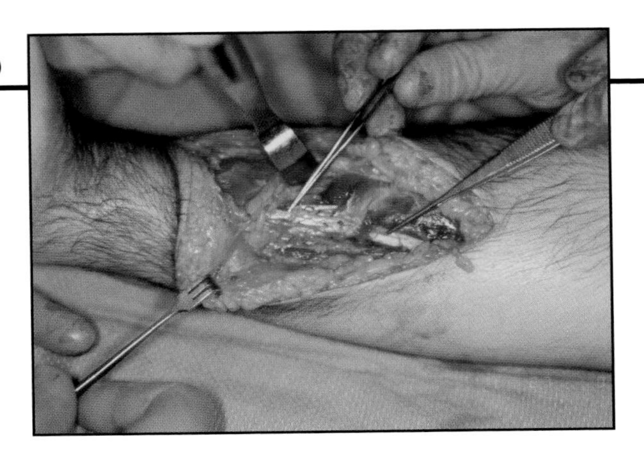

Production of a high-quality text like the Master Techniques series is the result of tremendous effort on the part of many dedicated specialists. First, we would like to again thank our contributors who were insightful and enthusiastic, as well as timely, with their chapters.

The team at Lippincott, Williams & Wilkins is replete with real champions: Robert Hurley, executive editor; Stacey Sebring, senior managing editor; Leah Hayes, managing editor. They have identified the need for the flexible and visual learning tool and perfected it with this entire series.

The base of operations for Lippincott, Williams & Wilkins is Baltimore, which was convenient because the center of the action for this volume is the Curtis National Hand Center at Union Memorial Hospital. Lyn Camire is an invaluable resource as our editor, serving our entire musculoskeletal group at Union Memorial Hospital; she does a great job in all facets of production and relations with publishers, editors, contributors, and artists. Day-to-day organization and execution on the part of Cynthia Johnson and Tori Wilson allowed us to complete the tasks related to the book.

Gary Schnitz again demonstrated why he is at the top of his field for medical illustration. His understanding of how to depict Hand Surgery in two dimensions for teaching purposes is unrivaled.

SERIES PREFACE

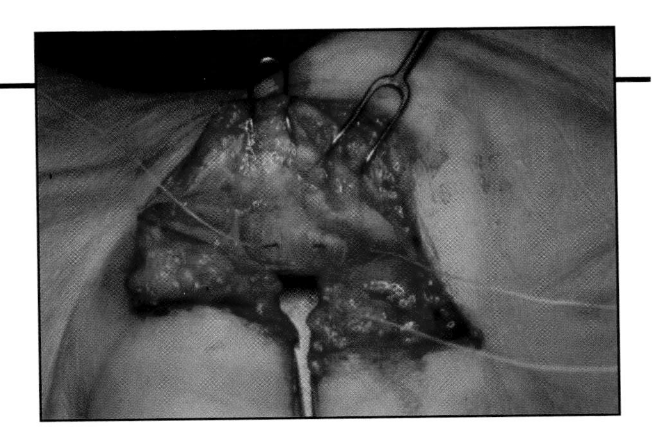

Since its inception in 1994, the Masters' Technique Series has become a well-accepted "must" for surgeons in training and in practice. The user-friendly style of providing and illustrating authoritative information on a broad spectrum of orthopedic techniques has filled a void in orthopedic education materials. The exceptional success of the series may be traced to the leadership of the original series editor, Roby Thompson, whose clarity of thought and focused vision sought "to provide direct, detailed access to techniques preferred by orthopedic surgeons who are recognized by their colleagues as 'masters' in their specialty" (Series preface, Volume I). The essential elements of success are clear. In addition to the careful selection of the master volume editor, the format of the presented material has almost become classic. I am personally rewarded by numerous comments by both residents and practicing orthopedic surgeons regarding the value of these volumes to their training or in their practice. The format has become a standard against which others are to be compared, "A standardized presentation of information replete with tips and pearls through years of experience with abundant color photographs and drawings to guide you step by step through the procedures" (Series preface, Volume II).

Eight second edition volumes are currently in print, and two more are in preparation. Building on the success of the current ten-volume series, we are in the process of expanding the texts to include an even broader range of relevant orthopedic topics. New volumes will appear on surgical exposures as well as peripheral nerve surgery. Other topics are being actively explored with an expectation that the series will expand to 15 titles over the next several years.

I am honored to be assuming the responsibility of the series editor. The true worth of this endeavor will be measured by the ongoing and ever-increasing success and critical acceptance of the series. I am indebted to Dr. Thompson for his inaugural vision and leadership as well as to the Masters' volume editors and to the numerous contributors who have been true to the style and to the vision. Ultimately, as is stated by the Mayo brothers, "The best interest of the patient is the only interest to be considered." It is hoped that the information in the Masters' Series equips the surgeon to realize this patient-centric view of our surgical practice.

Bernard F. Morrey, M.D.
Series Editor

PREFACE

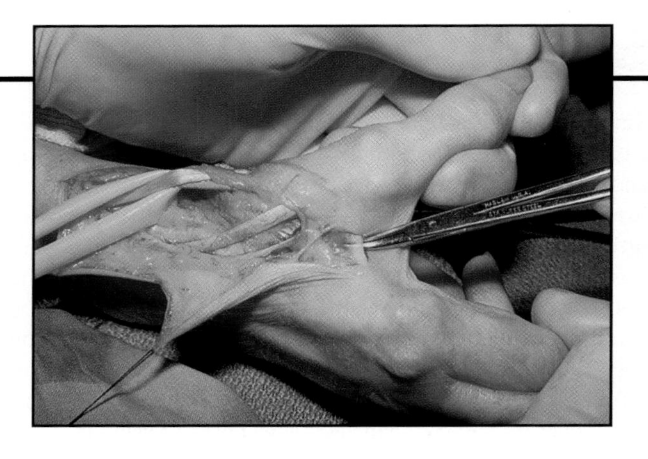

The intellectual and technical challenges of sophisticated hand surgery are practically unparalleled in the endeavors of the clinical sciences. Intimate knowledge of fine anatomy; well-planned and skillfully executed surgical exercises; and attention to detail before the operation, intraoperatively, and during rehabilitation are all required to maximize outcome.

Respect for time-tested techniques, with an open-minded approach to evolving surgical options, is demanded if a contemporary surgeon is to deliver the ultimate level of care to the wide array of patients seeking help for hand problems due to traumatic, congenital, inflammatory, neoplastic, or degenerative conditions.

The Master Techniques series has already risen to a unique niche in the dissemination of high-level surgical education. The initial edition of The Hand laid the groundwork for capturing the thinking and unique perspective that our distinguished colleagues have developed over years of practice. Students of Hand Surgery will see that this volume has further expanded the spectrum of procedures and pearls.

We credit the laureates who have contributed to this edition with concise words and vivid images. They have captured the salient points by recognizing the germinal components of the problems and the solutions. With tremendous photography and illustration strengthening the descriptions, the compendium of the written word and visual learning tools has resulted in an important contribution to our specialty.

Just as we shared the strong bond between mentor and pupil, we wanted to capture that singular experience for teaching and learning. To pass along our true thinking about our work, and ask our valued friends to do the same, is an honor. In this way, all the authors can feel the flexibility and intimacy that comes with disseminating knowledge from one colleague to the next in one of the best media we can imagine. All of the contributors appreciated the responsibility of accepting and completing these assignments and fulfilled them expertly.

All of those who worked on Master Techniques in Orthopaedic Surgery: The Hand hope that this volume connects with our readers in a way that makes it is a resource and stimulus for their own development. It is a text that is dynamic, not simply a moment frozen in our timeline of hand surgery, but a catalyst for greater discourse and creativity concerning the clinical tests that we all face.

Ultimately, there will be acceptance, inquiry, controversy and change in almost all of the views expressed herein. That is the nature of our specialty, and of all of medicine. For now, this is the best effort of many of the most dedicated and prolific contributors to our specialty, who also share a passion for teaching and life-long learning. We hope the book makes a positive impact on the practice of our readers and in the lives of their patients.

Thomas J. Graham, M.D.
James W. Strickland, M.D.

PART I

Fractures and Dislocations: The Digits

1

Open Reduction and Internal Fixation of the Tubular Bones of the Hand

Alan E. Freeland and Jorge L. Orbay

INDICATIONS/CONTRAINDICATIONS

It must be clearly understood that a majority of closed fractures of the tubular bones of the hand can be adequately managed by nonoperative methods. Open reduction and internal fixation (ORIF) is reserved for selected injuries, or for selected patients, for which the risk-benefit profile of the additional surgical morbidity is favorable.

Most closed, unstable diaphyseal fractures of the tubular bones of the hand can be treated by closed reduction and internal fixation (CRIF) using pins. However, there is a subset of complex fractures of the hand for which ORIF should be strongly considered. Irreducible fractures, displaced or unstable comminuted shaft fractures, hand fractures accompanied by polytrauma or other displaced fractures in the same hand or extremity are often identified as indications for ORIF. Open metacarpal and phalangeal diaphyseal fractures are the recognized candidates for open reduction and internal fixation. Fractures of the small bones involving the articular surfaces, whether or not they are associated with frank joint subluxation or dislocation, are typically indicated for definitive operative reduction and stabilization.

The reasons for open reduction and internal fixation of complex open fractures and those with bone loss are particularly compelling. Age, hand dominance, and functional requirements may impact the decision-making process in terms of the need for enhanced fracture stability. The perceived risk of patient noncompliance may be an indication for more secure internal fracture fixation. An operative approach provides an additional opportunity for wound- and intrinsic-muscle decompression when necessary.

Alan E. Freeland, M.D.: Department of Orthopaedic Surgery and Rehabilitation, University of Mississippi Medical Center, Jackson, MS

Jorge L. Orbay, M.D.: Miami Hand Center, Miami, FL

While any number of pinning configurations and techniques may be used for these fractures, interfragmentary screw and/or plate fixation provides substantially greater stability throughout the course of healing. The surgical science and techniques for application of these devices have improved, resulting in the ability to utilize them with minimal or no additional soft-tissue dissection when compared to modern pinning techniques. Stable fixation with indwelling hardware certainly allows earlier and more intensive rehabilitation, which encourages improved functional outcome.

Contraindications

Small fragment size, severe comminution, and poor bone quality may constitute relative contraindications to minifragment fixation. Although these methods may occasionally be appropriate for adolescents, they are rarely, if ever, indicated in children under the age of 10 years. Ultimately, the intangibles of judgment and experience may be the consummate determinant of the choice for fracture fixation. Resources, training, and familiarity with implants and techniques may also play deciding roles.

PREOPERATIVE PLANNING

Although anatomic fracture reduction is ideal, allowances may be made for minor deformities that cause only negligible or no functional impairment. Clinical and x-ray examinations help the surgeon to determine the presence and extent of anatomic deformity. Additionally, the patient's health status, vocational and avocational pursuits may determine the necessity for open reduction and internal fixation.

While some gross deformities requiring correction and stabilization are readily apparent, digital or wrist block may assist in this determination by allowing visualization of the injured digit moving throughout a complete or nearly complete arc of motion. Impingement upon or overlapping of an adjacent finger may be identified, as well as limitation of motion, malrotation, and compensatory joint postures.

Routine hand and digital x-rays can demonstrate shortening and angulation of the fracture, as well as its fracture pattern. Although conventional radiographs typically image the articular relationships adequately, magnified or oblique films may demonstrate an intra-articular fracture more precisely, and live fluoroscopy can be a useful aid in selected articular fractures to judge displacement. While rotational deformity may be seen or suggested by the radiographic appearance of the fracture, clinical examination is usually more accurate in evaluating this component of fracture deformity. Implant selection and configuration are matched to the fracture pattern to assure optimal fracture stability following reduction. This chapter deals with these choices.

SURGERY

The patient is placed supine on the operating table. The hand is placed in the midaspect of the hand table with the shoulder abducted approximately 70°. Hyperabduction of the shoulder is avoided so as to prevent brachial plexus traction injuries. The contralateral elbow and both heels are padded to avoid skin pressure on bony prominences and in areas of vulnerable neurovascular structures. Intravenous perioperative antibiotics may be administered at the discretion of the surgeon.

Local, regional, or general anesthesia is administered according to the needs and preferences of the patient, surgeon, and anesthesiologist. The anticipated time requirements of the procedure and the general health of the patient may impact the choice of anesthesia. Local or regional anesthesia may be preferable for procedures of shorter duration and for patients with compromised cardiopulmonary status.

Cast padding and a tourniquet are applied to the proximal arm or forearm. The upper extremity is prepared and draped in the usual sterile fashion. Exsanguination is performed with a 4-inch elastic bandage and the tourniquet pressure is elevated to 250 mm Hg. Adjustments in tourniquet pressure may be necessary in hypotensive or hypertensive patients to maintain tourniquet pressure at approximately 100 mm Hg above the systolic pressure.

An appropriate incision is selected to expose the metacarpal fracture site (Fig. 1.1). Branches of the dorsal sensory radial, ulnar and digital nerves are identified or avoided for protection, whenever possible. Proximal metacarpal shaft fractures may be approached by elevating the extensor mechanism in an effort to minimize scarring between the extensor tendon and the adjacent skin and bone. The distal metacarpal may be approached in the same manner or through an extensor tendon-splitting incision.

Dorsal incisions are standard for phalangeal fractures (Fig. 1.2). The Pratt incision may be centered over a phalangeal fracture at any level. The distal condyles are usually approached by an incision between the extensor slip and the lateral bands. Chamay has described an alternative approach to the distal condyles that elevates the central slip as a distally based flap.

The midaxial incision often is an excellent alternative for proximal or distal phalangeal metaphyseal fractures. There is slight difference between midaxial and midlateral incisions (Fig. 1.3). The midaxial incision connects the centers of rotation of the interphalangeal joints that are identified topographically by the dorsal extremes of the interphalangeal joint creases. The midlateral incision is made halfway between the dorsal and volar borders of the finger. The midaxial incision is thought to minimize mechanically stimulated scar formation during rehabilitation and is thus preferred. The lateral band and adjacent oblique fibers of extensor apparatus of the metacarpophalangeal joint may be excised from the midaxial approach to enhance fracture exposure and minimize postoperative extensor tendon adhesions.

Subperiosteal dissection protects the adjacent tendons, but extraperiosteal dissection is sometimes less traumatic and may maintain a more favorable biologic environment for

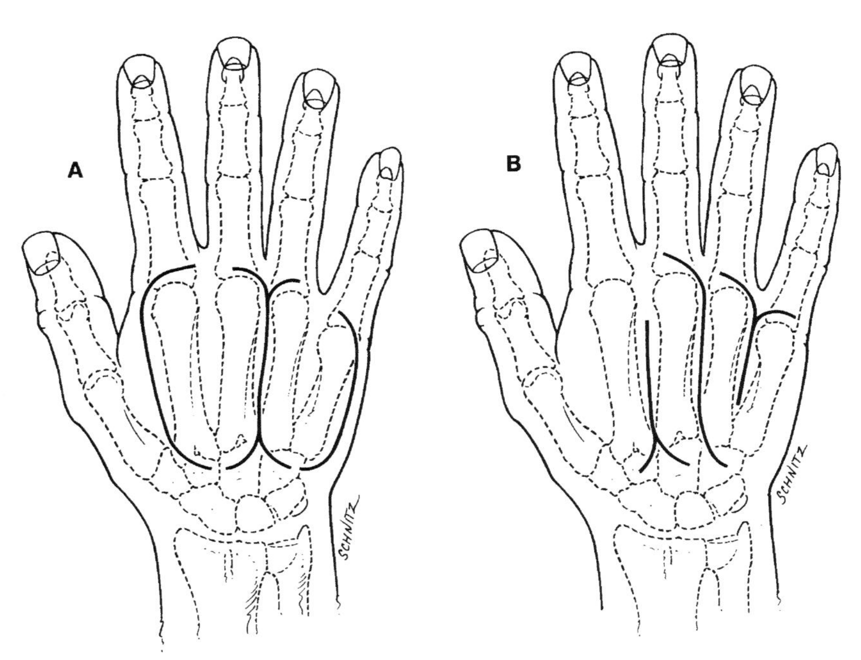

Figure 1.1. Longitudinal incisions are offset from the fractured metacarpal in an effort to spare the extensor tendon(s) from extensive scarring with contiguous skin and bone while providing adequate exposure of the fracture. **A:** Two adjacent diaphyseal fractures may be approached through a single incision that may be extended at either end. **B:** These are additional incision modifications for two adjacent metacarpal fractures proximally, distally, and at different levels. (With permission, from: Freeland AE, Geissler WB. Plate fixation of metacarpal shaft fractures. In: Blair WF, Steyers CM, eds. *Techniques in Hand Surgery.* Baltimore: Williams & Wilkins, 1996:257; Fig. 34-1.)

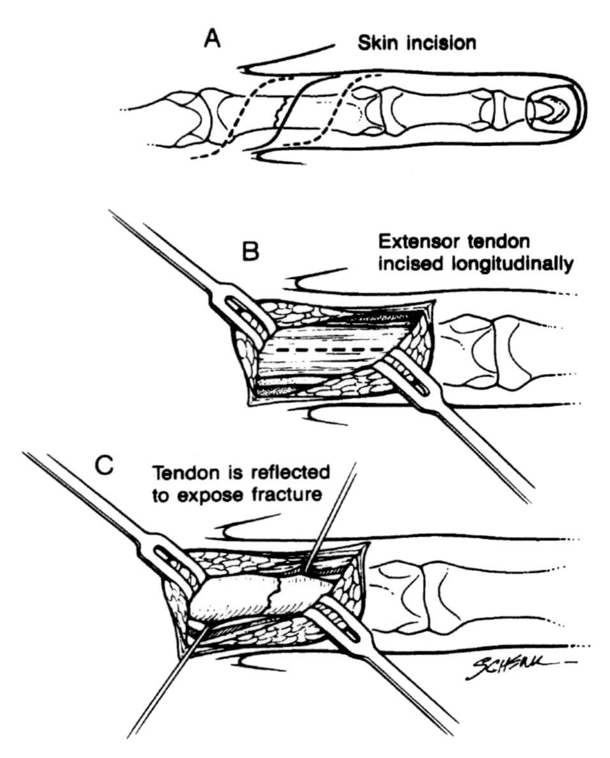

Figure 1.2. Dorsal approach to the proximal phalanx demonstrating: **A:** the skin incision; **B:** a longitudinal incision of the extensor tendon; and **C:** fracture exposure. (With permission, from: Pratt DR. Exposing fractures of the proximal phalanx of the finger longitudinally through the dorsal extensor apparatus. *Clin Orthop* 15:22–26, 1959; Fig. 2.)

healing. A bloodless, areolar layer exists between the undersurface of the extensor tendon and the dorsum of the metacarpal that can be easily exploited with minimal trauma, and, therefore, minimal adhesion development.

The fracture is exposed sufficiently to remove intervening soft tissue, clot, and any early callus to allow accurate fracture reduction and implant insertion. Pointed bone reduction

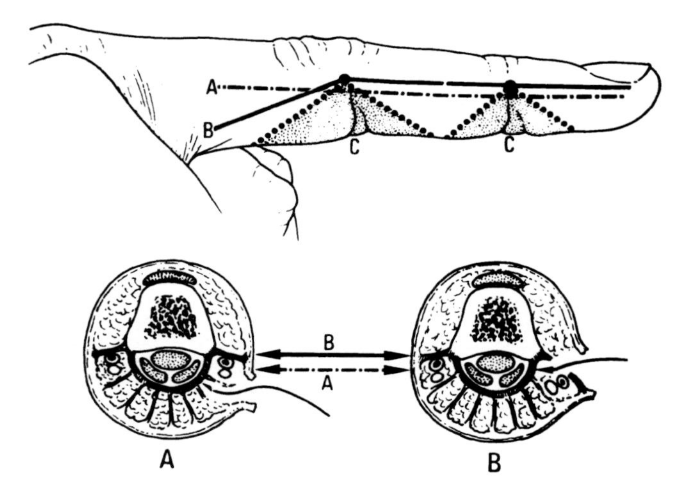

Figure 1.3. Mid-axial approach to the proximal phalanx. Line A indicates the mid-lateral line; line B, the mid-axial line; and line C, the interphalangeal flexion creases. The dotted line demonstrates a lateral view of a Bruner incision. The shaded areas indicate the areas of skin flaps that would be elevated by a Bruner incision. Bruner incisions extend to the center of rotation at the interphalangeal joints. (With permission, from: Littler JW, Cramer LM, Smith JW, eds. *Symposium on Reconstructive Hand Surgery.* St. Louis: CV Mosby, 1974:90; Fig. 8-4.)

forceps may facilitate fracture reduction and maintenance during implant application. The fracture should be anatomically or primarily reduced prior to implant insertion. Fracture reduction is monitored by direct visualization, but use of fluoroscopic guidance should verify anatomic reduction.

Although implant insertion will stabilize the fracture, reduction is not usually achieved by this maneuver. Provisional fixation with smooth wires, often placed in the location where eventual screws will be implanted, is an acceptable technique to hold fracture reduction and "simplify" certain patterns requiring more extensive work.

Digital alignment is evaluated throughout a passive arc of flexion and extension to assure proper rotational alignment. There should be no digital overlap and minimal-to-no impingement on adjacent fingers.

Tissues are intermittently irrigated to avoid desiccation. Miniplates are slightly bent over their entire length when used in the compression mode or contoured to the underlying bone surface when applied to neutralize or buttress the fracture.

Passive range of motion may be checked and recorded after implant application. Postoperative motion will not exceed the passive motion achieved at the time of surgery. Consequently, knowledge of the passive range of motion achieved at the time of surgery may serve as a guideline and goal for postoperative therapy.

When the periosteum can be reapproximated, it is sutured with fine resorbable sutures. The tourniquet is released and manual compression is applied over the incision for approximately 10 minutes. Further hemostasis and irrigation are accomplished. Drains are seldom necessary. The skin is reapproximated with fine interrupted sutures.

The wrist is positioned in 15°–20° of extension, the metacarpophalangeal joints in 50°–60° of flexion, and the interphalangeal joints in full extension or slight flexion. A soft, sterile, bulky, conforming hand dressing and overlying plaster splint are applied from below the elbow to support and protect the wrist and hand.

LONG OBLIQUE DIAPHYSEAL FRACTURES

A fracture line that equals or exceeds twice the diameter of the bone at the fracture site defines the "long oblique fracture" pattern. Such a fracture may be best treated by two or more mini-lag screws of appropriate length (Figs. 1.4 and 1.5). A miniscrew inserted perpendicular to the fracture line ("compression screw") has the greatest compression force, but its resistance to shear forces acting to displace the fracture along its surfaces decreases as it moves away from a perpendicular to the long axis of the bone. Conversely, a miniscrew placed perpendicular to the long axis of the bone has the greatest resistance to shear displacement ("neutralization screw"), but its compressive force lessens as it angles away from a perpendicular to the fracture surface.

There may be one or more points along the fracture at which its surface is parallel to the long axis of the bone. Miniscrews applied at these points have optimal compression and resistance to shear forces ("optimal screw"). Ideally, at least one miniscrew should have optimal resistance to shear displacement forces. The remaining miniscrew(s) may be placed in positions of optimal compression. Interlocking bony interstices may provide additional fracture stability.

The variables that are considered in the fixation of this pattern include the number of miniscrews, their orientation, their size (although the surgeon may elect to use different sizes in different locations of the fracture), whether or not to countersink the head, and whether or not additional compression is to be sought by overdrilling.

As a general rule, the surgeon can approximate the number of miniscrews that will safely and effectively secure the fracture by dividing the fracture length by the largest diameter of the bone within the confines of the fracture. When the fracture is twice the bone diameter, two miniscrews may be placed where the bone is divided into thirds. When the fracture length is three times the diameter of the bone, three miniscrews may be placed where the fracture is divided into fourths. Three miniscrews potentially increase the strength of fixation by 50% as compared to that provided by two miniscrews.

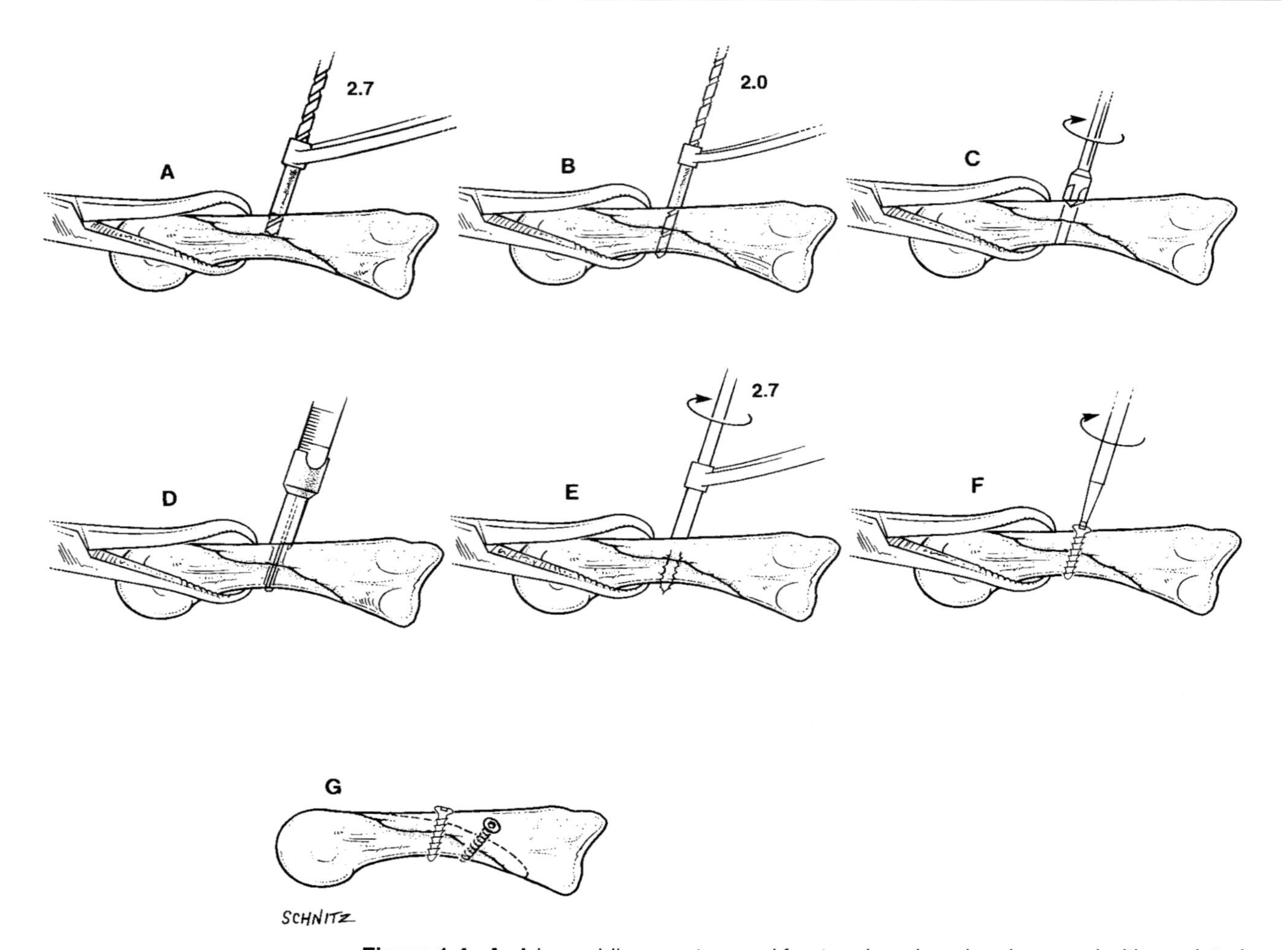

Figure 1.4. A: A long oblique metacarpal fracture is reduced and secured with a pointed reduction forceps. A gliding hole is drilled in the near cortex with a 2.7-mm drill. A drill guide is used to protect adjacent soft tissues and to prevent skating of the drill on the bone. **B:** The opposite end of a double-ended drill guide corresponds to the 2.7-mm diameter of the gliding hole. The drill guide is inserted in the gliding hole in the near cortex, and a 2.0-mm core hole is drilled concentrically through the opposite cortex. **C:** The countersink is rotated to fashion an area in the proximal half of the dorsal cortex to correspond to the screw head. **D:** A depth gauge determines the length of the screw hole. **E:** A 2.7-mm tap is used to thread the core hole of the distal cortex. A tap sleeve is used to protect adjacent soft tissues. This step is omitted when self-tapping screws are inserted. **F:** A self-tapping miniscrew is inserted. As it glides through the proximal hole, the head of the miniscrew engages the proximal cortex, creating compression at the fracture site as the screw threads purchase the distal cortex (lag screw effect). Note that a compression miniscrew is inserted perpendicular to the fracture. **G:** A second miniscrew is inserted using a similar technique to the first but in a plane perpendicular to the long axis of the bone, satisfying the need for maximum neutralization of shearing forces. (With permission, from: Heim U, Pfeiffer KM, eds. *Internal Fixation of Small Fractures, 3rd Edition.* New York: Springer Verlag, 1988:48; Fig. 24.)

Although this fracture work is delicate and the "tongue" of bone that is created by a long, oblique fracture is often gracile, overdrilling to enhance compression is a fundamental fracture fixation concept that is often considered or exercised. Great care is taken to keep the enlarged hole a safe distance from the fracture edge.

Countersinking the miniscrew head in the cortical diaphysis is advocated, as it prevents an irritating prominence under the skin and avoids interference with the overlying gliding tendons. Additionally, countersinking the miniscrew head into the bone minimizes the risk of fracture by engagement of the miniscrew head on the bone surface during screw tightening by distributing the force of the head over a larger surface area. The risk of fracture

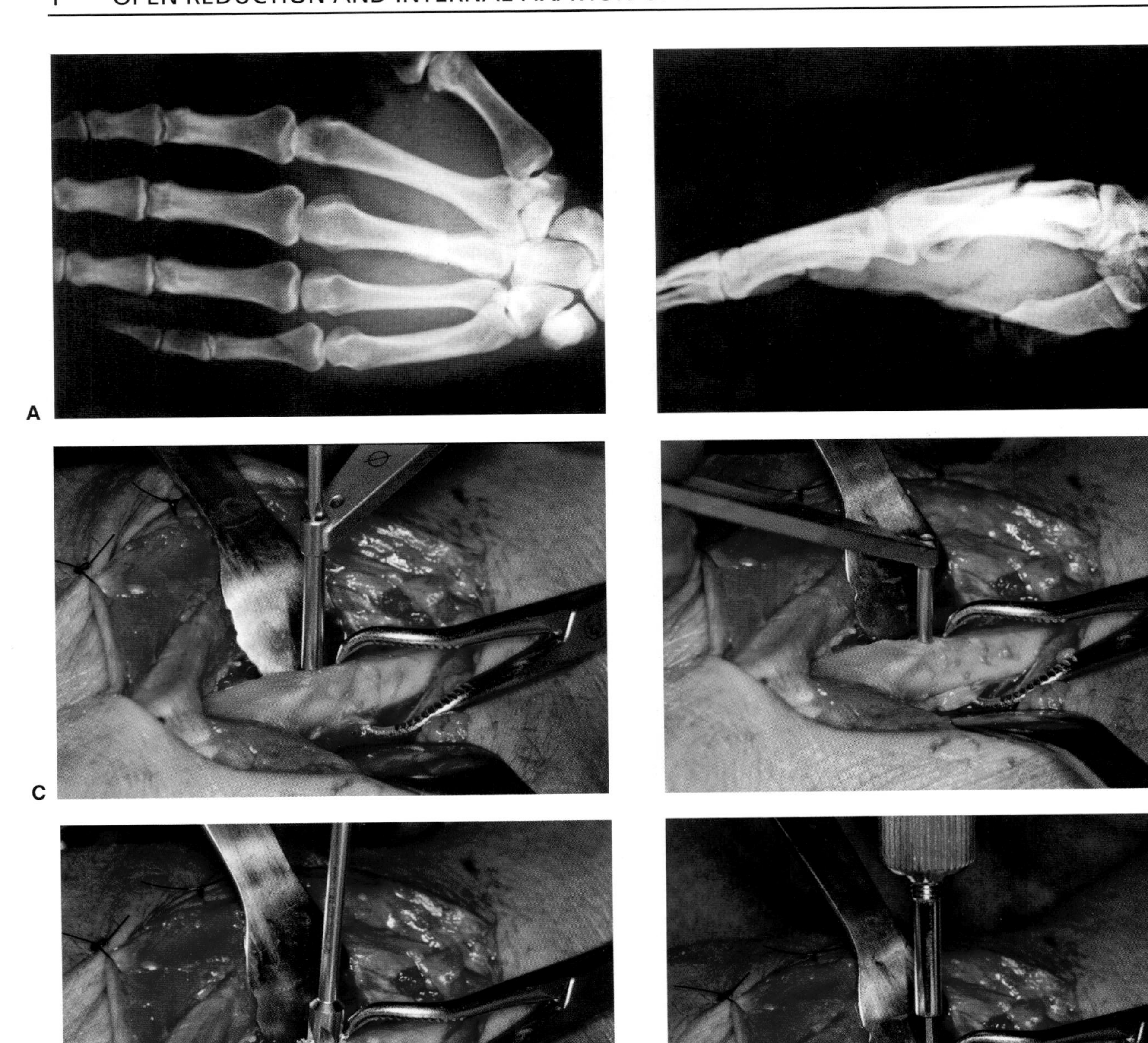

Figure 1.5. A, B: A displaced unstable long spiral fracture of the third metacarpal shaft. **C:** The fracture is reduced and secured with a pointed reduction forceps. A gliding hole is drilled in the near cortex with a 2.7-mm drill. A drill guide is used to protect adjacent soft tissues and to prevent skating of the drill on the bone. **D:** The opposite end of a double-ended drill guide corresponds to the 2.7-mm diameter of the gliding hole. The drill guide is inserted in the gliding hole in the near cortex, and a 2.0-mm core hole is drilled concentrically through the opposite cortex. **E:** The countersink is rotated to fashion an area in the proximal half of the dorsal cortex to correspond to the screw head. **F:** A depth gauge determines the length of the screw hole.

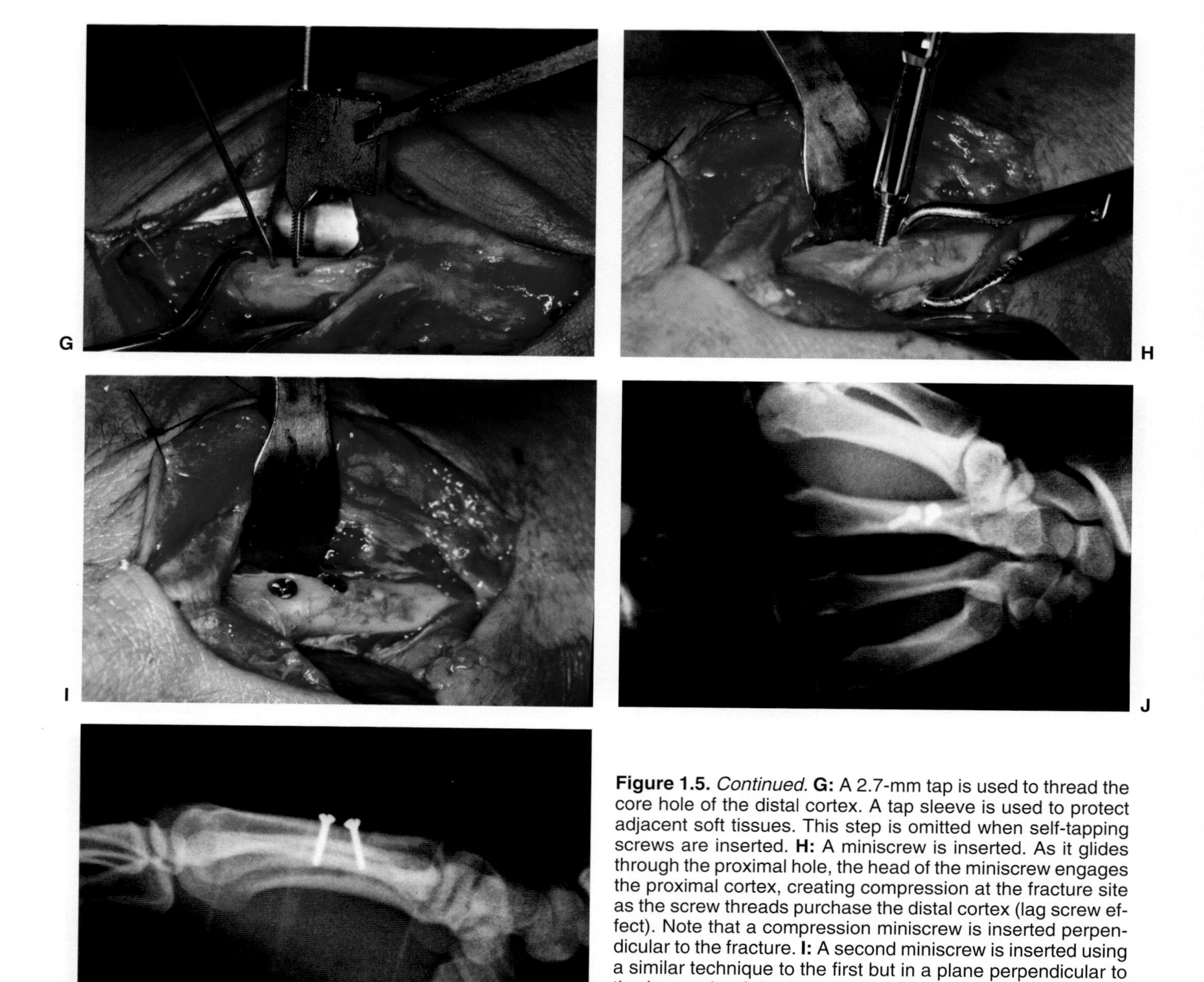

Figure 1.5. *Continued.* **G:** A 2.7-mm tap is used to thread the core hole of the distal cortex. A tap sleeve is used to protect adjacent soft tissues. This step is omitted when self-tapping screws are inserted. **H:** A miniscrew is inserted. As it glides through the proximal hole, the head of the miniscrew engages the proximal cortex, creating compression at the fracture site as the screw threads purchase the distal cortex (lag screw effect). Note that a compression miniscrew is inserted perpendicular to the fracture. **I:** A second miniscrew is inserted using a similar technique to the first but in a plane perpendicular to the long axis of the bone, satisfying the need for maximum neutralization of shearing forces. **J, K:** AP and lateral x-rays demonstrate an anatomic reduction of the fracture secured with two mini-lag screws.

through a screw hole is further minimized by keeping the ratio of the screw hole to bone diameter or to the nearest fracture edge over 3:1.

The surgeon will develop experience with applying pressure to optimally tighten the screw; overtightening a compression screw can sometimes propagate a fracture from the screw hole to a nearby edge of the initial fracture.

TRANSVERSE FRACTURES

Transverse (or nearly transverse) fractures of the tubular bones are treated either by pinning or by mini-compression plating techniques. The latter has advantages of anatomic reduction, enhanced stability, and avoidance of protruding hardware. Additionally, the plated fracture typically allows the confidence to begin an early aggressive-motion program.

Dorsal application of a 2.0 mm, 2.4 mm, or 2.7 mm straight miniplate with four to six holes is preferable for most diaphyseal fractures (Figs. 1.6 and 1.7). Mini-condylar, T-, or L-shaped plates are used with a similar compression technique for transverse fractures at the metaphyseal diaphyseal junction (Figs. 1.8 and 1.9). The miniplates are slightly bent to ensure uniform compression across the fracture site and at the bone cortex opposite the

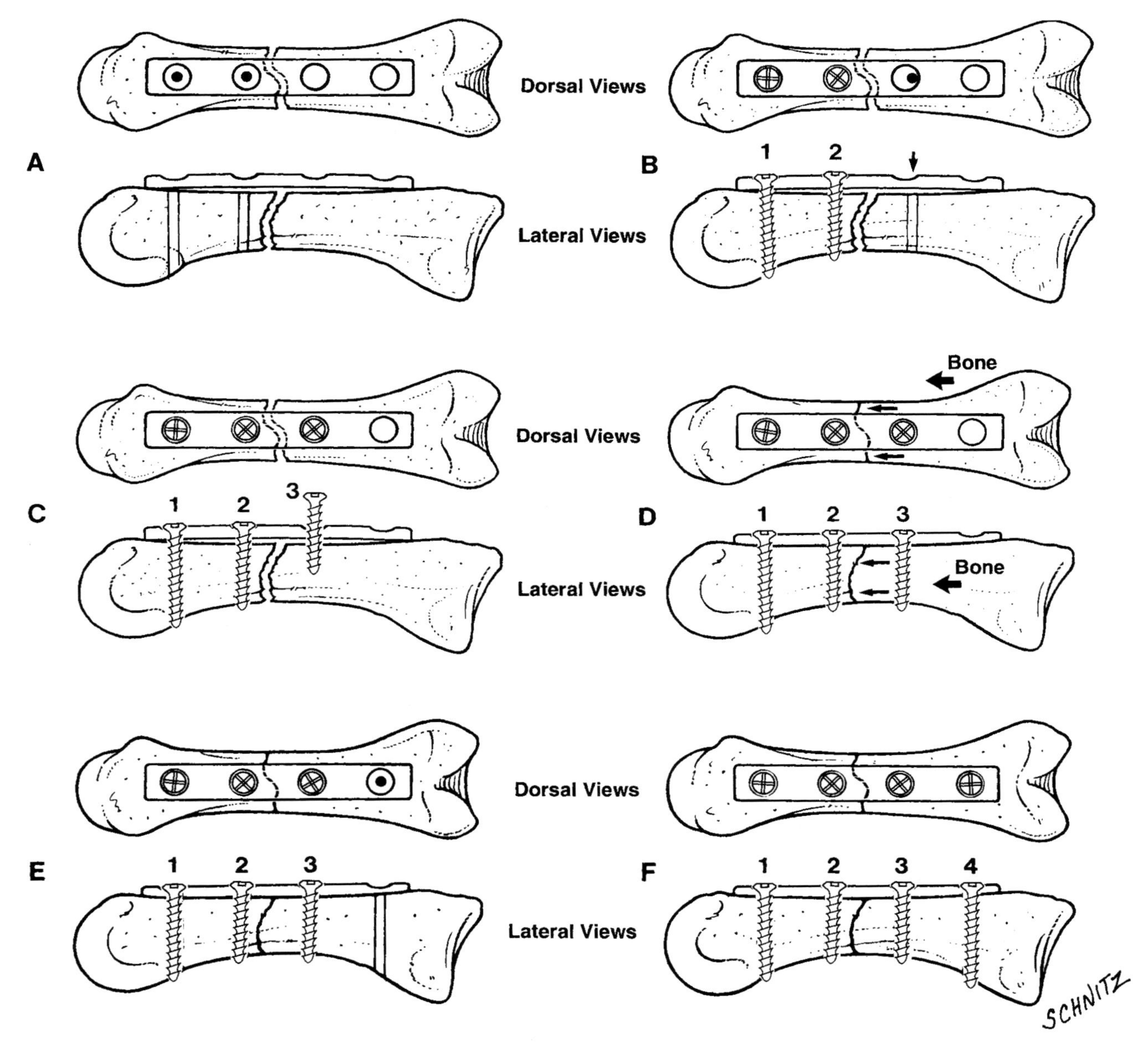

Figure 1.6. A reduced transverse metacarpal shaft fracture is diagrammed. **A:** Two drill holes are centered in the plate holes distal to the fracture. The miniplate has a graduated bend of approximately 5° centered at the middle of the miniplate with no acute bend or buckling of the plate, especially not at the level of the holes in the plate. **B:** Two neutral (centered in the plate holes and applying no force to the plate) miniscrews are inserted distal to the fracture. A drill hole is placed eccentrically away from the fracture in the miniplate hole just proximal to the fracture. **C:** A miniscrew is inserted into the eccentrically placed drill hole. **D:** The screw head engages the plate hole as the miniscrew is tightened, causing the fracture to compress as the plate moves proximally. **E:** A drill hole is centered in the remaining proximal plate hole. **F:** A neutral miniscrew is inserted, completing the fixation. The sequence of miniscrew insertion is numbered. (With permission, from: Heim U, Pfeiffer KM, eds. *Internal Fixation of Small Fractures, 3rd Edition.* New York: Springer Verlag, 1988:54–55; Figs. 31 and 32.)

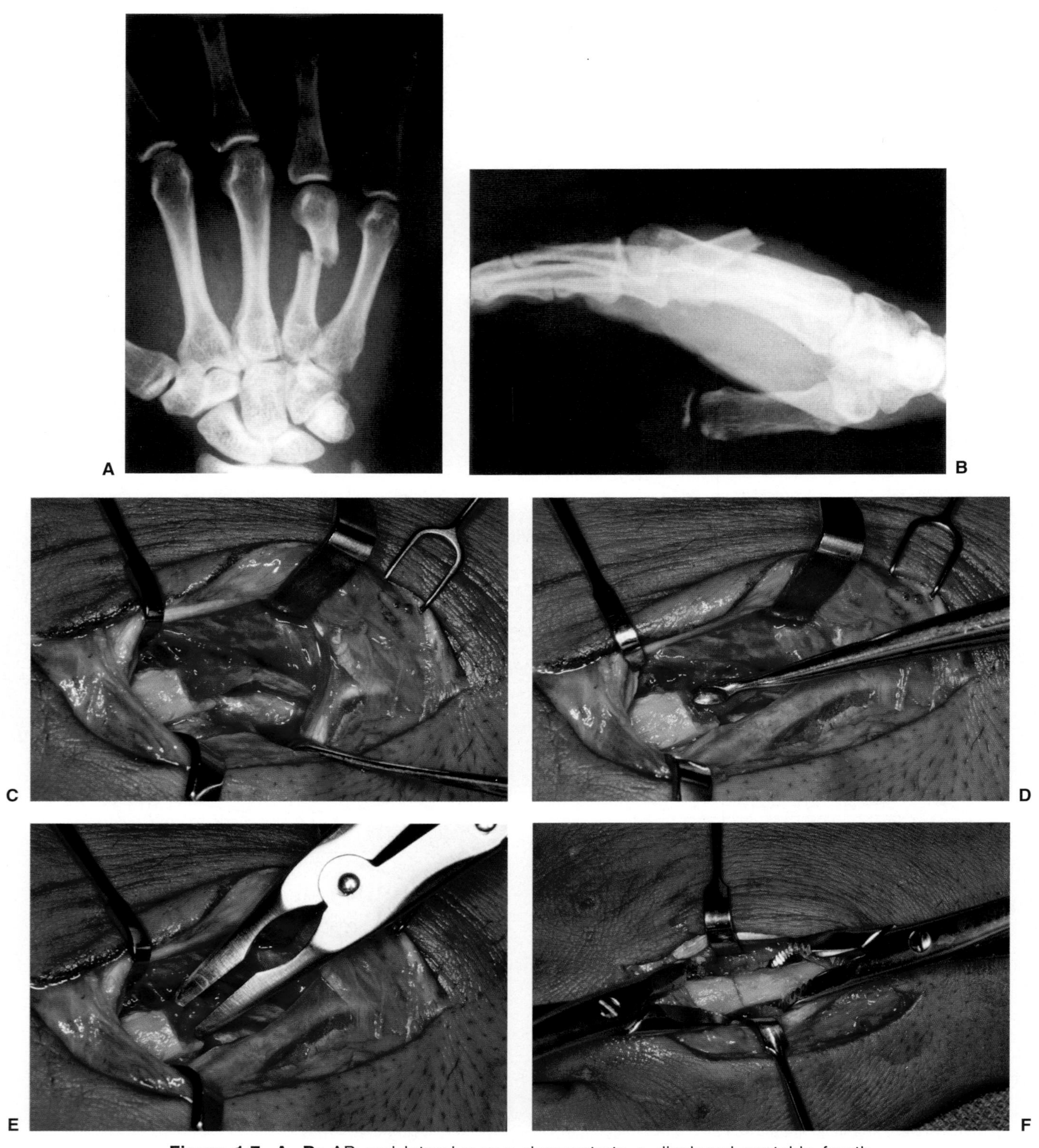

Figure 1.7. A, B: AP and lateral x-rays demonstrate a displaced unstable fourth metacarpal shaft fracture with shortening and angulation in both the AP and lateral planes. There was also rotational malalignment of the ring finger with digital flexion. **C:** The fracture has been exposed. **D, E:** A curette and rongeur are used to remove clot and granulation tissue at the fracture site. **F:** The fracture is reduced by manipulation and instrumentation using bone reduction forceps. Rotational alignment is checked with the fingers flexed into a fist.

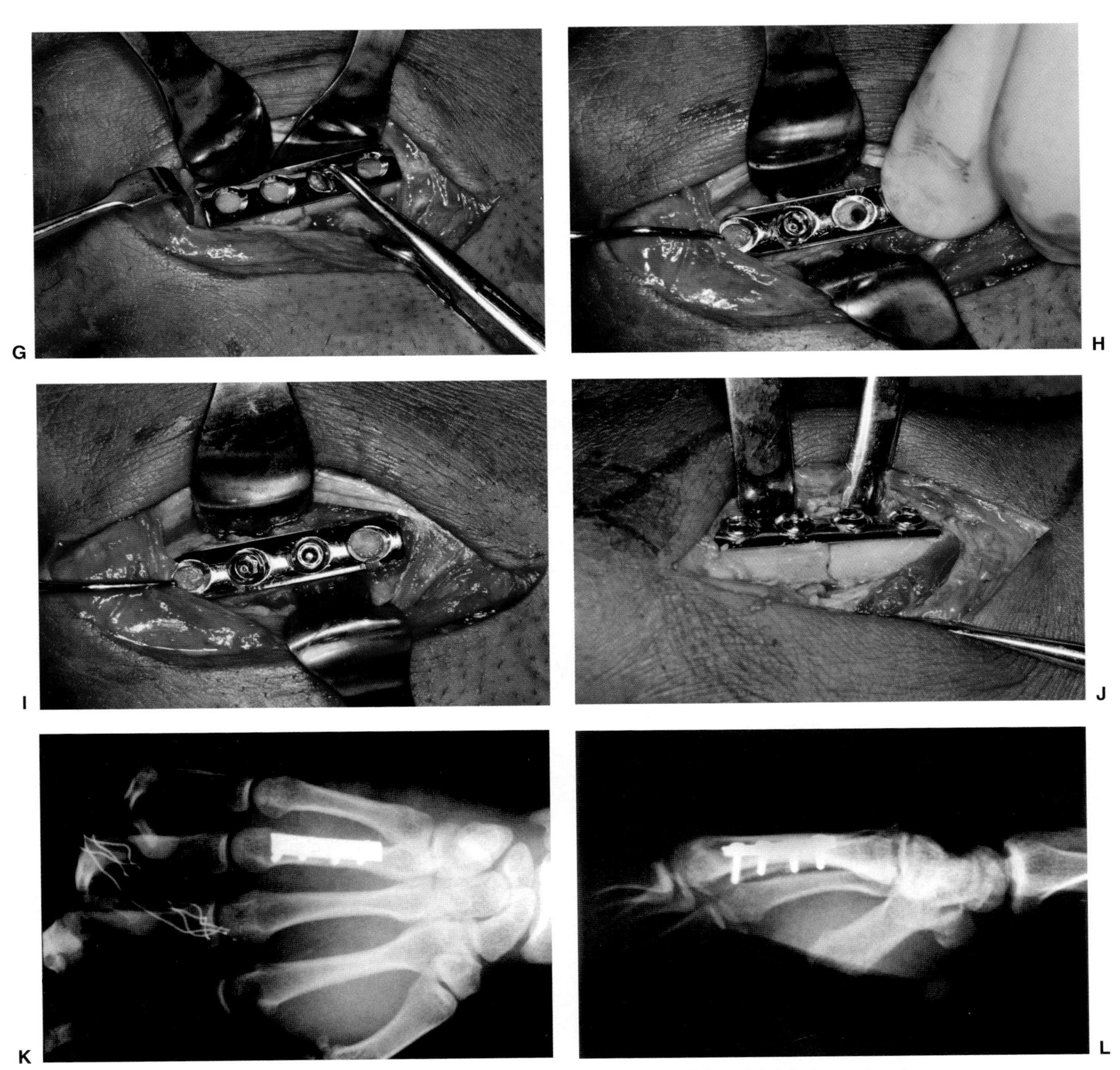

Figure 1.7. *Continued.* **G:** A four-hole slightly bent (5°) straight miniplate is centered over the fracture. **H:** The distal fracture fragment is initially secured with a neutral miniscrew inserted into the plate hole just distal to the fracture. An eccentric hole is drilled through the miniplate hole just proximal to the fracture. **I:** A second miniscrew is inserted into the eccentric drill hole. Engagement of the screw head with the plate hole has compressed the fracture. **J:** Two neutral miniscrews are inserted into the remaining plate holes to complete the construct. **K, L:** Postoperative anteroposterior and lateral x-rays demonstrate stable anatomic fracture fixation.

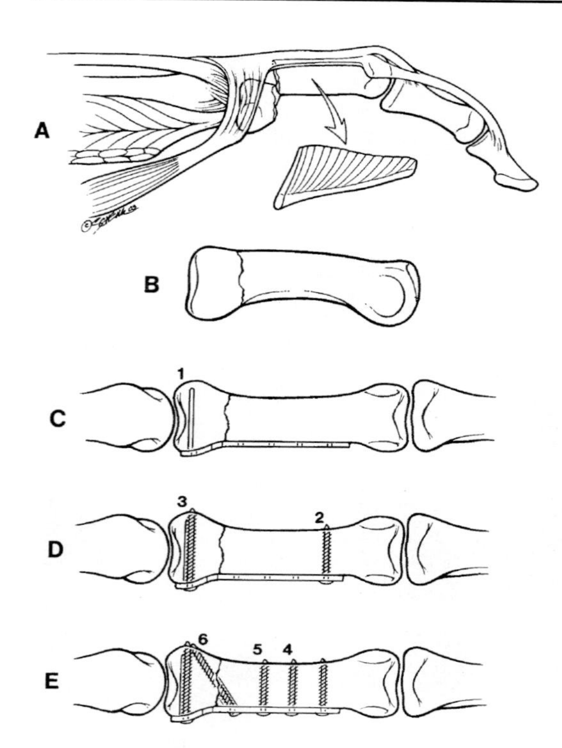

Figure 1.8. **A:** A displaced unstable transverse fracture at the base of a proximal finger phalanx is exposed by resecting one lateral band and the adjacent oblique retinacular fibers. **B:** The fracture is reduced. **C:** A mini-condylar plate is applied laterally by inserting its spike into a drill hole in the proximal metaphyseal fragment. **D:** The stem of the plate is aligned with the distal diaphyseal fragment and secured with a neutral miniscrew inserted through the most distal plate hole. A miniscrew is then inserted through the most proximal plate hole to secure the proximal metaphyseal fragment. Neutral miniscrews are inserted into the remaining distal plate holes in the plate stem. Finally, a mini-compression screw is inserted across the fracture to complete the fixation. (With permission, from: Freeland AE, Sud V, Lindley SG. Unilateral intrinsic resection of the lateral band and oblique fibers of the metacarpophalangeal joint for proximal phalanx fractures. *Techniques in Hand and Upper Extremity Surgery* 5:85–90, 2001; Figs. 3-5, p 87.)

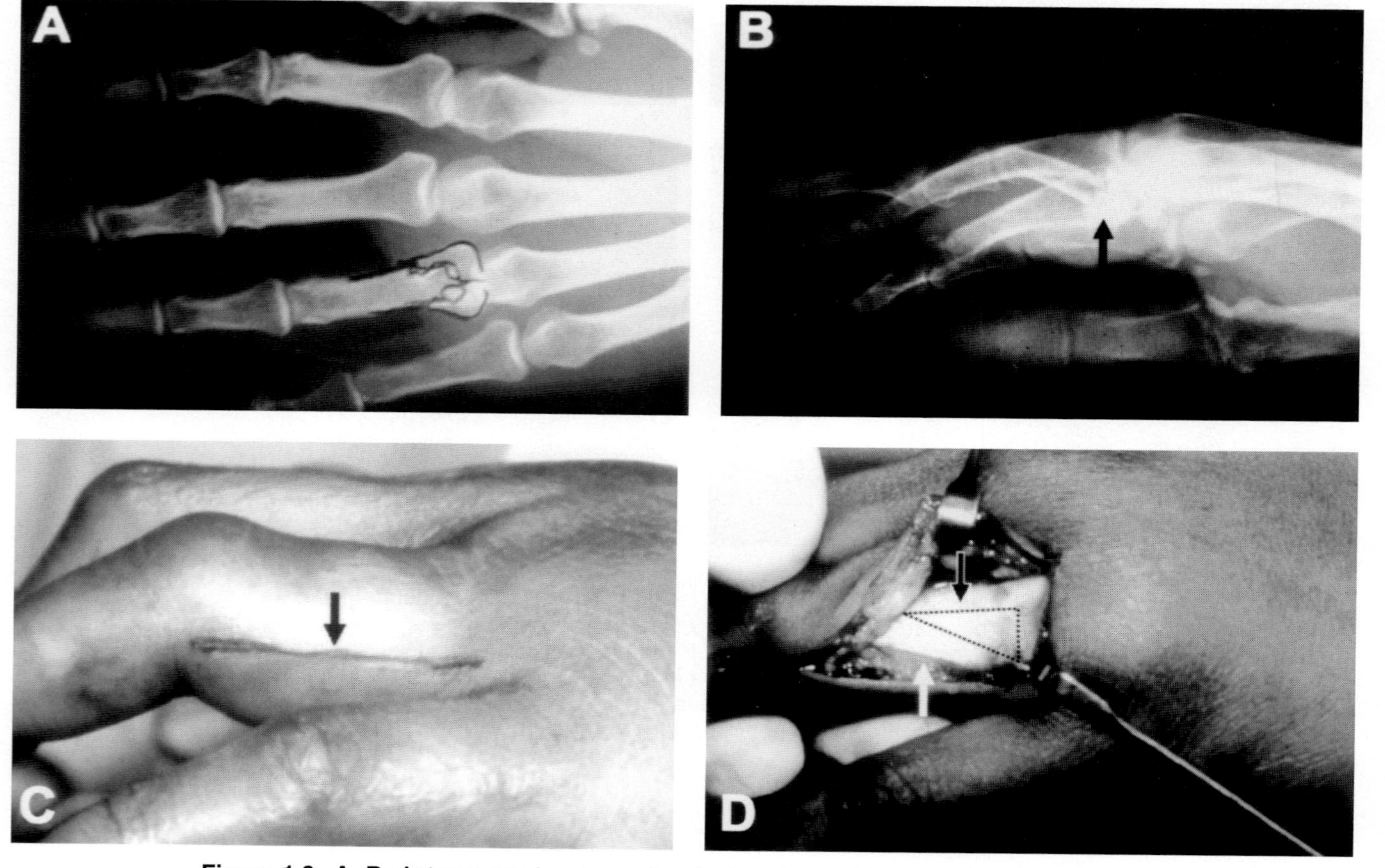

Figure 1.9. **A, B:** Anteroposterior views of a displaced unstable transverse fracture of the proximal phalanx of the ring finger with severe palmar angulation. **C:** A midaxial incision has been drawn on the ulnar side of the ring finger over the fractured proximal phalanx (*black arrow*). **D:** The central extensor tendon (*black arrow*), the oblique fibers (*black dotted triangle*), and the lateral band (*white arrow*) are identified.

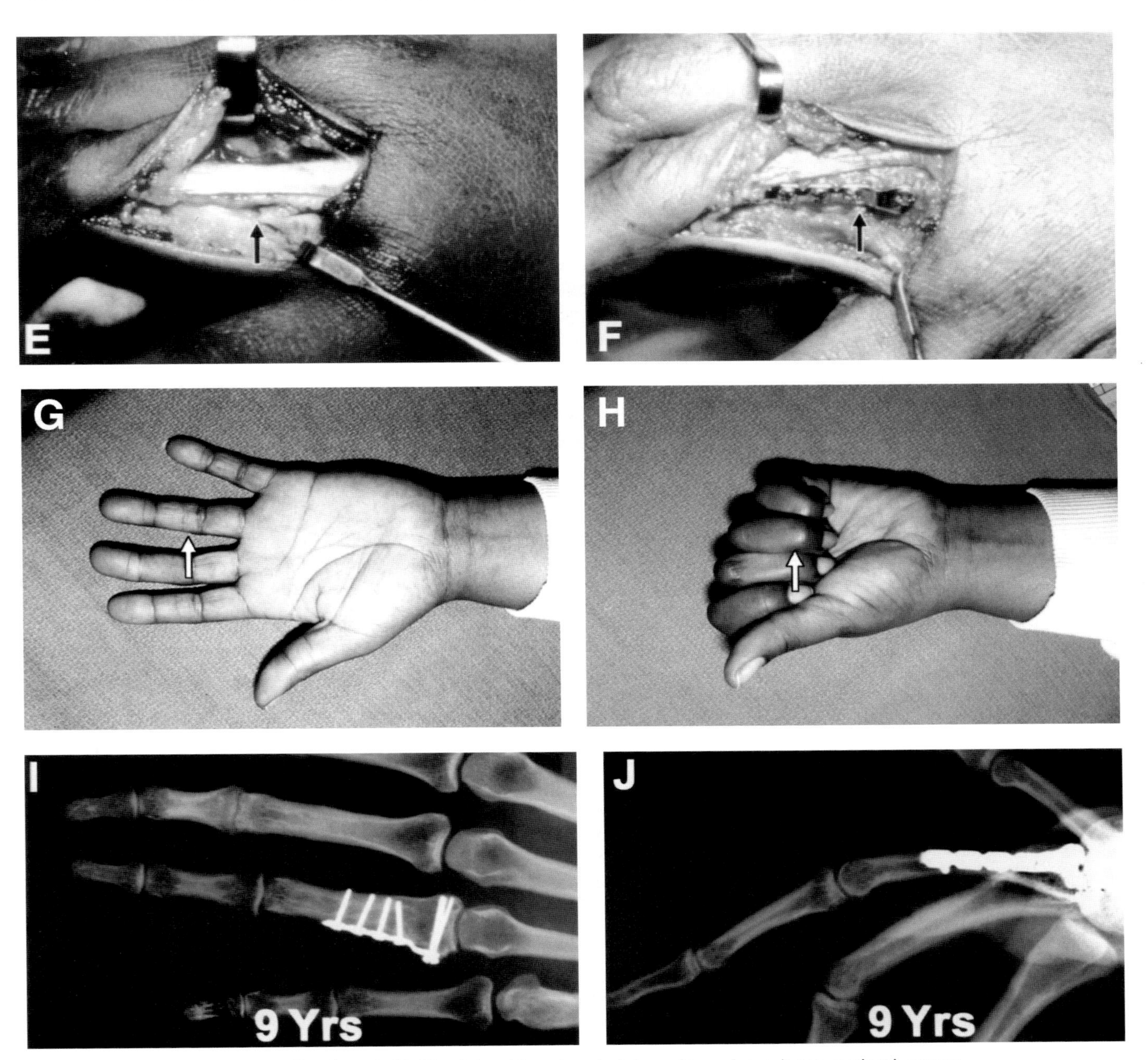

Figure 1.9. *Continued.* **E:** The lateral band and oblique fibers have been excised, exposing the phalangeal fracture (*black arrow*). **F:** The fracture has been reduced and stabilized with a mini-condylar plate (*black arrow*). **G, H:** Photographs demonstrate full recovery of extension and flexion of the ring finger.**I, J:** AP and lateral x-rays demonstrate complete healing of the fracture nine years after injury. (With permission, from: Freeland AE, Sud V, Lindley SG. Unilateral intrinsic resection of the lateral band and oblique fibers of the metacarpophalangeal joint for proximal phalanx fractures. *Techniques in Hand and Upper Extremity Surgery* 5:85–90, 2001; Fig. 6, 7, and 9, p 88–89.)

miniplate. The bend is spread across the entire miniplate by applying the bending irons at the ends of the miniplate. This technique avoids a sharply angled bend at a midplate screw hole that would weaken the miniplate owing to fatiguing forces.

SAGITTAL SHORT OBLIQUE DIAPHYSEAL FRACTURES

The length of the fracture is less than twice the diameter of the fracture in a short oblique fracture. The fracture plane should be noted. In diaphyseal fractures, it is usually preferable to place the miniplate dorsally. Sagittal short oblique fractures at the metaphyseal diaphyseal junction may be exceptions to this rule.

In short sagittal diaphyseal fractures, a mini-lag screw may initially be placed laterally in the compression mode outside the miniplate as shown in Figures 1.10 and 1.11. A five-hole mini-tubular plate may be applied dorsally in the neutralization mode to protect the outlying miniscrew from bending and torsional forces. If necessary, a mini-tubular plate may be bent to conform precisely to the contours of the underlying bone. A middle hole of the miniplate is centered over the outlying mini-compression screw, and no screw is placed in this miniplate hole.

T-shaped, L-shaped, or mini-condylar plates may be applied in the neutralization mode for sagittal short oblique fractures at the metaphyseal diaphyseal junction. Mini-condylar plates are often preferable because they are lower in profile and more precisely fit the bone than do T- or angled L-shaped miniplates. Mini-condylar plates are consequently less likely to obstruct tendon excursion or impede joint motion.

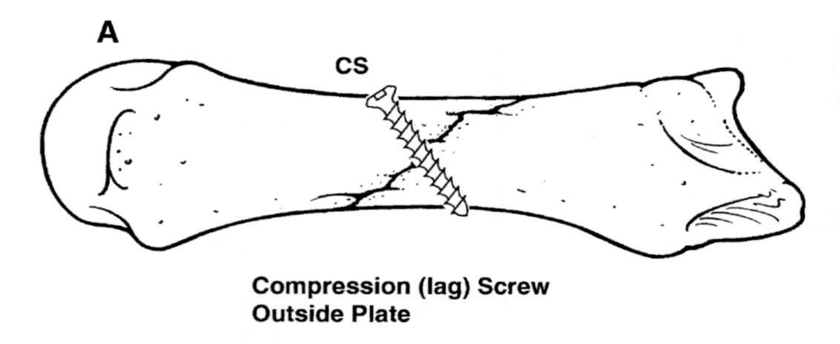

Dorsal Views of Metacarpals

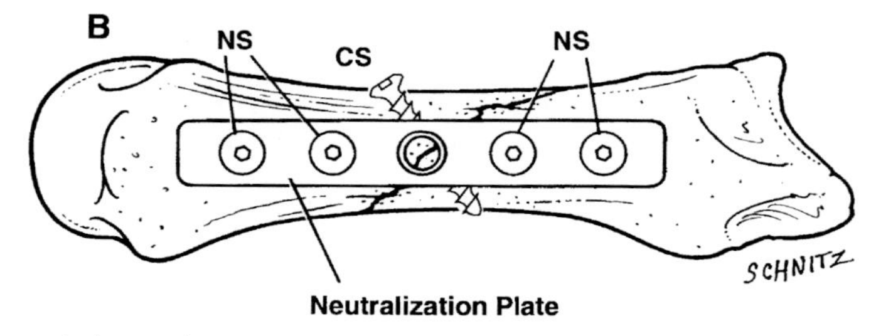

Figure 1.10. Dorsal views of a metacarpal. **A:** A compression miniscrew is first inserted across a short sagittal fracture. **B:** A straight miniplate is then centered dorsally to bridge the fracture and is secured with neutral screws (NS). The miniplate protects the compression screw (CS) from shearing, bending, and rotational forces: thus, it is called a neutralization miniplate. (With permission, from: Heim U, Pfeiffer KM, eds. *Internal Fixation of Small Fractures, 3rd Edition.* New York: Springer Verlag, 1988:58; Fig. 35.)

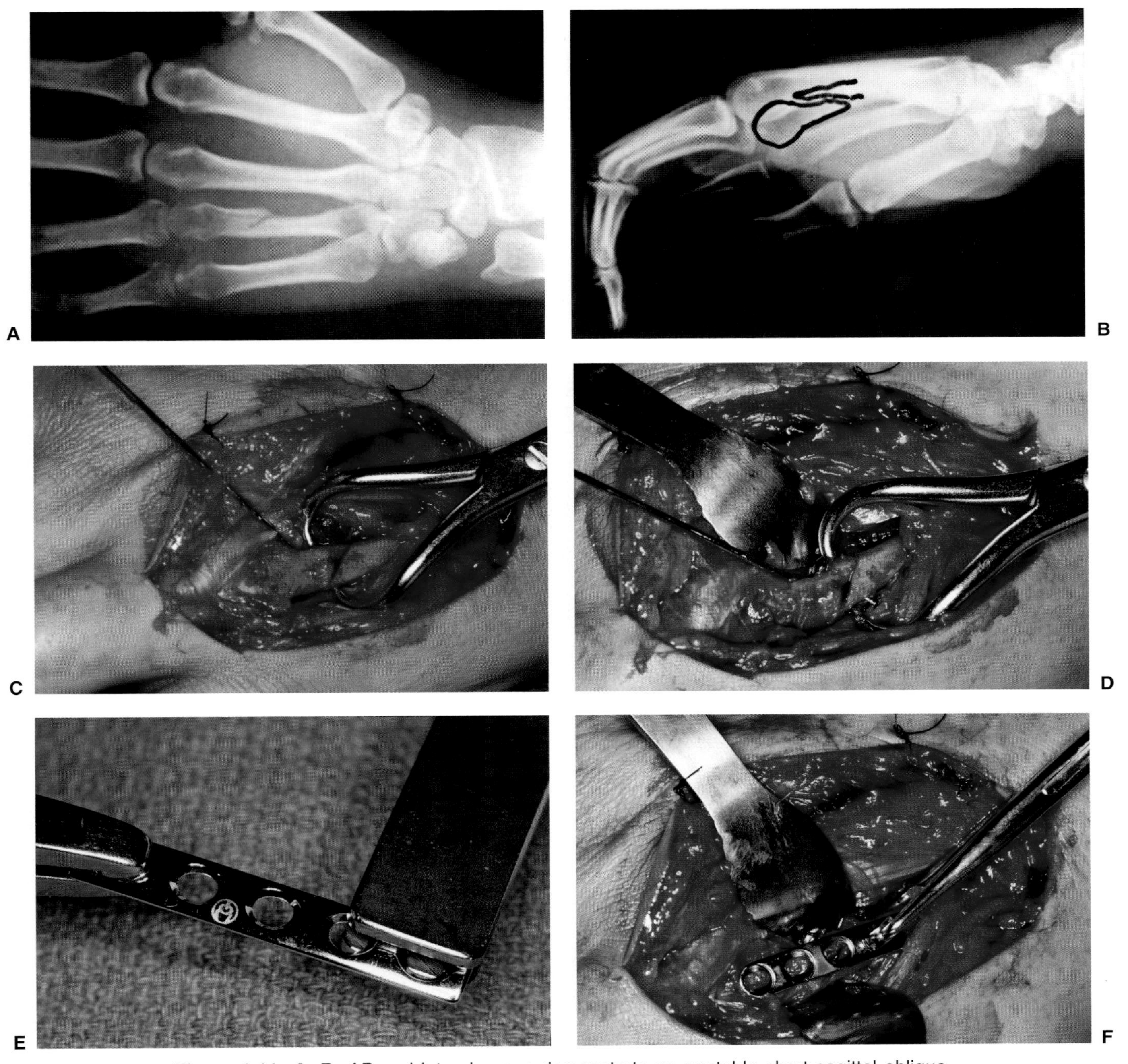

Figure 1.11. A, B: AP and lateral x-rays demonstrate an unstable short sagittal oblique fracture with rotational deformity and overlapping of the ring on the small finger on digital flexion. **C:** A short sagittal oblique metacarpal fracture is reduced and held in position by a pointed reduction forceps. A Kirschner wire is inserted across the distal portion of the fracture to add provisional stability and allow room for insertion of a compression miniscrew in the center of the fracture. **D:** A mini-compression screw is applied across the fracture as demonstrated in Figures 1.4 and 1.5. **E:** Bending irons are used to contour the miniplate so that it conforms to the dorsal cortex over the fracture. Reversing bends or twists of the miniplate may substantially diminish its fatigue strength. **F:** The miniplate is centered over the fracture and secured with a plate holding forceps applied over a screw hole in the miniplate to avoid or minimize plate damage.

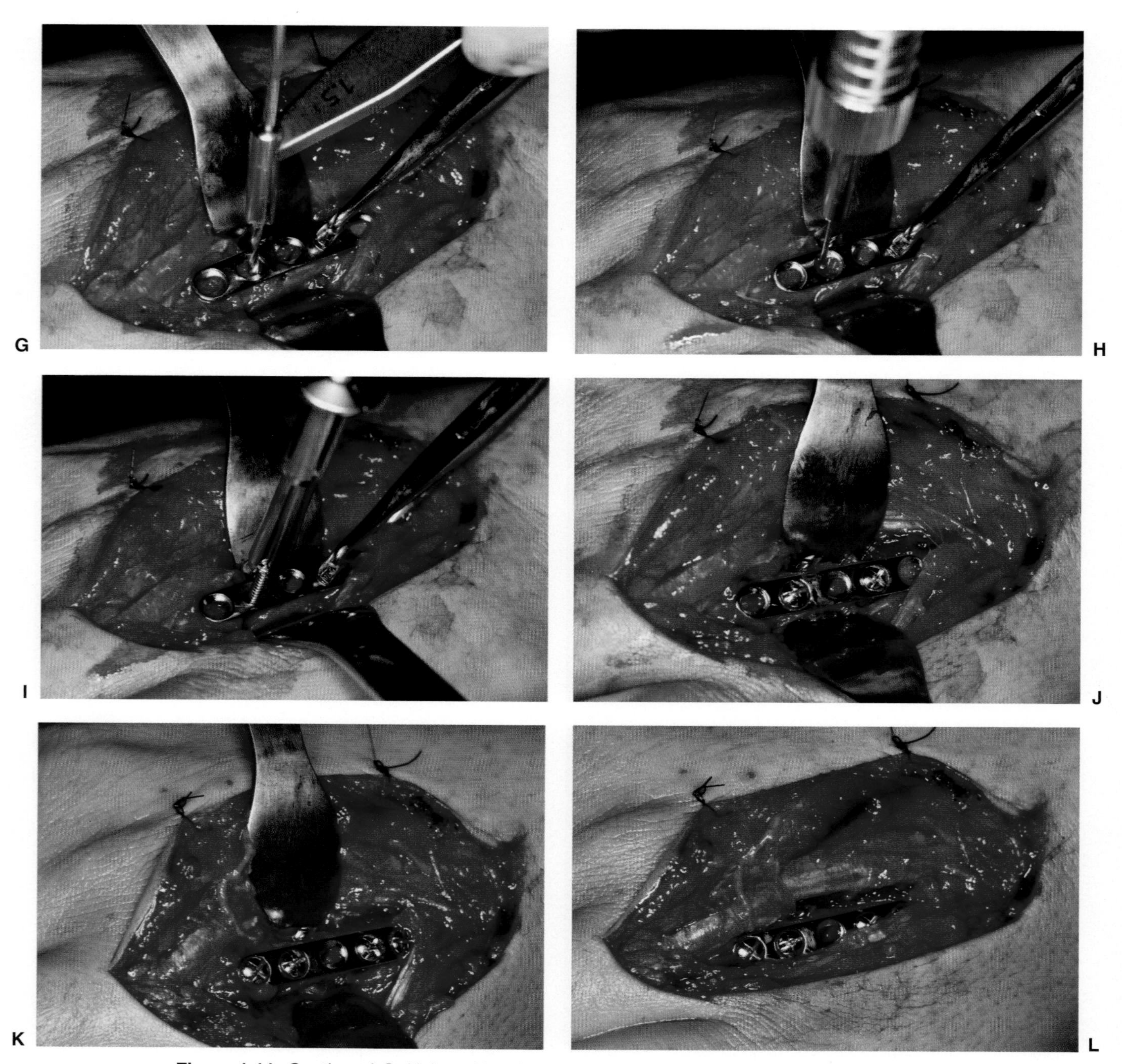

Figure 1.11. *Continued.* **G:** Holes with a diameter corresponding to the core diameter of the selected miniscrew are drilled into the center of the holes of the miniplate proximal and distal to the fracture. **H:** A depth gauge is used to determine the proper screw length. **I:** A self-tapping miniscrew is inserted into the plate hole distal to the fracture. **J:** Miniscrews now secure the miniplate proximal and distal to the fracture. The unfilled middle miniplate hole is directly over the mini-lag screw that is outside and adjacent to the miniplate. **K:** Two additional neutral miniscrews are inserted into the plate holes at both ends of the miniplate to complete the fixation. **L:** The retractor has been removed. The miniplate can still be visualized beneath the extensor tendon and overlying periosteum.

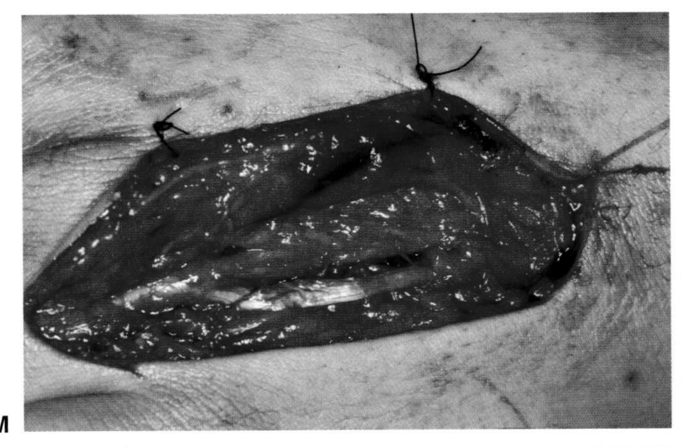
M

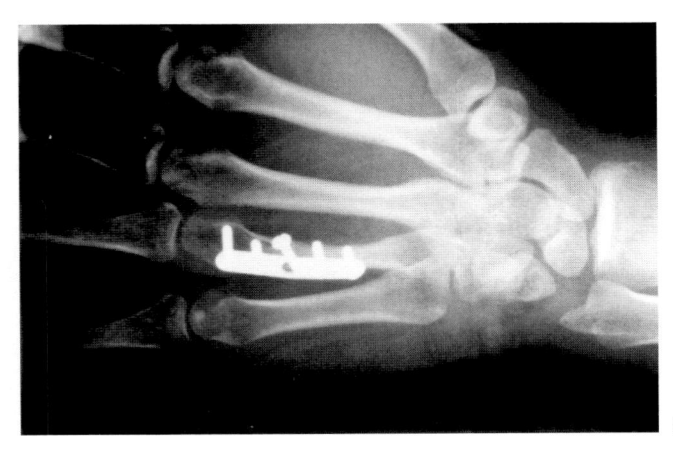
N

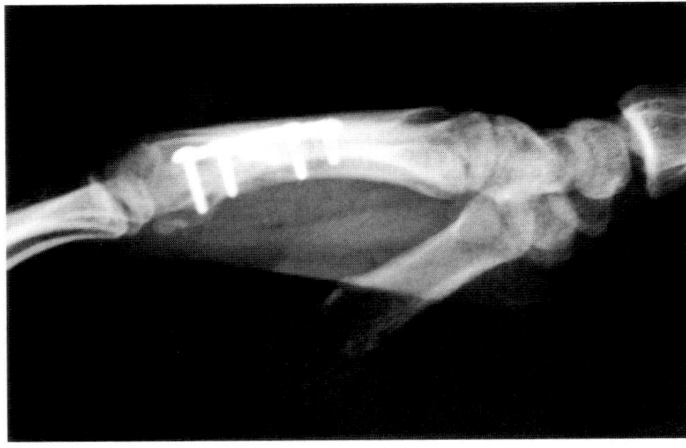
O

Figure 1.11. *Continued.* **M:** The periosteum has been repaired with fine resorbable sutures in an effort to further preserve the gliding function of the extensor tendon as it moves back and forth over the miniplate. **N, O:** Anteroposterior and lateral x-rays demonstrate stable anatomic reduction of the fracture.

CORONAL SHORT OBLIQUE DIAPHYSEAL FRACTURES

A mini-compression plate is applied to coronal short oblique fractures in the same fashion as for transverse fractures. Then, a mini-compression (lag) screw may be placed through a hole in the miniplate to provide further security (Figs. 1.12 and 1.13).

FRACTURES WITH SEVERE COMMINUTION OR BONE LOSS

In selected circumstances, significant comminution may result from high-energy closed mechanisms, or open fractures may be accompanied by bone loss. These challenging problems require advanced fixation techniques, including consideration of staged repair, hybrid fixation and bone grafting.

Mini-external fixation, spacer wires, transfixation wires, or combinations may be used to restore bone position at the time of initial surgery. Delayed primary or remote miniplate fixation and bone grafting (or synthetic graft material use) may be indicated when there is a lack of cortical contact directly opposite the miniplate, comminution, or bone loss. Compressed cancellous bone or synthetic substitutes may be used for partial or complete defects up to 1.5 cm in length. For larger defects, a corticocancellous graft may add stability to the fracture construct. The ipsilateral distal radius metaphysic (either volar or dorsal) is a suitable donor site with little additional morbidity.

Occasionally, the ipsilateral proximal ulna may be a suitable donor site, but this location has a slightly higher risk of traumatic fracture than the distal radius. Larger unicortical or tricortical grafts may be obtained from the iliac crest. Various bone "carpentry" techniques such as pegging, dowel and socketing, and mortising may be used (Figs. 1.14 and 1.15). A single mini-reconstruction plate may span both bone graft junctures, or two miniplates (one

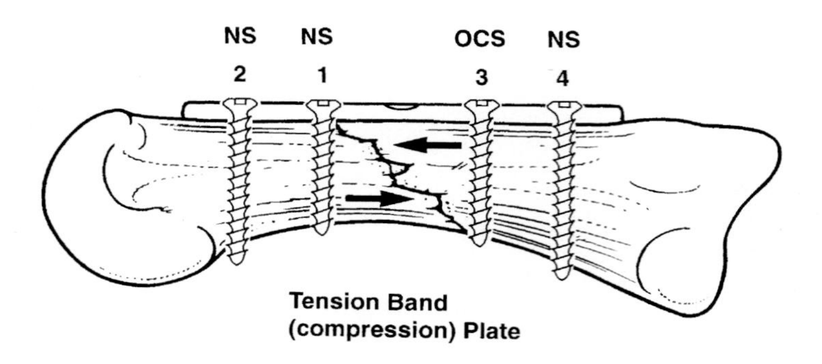

Lateral Views of Metacarpals

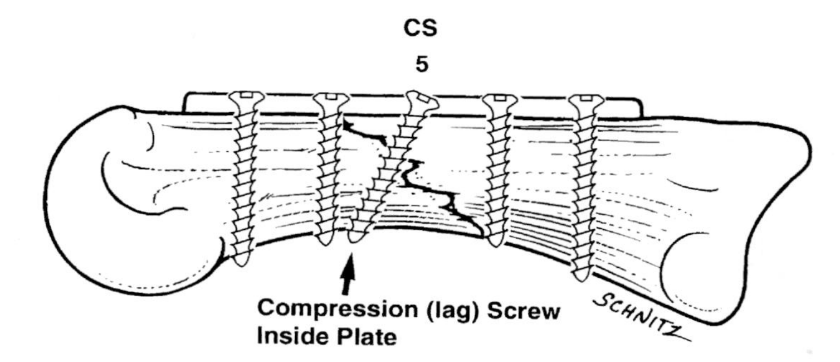

Figure 1.12. A: A dorsal miniplate is applied to compress a coronal short oblique metacarpal shaft fracture. It is essential to insert the offset compression screw (OCS) eccentrically away from the triangle of bone that is compressed into the axilla of the plate. **B:** A compression screw (CS) is then applied across the fracture. The sequence of screw insertion is numbered. (With permission, from: Heim U, Pfeiffer KM, eds. *Internal Fixation of Small Fractures, 3rd Edition.* New York: Springer Verlag, 1988:55; Fig. 32.)

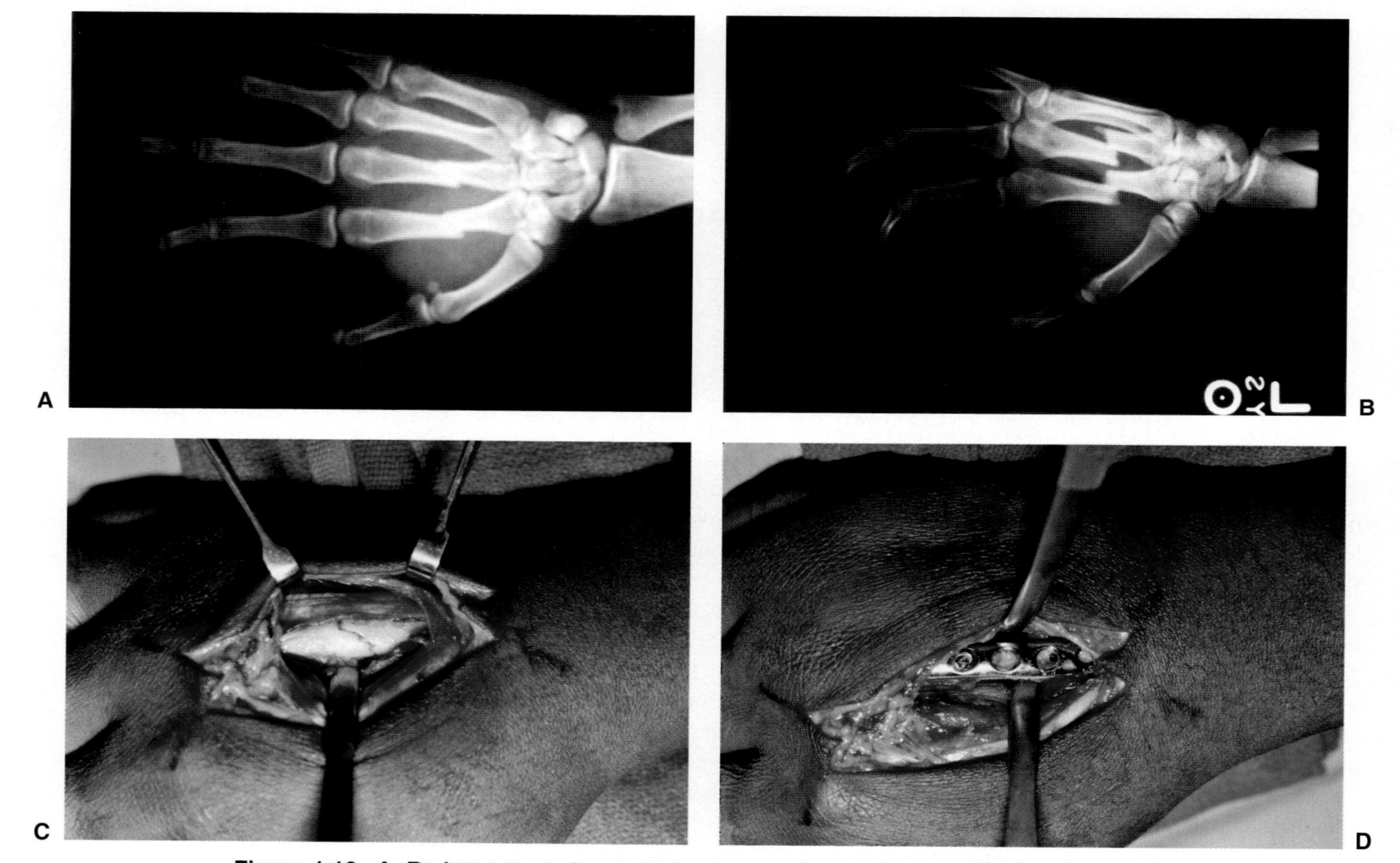

Figure 1.13. A, B: Anteroposterior and lateral x-rays demonstrate two displaced unstable metacarpal shaft fractures. The second metacarpal fracture is transverse and will be fixed with a compression miniplate. A miniplate applied by the technique demonstrated in Figure 1.12 will be applied to secure the short coronal oblique fracture of the third metacarpal shaft. **C:** The third metacarpal fracture is reduced. **D:** A five-hole straight miniplate with a graduated 5° bend is centered over the fracture. A neutral miniscrew is inserted into the distal fragment through the plate hole just distal to the fracture.

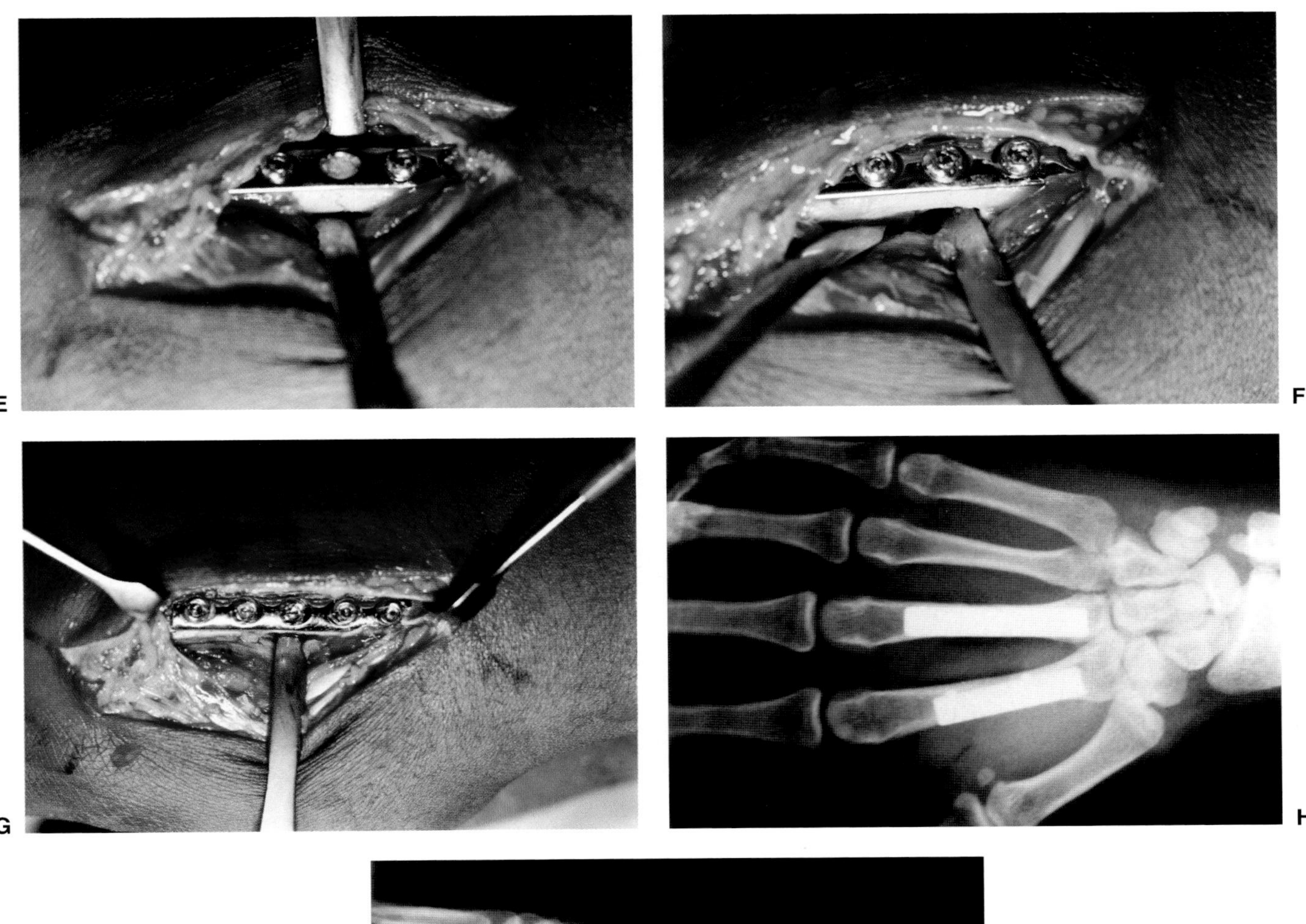

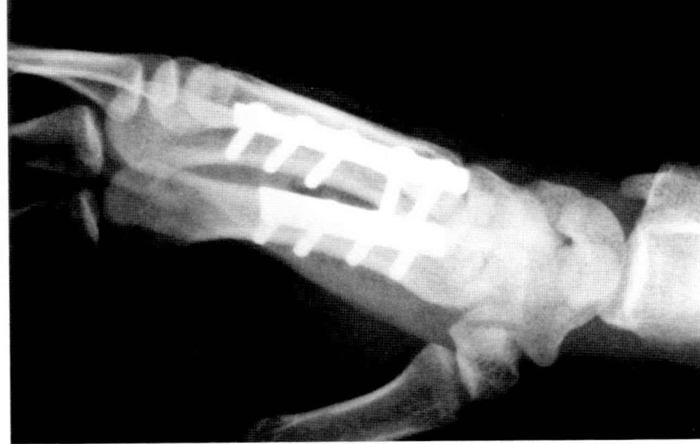

Figure 1.13. *Continued.* **E:** An offset or eccentric hole is drilled into the proximal fragment through the plate hole just proximal to the fracture. A miniscrew has been inserted. As the screw head engaged the plate hole, the distal triangle of the proximal fragment was compressed into the axilla between the distal fragment and the miniplate. **F:** A mini-compression screw was then inserted through the middle plate hole and across the fracture to enhance stability. **G:** Neutral miniscrews were added to the remaining proximal and distal plate holes to complete the fixation. **H, I:** Postoperative x-rays demonstrate anatomic alignment and stable fixation of both fractures. The transverse fracture of the second metacarpal shaft was restored with a four-hole straight miniplate while the coronal oblique fracture of the third metacarpal shaft was secured with a straight mini-compression plate with a mini-compression screw across the fracture through the middle plate hole. Both plates had a graduated 5° bend applied across the length of the plate and centered in the middle of the plate to assure uniform compression across the fracture site.

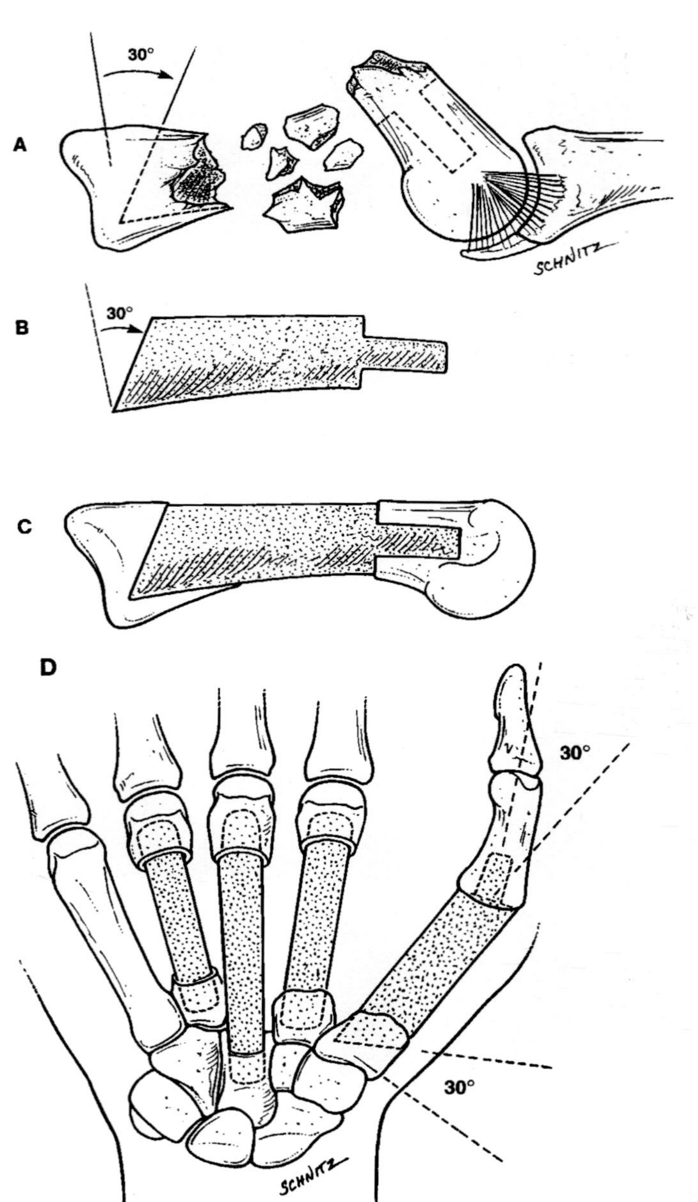

Figure 1.14. A: A mortise is constructed in the proximal metacarpal and a socket distally where bone loss intervenes. **B:** A corticocancellous bone graft is contoured to fit the mortise proximally and with a peg to fit distally. **C:** The bone graft is inserted into the prepared metacarpal. **D:** A variety of configurations of dowels or pegs (small dowels) in sockets and mortising may be used to securely bridge diaphyseal defects in tubular hand bones. (With permission, from: Littler JW. Metacarpal reconstruction. *J Bone Joint Surg* 29A:723–737, 1947; Fig 11, p 727.)

Figure 1.15. A: An AP x-ray demonstrates comminution, bone loss, and shortening of the third metacarpal following a close-range low velocity gunshot wound. **B:** The planned incision is diagrammed. The incision incorporates the wound of entry and is offset radially from the third metacarpal in an effort to minimize operative damage to the extensor tendons. **C:** The fracture is exposed and debrided. Two to three mm of shortening are allowed to avoid intrinsic muscle tightness resulting from muscle injury and to assure full motion at the metacarpophalangeal joint. A tricortical iliac bone graft is harvested, and the proximal and distal ends are shaped to fit into the prepared mortise-cut proximal and distal fractured metacarpal metaphyses. **D:** The bone graft is positioned with the cortical bone on the palmar side of the fracture. **E:** Two mini-condylar plates are inserted in the compression mode to secure the proximal and distal junctures between the bone graft and the fracture. The bone graft is also compressed against the stems of the miniplates with miniscrews inserted into the palmar cortex of the graft. This provides a more secure construct than if the cortex of the graft were secured directly under the plate with the cancellous bone on the palmar side. **F:** An AP x-ray demonstrates excellent fracture alignment and fixation of the fracture with firm apposition at the bone graft fracture junctions. **G:** An AP x-ray taken three years after injury demonstrates complete healing and incorporation of the bone graft. The patient achieved an excellent, unrestricted range of motion after plate removal and tenolysis.

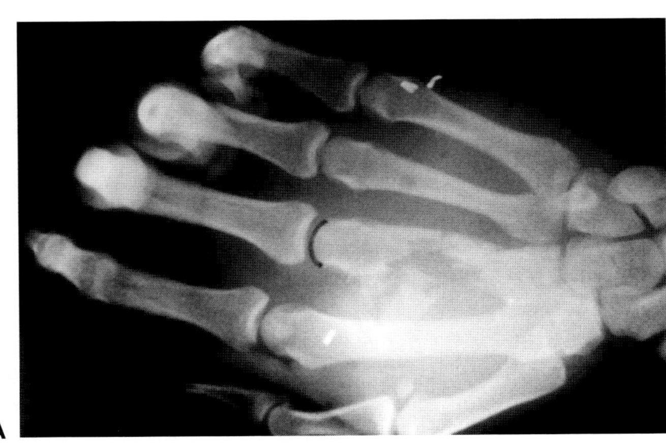

A

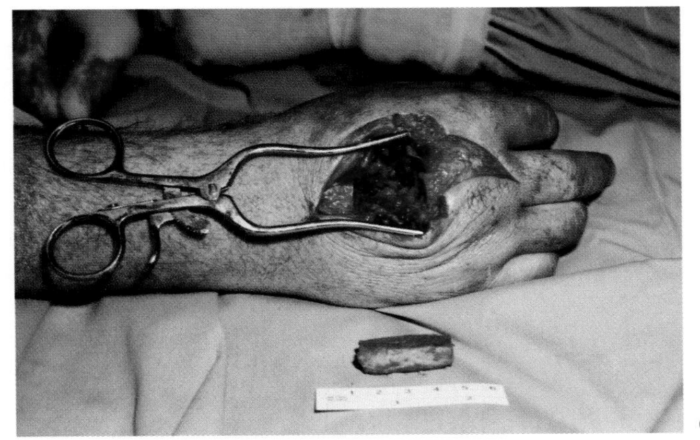

C

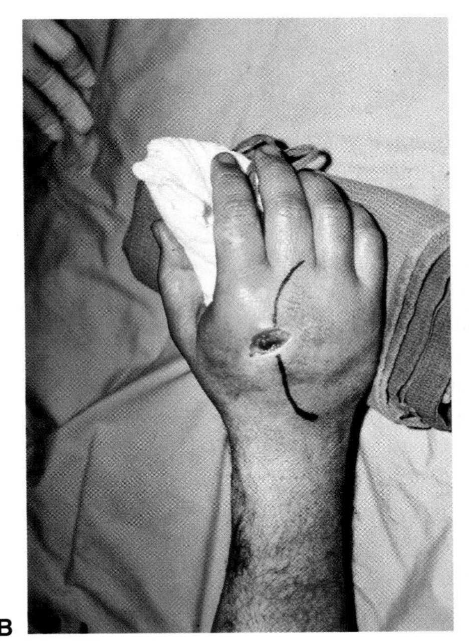

B

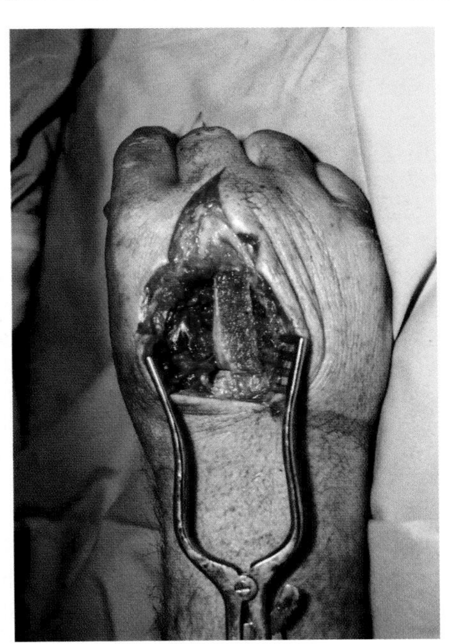

D

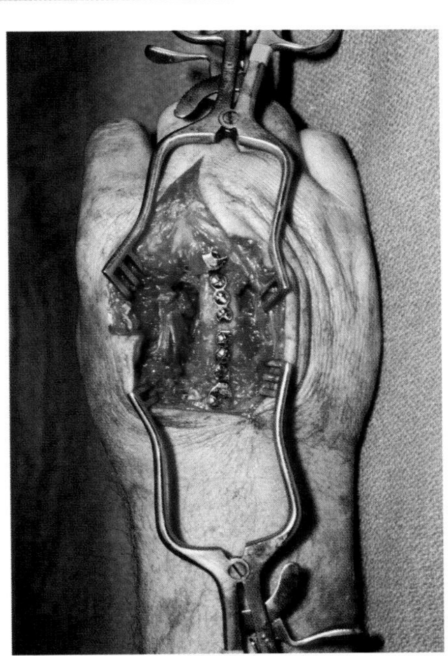

E

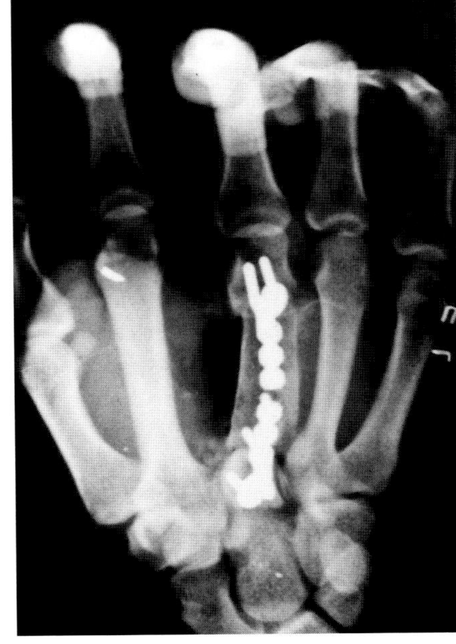

F

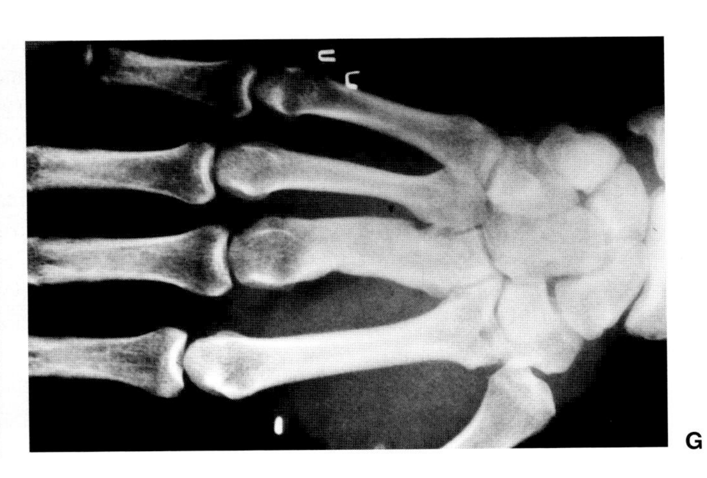

G

for each juncture) may be used. The miniplate selection and physiological application at the particular juncture where it is applied are determined by the configuration of the bone ends at that juncture, as previously described.

POSTOPERATIVE MANAGEMENT

Elevation of the hand above the elbow (and heart) helps to minimize swelling and edema in the immediate postoperative period. The patient is provided with a sling that may be worn during standing, walking, or sitting. Propping the hand on pillows on the arm of a chair may be a useful alternative to wearing a sling when sitting. The reclining patient may rest the hand on the abdomen, chest, or pillows. Ice may be used for up to 72 hours after surgery, but the container should not directly touch the skin. A layer of dry towels or suitable substitute should be used between the ice container and the skin. Ice should not be used if there is any history of cold sensitivity or Raynaud's phenomenon or disease. Appropriate pain medication is prescribed throughout the course of treatment.

The patient may move the fingers gently after surgery. Fingers that work together work best. The patient should be instructed on synchronous digital flexion and extension exercises, starting in the midrange of motion and progressing toward the extremes of full flexion and extension as swelling, tenderness, and pain diminish with time. There is no need to force this motion because a gain of 40° in the midrange of digital motion within the first four weeks after surgery usually prevents significant tendon adhesions. Adding synchronous synergistic wrist motion assists the flexors and extensors in achieving interphalangeal joint motion in a more timely and secure fashion. The hand is a "pump," so these digital actions will promote edema reduction, in addition to minimizing tendon adhesions.

The patient returns 3 to 7 days after surgery for inspection of the incision and digit. Local wound care, dressings, and protective splinting are continued as long as necessary. The splint may be removed to allow gradually progressive digital exercises. These exercises are encouraged every waking hour, may be cued to television commercials, and should not exceed the patient's pain tolerance. The importance of elevation should be reinforced.

The injured finger is often buddy-splinted to an adjacent finger for protection from snagging and to assist in rehabilitation. Tape and splints should be placed to avoid the flexor creases of the interphalangeal joints so as to avoid impeding motion.

Sutures may be removed at 7 to 10 days following surgery. Strength and conditioning exercises may be initiated when the local signs of pain, swelling, tenderness, redness, and heat have substantially receded or resolved, or when fracture callous is judged to be present on X-ray evaluation (approximately four weeks after surgery in uncomplicated cases). Dynamic splinting may be used for recalcitrant stiffness at this time.

Scar and edema management is performed concurrently with exercises during the course of rehabilitation. Elevation is the cornerstone of edema management. Digital motion, retrograde massage, elastic wrapping, compression pumps, and compression finger socks or gloves help to resolve swelling. Massage softens, mobilizes, and desensitizes scar tissue. Vibration therapy and soft plastics may assist in scar resolution. Specific desensitization programs may be useful for refractory cases.

Patients without hand-intensive vocations, especially those with nondominant hand injuries, are often able to return to work within 10 to 14 days after surgery. In contrast, manual workers must be well-healed, pain free (or nearly so), and have good return of function and endurance so that they may return to their jobs safely and productively. This may require up to 8 to 12 weeks after injury and surgery under the best of circumstances, and provided that there are no problems or complications. Light duty work may be negotiable for both heavy manual laborers and those with less hand-intensive vocations. Working to a level of "comfort and safety" may be the best way to express limitations to employers, as it allows the patient to make decisions about his or her own capability; "light duty" restrictions leave too much latitude for interpretation.

Good (i.e., 70%–84% of full normal finger motion) or excellent (i.e., 85%–100% of full normal finger motion) results in simple metacarpal shaft fractures treated with open reduction and internal fixation may be achieved in up to 80%–90% of patients. Owing to the tendency for proliferative and mechanically induced fibroplasia in the zone of the flexor tendon sheath, this figure drops to 60%–70% in phalangeal fractures. Thus, open reduction and internal fixation must be most prudently selected for phalangeal fractures. The thumb and middle and distal finger phalanges are much more forgiving of operative trauma than are the finger proximal phalanges and are better able to compensate for stiffness; good or excellent results may be expected in 80%–90% of these patients. In open fractures, additional motion may be lost commensurate with initial wound severity or complexity and bone comminution or loss.

Objectively, final digital motion has been the traditional measure of outcome. Generally, loss or recovery of strength, power, endurance, and functional activities parallel that of motion. Subjective outcome studies such as the Disabilities of Arm, Shoulder, and Hand (DASH) Evaluation give more insightful information about the patient's perception of the result. This type of outcome study, along with good communication regarding daily living, job, recreational, household, and child- or elder-care activities, will assist in achieving the best possible functional recovery and patient satisfaction.

COMPLICATIONS

The prevention of complications is certainly better than treatment whenever possible. Patients must recognize that a great deal of the outcome may be determined at the second of primary injury. Furthermore, the doctor and patient enter into the intimate relationship of considering surgery based upon a risk-benefit ratio. The risks of surgery are weighed against the benefit of anatomic reduction, enhanced stability, and early motion—all factors that are accepted as positive influences on functional outcome.

It is widely recognized that stiffness or contracture is a potential outcome of the injury itself and the subsequent surgery. Tendon and capsular adhesions can and do occur adjacent to the fracture site and may cause digital stiffness, as reflected by the recovery rates for the tubular hand fractures listed above. Patients appear to tolerate even moderate stiffness, however, provided that it is not accompanied by intolerable pain. A few patients may have an advanced contracture and may require tendon and/or joint capsular release. These patients are identified as surgical candidates only when their contractures are recalcitrant to appropriately aggressive rehabilitation.

The results of these releases are usually inversely proportional to the size of the original zone of injury. Contractures accompanying simple closed or open fractures are much more likely to respond favorably than are those due to crush. It is preferable, but not always possible, that the fracture be healed, the scar mature, and motion plateaued after an extensive therapy and rehabilitation program prior to undertaking adhesion or contracture release. Metal implants may be removed concurrently with soft tissue releases, provided that the fracture has adequately healed. Rarely, amputation may be necessary for a severely contracted finger, especially if it is painful or otherwise complicated; this consideration is almost always limited to the border digits (index and small rays).

Nonunion and malunion of simple fractures are rare (fewer than 1%). These complications are more likely to occur in fractures with comminution or bone loss (5%–6%). Implant loosening or breakage may occur, especially in cases of delayed union or nonunion. This type of occurrence may also lead to a loss of fracture alignment, but are most often associated with inadequate or poorly executed internal fixation.

The rate of infection is minimal with simple fractures but increases with injury severity, i.e., up to 5% with complex open fractures and 10% with digital replantations. Treatment is carried out with local wound care and systemic antibiotics. Stable fixation should be left in place until the fracture heals. If the fixation is not stable, it should either be revised or an alternative reconstruction procedure considered. Amputation may be necessary and prudent in severe cases, especially those complicated by osteomyelitis or joint sepsis.

Chronic scar- or nerve-mediated pain syndromes may occur. A "neuroma sign" (tingling or electric shock sensation at the point of impact of digital percussion) may signify the presence of a neuroma of a sensory nerve in an area of scar tissue. The dorsal sensory branches of the radial, ulnar, or digital nerves are most commonly involved. Resolution of pain with injection of local anesthesia at the site of the epicenter of the pain may lend further credence to this diagnosis. An aggressive therapy and desensitization may provide symptomatic relief. Steroid injections or nerve impulse suppressive medications are sometimes helpful. More often, the neuroma must be treated operatively by restoration with nerve grafting or transposition into bone, muscle, or non-impacted dorsal soft tissue in order to alleviate or resolve the patient's pain.

Chronic complex regional pain may occur, heralded by disproportionate pain, excessive and persistent swelling, dysvascular temperature, and color changes. Trophic signs such as smooth shiny skin, excessive sweating, brawny induration, loss of rugal pattern, and digital tapering may evolve. Firm fracture stabilization and avoidance of sensory nerve injury minimize this complication. Early recognition and treatment with neurosuppressive medications, sympathetic blocks, and vigorous therapy may be successful.

RECOMMENDED READING

1. Arzimanoglou A, Skiadaresis SM. Study of internal fixation by screws of oblique fractures in long bones. *J Bone Joint Surg* 34A:219–223, 1952.
2. Baratz ME, Divelbiss B. Fixation of phalangeal fractures. *Hand Clin* 13:541–555, 1997.
3. Buchler U, Fischer T. Use of a mini-condylar plate for metacarpal and phalangeal periarticular injuries. *Clin Orthop* 214:53–58, 1987.
4. Duncan RW, Freeland AE, Jabaley ME, et al. Open hand fractures: an analysis of the recovery of active motion and of complications. *J Hand Surg* 18A:387–394, 1993.
5. Freeland AE. *Hand Fractures: Repair, Reconstruction, and Rehabilitation*. Philadelphia: Churchill-Livingstone, 2000.
6. Freeland AE, Geissler WB. Plate fixation of metacarpal shaft fractures. In: Blair WF, ed. *Techniques in Hand Surgery*. Baltimore: Williams and Wilkins, 1996:255–264.
7. Freeland AE, Geissler WB, Weiss APC. Operative treatment of common displaced and unstable fractures of the hand. *J Bone Joint Surg* 83A:928–945, 2001.
8. Freeland AE, Jabaley ME. Hand and wrist fractures. In: Cohen M, ed. *Mastery of Hand and Reconstructive Surgery*, Volume 3. Boston: Little Brown, 1994:1508–1530.
9. Freelan, AE, Jabaley ME. Screw fixation of the diaphysis for phalangeal fractures. In: Blair WF, Steyers, CM eds. *Techniques in Hand Surgery*. Baltimore: Williams and Wilkins, 1996:192–201.
10. Freeland AE, Jabaley ME. Plate fixation of metacarpal fractures. In: Blair WF, Steyers CM, eds. *Techniques in Hand Surgery*. Baltimore: Williams and Wilkins, 1996:255–264.
11. Freeland AE, Jabaley ME. Stabilization of fractures of the hand and wrist with traumatic soft tissue and bone loss. *Hand Clin* 4:425–436, 1988.
12. Freeland AE, Jabaley ME. Open reduction internal fixation: metacarpal fractures. In: Strickland JW, ed. *Master Techniques in Orthpaedic Surgery: The Hand*. Philadelphia: Lippincott-Raven, 1988:3–33.
13. Freeland AE, Jabaley ME, Burkhalter WE, et al. Delayed primary bone grafting in the hand and wrist after traumatic bone loss. *J Hand Surg* 9A:22–28, 1984.
14. Freeland AE, Sennett BJ. Phalangeal fractures. In: Peimer CA, ed. *Surgery of the Hand and Upper Extremity*. New York: McGraw-Hill, 1996:921–937.
15. Freeland AE, Sud V, Lindley SG. Unilateral intrinsic resection of the lateral band and oblique fibers of the metacarpophalangeal joint for proximal phalanx fractures. *Techniques in Hand and Upper Extremity Surgery* 5:85–90, 2001.
16. Heim U, Pfeiffer KM. *Internal Fixation of Small Fractures*, 3rd ed. New York: Springer-Verlag, 1988.
17. Kozin SH, Thoder JJ, Lieberman G. Operative treatment of metacarpal and phalangeal shaft fractures. *J Am Acad Orthop Surg* 8:111–121, 2000.
18. Littler JW. Metacarpal reconstruction. *J Bone Joint Surg* 29A 723–737, 1947.
19. Littler JW. Hand, wrist, and forearm incisions. In: Littler JW, Cramer LM, Smith JW, eds. *Symposium on Reconstructive Hand Surgery*. St. Louis: Mosby, 1974:202.
20. Ouellette EA, Freeland AE. Use of the mini-condylar plate in metacarpal and phalangeal fractures. *Clin Orthop* 327:38–46, 1996.
21. Pratt DR. Exposing fractures of the proximal phalanx of the finger longitudinally through the dorsal extensor apparatus. *Clin Orthop* 15:22–26, 1959.
22. Stern PJ. Management of fractures of the hand over the last 25 years. *J Hand Surg* 25A:817–823, 2000.
23. Stern PJ, Wieser MJ, Reilly DG. Complications of plate fixation in the hand skeleton. *Clin Orthop* 214:59–65, 1987.
24. Strickland JW, Steichen JB, Kleinman WB. Phalangeal fractures: factors influencing digital performance. *Orthop Rev* 11:39–50, 1982.

2

Closed Pinning and Bouquet Pinning of Fractures of the Metacarpals

Lance A. Rettig and Thomas J. Graham

INDICATIONS/CONTRAINDICATIONS

The majority of isolated metacarpal fractures are effectively managed with closed reduction and splint immobilization in the safe position. However, a subset of metacarpal shaft or neck fractures cannot be reduced by closed means or are unstable after reduction. For these fractures, operative treatment is a consideration or a requirement.

Closed manipulation and percutaneous pinning is a surgical alternative for the transverse or short oblique diaphyseal metacarpal fracture that is reducible but cannot be maintained in plaster. Additional operative indications include multiple adjacent metacarpal fractures, fractures in the polytrauma patient, and metacarpal fractures associated with soft tissue injuries that preclude prolonged plaster immobilization.

In addition to conventional closed reduction and percutaneous pinning, the alternative of intramedullary or bouquet pinning is a valuable addition to the surgeon's portfolio of operative techniques. Bouquet pinning is best suited for unstable fractures in the distal metadiaphyseal or metacarpal neck region. The technique is most amenable for fracture fixation in the border digits (small and index). Additionally, bouquet pinning offers the reduction and stabilization capabilities that make it an attractive alternative for those special subsets of patients, athletes, surgeons, and upper extremity ambulators who need to minimize immobilization time. However, the desire of patients to realize the benefits of bouquet pinning and the success of this teaching in the hands of experienced surgeons are applying pressure to expand the indications beyond this selected group.

Lance A. Rettig, M.D.: Methodist Sports Medicine Center, Thomas A. Brady Clinic, Indianapolis, IN, and Indiana University, IN

Thomas J. Graham, M.D.: Department of Orthopaedic Surgery, The Curtis National Hand Center, Union Memorial Hospital, Baltimore, MD, and Departments of Orthopaedics and Plastic Surgery, Johns Hopkins University Hospital, Baltimore, MD

Few true contraindications exist to smooth wire stabilization of selected metacarpal fractures. Gracile metacarpal shafts, especially those with excessively narrow intramedullary canals, make either technique more challenging. Some patients, smaller females in particular, do not have a capacious intramedullary metacarpal canal, precluding bouquet pinning. Age is a consideration in patients with open physis.

PREOPERATIVE PLANNING

Physical examination should be directed toward assessing rotation, shortening, and angulation of the digit resulting from the metacarpal fracture. Anteroposterior, lateral, and oblique hand X-rays are important to help characterize the fracture and define the metacarpal anatomy.

When considering the technique of collateral recess pinning, special attention should be directed toward appreciating the morphology of the metacarpal head and neck region to rule out associated fractures and to familiarize the surgeon with the patient's unique anatomy. Reduction should be performed in all displaced metacarpal fractures because much can be learned about the relative stability of the fracture. An assessment of whether the fracture is the type that is suited for collateral recess pinning or bouquet pinning can be made on the basis of the radiographic and clinical data.

SURGERY

A myriad of configurations and techniques have been described for closed reduction and pinning of metacarpal fractures. These have included cross-pinning, transverse pinning to an adjacent intact metacarpal, longitudinal (intramedullary) pinning, or combinations of these patterns. Collateral recess pinning and bouquet pinning are described because of the technical challenge inherent in these fixation methods and their unique utility.

The operating room set-up is standard for surgery of the hand. The patient is supine with the affected extremity on a hand table. A padded pneumatic tourniquet encircles the proximal brachium. The anesthesia choices range from local (wrist block) and regional (including axillary and Bier block) to general endotracheal anesthesia.

Collateral Recess Metacarpal Pinning

Provisional closed reduction of the fracture is performed. The metacarpophalangeal joint of the fractured metacarpal is flexed to 90 degrees. A 0.045-inch or 0.062-inch Kirschner pin is manually positioned percutaneously onto the radial or ulnar collateral recess while maintaining the flexed posture of the metacarpophalangeal joint. The initial pin placement is completed by feel or stereognosis (Fig. 2.1A). Fluoroscopy is used to confirm appropriate placement at the deepest concavity of the collateral recess (Fig. 2.1B). A lateral view is also completed to evaluate the position of the wire in the sagittal plane.

Assessing initial pin position is critical to minimize the number of additional passes of the wire required to achieve fixation. Once the pin has been manually positioned in the collateral recess, the driver is positioned over the wire. The pin is captured at its flex point nearest the leading end of the Kirschner wire (Fig. 2.2A). The pin is then advanced into the shoulder of the metacarpal while the appropriate angle is established. One must consider the relationship of the pin to the metacarpal in both the sagittal and frontal planes prior to intramedullary placement of the wire. The Kirschner pin needs be positioned collinear with the long axis of the metacarpal within the sagittal plane (Fig. 2.2B). Alignment in the coronal plane requires that the pin be placed at an angle so that the leading edge of the wire crosses the fracture site within the confines of the intramedullary canal.

Fluoroscopy is repeated to check the overall alignment of the pin and its insertion site. The fracture site is visualized to check reduction. Once anatomic alignment of the fracture

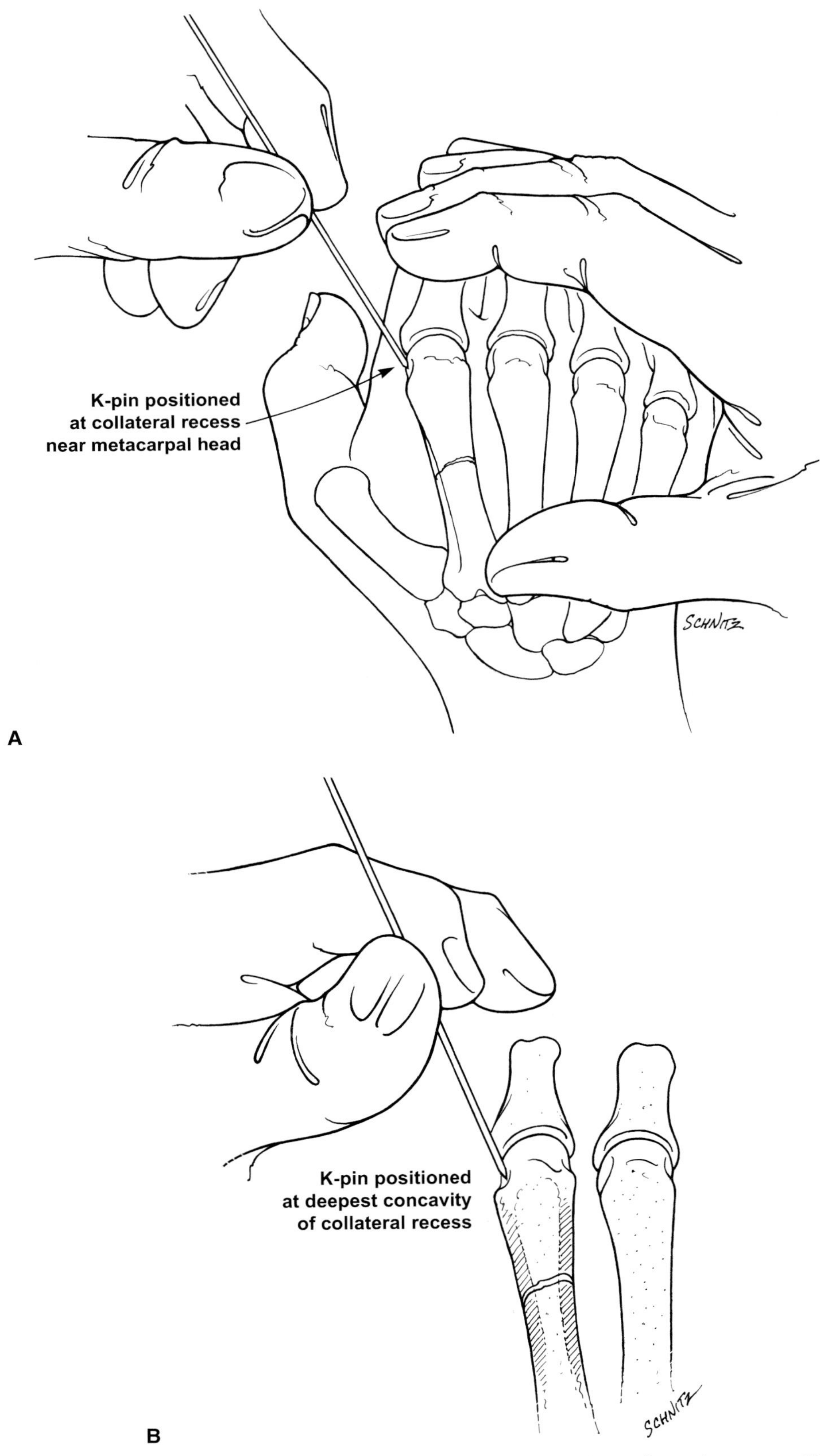

Figure 2.1. A: The Kirschner pin is manually placed into the collateral recess with the metacarpalphalangeal joint of the fractured metacarpal flexed to 90º. **B:** The smooth wire is placed at the deepest concavity of the collateral recess.

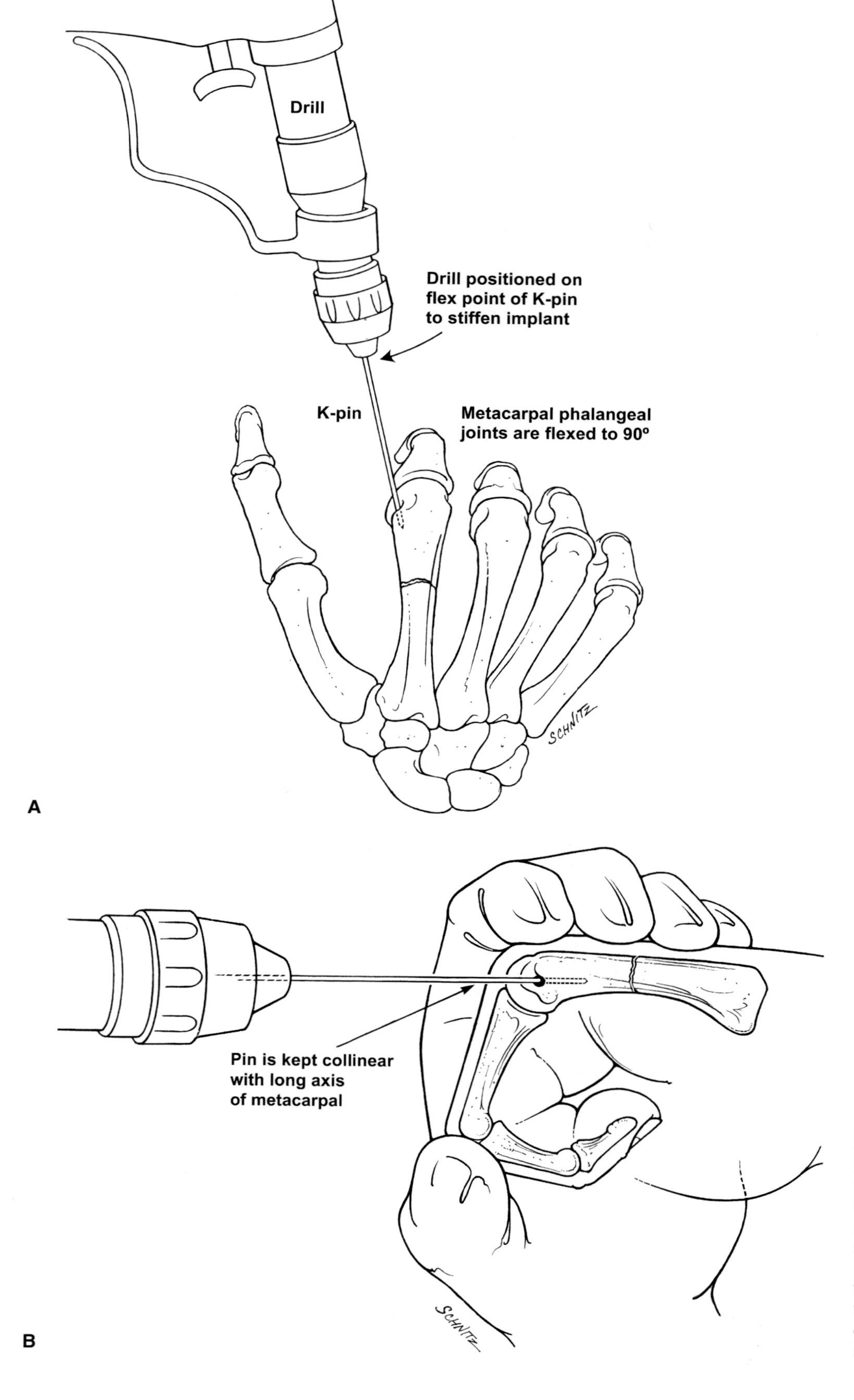

Figure 2.2. A: After manual positioning the Kirschner wire onto the collateral recess, the pin is captured at the flex point nearest the leading edge of the smooth pin. The metacarpophalangeal joint is maintained in a flexed position. **B:** Prior to pin advancement, the wire is positioned collinear with the long axis of the metacarpal shaft.

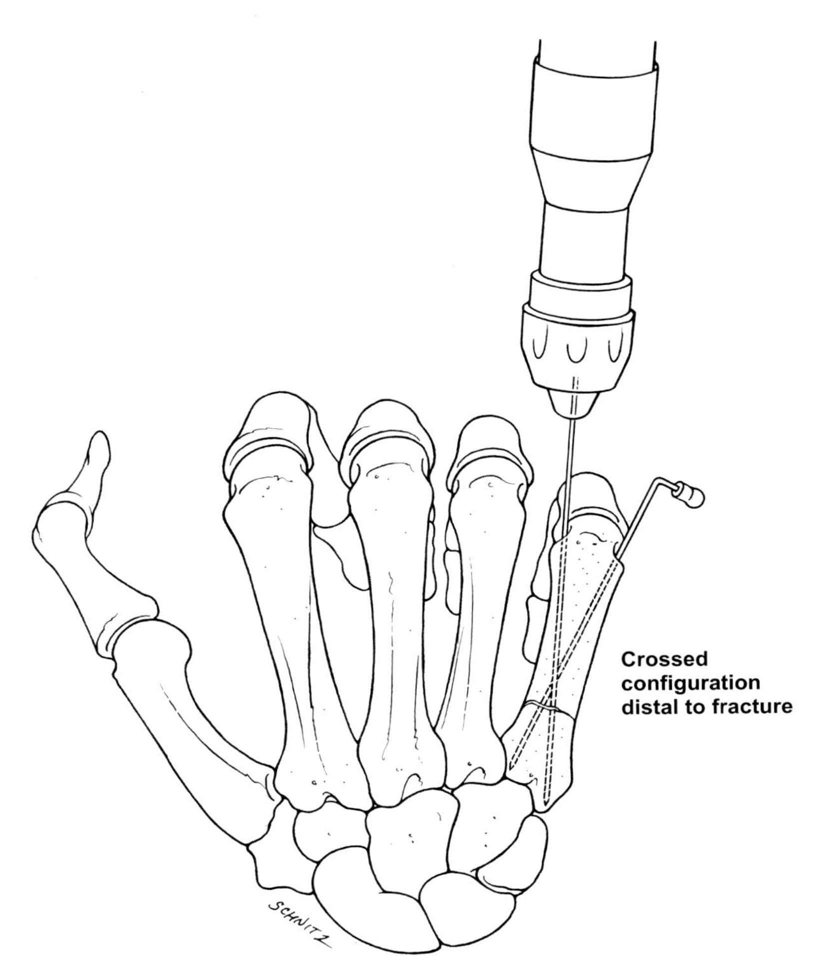

Figure 2.3. Ideally the collateral recess pins occupy a crossed configuration within the medullary canal with purchase in the proximal metacarpal metaphysis.

has been confirmed, the wire is advanced across the fracture, down the medullary canal, and into the proximal cortex. Ideally, proximal fixation is obtained with cortical purchase in the metacarpal base or metaphysis (opposite cortex from initiation point) (Fig. 2.3). Crossing the carpometacarpal (CMC) joint to allow the pin to reside in the distal carpus is typically not problematic (Fig. 2.4).

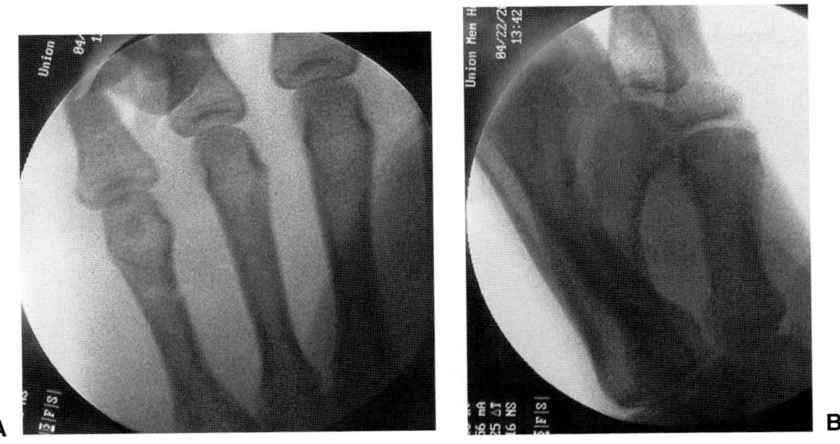

Figure 2.4. A, B: Preoperative flouroscan views of a 16-year-old elite lacrosse player who presented with a middle 1/3, distal 1/3 diaphyseal small finger metacarpal fracture difficult to control by closed means. Clinically, he was found to have metacarpal head prominence within the palm of his stick-handling extremity. Bouquet pinning was considered for these reasons.

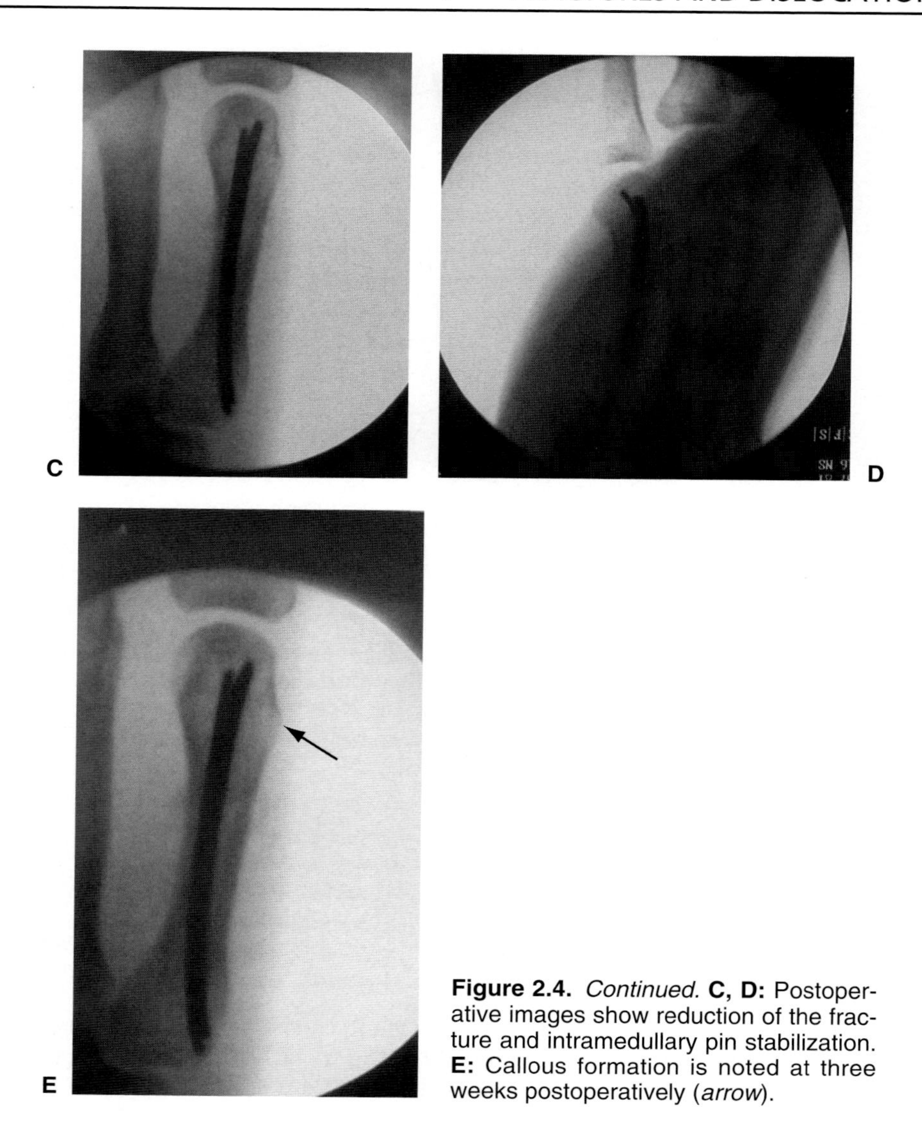

Figure 2.4. *Continued.* **C, D:** Postoperative images show reduction of the fracture and intramedullary pin stabilization. **E:** Callous formation is noted at three weeks postoperatively (*arrow*).

Maintenance of fracture reduction and pin placement is confirmed with intra-operative imaging. A second pin of the same caliber is placed in the opposite collateral recess using the previously discussed technique. Often the two pins obtain a crossed configuration proximal to the fracture site. With the pins in place, the stability of the fracture fixation and the rotational alignment are assessed. The pins are bent at 90° and cut (Fig. 2.5). A bulky dressing and protective splint is applied.

When performing pinning of more than one metacarpal, the most radial metacarpal fracture should be addressed initially. This will facilitate subsequent pin placement in moving from a radial to ulnar direction.

Bouquet Pinning of the Fifth Metacarpal

The incision is distant from the distal metacarpal fracture site. It is made at the glaborous border over the tubercle of insertion of the extensor carpi ulnaris (ECU) tendon (Fig. 2.6). The length of the incision may vary with patient size, but 2.0 cm to 3.0 cm is standard. Care must be exercised to avoid damage to smaller arborizations of the dorsal sensory branch of the ulnar nerve. Typically, the main sensory branch crosses the midaxis, an imaginary line drawn between the ulnar styloid and the ECU tubercle, about halfway between these struc-

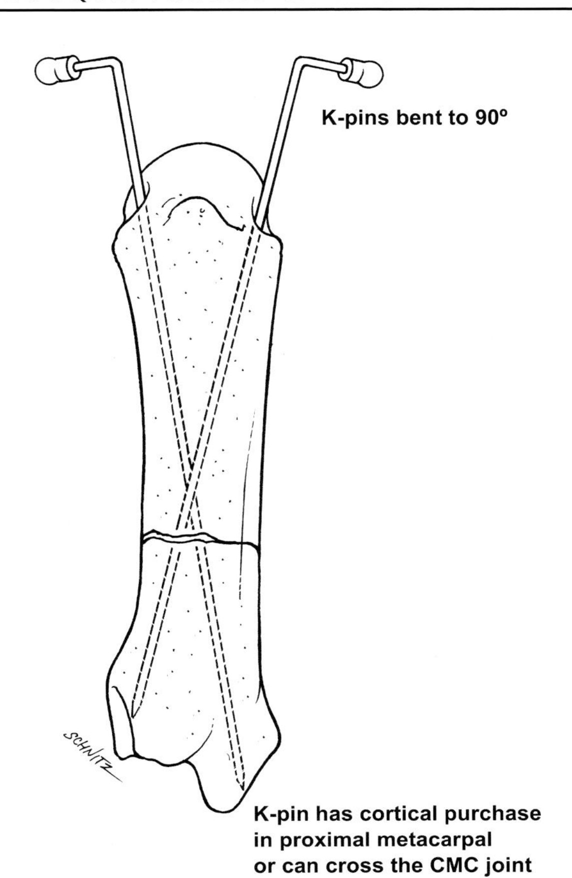

Figure 2.5. Kirschner wires are bent and cut after flouroscopic confirmation of the collateral recess pins.

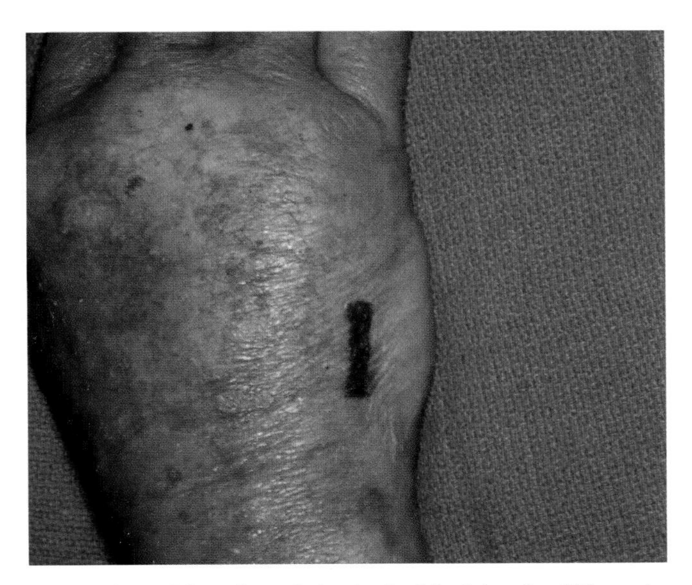

Figure 2.6. The length and location of the typical incision for fifth metacarpal bouquet pinning is shown.

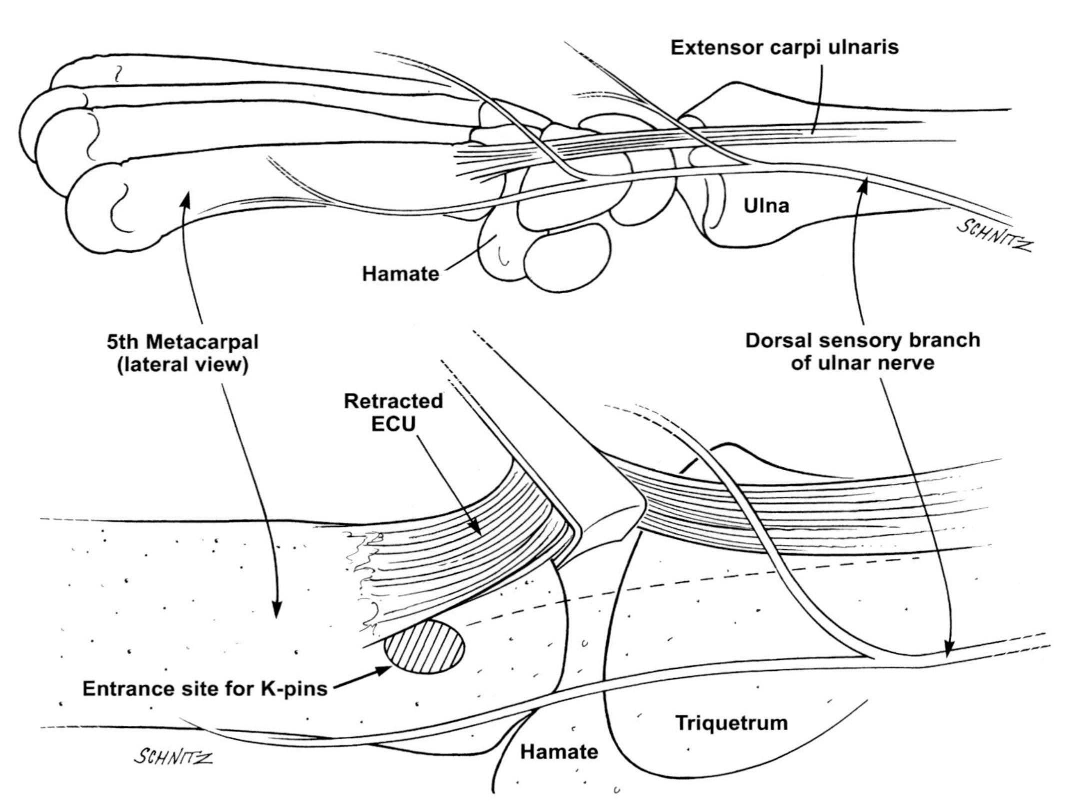

Figure 2.7. The diagram illustrates the course of the dorsal sensory branch of the ulnar nerve and its proximity in the approach utilized for small finger metacarpal bouquet pinning. A retractor is placed deep to the extensor carpi ulnaris and is retracted radially.

tures. Thus it is conceivable that handling of the nerve will be necessary, even through such a limited incision (Fig. 2.7).

Because a relatively volar starting point is desired, the ECU tendon should be reflected dorsally, but splitting the insertion as it fans to a broader area is acceptable. There is a small area of prominence, a "shoulder," at the ulnar metacarpal base that presents a convexity relative to the juxta-articular margin at the carpometacarpal joint and the remainder of the metaphysis; it is at this area, or just proximal to it, that the intramedullary canal should be entered (Figs. 2.8A, B). Use of fluoroscopy to locate the entry site is recommended to avoid potential pitfalls (Fig. 2.8C). If the cortical window is made too proximal, intra-articular fracture into the CMC joint could result. More commonly, the entry is too distal, which makes introduction of the pin arduous as it has difficulty bypassing the narrow isthmus.

Cortical perforation can be accomplished with hand tools or power drills. After initial opening of the canal, the entry site is best enlarged with curettes. Because the direction of the tools entering the canal influence the tract taken by the fixation pins, the introitus should be machined with the most acute angle possible (Fig 2.9). Although the integrity of the metacarpal base must be maintained, the portal of entry must be large enough to accommodate the desired number of pins (usually three). The size of the hole is approximately 4–6 mm in diameter. The portal is made ovoid to minimize the chance for fracture propagation due to this stress riser.

While the skin edges and ECU are retracted, access to the canal should be unrestricted, and attention is turned to preparation of the pins for insertion. To minimize tourniquet time, the pins can be prepared ahead of time, with some consideration of the individual patient's anatomy. Most commonly a 0.045 -inch smooth wire is the implant of choice. Occasionally, a 0.062-inch wire may be required for extremely large hands. The 0.035-inch wire can be used for gracile metacarpals or for secondary or supplemental pins after instrumenting the canal with a 0.045-inch wire.

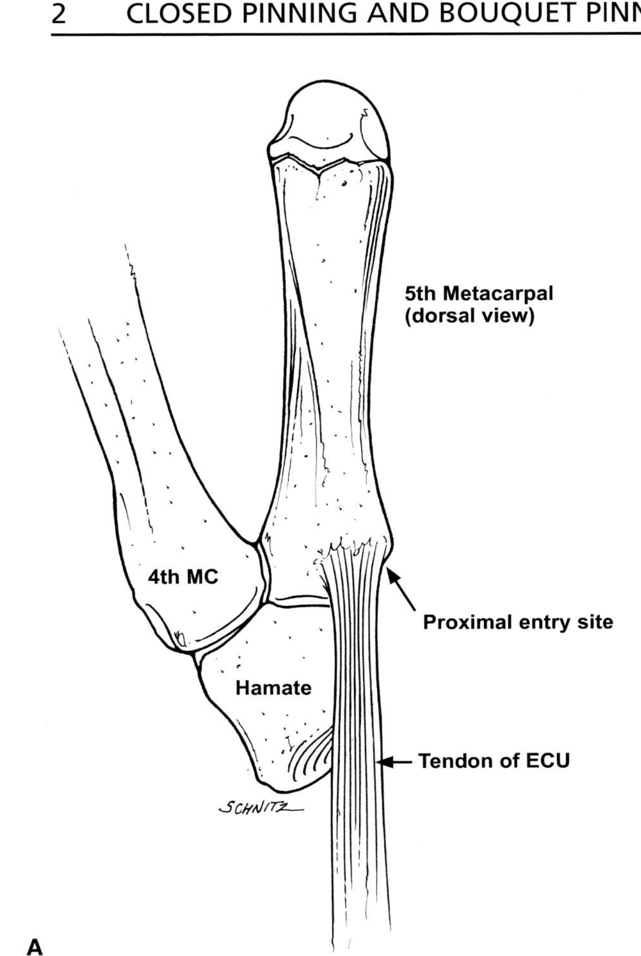

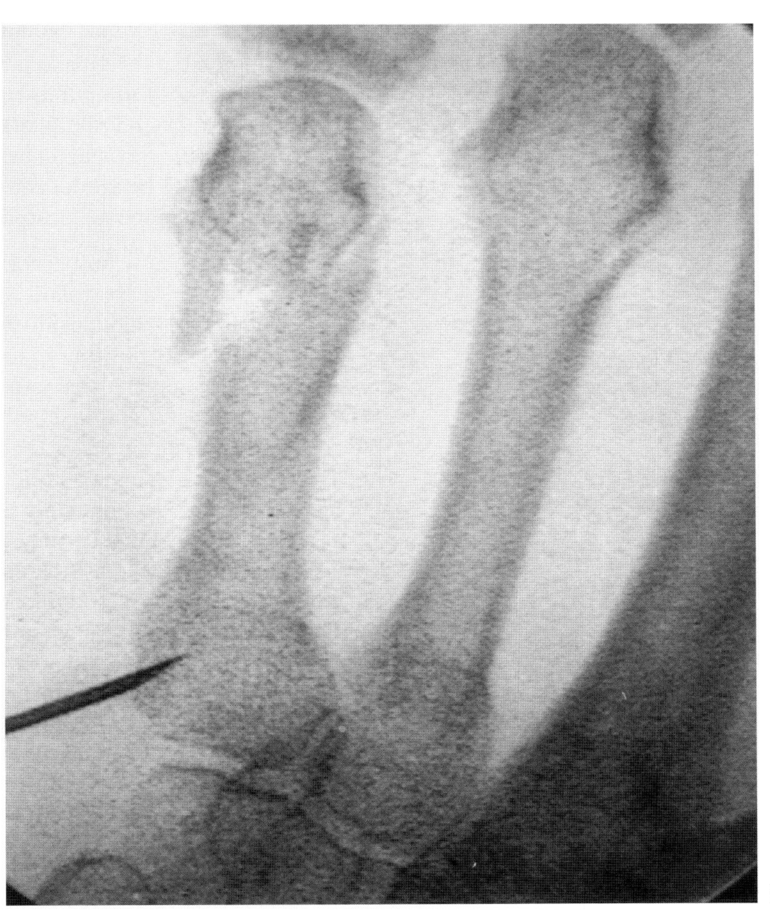

Midline axis of 5th metacarpal
Lateral view of hamate
Entrance site
for K-pins
SCHNITZ
B

Figure 2.8. A: The entrance site is located just proximal to the convexity at the base of the small finger metacarpal. **B:** A sagittal plane view of the fifth metacarpal shows the close proximity of the cortical window to the juxta-articular margin. The length of the portal measures approximately 4–6 mm. **C:** With the use of intra-operative image intensification, the starting point can be localized with a hypodermic needle.

The next three steps are critical to successful bouquet pinning:

1. ***Cut the sharp tips off the pins***. Leaving the sharp tip may create a second perforation in the cortex. The additional cortical defect often captures the pin on subsequent passes, complicating the procedure.
2. ***Bend the pin throughout its length***. The pin is contoured with a gentle bend along its entire body. The best way to describe the bend is to liken it to a catenary or a telephone

wire between two points. Minor adjustments are made to conform to the individual canal morphology, but the typical prebend as described will suffice for the majority of pins.

3. ***Deflect the tip of the pin at its leading end***. The creation of a bend allows the pin to "bounce off" the endosteum of the canal and gives the pin direction. The secondary bend is performed in the same plane as the primary arc, but is placed about 3 mm from the end of the pin to be introduced into the canal _ the end that will eventually reside distal to the fracture in the metacarpal head (Fig. 2.10).

After the correct pin morphology is created, the pin is introduced into the intramedullary canal. The pin is best controlled with two large needle holders that can be used to advance the implant and reorient it inside the canal. This will allow for controlled progression of the pin and optimize its position in the metacarpal head. The position of the terminal bend is inferred from the greater arc of the pin, directing the tangential contact of the pin with the endosteum and determining that the "bouquet" can reliably be accomplished by paying attention to the three-dimensional characteristics of the bent pin.

There are two useful techniques that can facilitate the procedure. First, using one needle holder to advance the pin, while the second is grasping nearer the insertion site, serves to "stiffen" the implant and permit easier passage (Fig. 2.11). Second, radial-deviation of the hand (for fifth metacarpal fractures, or ulnar deviation for second metacarpal fractures) makes pin introduction more facile.

The senior author has reluctantly used as few as two pins to stabilize a fifth metacarpal head fracture in a small patient with a gracile canal. However, we advocate the use of at least three pins in most circumstances. The maximum number we have used is six pins (a combination of 0.035-inch and 0.045-inch wires in a large male patient).

Viewing the fracture under biplanar image intensification to ensure reduction is crucial. Before passing the leading edge of the pin across the fracture site, a manual reduction maneuver must be performed (Fig 2.12). Perforation of the pin through the (dorsal) cortex of the shaft or through the fracture site must be guarded against. If these difficulties occur, par-

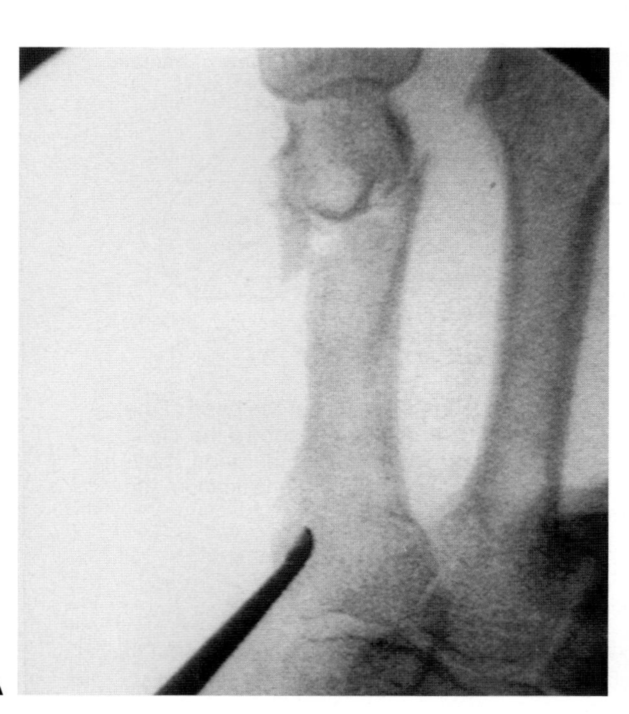

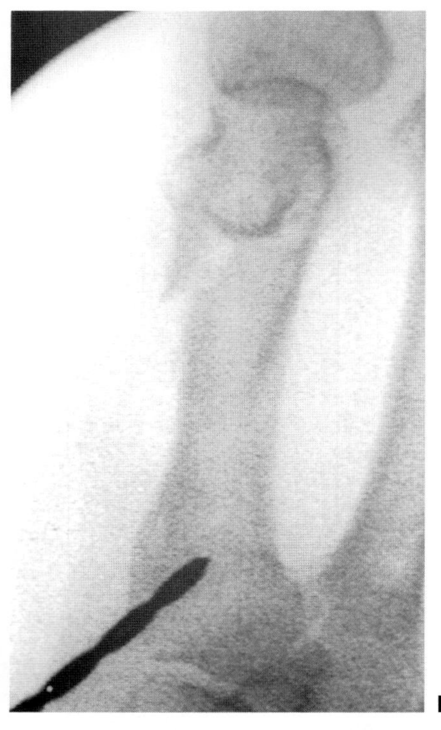

Figure 2.9. A: The canal is entered with a drill or awl. The starting point and direction of cortical perforation are both critical elements for eventual success. **B:** It is helpful to create a conduit in the metaphyseal bone of the metacarpal base that influences the direction of the pin.

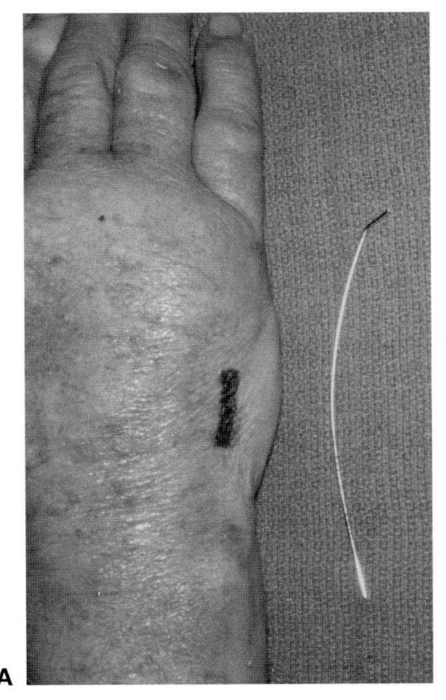

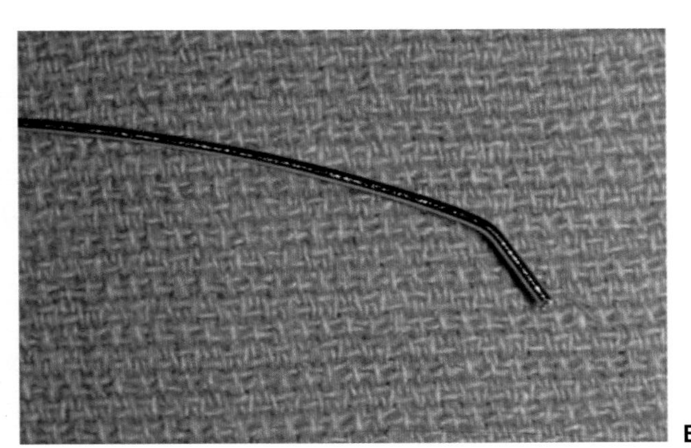

Figure 2.10. **A:** The pin adjacent to the hand is prebent for the specific reasons described in the text. **B:** A secondary bend is fashioned in the same plane as the primary arc, placed 3 mm from the end of the leading edge of the pin.

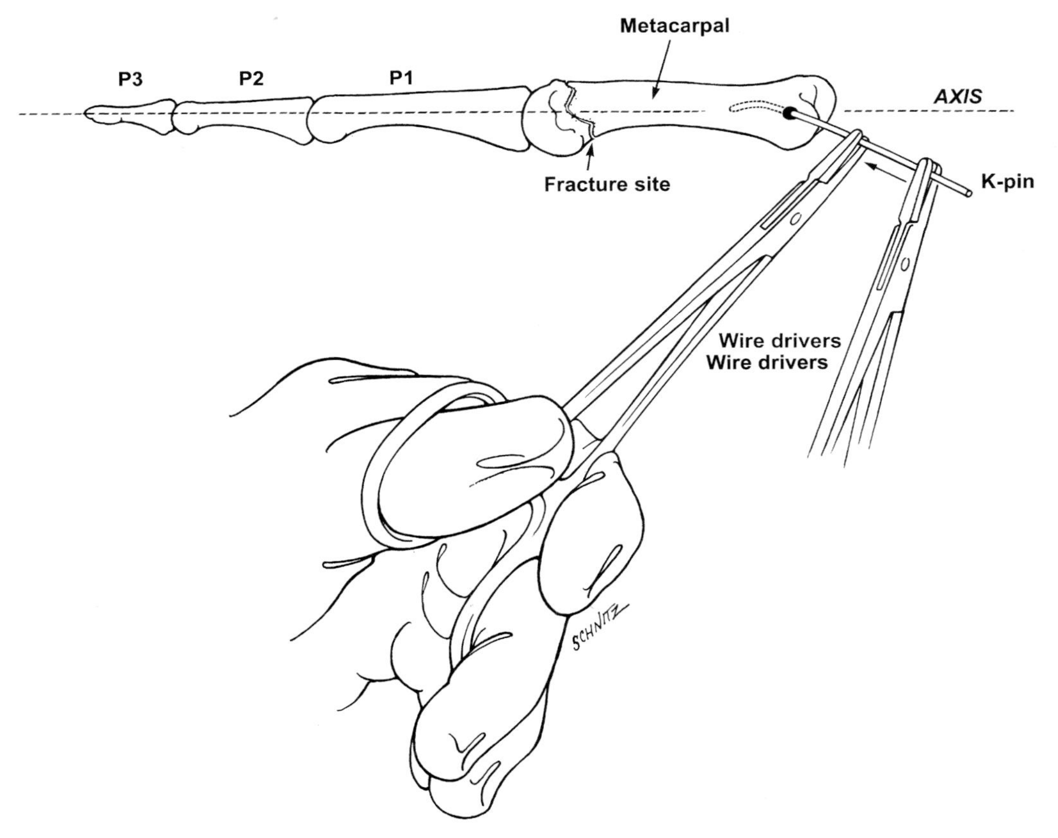

Figure 2.11. The passage of the pin within the metacarpal canal is facilitated by the surgeon positioning the two needle holders as depicted in the illustration.

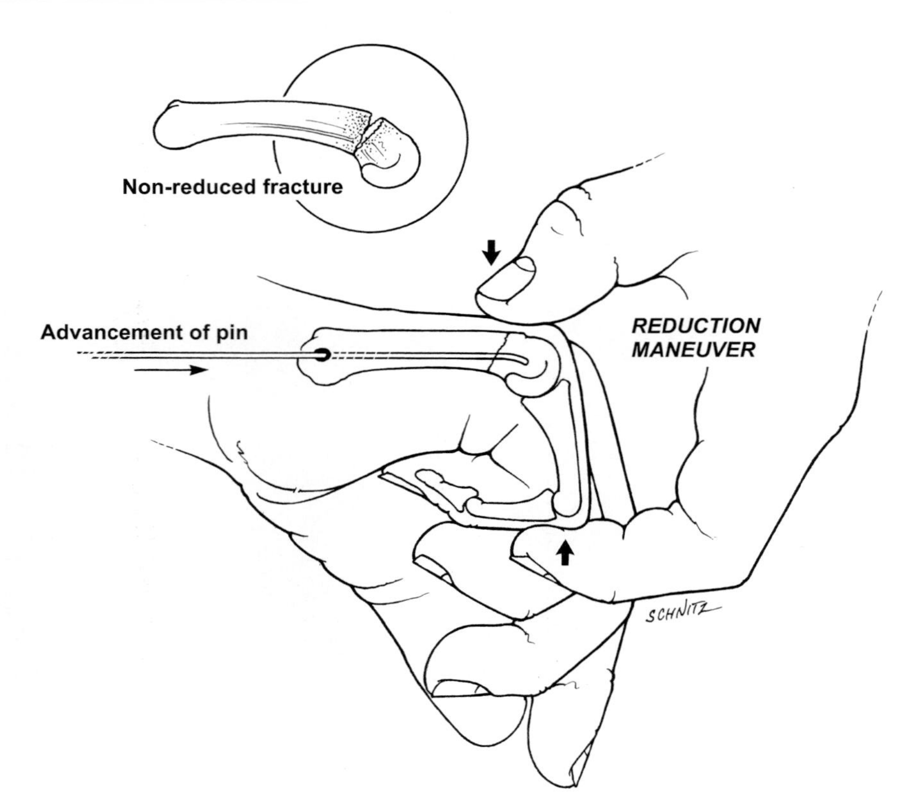

Figure 2.12. A reduction maneuver is performed before passing the wire across the fracture site.

tial or complete removal of the pin from the canal and reorientation by utilizing the two needle holders will usually rectify the problem. At times, two or more pins may act as a "track" for subsequent pin insertions; typically this is beneficial, yet this arrangement can also preclude placement of the pin in the desired location (Fig. 2.13).

Once the fracture has been reduced and the pins placed, the ends are cut as close to the canal as possible (Fig. 2.14). The pins can be advanced slightly with a bone tamp, provid-

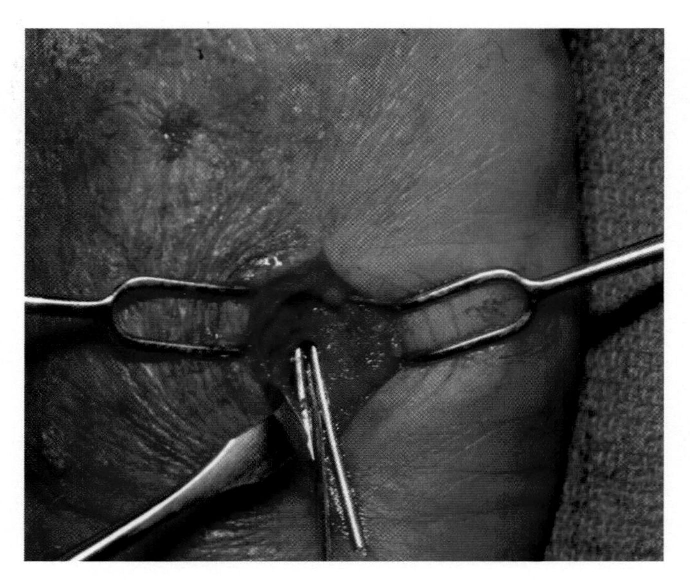

Figure 2.13. The proximal ends of the inserted pins are left slightly long to make the track that allows subsequent pins to be inserted more easily.

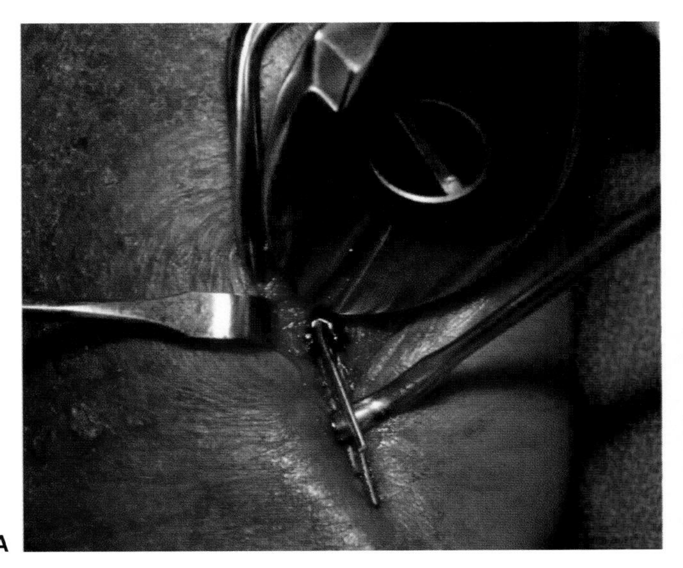

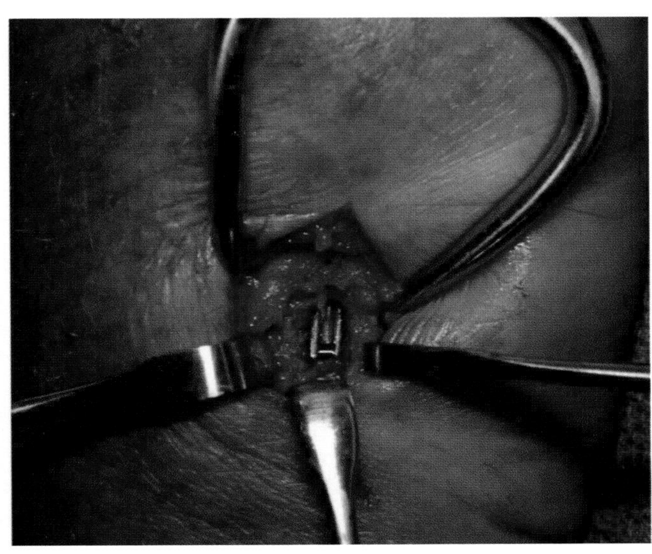

Figure 2.14. A: A retractor assists in delivering the inserted pins into the jaws of the wire cutter. **B:** The wire ends naturally recess into the metacarpal canal and can be further secured by gentle bone tamp use.

ing there is enough room at the distal aspect of the metacarpal head. The proximal ends of the pins reside in the canal and are sometimes locked into position by the proximal lip of the cortical perforation (Figs. 2.15 and 2.16).

The soft tissues are closed over the cortical defect. The skin is closed with a nylon suture. A bulky dressing is applied to the level of the proximal interphalangeal joint (PIP) that restricts metacarpophalangeal (MCP) joint motion only slightly.

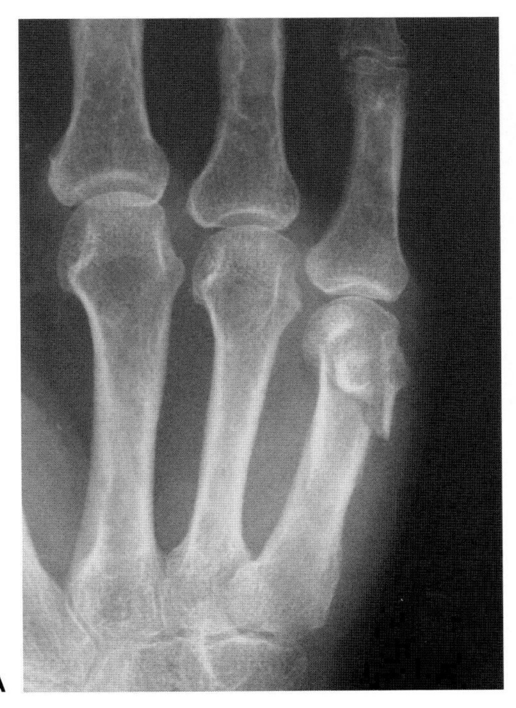

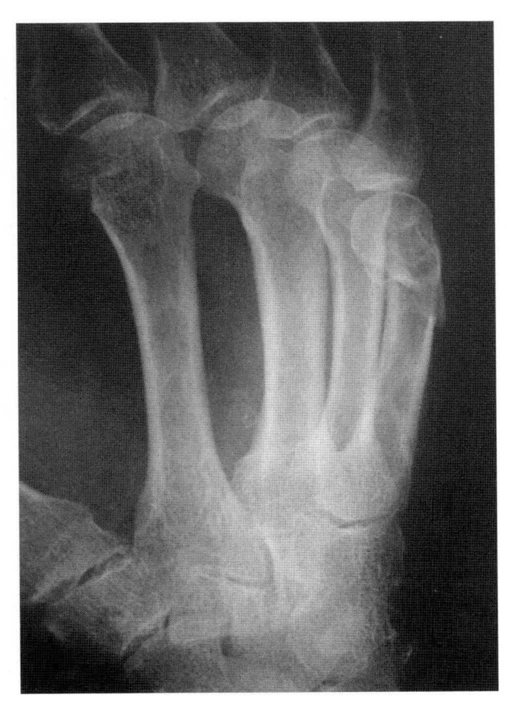

Figure 2.15. A case of an upper extremity ambulatory patient who sustained a fracture of the fifth metacarpal neck in a fall. **A, B:** AP and lateral x-rays of the patient's hand.

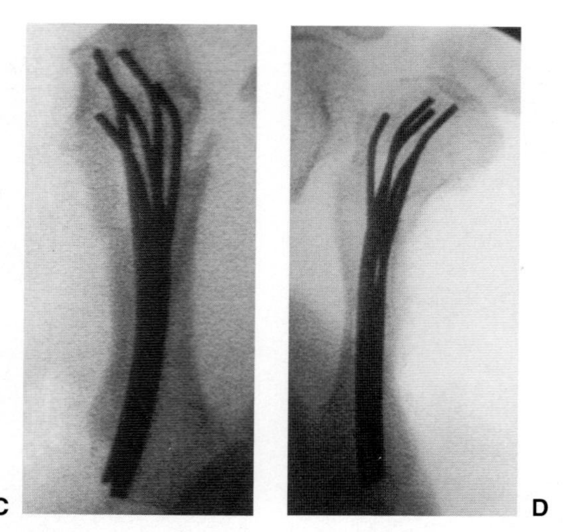

Figure 2.15. *Continued.* **C, D:** The intra-operative images from the fluoroscopy unit after bouquet pinning.

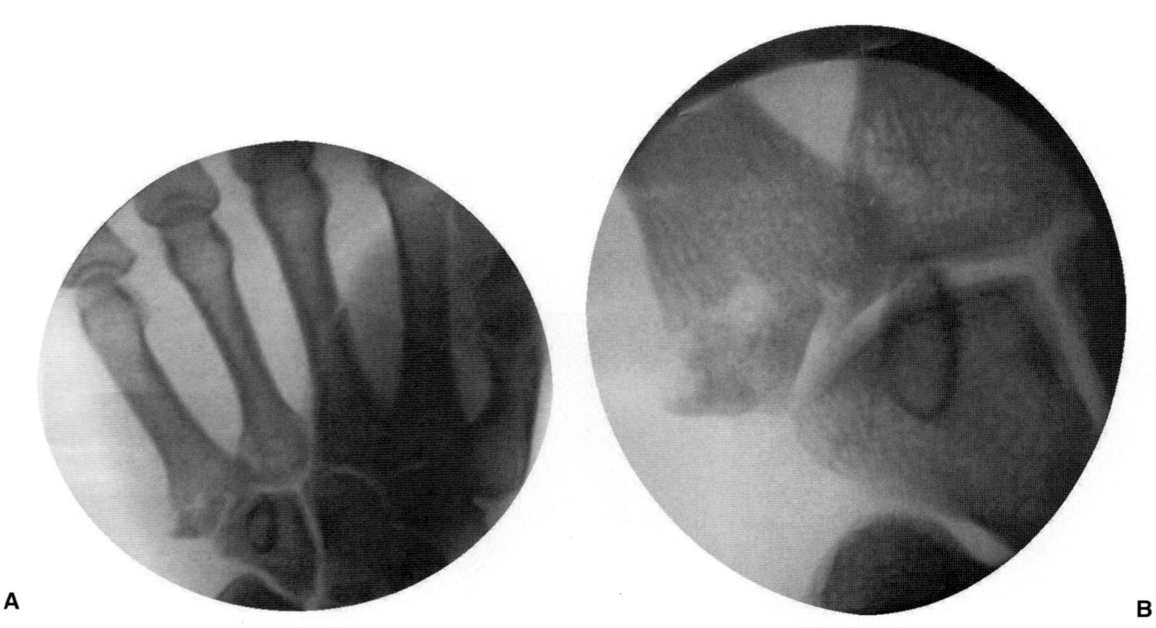

Figure 2.16. A: The preoperative radiographs shown are of a 25-year-old male professional baseball player who sustained a closed carpometacarpal (CMC) fracture dislocation of the left hand after a diving catch. **B:** Note the displaced fracture of the small finger metacarpal base.

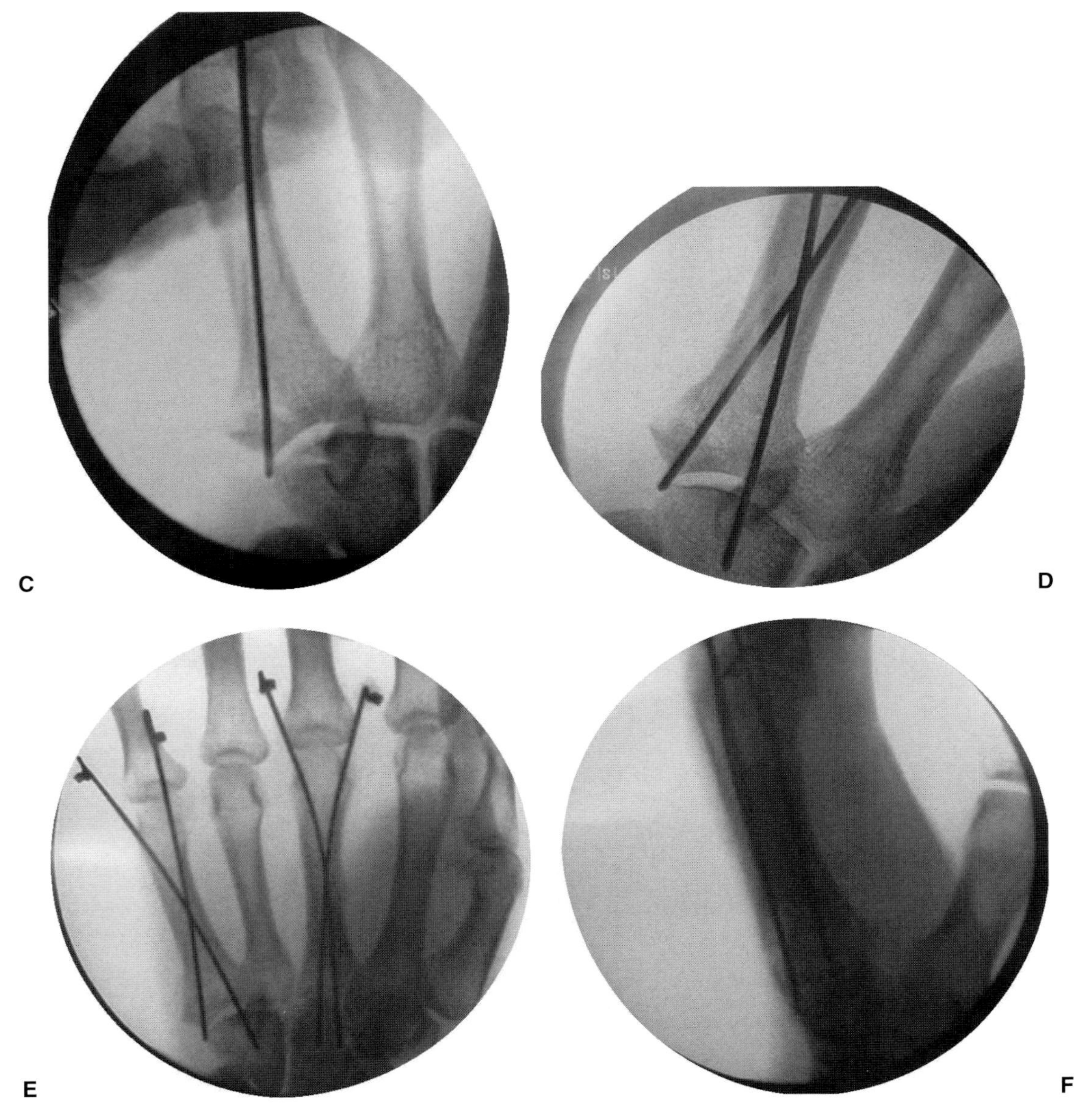

Figure 2.16. *Continued.* **C:** After closed reduction of the small finger metacarpal base fracture, the fragment was stabilized with a 0.045 smooth wire placed from the radial collateral recess. **D:** A second pin was placed from the ulnar collateral recess across the CMC joint for added stability. **E, F:** Stabilization of the long finger metacarpal shaft fracture was achieved with collateral recess pinning. Both the radial and ulnar recess wires were advanced across the CMC joint to secure fixation of the long finger metacarpal diaphyseal fracture.

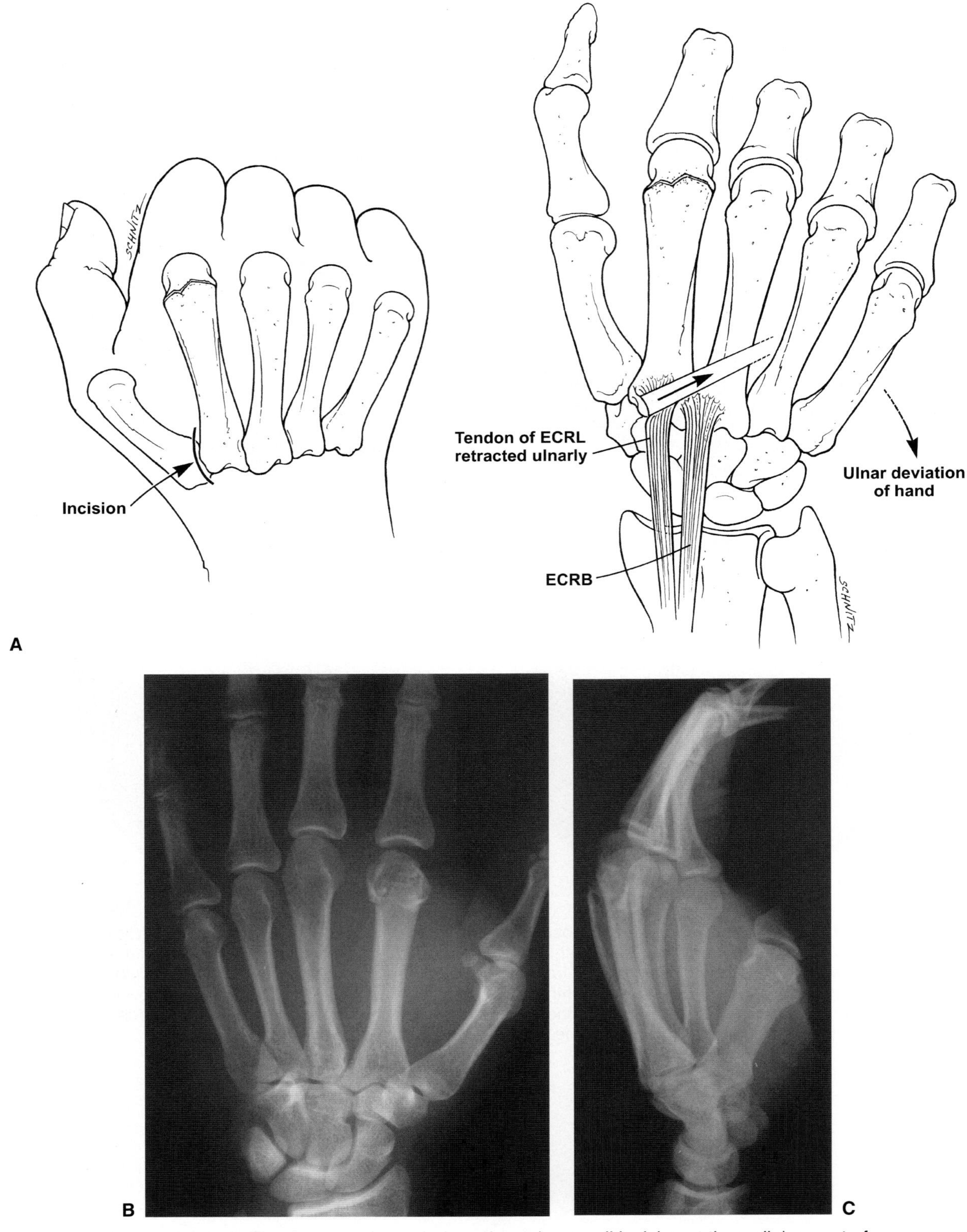

Figure 2.17. A: The exposure is carried out through a small incision at the radial aspect of the second metacarpal base. Bouquet pinning of the index metacarpal requires elevation of the extensor carpi radialis longus at the radial aspect of the metacarpal. Ulnar deviation of the wrist helps to access the metacarpal base. A case of an index finger metacarpal fracture that initially failed closed reduction. **B, C:** The AP and lateral x-rays of the patient's hand.

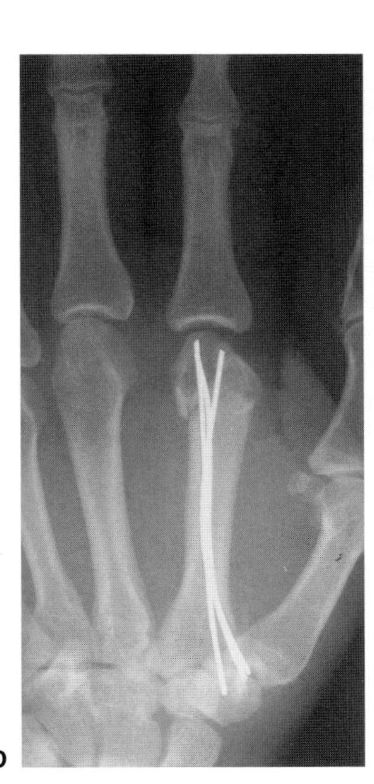
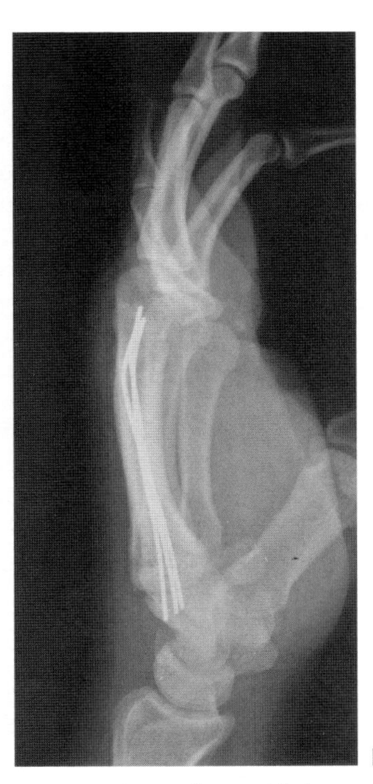
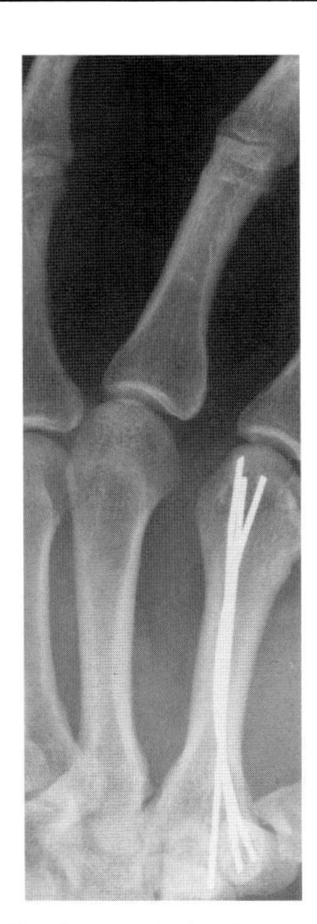

Figure 2.17. *Continued.* **D–F:** Intra-operative radiographic images after bouquet pinning.

Bouquet Pinning of the Index Finger Metacarpal

The technique for index finger metacarpal pinning is very similar to that of fifth ray fixation. The palpable base is exposed with care to avoid injury to the cutaneous nerve branches. The fibers of the extensor carpi radialis longus (ECRL) are elevated or split at the radial aspect of the metacarpal base. The remainder of the steps reflects those described above. As previously mentioned, ulnar deviation of the wrist can help facilitate passage of the pin (Fig. 2.17).

POSTOPERATIVE MANAGEMENT

Bouquet pinning is performed to obtain stable fixation in a reduced position so that early motion may be initiated. We have allowed some patients (upper extremity ambulators, unilateral amputees, and surgeons) to utilize the operated hand to their level of comfort almost immediately after surgery. The patient is maintained in the soft post-surgical dressing for one to two weeks. Most patients should expect to have enough pain control to initiate mobilization within the bulky dressing during the first week.

Sutures are removed at 10 to 14 days, at which time radiographs are obtained and rigid immobilization is discontinued in nearly all patients. Interval splinting with intermittent motion is permitted. A terminal visit with x-rays is done at four to six weeks postoperatively, at which time callus has been uniformly seen and the position of the fracture fragments has been maintained.

Metacarpal fixation with collateral recess pinning requires approximately four weeks of immobilization in a safe-position splint; in most patients, the PIP joint can be free. Therefore, an extended period of splint immobilization is required. At four to five weeks, the pins are routinely removed in the office. If radiographic findings are consistent with fracture consolidation, the patient is placed into a removable thermoplast splint.

REHABILITATION

Following bouquet pinning, a program of active and active-assisted motion commences as comfort permits, usually about three to seven days after surgery. A removable, short arm, safe-position orthosis is furnished to immobilize the hand during the intervals between exercise sessions. Passive range of motion commences at three to four weeks following stabilization when clinical and radiographic union is achieved. It is logical to begin strengthening when motion recovery exceeds 50% to 75% of normal. The majority of patients are able to return to heavy-labor vocations at the eighth week postoperative period.

Patients undergoing collateral recess pinning follow a supervised therapy program. Because pin stability and pin tract infections are concerns, appropriate immobilization is required when the pins are indwelling. This is usually accomplished with an initial three to four weeks of rigid immobilization followed by interval splinting. Careful motion of adjacent digits and even other digital segments of the operated ray can be pursued. At one month postop after pin removal, an active and active-assisted motion protocol of the distal interphalangeal (DIP), PIP, and MCP joints is initiated. The patient is maintained in an orthosis for an additional two weeks. With clinical and radiographic signs of healing, the splint is gradually weaned.

RESULTS

Collateral Recess Pinning

Because the patient can pursue a program of interphalangeal motion and no direct manipulation of these levels is undertaken, the PIP and DIP joints usually recover motion rapidly. A program of blocked flexion and intrinsic stretching can assist in accelerating the functional return.

The MCP joints are initially limited in motion. The most frequent presentation is that of extension lag, which sometimes exceeds 30 degrees. This result is likely due to the influence of the fracture callus and the extensor penetration by the pins. Because the collateral ligaments are held at their greatest length during pin insertion, the lag is probably not related to capsuloligamentous contracture. The extensor has relatively little excursion through the composite motion arc (compared to the flexors), which may help to explain this phenomenon.

Flexion usually returns rapidly and heralds greater functional capability, such as grasping, that is key for strengthening tasks. As long as the fracture is believed to be clinically united, the pursuit of MCP motion can be aggressive. In addition to night splinting in extension and any active motion, intrinsic stretching and even dynamic splinting is reasonable.

Eventually, buddy-taping to an adjacent normal digit can assist in promoting a greater arc of motion. Return to contact activities is safe if comfort and reasonable function has been demonstrated. This is typically between the sixth and eighth postoperative week, or the third to fourth week after the pins have been discontinued.

Our experience with collateral recess pinning now exceeds 100 patients. To date, we have not experienced any major complications, and healing of the fractures has been seen in all patients, including multiple-fracture cases.

Pin tract infections have occurred in less than 5% of patients and have been treated with pin removal, local wound care, and oral antibiotics. We have not seen any cases of septic arthritis. Although it is difficult to categorize patients on whom this technique has been employed, we can state that no significant motion limitation, strength compromise, or repeat surgery has been associated with the subgroup of patients treated for closed fractures.

Because we employ this technique for even more complex injuries, including open fractures and combined injuries (skin, bone, tendon, nerve, and vessel), revision or salvage surgery has been employed in some cases to maximize results. We have not found any untoward sequelae related to this fixation method.

Collateral recess pinning deserves a place in the armamentarium of almost any surgeon handling fractures of the tubular bones of the hand because of its unique versatility and capability to solve challenging fractures from the area of the distal metacarpal through complex CMC fracture-dislocations. As with many specialized surgical procedures in the hand, there is a learning curve and an element of feel involved. We have observed that these modest obstacles are easily overcome, allowing the surgeon the satisfaction of being able to offer a minimally invasive technique that imparts great stability to even the most challenging fracture and fracture-dislocation patterns involving the metacarpals.

Bouquet Pinning

This technique ranks among the favorites of any surgeon who has been introduced to it and utilizes it on a regular basis, and patient satisfaction is routinely high. The ability of bouquet pinning to reduce fractures, stabilize them rigidly, and permit early motion is unparalleled. The opportunity to operate away from the joints of the osteo-articular column of the hand, where there is such a premium on flexibility, is tremendously attractive.

We have now employed the bouquet-pinning technique in over 100 patients. Over 90 of those cases have involved the fifth metacarpal. To date, there have been no significant complications. We have noted no iatrogenic nerve injuries, hardware migrations, loss of reduction, infections, or need for repeat surgery. Even in cases of complex fracture patterns of open injuries (six cases), this technique has proven complication-free.

One of the most impressive observations about this tool is the abundant fracture healing response that accompanies pin placement. Often early callus is seen on radiographs at initial postoperative visits between 10 and 14 days after surgery. Most patients already have recovered between 50% and 75% of their composite motion at the MCP, PIP, and DIP joints by that first visit because the bulky dressing has not restricted their motion.

We performed this technique in four in-season professional athletes, and all have returned to play in contact sports between the second and fourth postoperative week. Two surgeons returned to the operating room within one week of bouquet pinning.

The only clinical issue we have encountered is a lingering (six- to eight-week) soreness at the incision site. This appears to be related to the difficulty with which the initial access to the canal was gained. This predictable sequelae responds to aggressive scar massage and initial pad protection if early contact is required by the patient's vocation or avocation. We have not encountered pin migration or need for pin removal because we place the proximal pin ends within the metacarpal shell.

We strongly advocate adding this procedure to the portfolio of options for patients with metacarpal neck fractures and selected patients with other patterns of distal metacarpal injury. The procedure has been performed mainly by hand surgeons, but it can be mastered by all who operate on the hand. Meticulous technique, strict adherence to the process of pin preparation and insertion, and the confidence to allow patients to pursue early motion should yield good results for almost all patients where the technique is indicated.

COMPLICATIONS

Bouquet intramedullary pinning of metacarpal fractures yields few postoperative complications. Reported complications are dorsal ulnar sensory nerve embarrassment, reflex sympathetic dystrophy, infection, and discomfort at the base of the operated metacarpal, yet these untoward occurrences are infrequent.

Injury to the dorsal ulnar sensory nerve can be avoided with careful attention to surgical dissection and awareness of local anatomy. The few reported cases of reflex sympathetic dystrophy have been associated with crush injuries and multiple metacarpal fractures. Some complications can occur as a result of technical error. Penetration of the wire through the metacarpophalangeal joint, extensor tendon rupture secondary to proximal protrusion of the wire, and secondary displacement of the fracture after early wire removal have been reported. In our practice, hardware removal is not advocated.

Although rare for closed pinning of metacarpal fractures, nonunion has been reported.

Malunion, including rotational malalignment, shortening, and dorsal angulation of the fracture is a potential complication for collateral recess pinning. Loosening and pin-tract infection are disadvantages with the use of closed manipulation and pin fixation of metacarpal fractures.

RECOMMENDED READING

1. Calder JDF, O'Leary S, Evans SC. Antegrade Intramedullary Fixation of Displaced Fifth Metacarpal Fractures. Injury. *Int J Care Injured* 31:47–50, 2000.
2. Foucher G. Bouquet Osteosynthesis in Metacarpal Neck Fractures: A Series of 66 Patients. *J Hand Surg* 20A: S86–S90, 1995.
3. Frere G, Hoel G, Moutet F, et al. Fractures of the Fifth Metacarpal Neck. *Ann Chir Main* 1(3):221–226, 1986.
4. Green DP, Rowland SA. Fractures and dislocations in the hand. In: Rockwood CA Jr, Green DP, Bucholz RW, eds. *Fractures in Adults*. 3rd ed. Philadelphia: JB Lippincott, 1991:411–562.
5. Gonzalez MH, Hall RF. Intramedullary fixation of metacarpal and proximal phalangeal fractures of the hand. *Clin Orthop* 327:47–54, 1996.
6. Manueddo CA, Della Santa D. Fasciculated intramedullary pinning of metacarpal fractures. *J Hand Surg* 21B:2:230–236, 1996.
7. Stern PJ. In: Fractures of the metacarpals and phalanges. Green DP, ed. *Operative Hand Surgery*, 3rd ed. New York: Churchill Livingstone, 1993;695–758.
8. Varela CD, Carr JB. Closed intramedullary pinning of metacarpal and phalanx fractures. *Orthopedics* 13:213–215, 1990.

Classification of Fracture Type

Unicondylar fractures occur in four common patterns, each reflective of the magnitude and direction of force applied to the joint (Fig. 3.3).

Type I fractures involve a short fracture surface oblique to both frontal and sagittal planes. The fracture exits just proximal to the collateral ligaments, providing little fragment area for internal fixation proximal to the ligament origins. The oblique fracture plane renders this fracture pattern highly unstable. Deformity occurs in a single plane oblique to both frontal and sagittal planes. It is most simply described as lateral angulation and rotational malalignment.

Type II fractures involve a long, oblique fracture line in the sagittal plane. The longitudinal nature of this fracture also renders it extremely unstable. The long fracture surface, however, makes it more facile to stabilize with interfragmentary fixation.

Type III fractures involve a dorsal coronal fragment, usually small, produced by an axial compression injury associated with dorsal joint dislocation. The dorsal aspect of one condyle is impacted and displaced by the middle phalanx as it dislocates. This class of dorsal coronal fractures is least likely to interfere with PIP joint motion. Most dorsal fracture fragments are best treated by surgical excision. When the fracture projects into the joint at a point equal to or greater than the midpoint of the anteroposterior condylar diameter, internal fixation is required.

Type IV fractures involve a palmar coronal fragment, also small, and created by an axial compression injury associated with volar joint dislocation. Nearly all Type IV volar coronal fractures interfere with PIP joint flexion, and most require open treatment. Large fragments are reduced and internally fixed. Smaller fragments may be excised, if concentric reduction can be maintained throughout the arc of PIP flexion.

Open treatment is indicated when an anatomic reduction cannot be achieved or maintained by closed methods. Although there exists no data on the correlation between ultimate

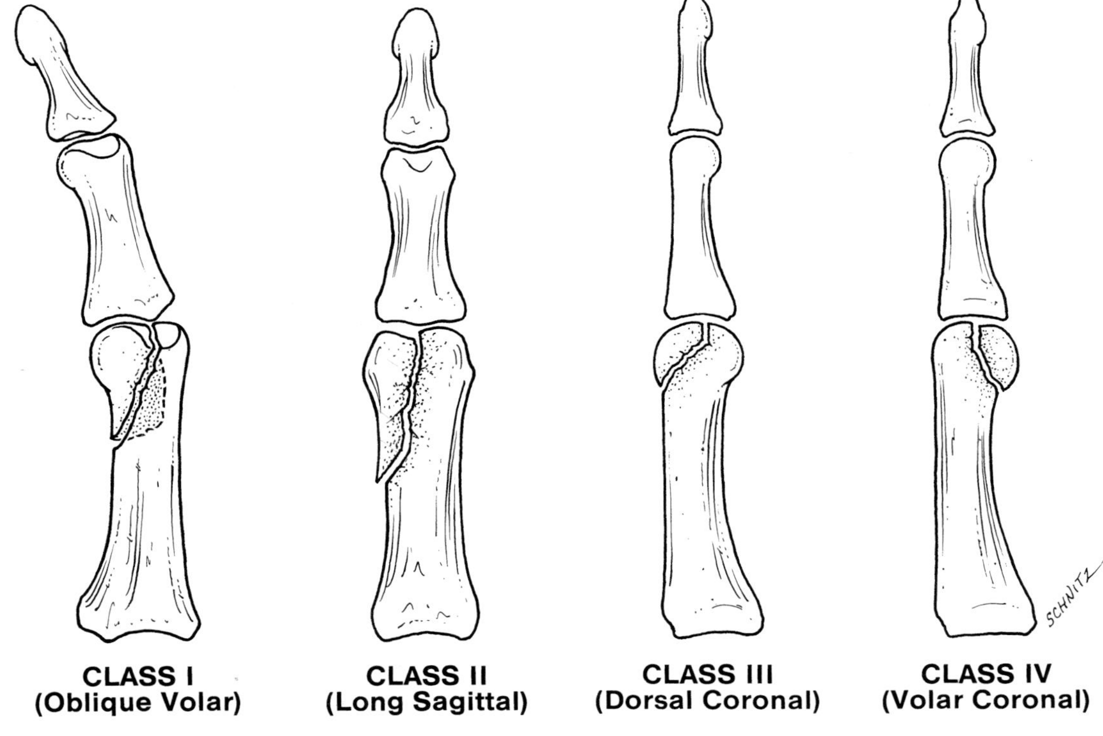

Figure 3.3. Classification of unicondylar proximal phalangeal fractures. (With permission, from: Weiss AC, Hastings H. Distal unicondylar fractures of the proximal phalanx. *J Hand Surg* 18A:594–599, 1993.)

fragment displacement and accelerated arthrosis or instability, residual articular incongruity exceeding 1 mm would be poorly tolerated and likely demand anatomic reduction and internal fixation. Open reduction is indicated in all open displaced fractures and most all fractures that present after remote trauma (between the second and sixth week after injury).

All Type I and Type II fractures are inherently unstable and, when displaced, require internal fixation. There are no absolute contraindications to operative management other than poor health or inability of the patient to cooperate with operative management and postoperative rehabilitation.

Nearly all Type III fractures require excision of the dorsal unstable fracture fragment. Operative management is contraindicated in fractures that are nondisplaced or minimally displaced and that may heal by bony union or fibrous stabilization after a short period of digital immobilization. Nearly all Type IV fractures require operative management. There are no contraindications to operative management other than when the fracture is inconsequentially small.

PREOPERATIVE PLANNING

Radiographic Evaluation

All patients with PIP-joint fractures and fracture-dislocations should be evaluated by anteroposterior (AP), lateral, partially supinated oblique, and partially pronated oblique radiographs. The oblique radiographs are particularly important to identify correctly the fracture plane and the extent of comminution in the most common Type I short volar oblique fractures. Magnification radiographs are particularly helpful in providing improved visualization of small fracture fragments. Radiographs should also include the distal interphalanged joint (DIP), which is frequently involved by fracture as well. The use of live fluoroscopy in evaluating, and later repairing, these injuries can be invaluable.

Clinical Evaluation

The neurovascular examination is usually normal, but objective and subjective observations should be recorded. Inspection of the skin, particularly at the level of the PIP flexion crease, would indicate whether the fracture was open before provisional reduction "in the field."

The location and extent of PIP joint swelling are noted. Particular attention should be paid to assessment of axial and rotational alignment. Depression of one of the proximal phalangeal condyles can sometimes introduce a subtle angulation that is best appreciated when full digital extension is attempted.

Type III dorsal and volar coronal fractures present with relatively undisturbed alignment. Both Type I oblique volar and Type II long sagittal fractures, when displaced, produce angular deformity. Displaced Type I oblique volar fractures also present rotational deformity, which is best assessed in PIP flexion. Active range of motion should be documented, including extension and flexion deficits.

SURGERY

Anesthesia

General or regional anesthesia is administered. While treatment can be accomplished in a cooperative patient under a wrist or digital block, an axillary block is preferred for relaxation of the extensors and flexors. After extremity preparation and draping, the arm is exsanguinated and an upper-arm brachial tourniquet inflated to a pressure of 250 mm Hg.

Type I: Oblique Volar

Closed Reduction & Percutaneous Pinning. Acute fractures may be reducible by closed means. When anatomic reduction is achieved, it is best maintained by percutaneous Kirschner-wire fixation. I believe Type I fractures occur from a force applied to the partially flexed PIP joint, which imparts a tension force to the condyle through the collateral ligaments (Fig. 3.3). After injury, the fracture fragment settles back proximally and palmarly. In radial unicondylar fractures, the digit appears rotated into pronation and axially deviated in a radial direction. Reduction, therefore, is achieved by supination and ulnar deviation.

Conversely, ulnar unicondylar fractures present a combined deformity represented in part by supination and ulnar deviation. Reduction is accomplished by pronation and radial deviation. The fractured articular surface must be compressed together by an externally placed fracture-reduction forceps. Most commonly, I use an Ikuta (W. Lorenz, Jacksonville, FL, U.S.A.) or Stag Beetle (Synthes, Inc., Paoli, PA, U.S.A.) forceps. Placement of the fracture-reduction forceps and assessment of reduction are best achieved by using a computer-enhanced fluoroscopic device, which provides high-quality magnification images with minimal to no radiation exposure to the operating surgeon. Anatomic joint reduction must be obtained with residual articular step-off less than 1 mm. If this can be obtained, reduction is secured by the use of percutaneous Kirschner wires. A minimum of two Kirschner wires is required to prevent redisplacement; a single Kirschner wire is *not* sufficient.

Depending on the fracture fragment size, either 0.028-inch or 0.035-inch Kirschner wires are chosen. The central and dorsal portions of the fracture fragment invariably contain thin, weak, cortical elements and thus provide poor fixation. The best fixation area lies distal and palmar. Accordingly, Kirschner wires should be inserted from the contralateral dorsal side of the intact condyle proximal to the collateral ligament and advanced into the palmar distal aspect of the fractured condyle. During insertion, the PIP joint is held in extension, which relaxes and slightly dorsally displaces the conjoined lateral bands. The Kirschner wires are inserted just volar to the conjoined lateral band and directed obliquely toward the palmar aspect of the fractured condyle.

Alternatively, the Kirschner wires may be inserted from the palmar-lateral aspect of the fractured fragment, advanced through the intact condyle, and withdrawn to the proper length. Kirschner wires are cut off percutaneously outside the intact condyle. A light compressive dressing and digital splint are applied. Definitive AP, lateral, and oblique radiographs are obtained as permanent documentation of the Kirschner-wire positions and fracture reduction.

Open Reduction and Internal Fixation. Fracture exposure is obtained through a midaxial approach, based on the side of the fractured or depressed condyle (Fig. 3.4) with incision of the transverse retinacular ligament (Fig. 3.5). The conjoined lateral bands and central tendon are retracted dorsally (Fig. 3.6). A dorsal capsulotomy will expose the articular fracture component (Fig. 3.7). Interposed hematoma, soft tissue, or early callous formation are removed from the fracture by a small elevator or scalpel. It is most important to prepare the articular osteochondral surfaces for perfect apposition. The unicondylar fracture fragment is manipulated into reduction by a small skin or bone hook, or reduction is held provisionally by either a reduction forceps (Fig. 3.8) or 0.018-inch Kirschner wire. The Kirschner wire should be placed intentionally in a position other than where the desired lag screw fixation is to be accomplished subsequently. The best Kirschner-wire position is distal and close to the joint. The position for screw fixation is identified. Usually, a single screw is used and positioned to pass through the center of the fracture surface or just slightly distal to its center.

With a larger unicondylar fracture component, the screw may be placed safely at the proximal origin of the collateral ligament. Smaller fragments require screw fixation more distally, which, if larger screws are used, can interfere with the collateral ligament (Fig. 3.9A). More distal screw placement requires that the collateral ligament be handled by one of two methods. First, the collateral ligament can be partially elevated subperiosteally from proximal to distal (Fig. 3.9B) to allow screw placement in the proximal part of the fracture fragment. Second, and preferentially, 1.0-mm or 1.3-mm screws can be placed distal to the

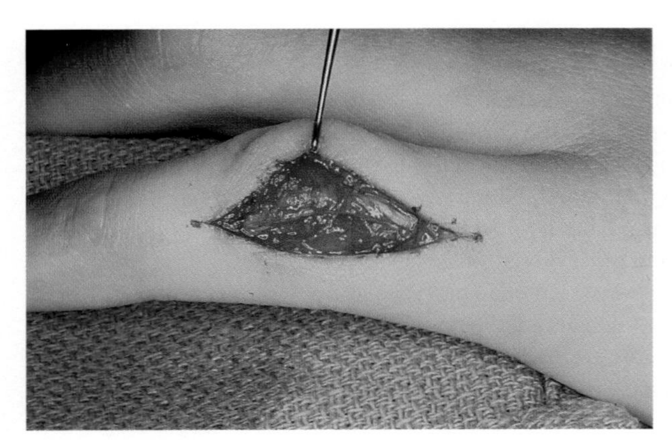

Figure 3.4. Dorsoradial approach.

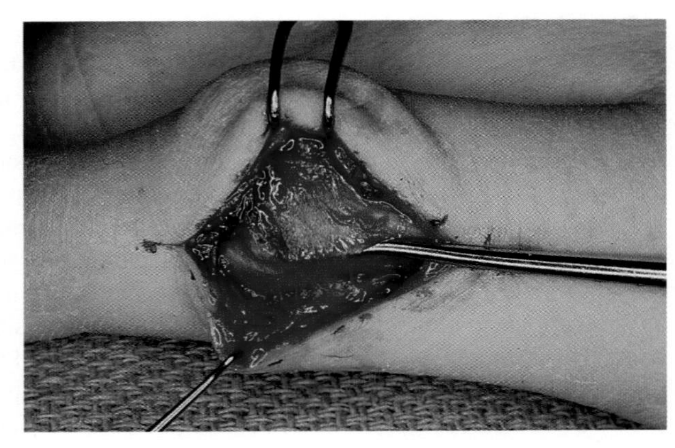

Figure 3.5. Exposure and release of transverse retinacular ligament. Probe is placed underneath transverse retinacular ligament.

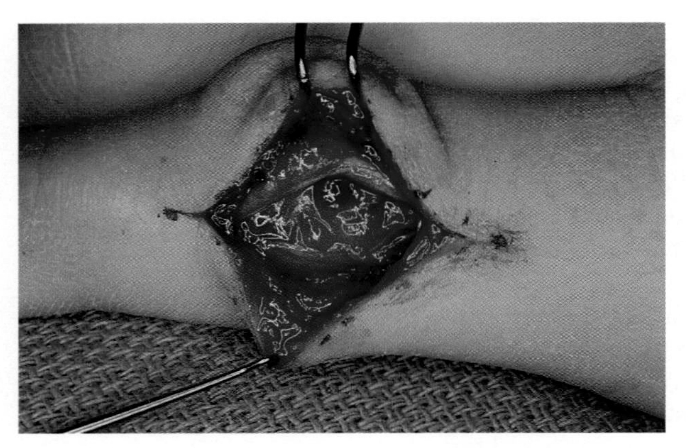

Figure 3.6. Dorsal retraction of conjoined lateral band and central tendon to expose dorsal capsule.

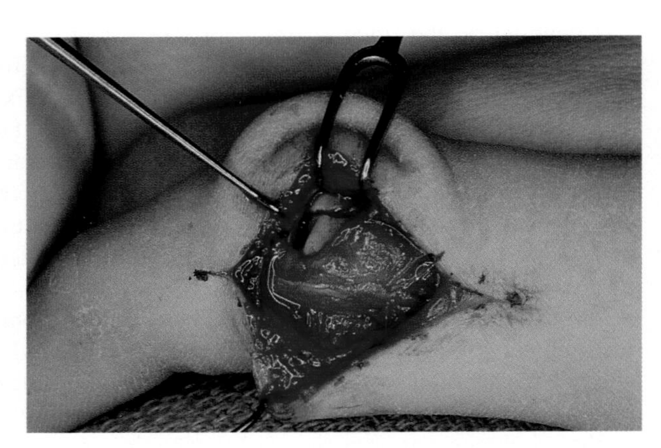

Figure 3.7. Dorsal capsulotomy allows for intra-articular fracture exposure.

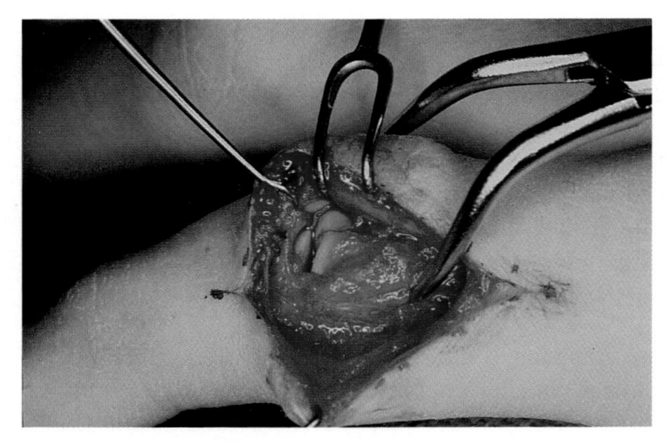

Figure 3.8. After debridement of fracture hematoma, the fracture is anatomically positioned and provisionally held by a Stag Beetle forceps.

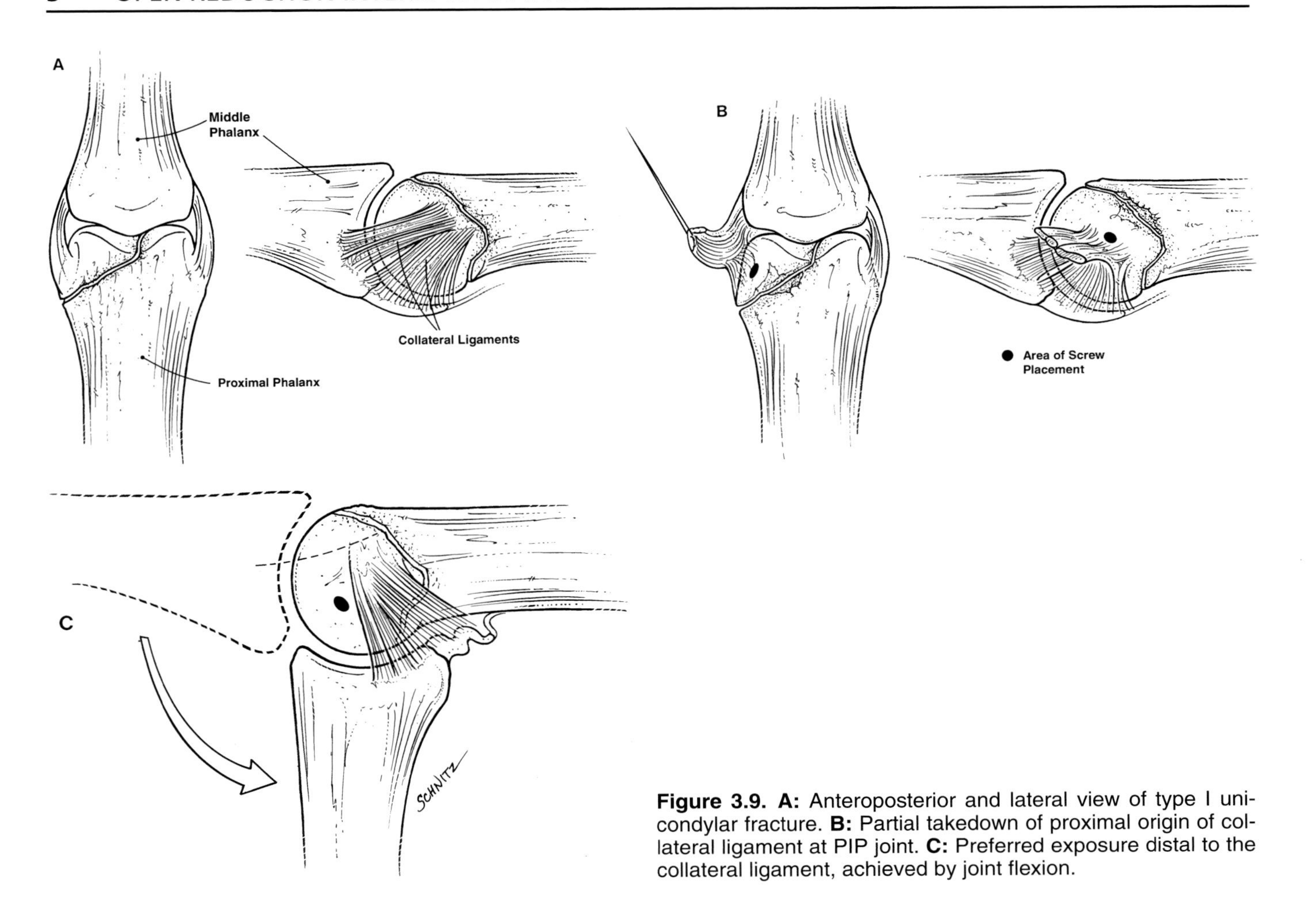

Figure 3.9. A: Anteroposterior and lateral view of type I unicondylar fracture. **B:** Partial takedown of proximal origin of collateral ligament at PIP joint. **C:** Preferred exposure distal to the collateral ligament, achieved by joint flexion.

collateral ligament in flexion. The small screw head size allows recession flush to the bone surface, which avoids collateral ligament interference (Figs. 3.9C).

Stabilization by Miniscrew or Microscrew Fixation

Stable fixation by use of a single screw requires interfragmentary compression to impart friction between fracture surfaces. Either 1.0-mm or 1.3-mm screws are used; 1.0-mm screws are preferred. Both screws provide small heads that can be recessed flush to the surface of the bone.

The fracture is reduced and provisionally held by reduction forceps or temporary 0.028-inch Kirschner wires. Joint flexion allows for exposure of almost the entire lateral surface of the condyle to be fixed. For a 1.0-mm screw, a 0.76-mm drill is passed across the fracture and aimed slightly proximal so as to exit proximal to the opposite collateral ligament origin (Figs. 3.10A, 3.10B, and 3.11A). The depth is measured (Figs. 3.10C and 3.11B) and the near fragment overdrilled with a 1.0-mm drill (Figs. 3.10D and 3.11C). A self-tapping 1.0-mm screw is inserted to compress the fracture fragment (Figs. 3.10E and 3.10F). The 1.0-mm screw size allows for placement of at least two screws in even small unicondylar fracture fragments (Figs 3.10G, 3.11 D–F, and 3.12 A–G).

For a 1.3-mm screw, the same sequence is followed, pre-drilling with a 1.0-mm drill and overdrilling at the near cortex with a 1.3-mm drill. The smaller head profiles of both the

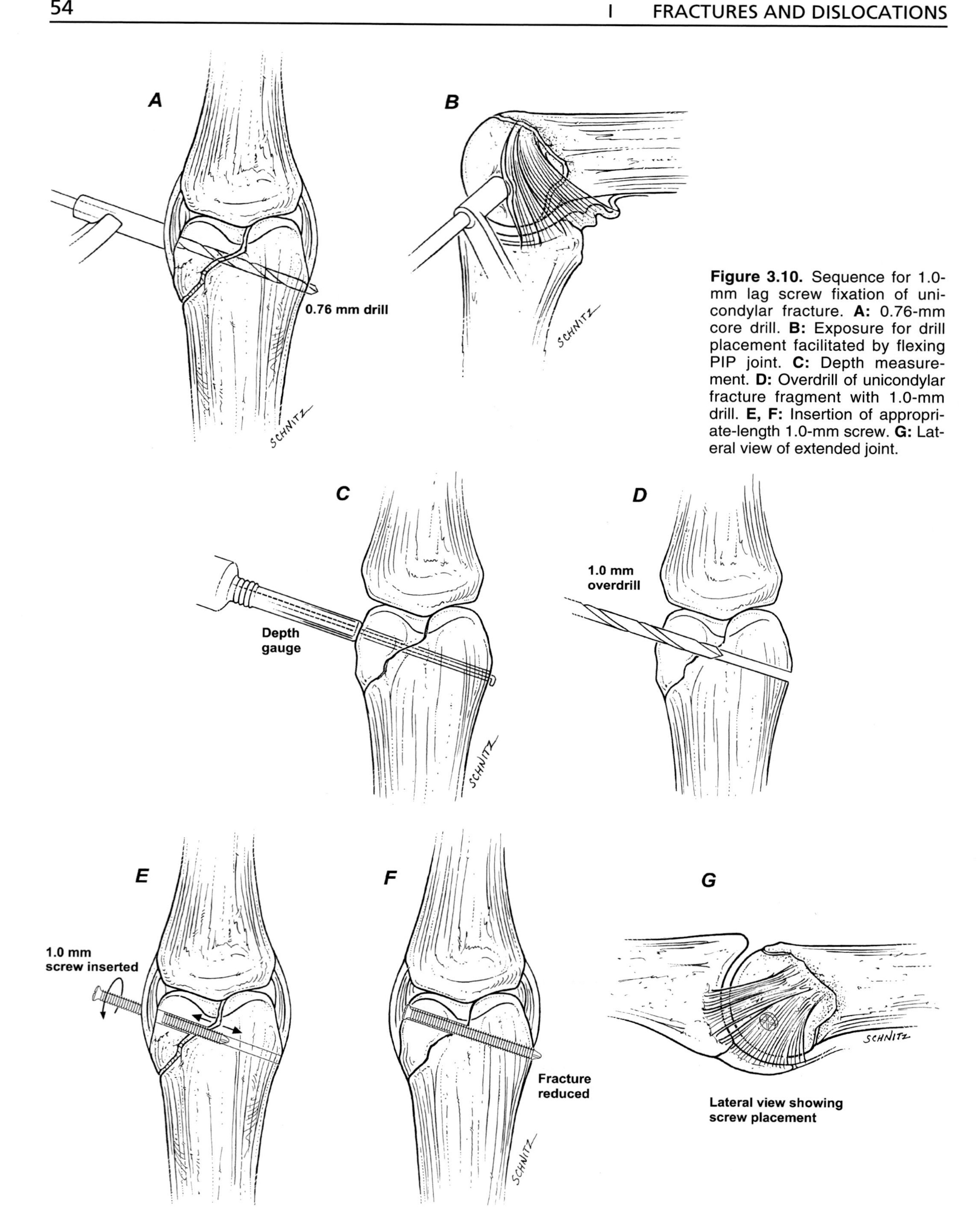

Figure 3.10. Sequence for 1.0-mm lag screw fixation of unicondylar fracture. **A:** 0.76-mm core drill. **B:** Exposure for drill placement facilitated by flexing PIP joint. **C:** Depth measurement. **D:** Overdrill of unicondylar fracture fragment with 1.0-mm drill. **E, F:** Insertion of appropriate-length 1.0-mm screw. **G:** Lateral view of extended joint.

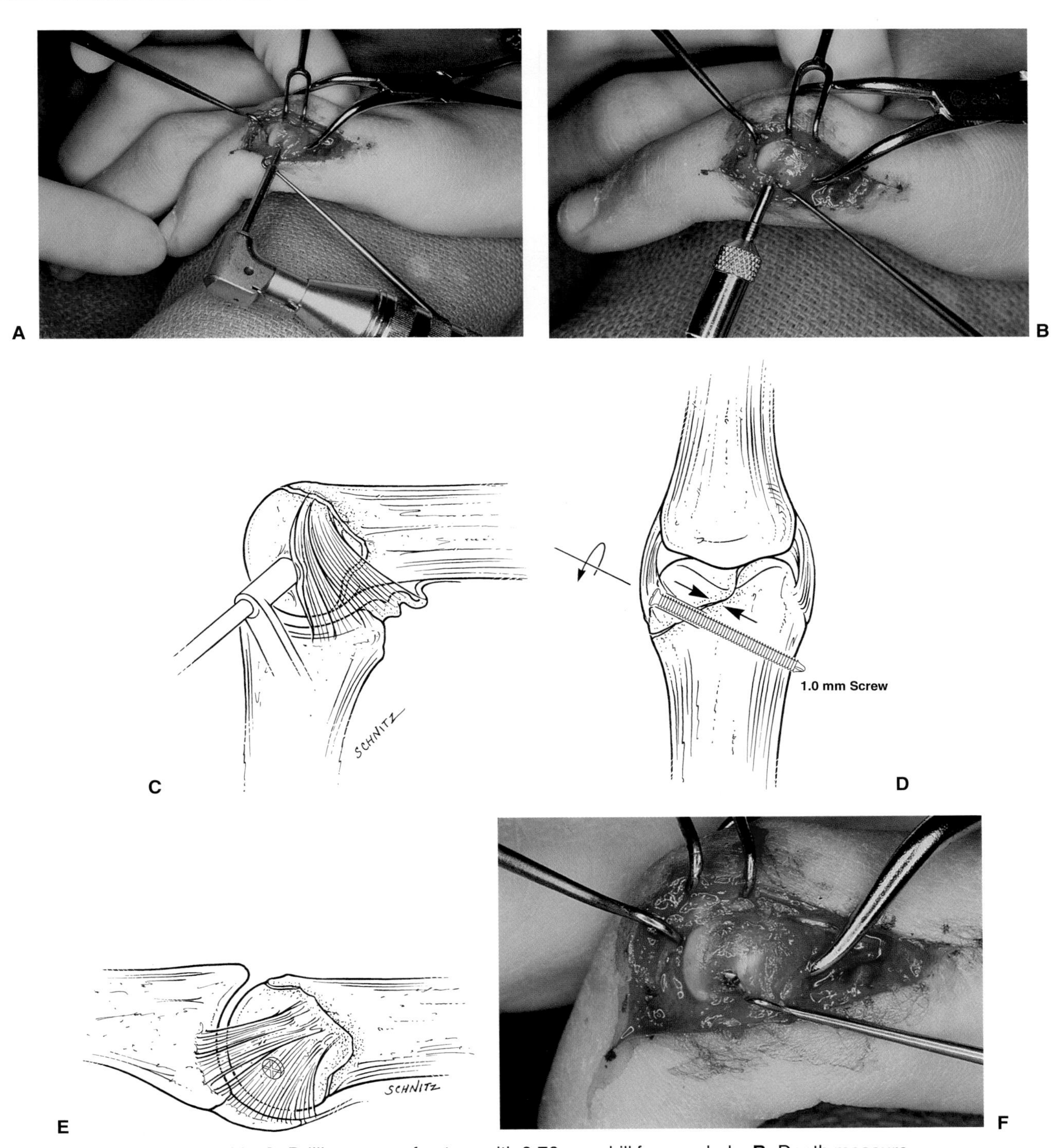

Figure 3.11. **A:** Drilling across fracture with 0.76-mm drill for core hole. **B:** Depth measurement. **C:** Overdrilling of fracture fragment with of 1.0-mm drill for gliding hole. **D:** Screw position on anteroposterior view. **E:** Screw position on lateral view with screw head recessed flush to bone surface underneath collateral ligaments. **F:** Clinical appearance after screw fixation.

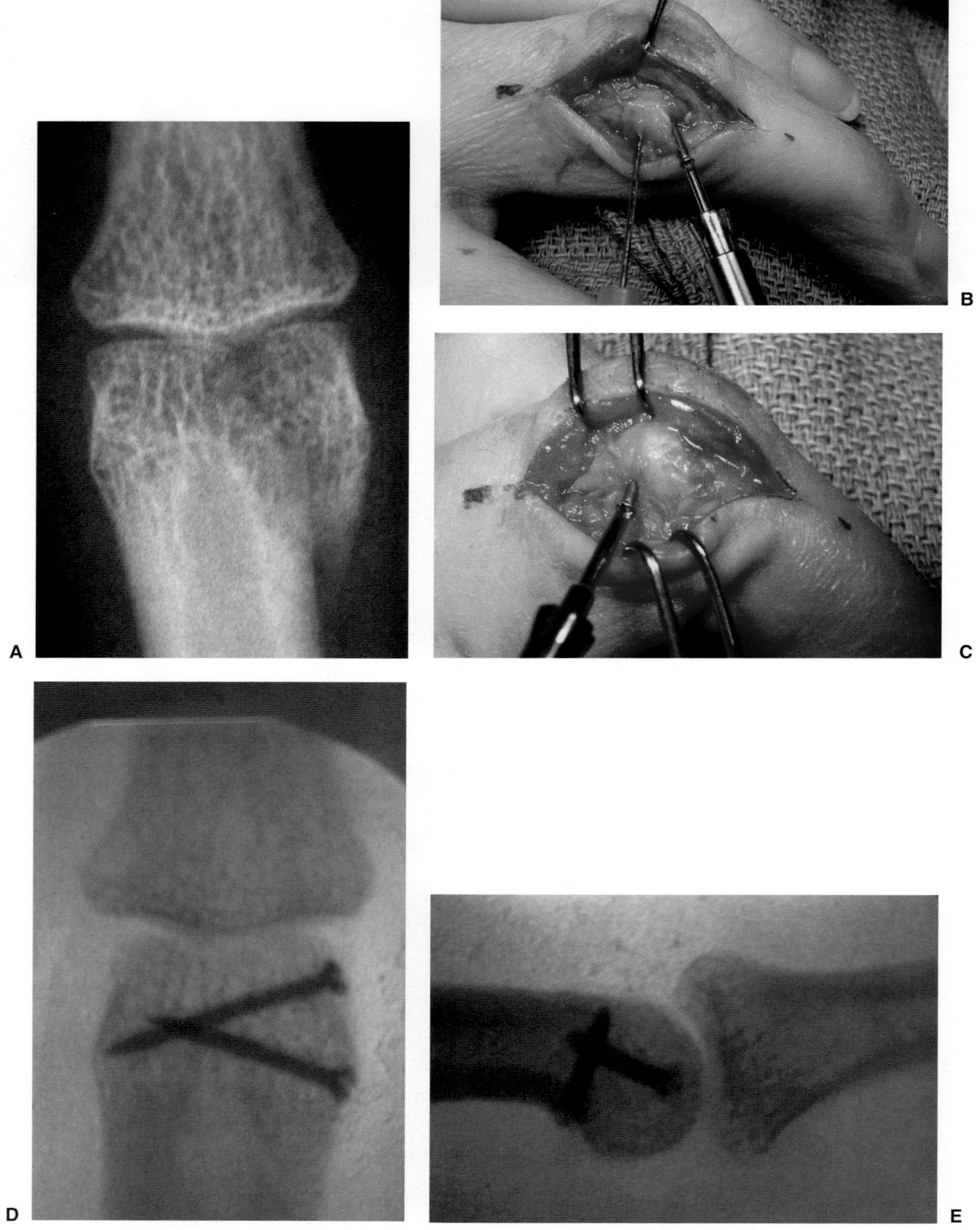

Figure 3.12. Larger Type 1 unicondylar fracture–two-screw fixation. **A:** Anteroposterior radiograph. **B:** Placement of distal screw. **C:** Placement of proximal screw. **D:** Anteroposterior radiograph after fixation.

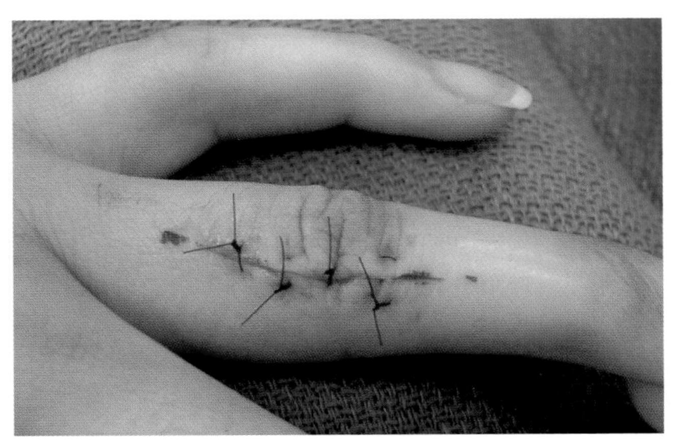

F

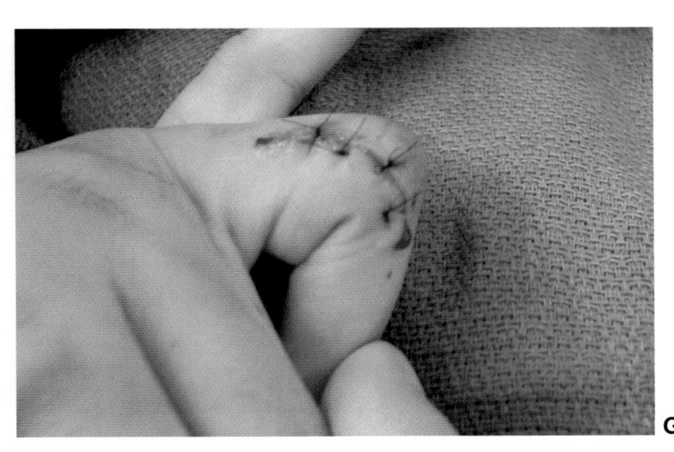

G

Figure 3.12. *Continued.* **E:** Lateral radiograph after fixation. **F:** Wound closure and extension. **G:** Fixation in flexion.

1.0-mm and 1.3-mm screws allow them to be placed distal to and irrespective of the collateral ligament as the collateral ligament will freely glide over them after insertion.

Some small unicondylar fragments can alternatively be fixed from the opposite side (Fig. 3.13). After provisional 0.028-inch Kirschner-wire fixation, a 0.76-mm drill is passed through the unicondylar fragment, across the fracture, and out the intact condyle. Depth is measured and the intact condyle drilled from the opposite side with a 1.0-mm drill to the fracture plane to create a gliding hole. An appropriate-length screw is inserted from the intact condyle and into the fractured condylar fragment. With larger screws, this is less likely to lead to fragmentation of the small unicondylar fragment. Protrusion of the screw tip can interfere with collateral ligament motion. In most cases, the use of 1.0-mm screws has made this technique obsolete.

Following fixation, the joint is visually inspected to confirm anatomic articular reduction. The extensor mechanism is repositioned without requirement for suture (Fig. 3.14A, B).

Closure. The skin is closed with monofilament 5-0 nylon. A light compressive dressing is applied with a small volar splint to maintain the interphalangeal joints in extension.

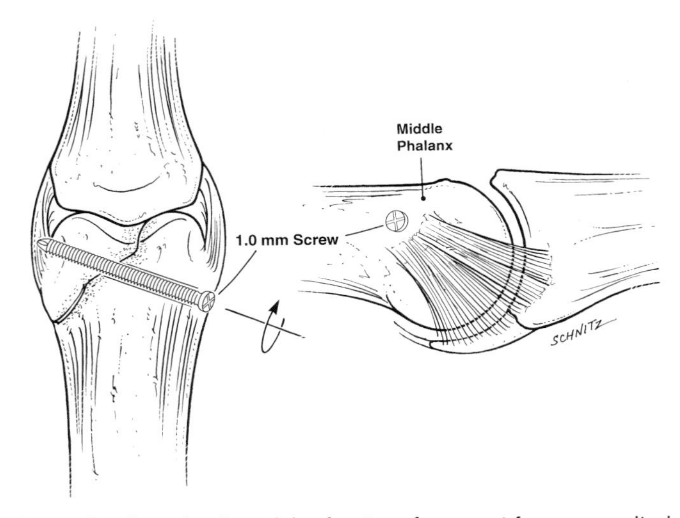

Figure 3.13. Screw fixation of unicondylar fracture fragment from opposite intact condyle.

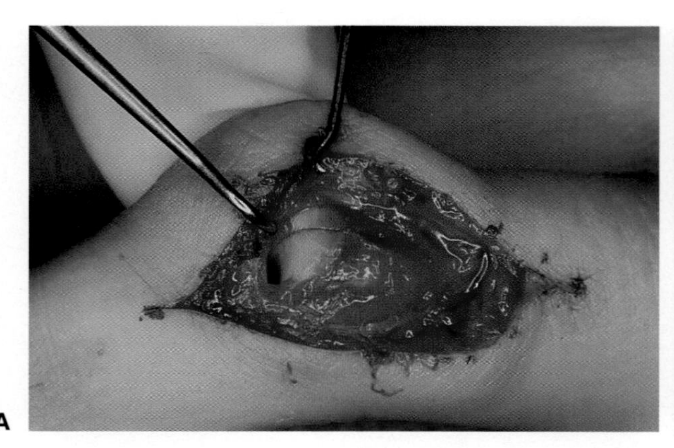

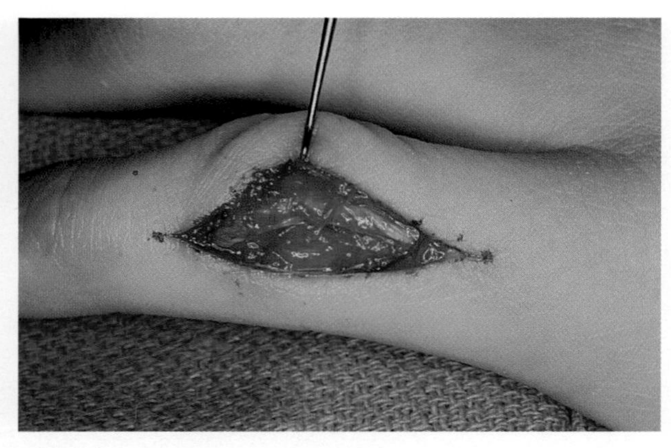

Figure 3.14. **A:** Appearance of articular surface following reduction and fixation. **B:** Repositioning of extensor mechanism.

POSTOPERATIVE MANAGEMENT

Kirschner-Wire Fixation

The initial operative dressing is removed within 3 to 5 days, and a lower-profile thermoplastic splint is applied volarly to immobilize the PIP joint alone in extension. Active range-of-motion exercises are initiated and performed at least 6 times a day. The Kirschner wires are removed at 3 weeks. Some protection from sports and work activities is needed for an additional 3 weeks and usually is best accomplished by buddy-tape immobilization to an adjacent digit.

Screw Fixation

The initial operative dressing is removed at three days. A light compressive dressing is applied, and active range of motion is encouraged. No protection other than buddy-tape splinting to an adjacent digit is needed. A thermoplastic extension splint is used at night. Normal, unrestricted activities are allowed at 6 weeks. It is expected that the normal flexion will be achieved at both the PIP and DIP joints. Frequently, the PIP joint will have a 5- to 10-degree extension deficit.

COMPLICATIONS

Active Extension Deficit

Problems with Extensor Lag/Passive Flexion Contracture. Immobilization of the digit between exercises for the first three weeks should be in a position of full PIP joint extension, which will prevent development of a passive flexion contracture; however, it does not always prevent development of an extensor lag. Mild extensor lags of less than 20 degrees are addressed by active range-of-motion exercises, especially active interphalangeal extension from a position of metacarpophalangeal joint flexion. Functional electrical stimulation may be helpful.

Passive flexion contractures greater than 30 degrees should be avoided by early stabilization and mobilization of these injuries, but when they occur, they are treated by use of a dynamic dorsal extension splint. Passive flexion contractures greater than 10 degrees and less than 30 degrees are treated with a safety-pin, or Capener-type, splint. Those less than 10 to 15 degrees are treated with an LMB splint (LMB Hand Rehabilitation Products, San Luis Obispo, CA, U.S.A.). Active extension exercises are best facilitated by blocking the metacarpophalangeal joint in slight flexion, which augments the power of the extensor digitorum communis at the PIP joint.

Passive Flexion Contracture

Flexion Deficit/Extension Contracture. Flexion deficits are best addressed by active flexion exercises. Use of a metacarpophalangeal joint-flexion block splint will better concentrate flexion forces at the PIP joint. If significant progress is not made by 5 to 6 weeks postoperatively, dynamic flexion splinting is added. Putty for strengthening may be added at 4 weeks for injuries with long fracture surfaces and at 6 weeks for short, limited fracture surfaces.

Loss of Reduction

Loss of reduction is most often associated with an insufficient number of Kirschner wires or faulty technique in screw fixation. Two or more Kirschner wires are required. At least one wire should purchase the palmar distal aspect of the fracture fragment. Loss of reduction usually occurs slowly. Once identified, open reduction is required to restore anatomic joint congruity and provide for stable fixation. If open reduction is required, fixation is best accomplished by use of microscrew fixation: 1.0- or 1.2–mm AO microscrews are used.

Larger fragments may be fixed with 1.5-mm lag screws. A dorsoradial approach is used. The transverse retinacular ligament is incised, the conjoined lateral band and central tendon retracted dorsally, and the fracture identified. Callus is removed from the fracture surfaces to allow for anatomic repositioning of the fragment. Reduction is maintained by definitive lag-screw fixation.

Pin-Tract Infection

Early pin-tract cellulitis is treated by a period of immobilization and oral antibiotics, usually an oral cephalosporin. Infections that occur after the second week are handled by removal of the offending pins and continued splint immobilization until the 3-week postoperative point has been reached.

Inadequate Reduction

Incomplete reduction results from inadequate clinical and radiographic assessment of the initial operative reduction. This may occur when large fluoroscopic devices are used that deliver very small images. During fluoroscopy, the digit should be positioned close to the emitting beam to magnify the image. Lateral, AP, partially supinated, and partially oblique views must be obtained and carefully assessed. Capsulotomy should always provide for adequate confirmation of anatomic articular reduction.

One region where inadequate or lost reduction may be particularly impactful from a functional standpoint is in the subcondylar recess. When this area is "crowded" by bone fragments or callus, the volar lip of the middle phalanx can be blocked from the end of its flexion arc. Great care must be taken to restore the anatomy in this area.

RECOMMENDED READING

1. Bowers WH. The proximal interphalangeal joint volar plate. II. A clinical study of hyperextension injury. *J Hand Surg* 6:77–81, 1981.
2. Bowers WH, Wolf I, Nehil I, et al. The proximal interphalangeal joint volar plate. I. An anatomical and biomechanical study. *J Hand Surg* 5:79–88, 1980.
3. Eaton RG. *Joint Injuries of the Hand.* Springfield, IL: Charles C. Thomas, 1971:3–34.

4. Hastings H, Carroll C. Treatment of closed articular fractures of the metacarpophalangeal and proximal interphalangeal joints. *Hand Clin* 4:503–527, 1988.
5. Kiefhaber TR, Stern PI, Grood ES. Lateral stability of the proximal interphalangeal joint. *J Hand Surg* 11A:661–669, 1986.
6. Kuczynski K. The proximal interphalangeal joint: anatomy and causes of stiffness of the fingers. *J Bone Joint Surg* 5013:656–663, 1968.
7. Kuczynski K. Less-known aspects of the proximal interphalangeal joints of the human hand. *Hand* 7:31–33, 1975.
8. Weiss AC, Hastings H. Distal unicondylar fractures of the proximal phalanx. *J Hand Surg* 18A:594–599, 1993.

4

Hemi Hamate Resurfacing Arthroplasty for Salvage of Selected Fracture-Dislocations of the Proximal Interphalangeal Joint

Hill Hastings II

INDICATIONS/CONTRAINDICATIONS

Dorsal fracture-dislocations of the proximal interphalangeal (PIP) joint with palmar margin fractures are classified according to stability. Those with less than 30% articular involvement at the base of the middle phalanx tend to be stable and congruent through a full arc of motion. A critical threshold exists at 42% volar articular involvement, beyond which the joint becomes increasingly unstable. Joint reduction is tenuous with articular involvement of 30–50% and usually requires increasing degrees of flexion to maintain stability.

Beyond 50% articular involvement, the joint becomes markedly unstable, almost always requiring some type of operative intervention to reassociate the joint and promote functional range of motion. Since the collateral ligaments do not contribute to dorsal-palmar stability, the PIP joint is unstable in all positions of flexion when 65% or more of the articular surface is damaged.

As described in other chapters, volar plate arthroplasty (VPA) is a logical choice for reconstruction of PIP fracture-dislocations when volar resurfacing can be accomplished in cases in which adequate dorsal bone stock of the middle phalanx has survived. However, in some more severely injured joints with inadequate osseous architecture to support VPA, hemi hamate resurfacing is an attractive salvage alternative.

Hill Hastings II, M.D.: Orthopaedic Surgery, Indiana University Medical Center, Indiana Hand Center, Indianapolis, IN, and Orthopaedic Surgery, St. Vincent's Hospital, Indianapolis, IN

Hemi hamate resurfacing arthroplasty is indicated for the following:

1. comminuted unstable PIP palmar lip fractures with dorsal dislocation of the joint;
2. comminuted lateral plateau fractures of the base of the middle phalanx; and
3. salvage after failed external fixation, open reduction internal fixation, or palmar plate arthroplasty for complex fracture-dislocations of the PIP joint.

Contraindications include inability of the patient to comply with postoperative therapy and articular cartilage defect or significant alteration of the articular morphology of the distal condyles of the proximal phalanx. This includes substance defects in which part of the condyle is missing, malaligned, or affected by degenerative arthritis.

PREOPERATIVE PLANNING

Acute and subacute injuries will usually have mild to moderate swelling about the PIP joint. Palmar fracture of the base of the middle phalanx (P2) can be associated with significant impaction on one side of the joint. This may lead to a clinical deviation and rotational deformity of the digit. Mechanism of the injury by axial load at times will also damage the distal interphalangeal joint (DIP), and careful clinical and radiographic assessment is indicated to rule out a tendinous or bony mallet deformity. Range-of-motion measurements should be recorded for both PIP and DIP joints.

Obtain anteroposterior (AP) and lateral x-rays of the PIP joint. Another very useful technology for understanding the joint relationships at the PIP joint, particularly as the joint is taken through a range of motion, is live fluoroscopy. Fluoroscopic evaluation allows visualization at an infinite number of angles, better visualization of the subcondylar fossa, and detection of subtle changes in concentric reduction and joint tracking.

A properly reduced joint will have concentric matching surfaces on lateral radiographs. Any relative widening of the dorsal portion of the joint surface compared with the palmar portion suggests subluxation. An inability to visualize both condyles of the proximal phalanx as a single, aligned unit suggests a geometric or morphological change on the P1 side of the joint (double "C" sign).

PIP joint subluxation on lateral radiographs will present as a "V" sign (Fig. 4.1). The AP radiographs will best show whether or not one plateau of the articular base of the middle phalanx is more impacted than the other (Fig. 4.2). Lateral radiographs will best show the extent of volar articular involvement (Fig. 4.3). Frequently, one facet will have a greater percentage of involvement than the other, and this may be best detected with an oblique radiograph. In most cases, radiographs will tend to underestimate the amount of articular fracture involvement, which is why fluoroscopy can be so valuable.

SURGERY

Positioning, Draping, and Organization of the Operating Room

A general or regional block anesthetic is administered. Position the patient supine on the operating table, with the involved extremity supported by a hand table. Apply a brachial tourniquet. Sterilely prep and drape the arm to the tourniquet level. When available, the arm of a small fluoroscopic unit is draped for later fluoroscopic assessment.

Make a modified palmar Bruner or midaxial incision. I favor the former, which is accomplished by incising in a line extending from the palmar digital flexion crease proximally to the DIP flexion crease distally (Fig. 4.4). Elevate skin and subcutaneous tissue with a No. 15 surgical blade superficial to the neurovascular bundle adjacent to the apex of the Bruner incision (Fig. 4.5). Once midline is reached, continue the plane of dissection along the palmar surface of the flexor sheath over to the opposite neurovascular bundle. Leave the opposite neurovascular bundle intact within the retracted flap. Place 4-0 nylon

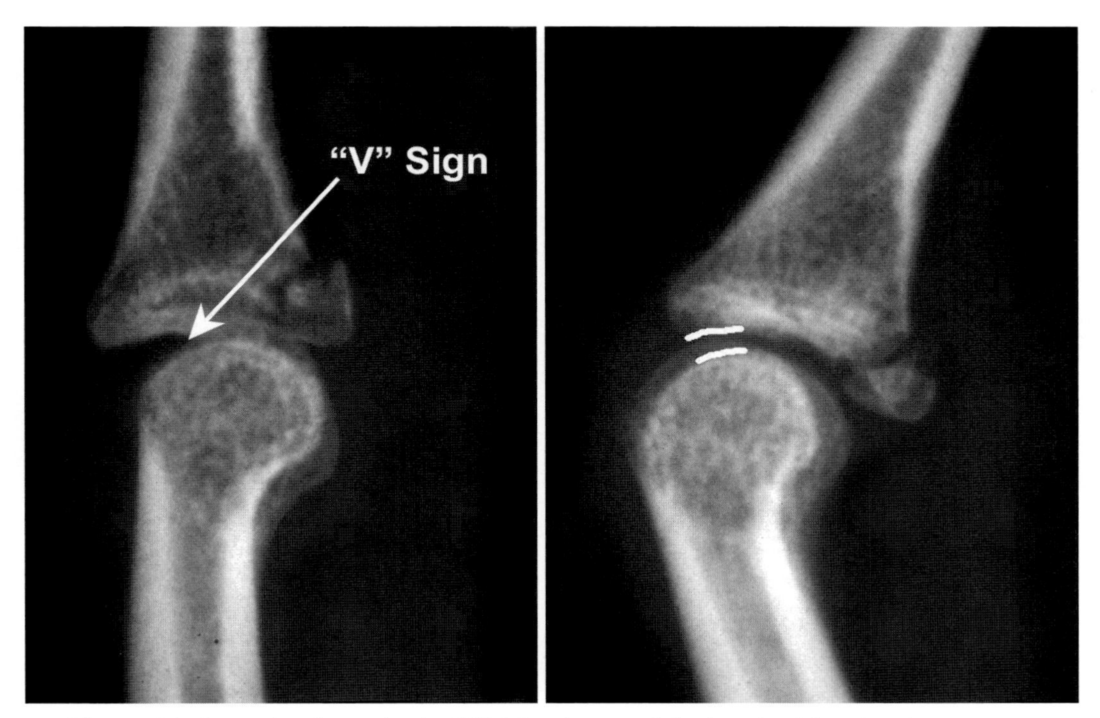

Figure 4.1. Lateral radiograph of a PIP joint shows subtle dorsal subluxation, best recognized by dorsal joint widening termed the "V-sign."

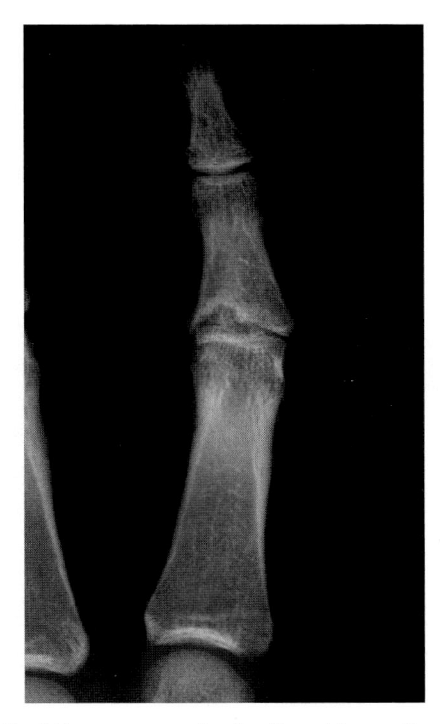

Figure 4.2. AP x-ray reveals significant impaction of the ulnar plateau at the articular base of the middle phalanx.

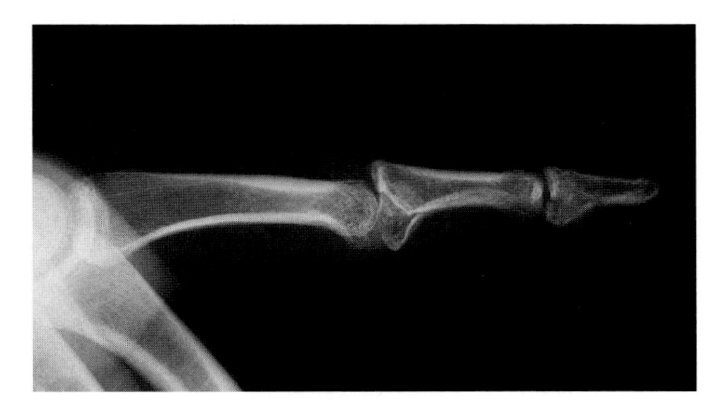

Figure 4.3. Lateral radiograph shows significant volar impaction and dorsal dislocation of the middle phalanx.

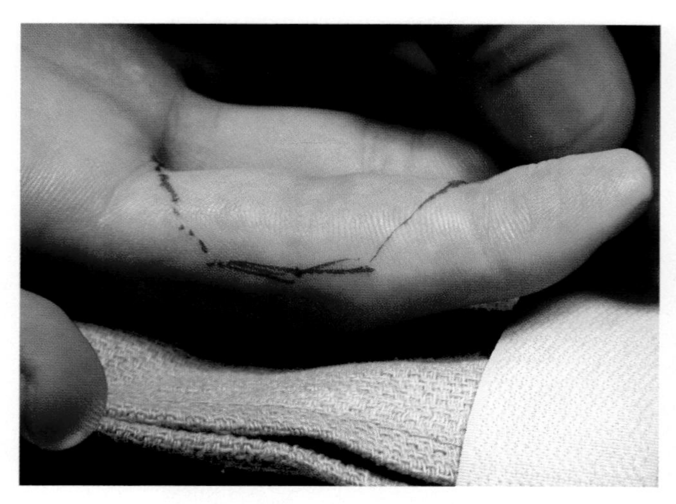

Figure 4.4. Midaxial incision is made across the PIP joint extended distally and proximally in a modified Bruner fashion.

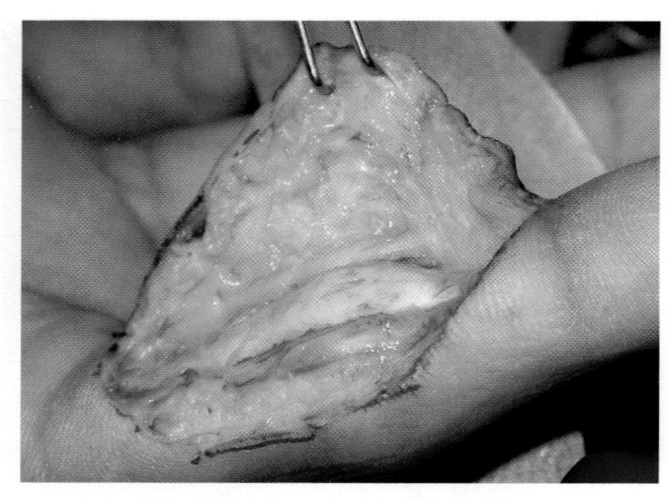

Figure 4.5. Elevation of palmar skin and subcutaneous tissue superficial to the radial nerve vascular bundle and flexor tendons. The ulnar nerve vascular bundle is included within the retracted flap.

suture stays in the flap to maintain its retraction during the operative procedure; it is usually easiest to suture the flap to the dorsal skin of the digit.

Create a window in the flexor sheath between the A2 and A4 pulleys. To do so, longitudinally incise the tendon sheath unilaterally at its dorsal margin between the A2 and A4 pulleys. Use a pair of small scissors or careful sharp dissection to transversely incise the sheath along the distal edge of the A2 pulley proximally and the proximal edge of the A4 pulley distally. Retract the rectangular flap to the opposite side.

Incise the juncture of the accessory collateral ligament into the volar plate longitudinally from proximal to distal on either side of the flexor tendon sheath (Fig. 4.6). Extend these longitudinal incisions distally to the proximal edge of the A4 pulley. Retract the flexor digitorum superficialis (FDS) and flexor digitorum profundus (FDP) away from midline (Fig. 4.7) and transversely incise the volar plate insertion from the P2 base. Retraction of the

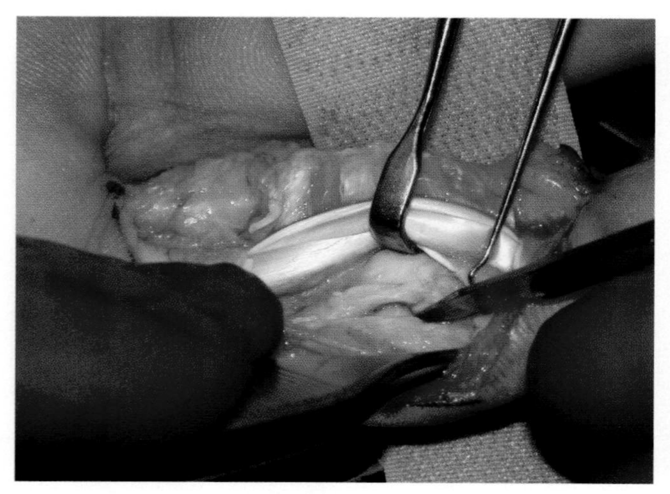

Figure 4.6. Longitudinal incision is made at the lateral margin of the volar plate on either side of the flexor tendon, dividing the attachment of the accessory collateral ligament to the volar plate on each side of the joint.

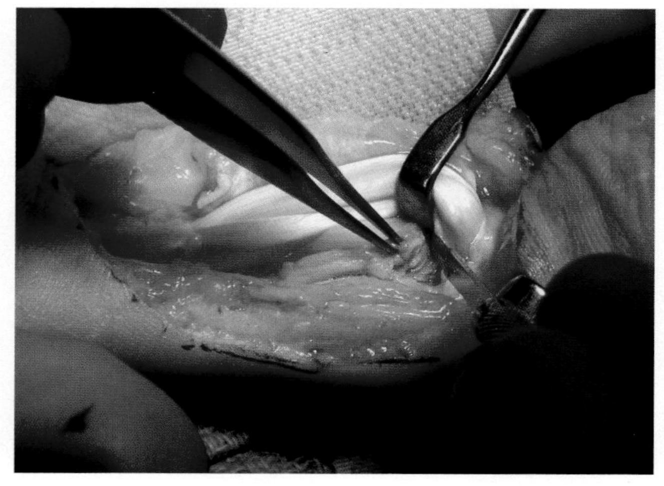

Figure 4.7. Flexor tendons are retracted to allow transverse incision at distal volar plate insertion.

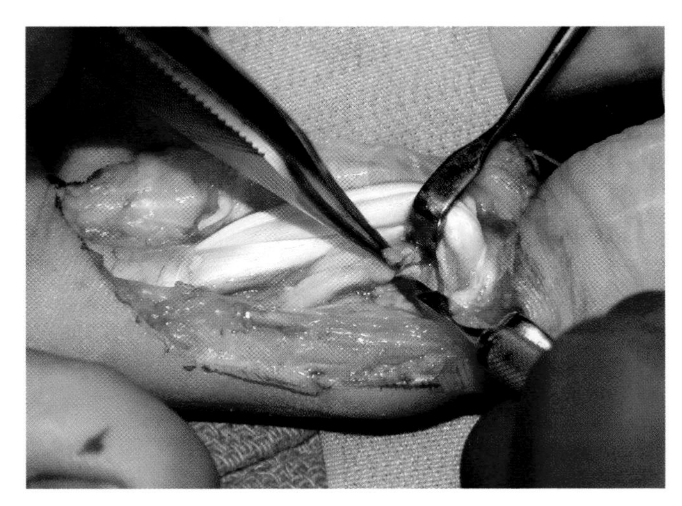

Figure 4.8. The volar plate is sharply elevated from distal to proximal.

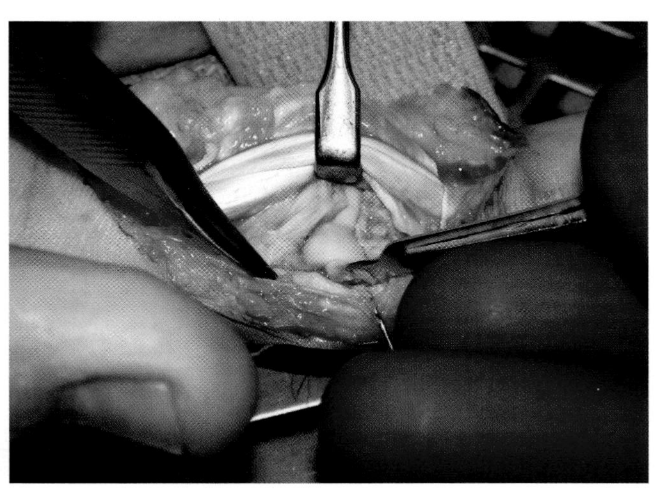

Figure 4.9. The radial and ulnar collateral ligaments are subperiosteally released from their proximal phalangeal origin.

FDS and FDP tendons to opposite sides is usually required to complete the transverse limb of the volar plate dissection without injury to the contents of the sheath. Elevate the volar plate from distal to proximal with a No. 15 surgical blade or No. 69 Beaver blade (Fig. 4.8). The volar plate remains attached proximally by its "checkrein" ligament origin.

Expose the articular surfaces of the head of the proximal phalanx and the base of the middle phalanx by obtaining complete hyperextension of the PIP joint ("shotgun maneuver"). This is achieved by subperiosteal release of the proper collateral ligament origins from the head of the proximal phalanx (Fig. 4.9). Position the surgical blade in the sagittal plane and sweep it from dorsal to palmar along the undersurface of the collateral ligament origin, detaching it from the proximal phalanx. Hyperextend the PIP joint (Figs. 4.10 and 4.11). In subacute or late cases, there may be dorsal capsular contracture and/or extensor adhesions that require lysis with a Freer elevator or formal sharp release. Evacuate any bony or fibrous tissue in the subcondylar fossa that may later impinge on the hemi hamate graft and limit extreme flexion.

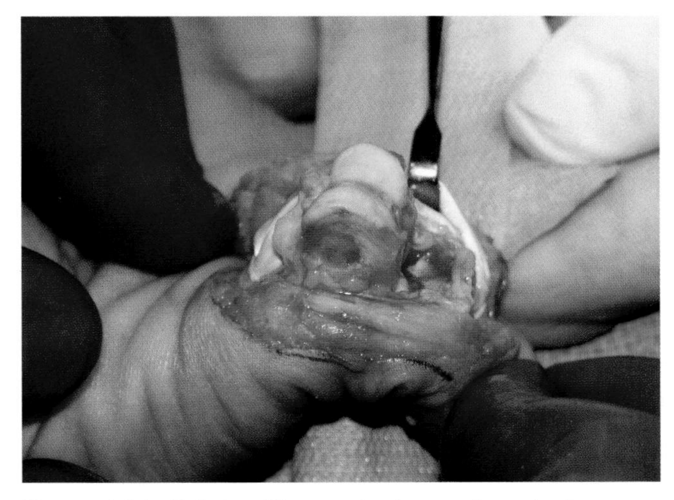

Figure 4.10. Collateral ligament release allows for hyperextension of the joint to expose the articular base of the middle phalanx. Note the severe articular comminution and impaction.

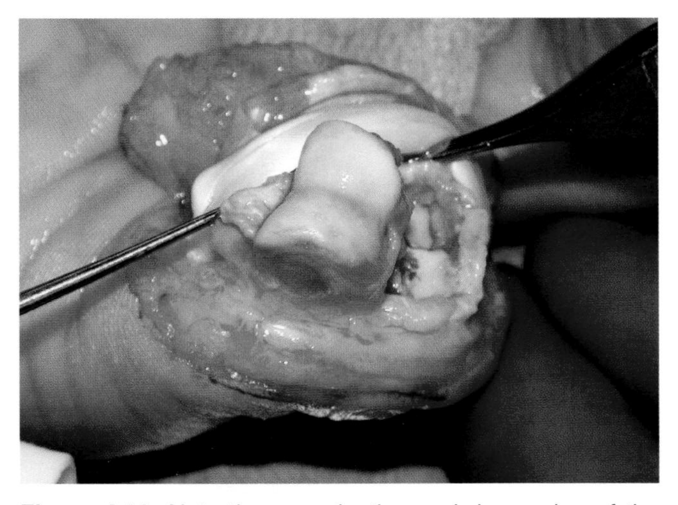

Figure 4.11. Note the comminution and depression of the volar middle phalangeal articular base.

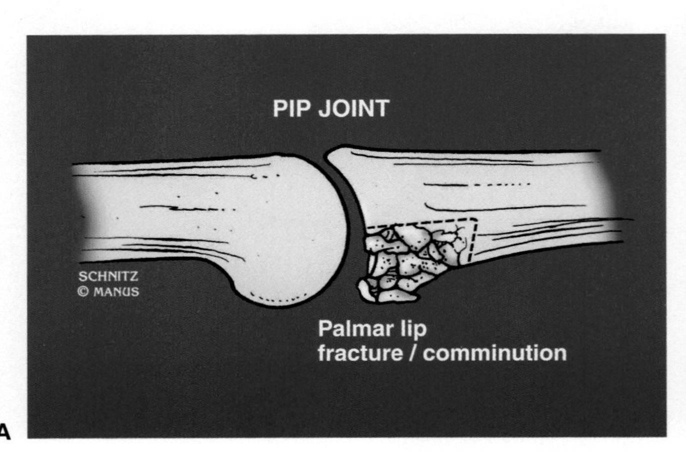

A

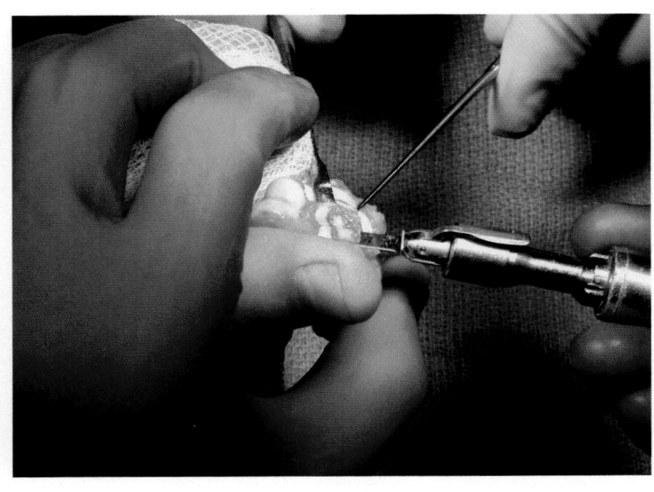

B

Figure 4.12. **A:** Depiction of the area of comminuted articular base to be resected. **B:** A 4-mm oscillation saw is used to resect the comminuted articular fragments and create a box-like recipient defect.

Preparation of the Articular Base of Middle Phalanx

Excise the depressed portion of the articular surface with hand tools or a 4-mm oscillating saw to create a box-like recipient defect (Fig. 4.12, A and B). Often, the fracture plane is not perfectly situated in the coronal plane, involving more of the volar surface on one plateau than the other. For ease of surgical reconstruction, the defect is simplified to match the perfect coronal plane to accept the graft.

Measure the dimensions of the recipient defect. This includes particularly the width of the articular surface defect, the dorsal-to-palmar height, and the proximal-to-distal length (Fig. 4.13).

Harvesting of Hamate Osteochondral Graft

Make a longitudinal incision, centered over the articular base of the fourth and fifth metacarpals (Fig. 4.14). Mobilize dorsal veins and protect the dorsal sensory branches of

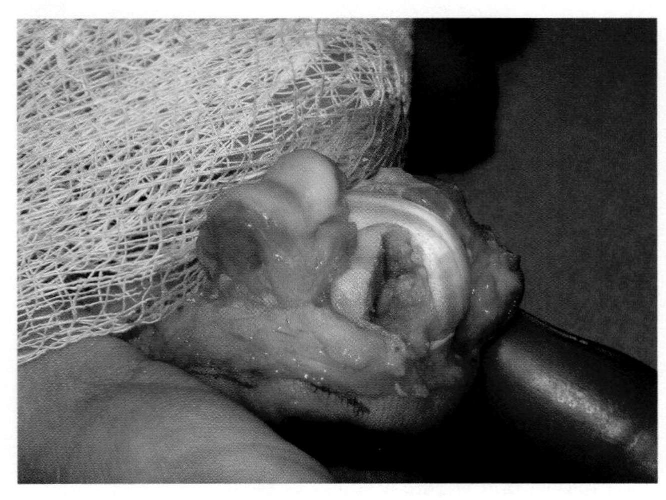

Figure 4.13. Final appearance of the recipient defect.

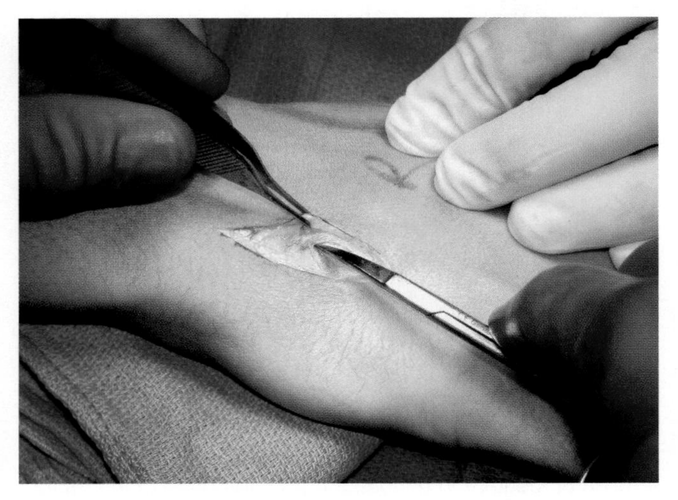

Figure 4.14. Longitudinal incision over the fourth and fifth carpometacarpal joints with mobilization of dorsal sensory branches of the ulnar nerve.

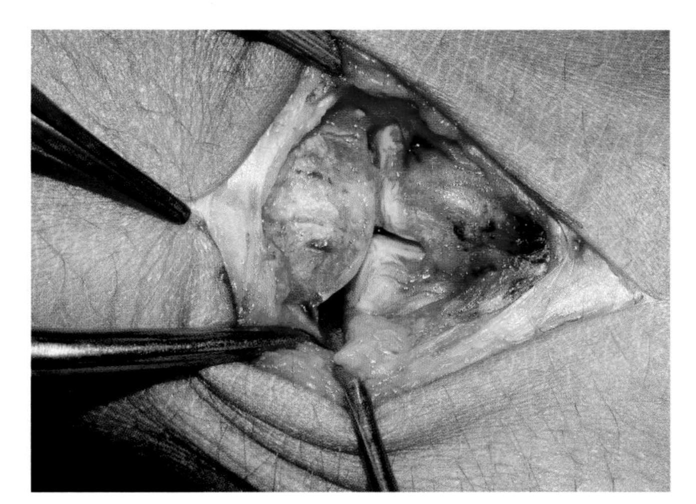

Figure 4.15. Exposure of the fourth and fifth carpometacarpal joints between the extensor digitorum communis of the ring finger and the extensor digiti quinti tendons.

the ulnar nerve. Retract the common and proper extensors of the fifth digit (extensor digitorum communis of the small finger [EDCV] and extensor digiti quinti [EDQP]) ulnarly and the extensor digitorum communis of the ring finger radially. Incise the capsule over the carpometacarpal joint and sharply elevate the capsule away from the hamate-fourth metacarpal and hamate-fifth metacarpal articulations (Fig. 4.15).

With a marking pen, measure and draw the donor graft template to match the measurements of the recipient defect (Fig. 4.16, A and B). Liberate the hamate graft with a 4-mm saw, cutting to the dimensions of the template and taking care to cut to the appropriate depth. Remove a 2-mm section of hamate along the proximal cut, down to the depth of the dorsal-volar height of the required graft. Use a small osteotome to create a coronal plane cut from within the joint, with the osteotome directed distal to proximal. The articular surface cut begins at the appropriate distance within the joint that matches the dorsal-to-palmar articular surface needed. The cut is directed distal-dorsal to proximal-volar, such that the more proximal part of the osteochondral graft is slightly thicker than that at the articular margin (Fig. 4.17). As the cut is being made, be sure to apply a moistened surgical sponge directly over the hamate so that it is contained and is not lost from the wound when it becomes free. Removal of a proximal hamate section minimizes the chance of a propagated fracture of the hamate body by creating a stress riser in the appropriate place and helps to

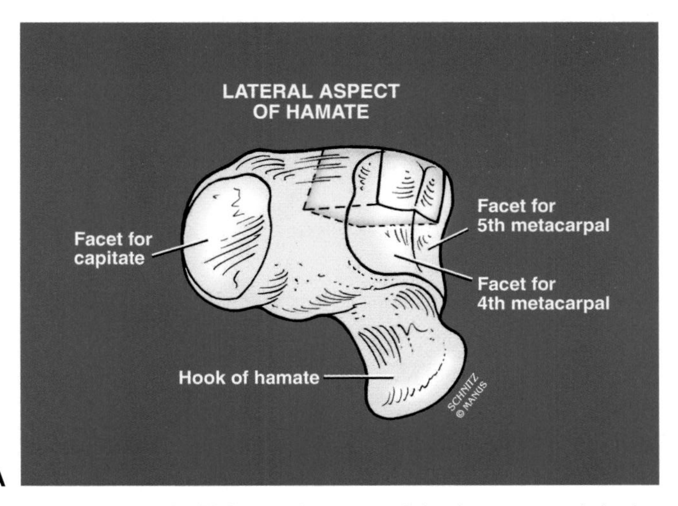

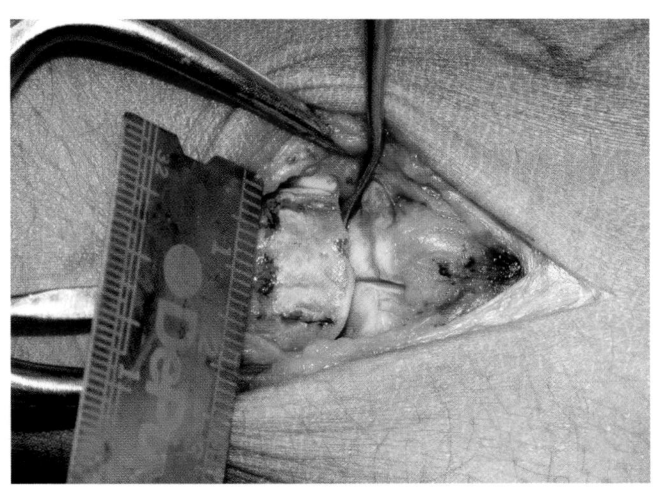

Figure 4.16. A: Bi-faceted nature of the hamate and depicted graft location. **B:** Measurement and marking of the donor graft.

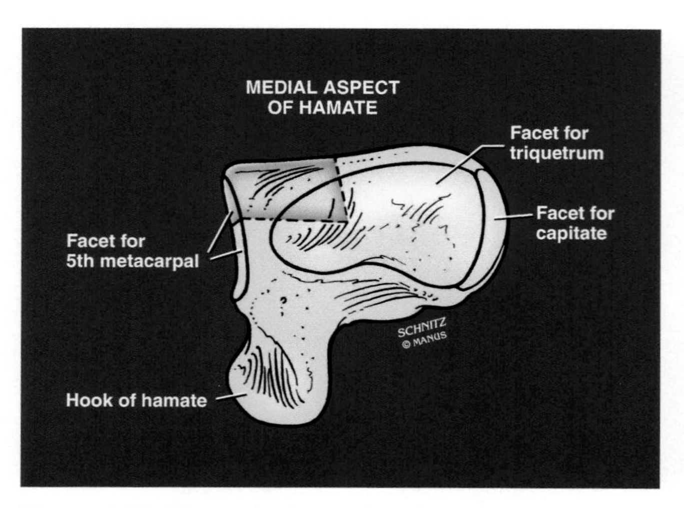

Figure 4.17. Planes for harvesting the osteochondral graft from the hamate (sagittal view).

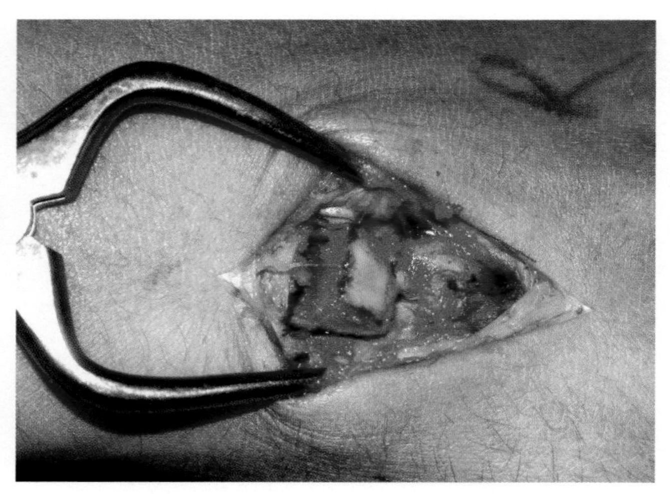

Figure 4.18. Appearance of the harvested osteochondral hamate graft.

avoid losing the graft by channeling "ejection forces" when the graft is finally free (Fig. 4.18).

Pack the donor defect with a Gelfoam sponge. Close the capsule with 4-0 braided nylon suture and the skin with interrupted 5-0 nylon suture (Figs. 4.19 and 4.20).

Shaping the Osteochondral Graft

The graft can be trimmed down to a smaller dimension as needed or the recipient defect can be enlarged slightly so that the two components match. I recommend that the cuts be made with a 4-mm power oscillating saw to maximize control of the geometry of the graft.

It is critical for successful reconstruction to "tip" the graft to restore the proper palmar lip and buttress to the middle phalanx (Fig. 4.21). It is easiest to trim the graft to the appropriate medial-lateral width first, followed by trimming to the appropriate dorsal-palmar height. Position the graft into the recipient defect, and finally trim the distal surface to adjust the length of the graft such that the articular surfaces match perfectly. Final length ad-

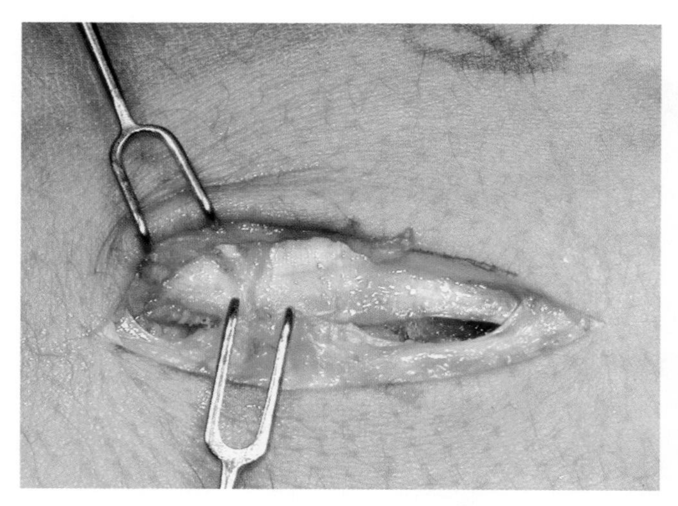

Figure 4.19. Closure of fascia and capsule over the carpometacarpal joint.

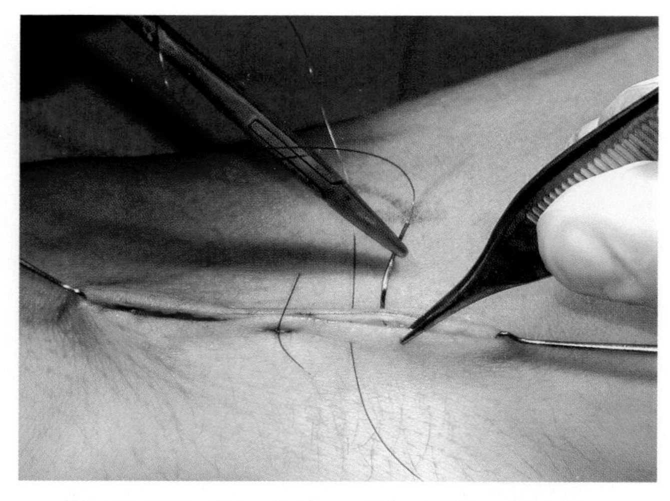

Figure 4.20. Skin closure with monofilament nylon.

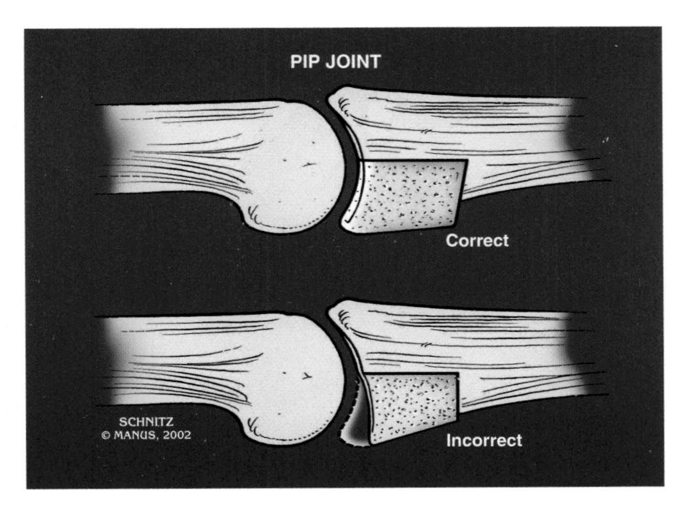

Figure 4.21. Examples of correct and incorrect orientations of graft.

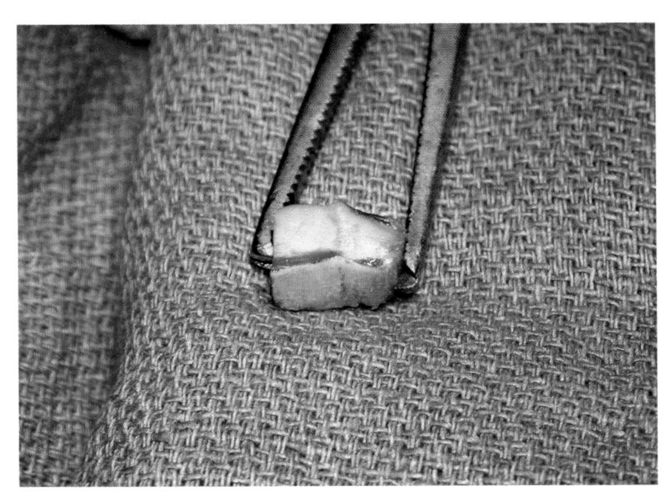

Figure 4.22. Appearance of the osteochondral graft. Note the bi-faceted appearance of the joint surface.

justment is usually made through small adjustments to both the recipient bed and the graft (Fig. 4.22).

Provisionally fix the graft with 0.028-inch Kirschner wires in the central and proximal part of the graft (Fig. 4.23).

Definitive fixation is accomplished with three 1.0-mm lag screws (Fig. 4.24). Make two 0.76-mm drill holes in the more distal medial and lateral portions of the graft (Figs. 4.25 and 4.26). Measure the depth of the required screws (Fig. 4.27). Make a 1.0-mm gliding-hole to the depth of the graft and insert a self-tapping screw of an appropriate length in each hole (Fig. 4.28). Remove the provisional Kirschner wire and place a similarly prepared third screw through its hole.

Reduce the PIP joint and ensure that correct rotational alignment exists and that the joint is stable through a full arc of motion. With the graft appropriately positioned, it should be stable all the way to full extension.

Assess the joint under fluoroscopy to determine that the screws are of proper length and position. Confirm congruent stability of the joint through a full arc of motion. Reattach the

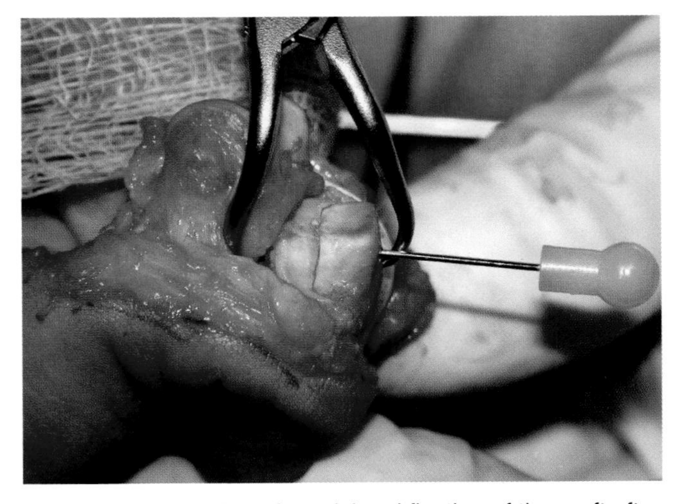

Figure 4.23. Position of provisional fixation of the graft after trimming the graft to fit the recipient defect.

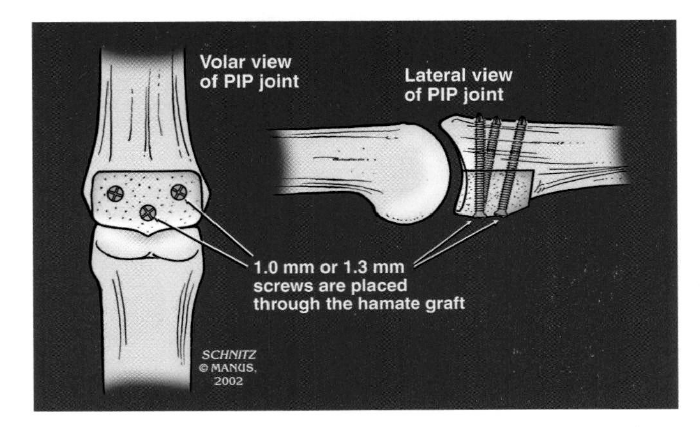

Figure 4.24. Artist's illustration of positions for screw fixation.

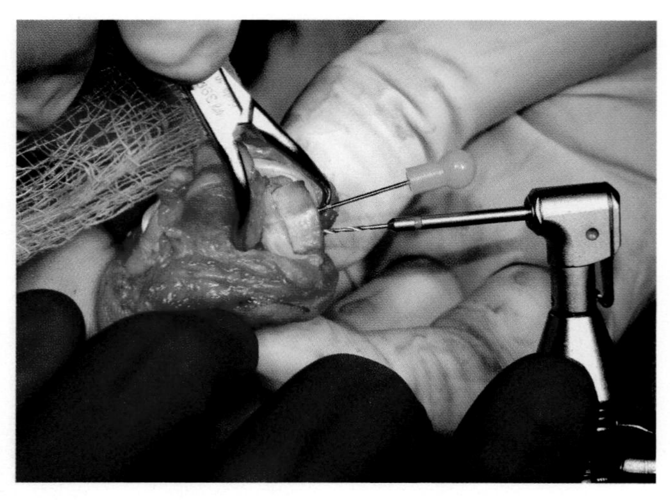

Figure 4.25. A 0.76-mm drill hole for placement of a 1.0-mm screw.

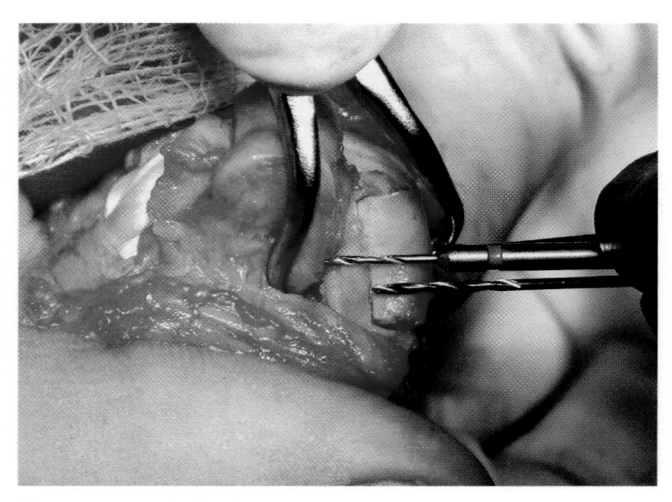

Figure 4.26. Drills show corresponding depths of a 0.76-mm drill for the core hole and a 1.0-mm overdrill for the gliding hole.

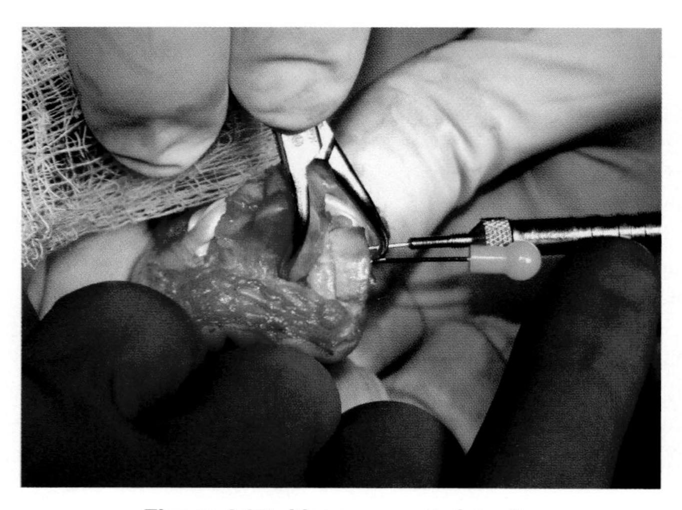

Figure 4.27. Measurement of depth.

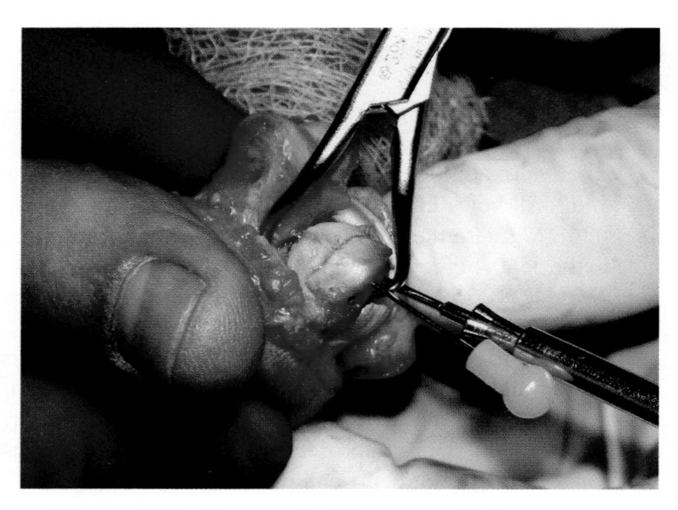

Figure 4.28. Placement of the second 1.0-mm screw.

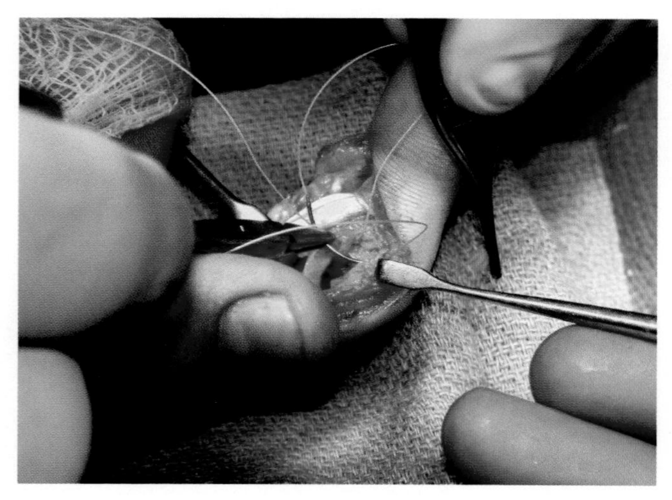

Figure 4.29. Repair of the volar plate on each lateral side.

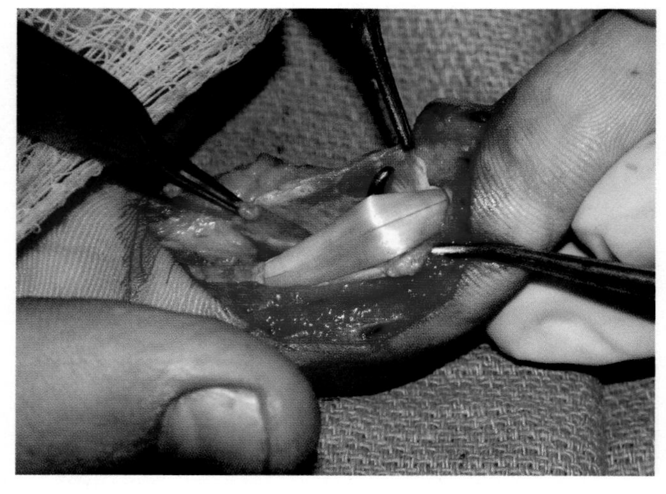

Figure 4.30. Transposition of the flexor tendon sheath flap deep to flexor tendons.

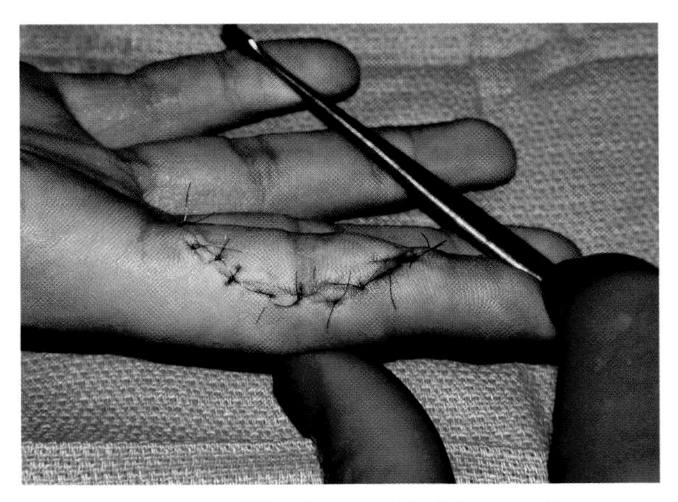

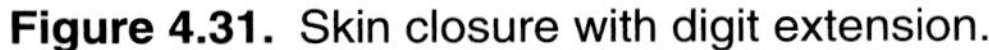

Figure 4.31. Skin closure with digit extension.

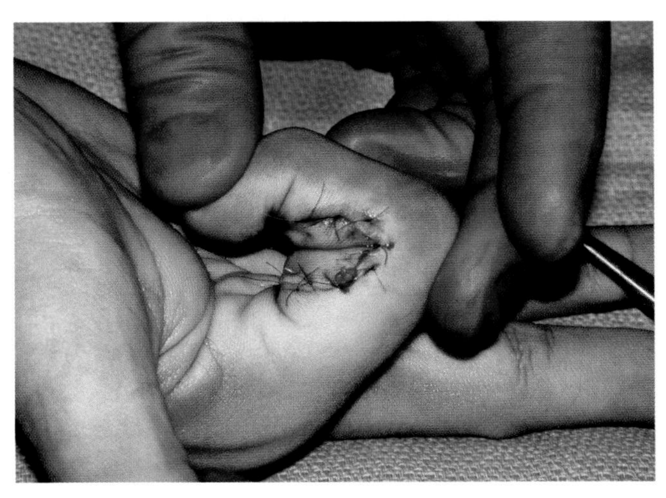

Figure 4.32. Passive flexion after wound closure.

volar plate to its medial and lateral distal margins. The volar plate is usually not excessively thickened or foreshortened. Its repair is critical to prevent hyperextension and swan-neck postoperative deformity. The joint should stably flex and extend fully. Use 4-0 braided nylon sutures to fix the medial and distal margins of the volar plate to the confluence of soft-tissue insertion of the collateral ligament and the beginning of the A4 pulley (Fig. 4.29). Transpose the flexor sheath flap deep to the flexor tendons to reinforce the volar plate repair and further separate the flexor synovial environment from the graft (Fig. 4.30). Tack the flexor sheath back to the soft tissues deep to the opposite neurovascular bundle. Close the skin with 5-0 monofilament nylon (Figs. 4.31 and 4.32).

POSTOPERATIVE MANAGEMENT AND REHABILITATION

On completion of the operation, apply a short-arm, bulky supportive dressing and volar splint, holding the wrist in 30 degrees of dorsiflexion, with the metacarpophalangeal joints in flexion and the interphalangeal joints in 20-degree extension.

Remove the dressing on the third to fifth postoperative day to initiate active and passive range-of-motion exercises. Apply a light compressive dressing with Coban to control edema. Mold an Orthoplast dorsal block splint to maintain the PIP joint in 20 degrees of flexion. Initiate active and passive complete flexion beyond this point. If the patient is unable or it is too painful to flex the digit fully, at least fingertip to palm, administer a digital block to assist with initiation of range-of-motion therapy. Instruct the patient to perform active and passive flexion and extension exercises a minimum of six times per day.

At 10 to 14 days, remove the sutures. At 4 weeks, discontinue the dorsal block splint. At 6 weeks, any residual passive flexion contracture at the PIP joint is addressed by dynamic extension splinting. Care should be taken to avoid hyperextension deformity.

Obtain postoperative radiographs at 10 to 14 days and AP and lateral projections at 6 weeks (Fig. 4.33). Additional useful x-rays include both an extension lateral and a flexion lateral to assess the congruency of the joint through an arc of motion (Figs. 4.34 and 4.35). Initiate formal strengthening exercises with putty at 6 weeks and with a string or rubber-band-resistance grip-strengthening device at 8 weeks.

Advise patients that the operation should restore a stable, well-aligned PIP joint. It should allow for a functional arc of motion, with flexion past 90 degrees, in many cases. We anticipate gaining nearly full extension, but advise the patient that it is not uncommon to have a 15- to 20-degree extension deficit at final outcome. Healing of the graft requires 6 weeks, and for this reason strengthening and forceful use are not allowed until after that period. Fully unrestricted use should be anticipated by 12 weeks.

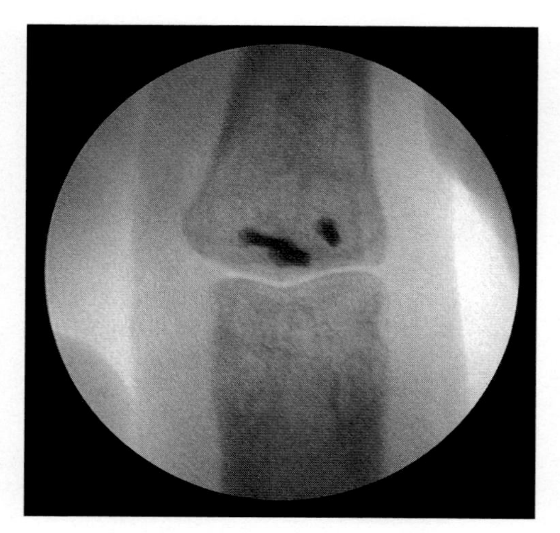

Figure 4.33. Postoperative AP x-ray.

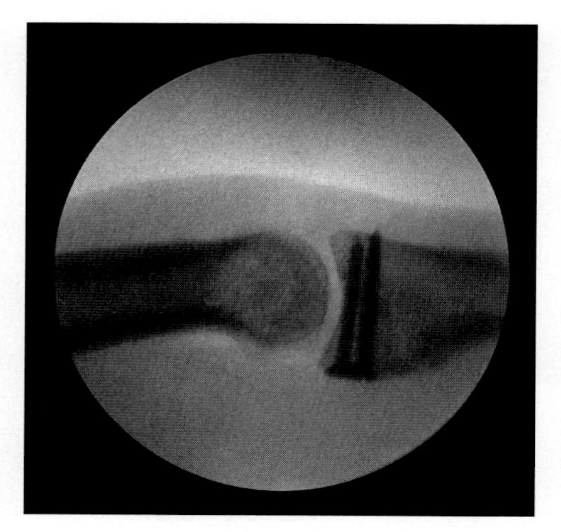

Figure 4.34. Postoperative lateral x-ray in extension.

RESULTS

The majority of patients have no symptoms at the donor site. A 100% union rate of the osteochondral graft has been seen, with no resorption, in our series. In two separate clinical trials, average motion at the PIP joint was 20 degrees of extension through 97 degrees of flexion, and at the DIP joint, 1 degree of extension and 60 degrees of flexion. Grip strength averaged 98 pounds (81% of the comparison side). In a more recent series by Williams et al., the average arc of motion at the PIP joint was 87 degrees (range, 65–100 degrees), with an average flexion contracture of 9 degrees (range, 0–25 degrees). Average grip strength was 85% on the opposite side. My longest follow-up to date is 8.5 years with normal maintenance of joint space without evidence of degenerative change (Fig. 4.36, A–C). PIP range of motion was 5 degrees of extension and 105 degrees of flexion, with DIP extension 0 degrees and flexion 90 degrees (Fig. 4.37, A and B).

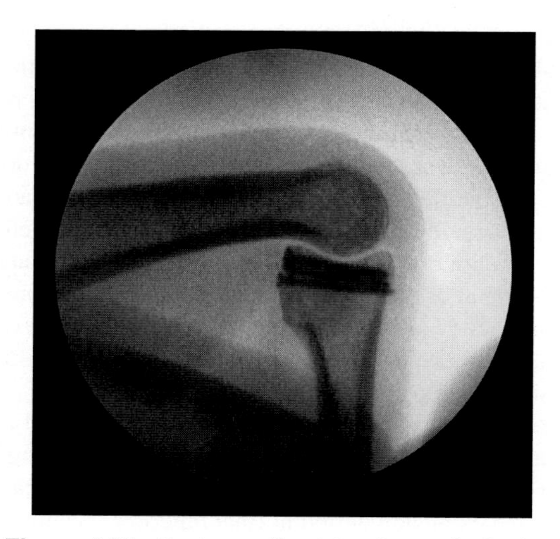

Figure 4.35. Postoperative lateral x-ray in flexion.

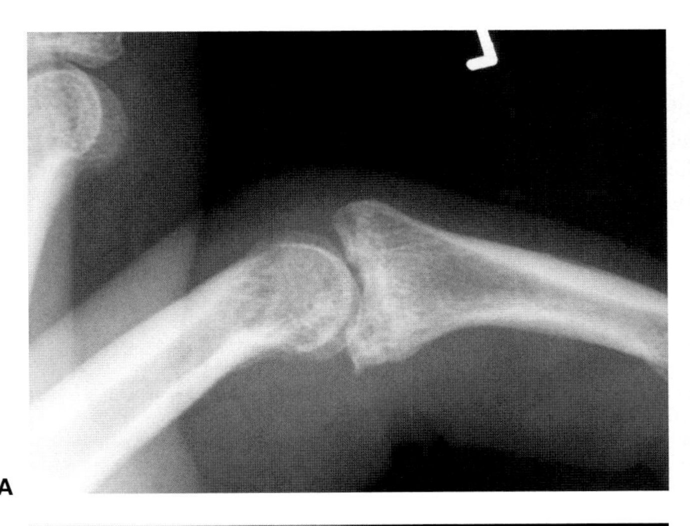

A

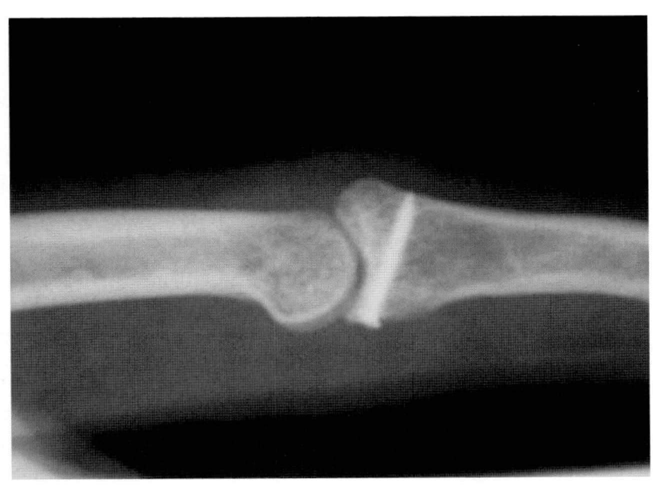

B

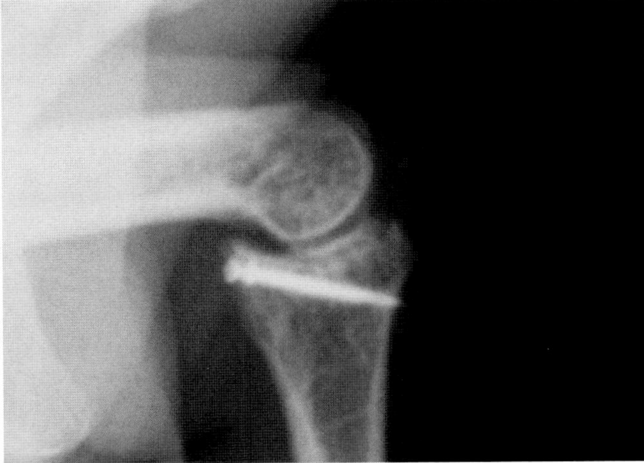

C

Figure 4.36. **A:** Lateral radiograph 5 months and 3 weeks after injury. **B:** Lateral radiograph in extension 8.5 years after hemi hamate resurfacing arthroplasty reconstruction. **C:** Lateral radiograph in flexion 8.5 years after hemi hamate resurfacing arthroplasty reconstruction.

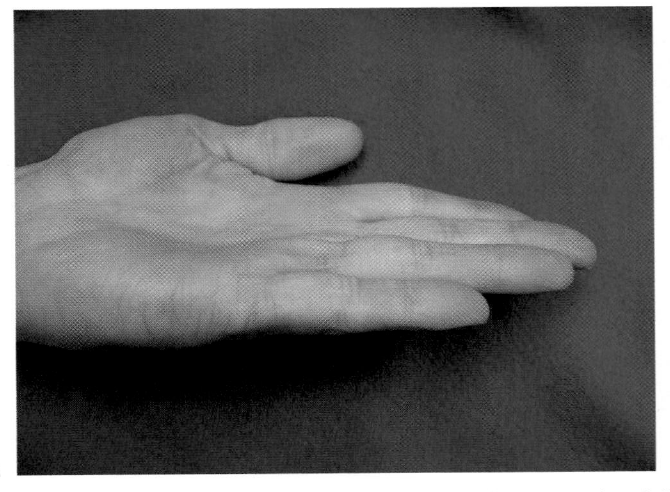

A

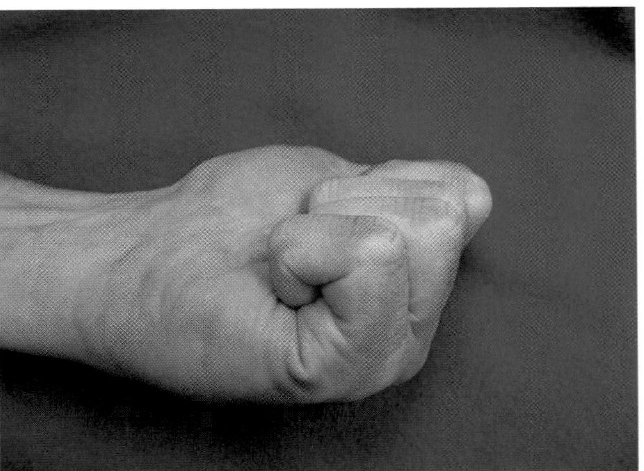

B

Figure 4.37. **A:** Postoperative extension 8.5 years after reconstruction. **B:** Postoperative flexion 8.5 years after reconstruction.

COMPLICATIONS

Complications have resulted from progressive arthrosis secondary either to excessive articular damage to the head of the proximal phalanx or to failure to technically restore an adequate palmar buttress to the middle phalanx. Swan-neck deformity can occur from inadequate repair of the volar plate or failure to protect the volar-plate repair.

RECOMMENDED READING

1. Boulas HJ, Herren A, Buchler U. Osteochondral metatarsophalangeal autografts for traumatic articular metacarpophalangeal defects: a preliminary report. *J Hand Surg* 18A:1086–1092, 1993.
2. Eaton RG, Malerich MM. Volar plate arthroplasty of the proximal interphalangeal joint: a review of ten years' experience. *J Hand Surg* 15A:260–268, 1980.
3. Gross AE, McKee NH, Pritzker KPH, et al. Reconstruction of skeletal defects at the knee: a comprehensive osteochondral transplant program. *Clin Orthop* 174:96–106, 1983.
4. Hamlet WP, Hastings H II. Critical assessment of PIP joint stability after palmar lip fracture dislocations. Paper presented at: 56th Annual Meeting of the American Society for Surgery of the Hand, October 4–6, 2001, Baltimore, MD.
5. Hasegawa T, Yamano Y. Arthroplasty of the proximal interphalangeal joint using costal cartilage grafts. *J Hand Surg* 17B:583–585, 1992.
6. Hastings H II, Carroll C IV. Treatment of closed articular fractures of the metacarpophalangeal and proximal interphalangeal joints. *Hand Clinics* 4(3):503–527, 1988.
7. Hastings H, Stern PJ, Capo JT, et al. Hemicondylar hamate replacement arthroplasty (HHRA) for PIP fracture/dislocations. Paper presented at: 54th Annual Meeting of the American Society for Surgery of the Hand, September 2–4, 1999, Boston, MA.
8. Katsaros J, Milner R, Marshall NJ. Perichondral arthroplasty incorporating costal cartilage. *J Hand Surg* 20B:137–142, 1995.
9. Williams RMM, Hastings H, Kiefhaber TR. Use of the Hemi Hamate Autograft in PIP Fracture/Dislocation. In: Weiland AJ, ed. *Techniques in Hand & Upper Extremity Surgery* 6(4):185–192, 2002.

5

Volar Plate Arthroplasty for Acute and Chronic Proximal Interphalangeal Joint Fracture/Subluxation

Matthew M. Malerich and Richard G. Eaton

INDICATIONS/CONTRAINDICATIONS

Volar plate arthroplasty (VPA) is used to resurface the middle phalangeal articulation of the proximal interphalangeal (PIP) joint in acute, subactute, and salvage situations. Indications include acute fracture-subluxation or fracture-dislocation of the PIP joint with comminution or impaction of 40% to 60% of the middle phalangeal articular base (Figs. 5.1 and 5.2). VPA is perhaps most often elected as a reconstructive procedure in chronic fracture-subluxation with a malunion of the articular surface (Figs. 5.3 and 5.4) and in cases of osteoarthritis resulting from PIP joint injury (Figs. 5.5, 5.6, and 5.7, A and B).

A viable articular surface of the proximal phalanx is a prerequisite for VPA. If there is significant incongruity, advanced arthrosis, angular deformity, telescoping, and/or loss of bone stock that would make open reduction and internal fixation or the VPA unfeasible, one should consider other reconstructive options (fusion, implant arthroplasty, autograft reconstruction).

PREOPERATIVE PLANNING

Examination of the involved finger will reveal translational instability of the PIP joint and crepitus in acute injuries. Most often, an extension contracture and limited arc of mo-

Matthew M. Malerich, M.D.: Department of Orthopaedic Surgery, University of California Irvine, Orange, CA

Richard G. Eaton, M.D.: Department of Surgery, Columbia University, New York, NY, and C.V. Starr Hand Service, St. Luke's–Roosevelt Hospital, New York, NY

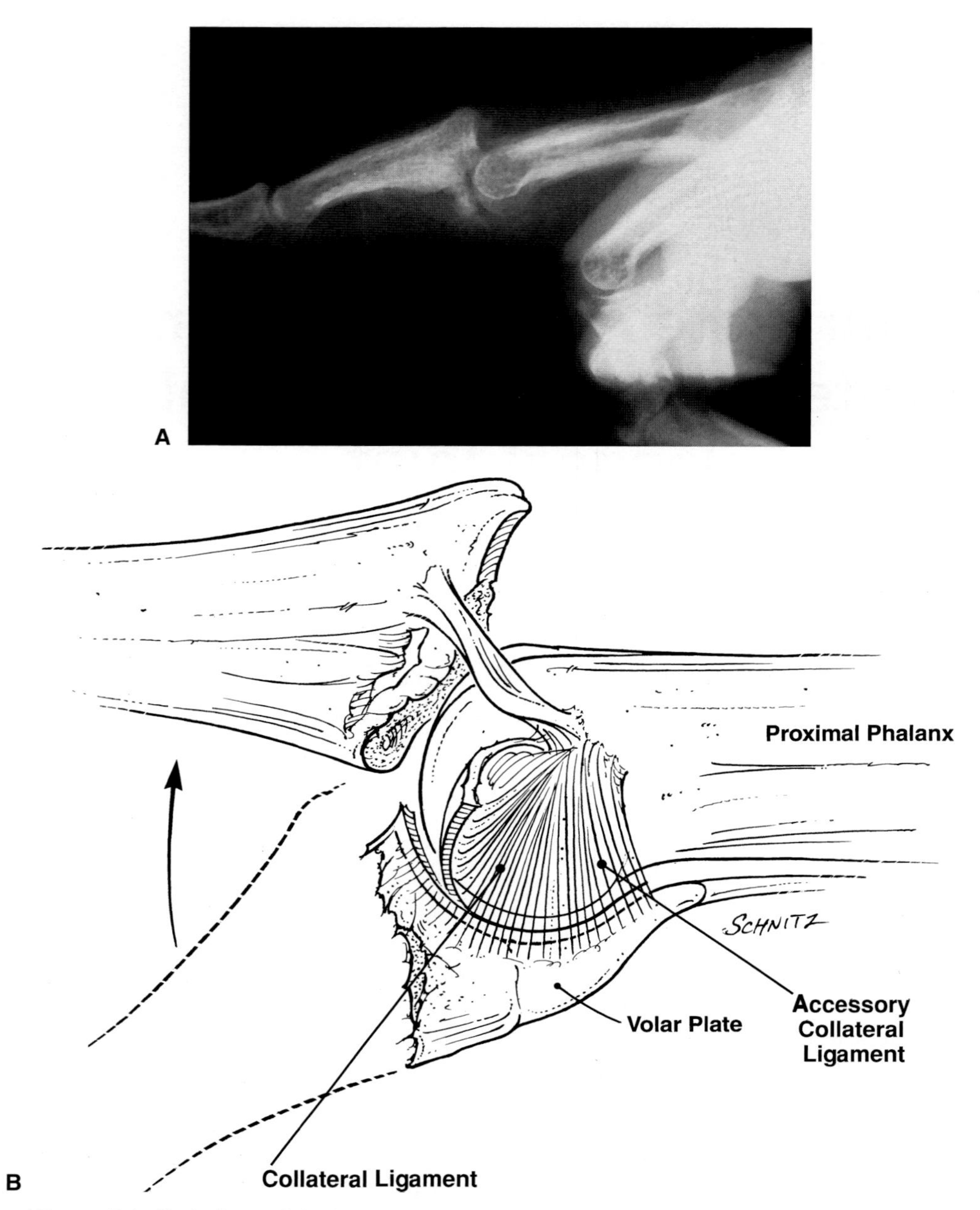

Figure 5.1. Pathology of the injury demonstrating loss of collateral ligament support to the joint, producing the marked instability in this injury.

tion accompany a chronic PIP fracture-dislocation. Loss of distal interphalangeal joint (DIP) flexion is seen in some chronic injuries, but extensor side fibrosis can just as easily lead to mild DIP lag.

Careful palpation will confirm dorsal displacement of the base of the middle phalanx with respect to the articular surface of the middle phalanx. Anteroposterior (AP) and lateral x-rays of the PIP joint are usually sufficient to characterize the injury; oblique films may better characterize some deformities, and live fluoroscopy is very helpful when assessing conguity through the arc of motion. The AP view will help delineate asymmetric impaction. The lateral view reveals the degree of comminution, the amount of joint surface involved, and any "hinging" the leading edge of the middle phalanx base may demonstrate due to the incompetent volar lip.

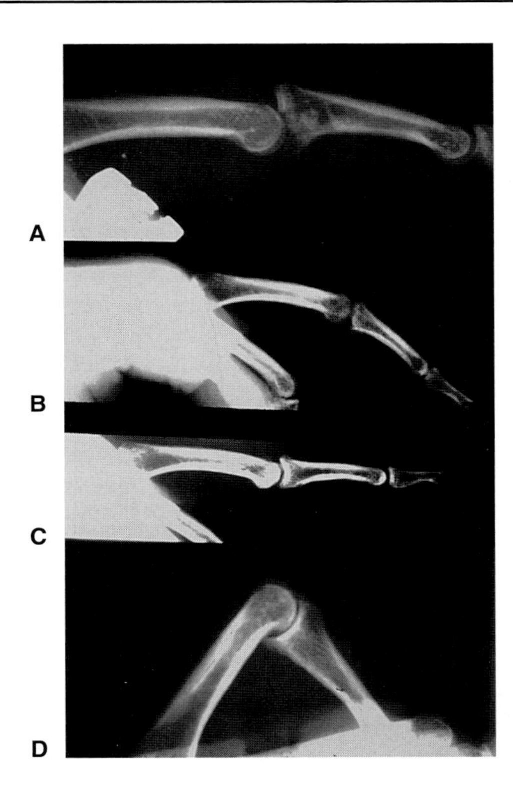

Figure 5.2. Radiographic sequence showing remodeling of the PIP joint over 11 years. **A:** Initial fracture of subluxation. **B:** Six-month postoperative film. **C:** Extension x-ray 11 years postoperatively showing remodeling of the volar lip of the middle phalanx. **D:** Flexion x-ray 11 years postoperatively.

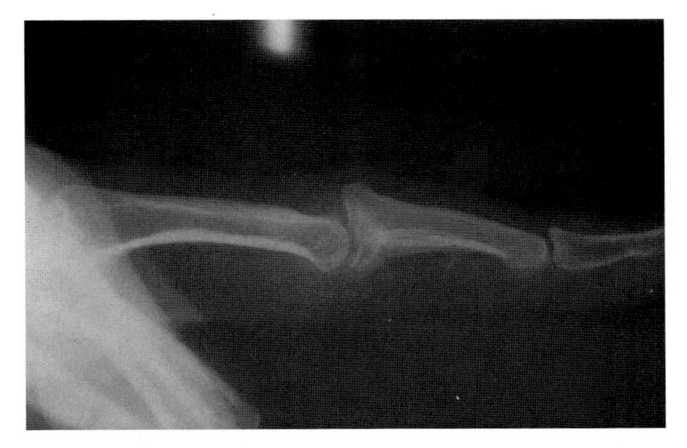

Figure 5.3. Eight-month-old ring finger malunion in a 19-year-old female patient.

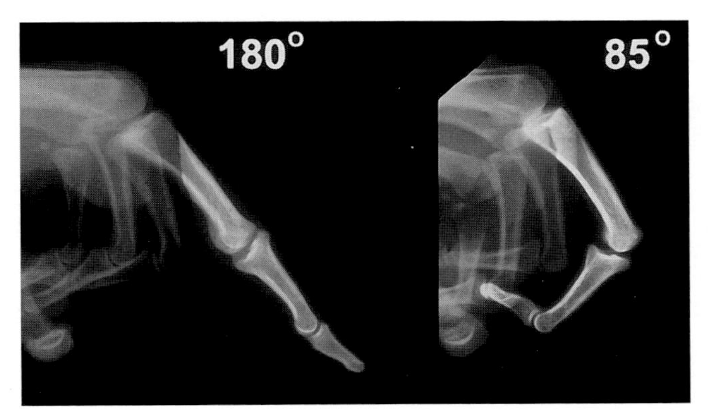

Figure 5.4. Eighteen-month follow-up demonstrating PIP joint motion. Some remodeling is evident.

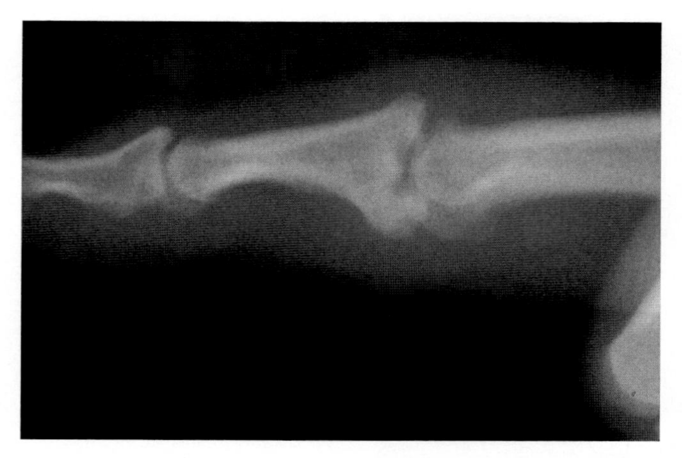

Figure 5.5. One year after injury to the right index finger in a 34-year-old police officer. Preoperatively, the patient has 20 degrees of active motion with pain. Posttraumatic osteoarthritis is present. Proximal phalanx articular contour is intact.

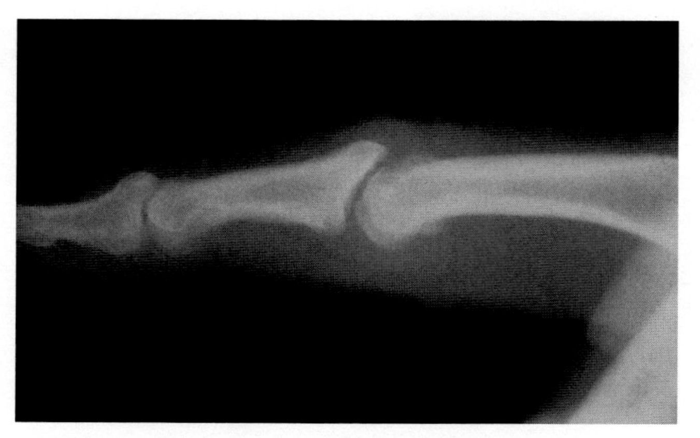

Figure 5.6. Fourteen months after arthroplasty with little remodeling evident.

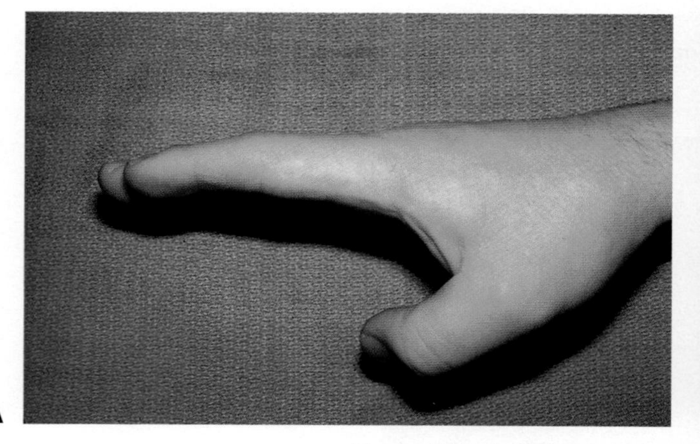

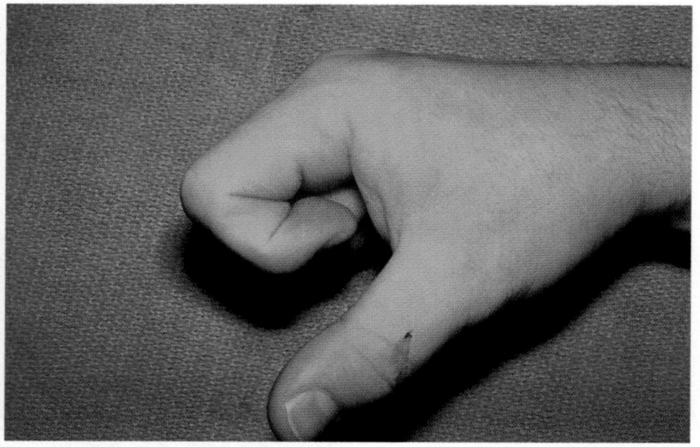

Figure 5.7. A, B: Range of motion 14 months postoperatively.

SURGERY

The procedure can be performed under general or regional anesthesia. If a Bier block is used, a supplemental wrist or intermetacarpal block is suggested. Intraoperative image intensification is useful to assess the joint reduction, along with Kirschner (K) wire placement.

The PIP joint is approached volarly through a radially based flap (Fig. 5.8). The flexor sheath is excised from the A2 to the A4 pulleys. The flexor tendons are retracted and the volar plate is cut along its lateral margins and detached as far distally as possible. Care is taken to respect the volar plate attachment to any fracture fragments, especially those containing any articular surface. Carefully disimpacting of the middle phalangeal fracture fragments and liberating the volar plate are recommended.

The neurovascular bundles are retracted laterally, the collateral ligaments are incised vertically, and the joint is opened like a "shotgun" (Fig. 5.9). All but the distal 20% of the collateral ligaments are now excised (Fig. 5.10). The joint can now be reduced and full passive range of motion should be possible. If full flexion is not present, a dorsal capsular release will be needed. Additionally, limited extensor tenolysis can be performed through the hyperextended joint or by accessing the dorsum of the digit through the original incision. In either case, careful dissection or use of a Freer elevator must accompany exceptional three-dimensional anatomic appreciation so that adjacent structures are not compromised.

With this exposure, open reduction and internal fixation of the fracture should be done, if feasible (Fig. 5.11); this is possible in slightly more than 50% of cases, in my experience, even in chronic injuries. Since the pins will be placed from volar to dorsal in this shotgun position, I avoid tenting the skin and spearing the lateral bands by marking the skin at the extensor tubercle of the proximal phalanx with the joint reduced, and I aim my 0.028 K-wires through these two confluent exit points. The pins are cut and bent dorsally for later removal. The distal lateral volar plate margins are then sutured to the distal collateral ligament stumps.

If open reduction cannot be performed, I now proceed with the VPA.

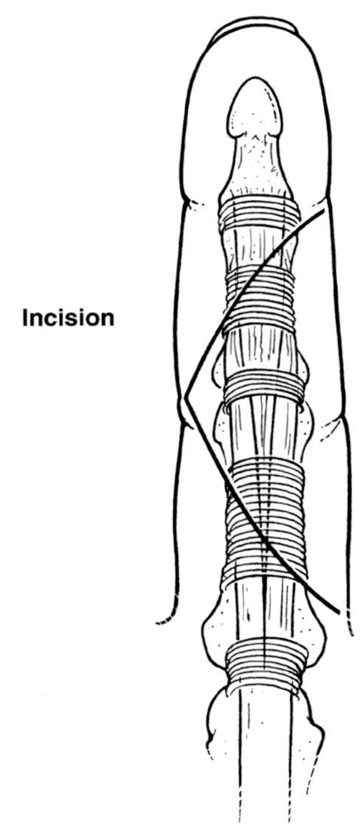

Figure 5.8. Skin incision.

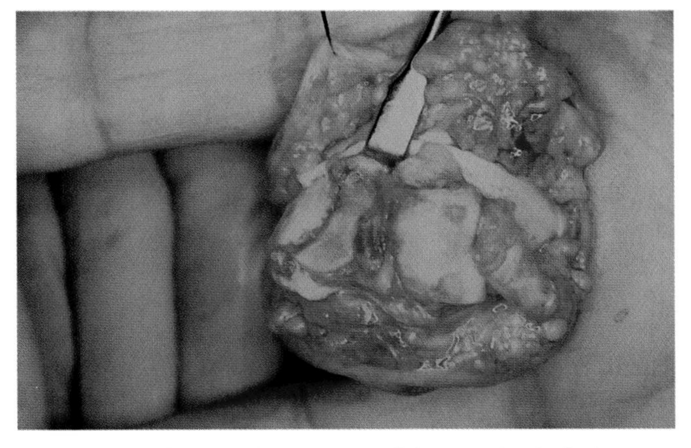

Figure 5.9. "Shotgun" exposure of the proximal phalanx articular surface at right and a large volar depression fracture in the middle phalanx at left.

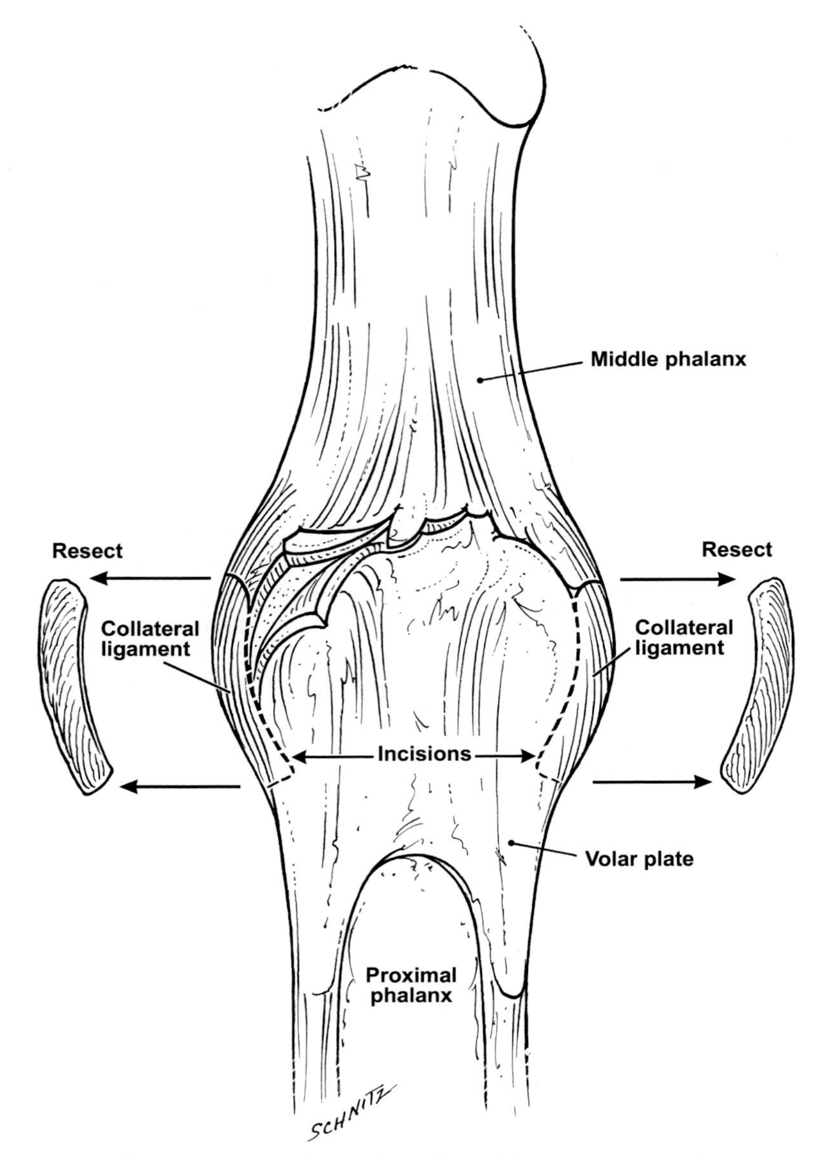

Figure 5.10. Portion of the collateral ligament resected.

There is usually an asymmetric impaction defect in the base of the middle phalanx (Fig. 5.12). It is necessary to create a symmetrical trough of sufficient depth to allow the thickness of the volar plate to fill the defect (Fig. 5.13). A common mistake is to remove too much bone or impacted cartilage.

A 3-0 Prolene "baseball stitch" is placed in the volar plate (Fig. 5.14). I begin this stitch in one distal lateral margin, securing the body of the volar plate, including a transverse pass at its proximal extent, then exit at the opposite distal lateral margin. I then place two 4-0 nylon margin sutures in the volar plate and pass them through the distal collateral ligament stump to be tied later (Fig. 5.14B).

Two Keith needles are loaded into a K-wire driver and drilled through the lateral margins of the symmetrical trough to pass the pull-out stitch dorsally through a padded button (Figs. 5.15 and 5.16). The "checkrein" proximal extensions of the volar plate may occasionally need to be released at this time if the volar plate does not fill the defect or if joint extension is restricted (Fig. 5.14B).

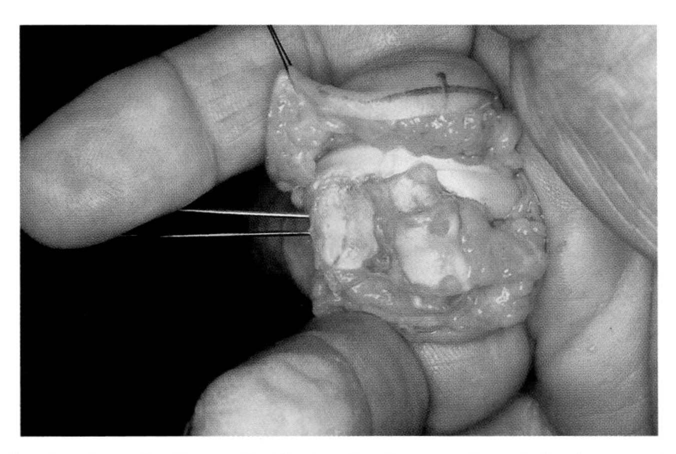

Figure 5.11. Anatomic reduction with K-wire fixation made relatively easy because of exposure.

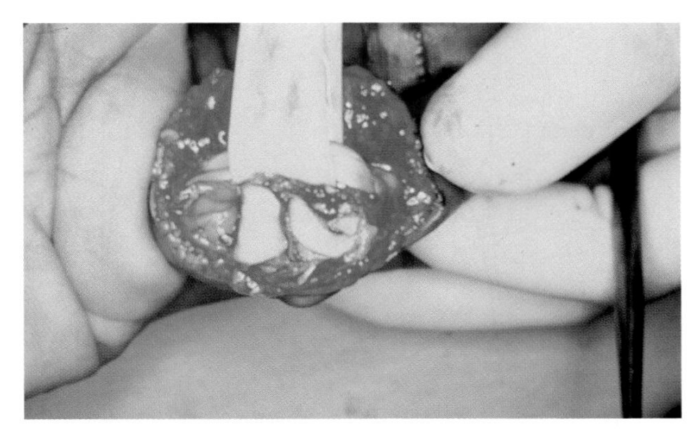

Figure 5.12. Intraoperative photograph of the PIP joint opened in the "shotgun" manner exposing the pathology. Note the asymmetric impaction in the middle phalanx articular surface.

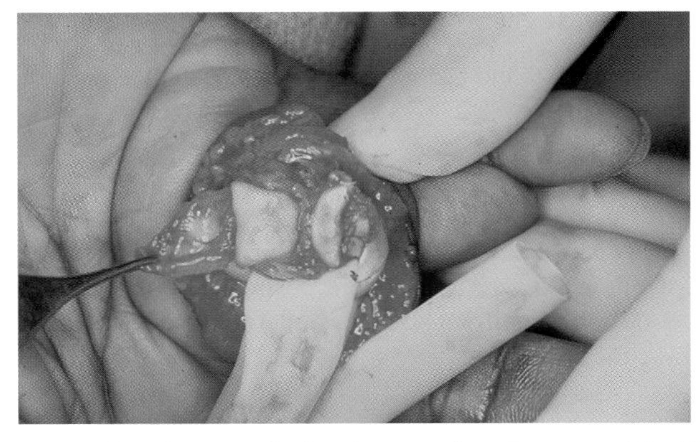

Figure 5.13. Intraoperative photograph showing creation of a symmetrical trough to prevent angular malalignment of the joint.

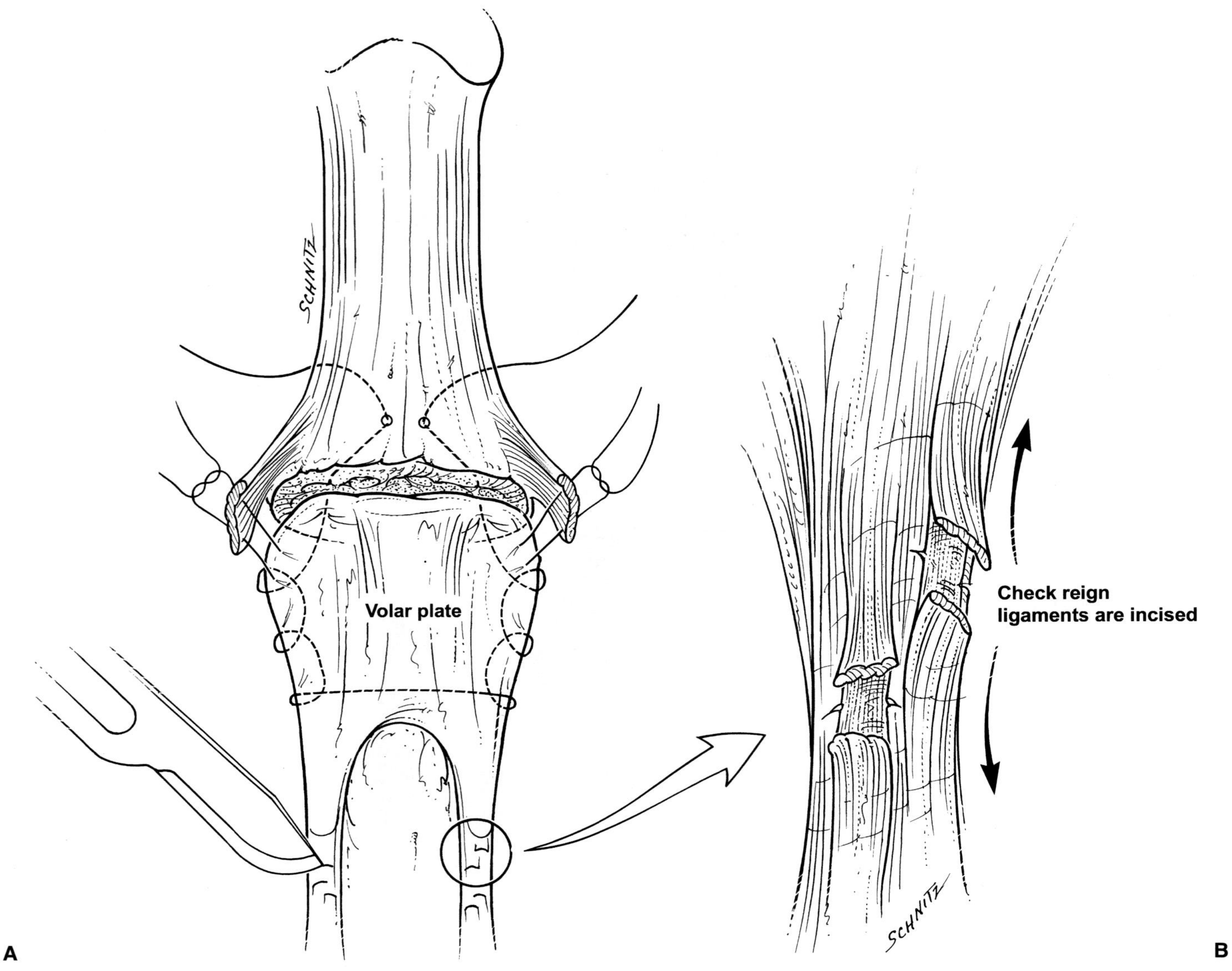

Figure 5.14. A: Pull out suture 2-0 or 3-0 Prolene passed through the volar plate as shown. **B:** Release check-rein ligaments if needed to ensure adequate mobilization of the volar plate and to allow complete passive extension of the PIP joint. Suture the lateral margin of the volar plate to the distal stump of the collateral ligament.

The joint is now pinned in slight flexion (20–30 degrees) as shown (Fig. 5.16) using C-arm control in the AP and lateral planes to confirm a concentric reduction between the remaining joint surfaces and the desired location of the pin. Once reduction is confirmed, the 3-0 Prolene pull-out suture is tied, followed by the two 4-0 nylon margin sutures, completing the arthroplasty.

POSTOPERATIVE MANAGEMENT

The K-wire is removed at 3 weeks, and range of motion with an extension block splint is initiated. The pull-out suture is removed at 4 weeks. Dynamic extension splinting should be used at 6 weeks if complete extension is not possible. Swelling may persist for 6 to 10 months.

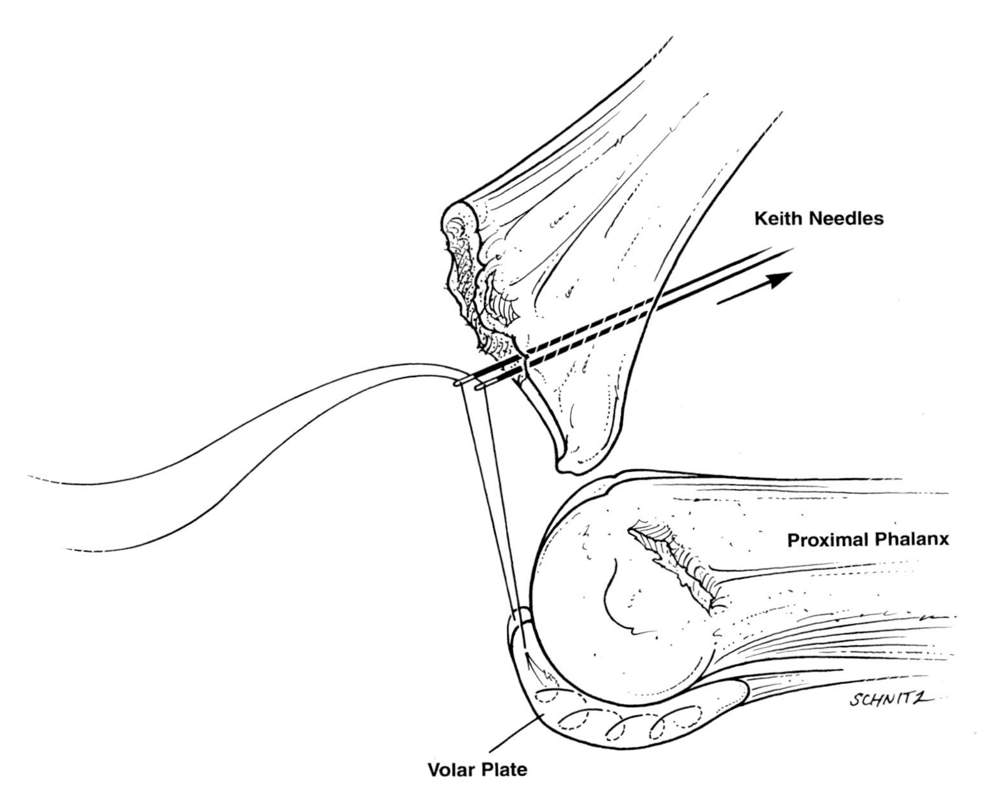

Figure 5.15. Sutures passed as shown through lateral margins of the defect and exiting dorsally.

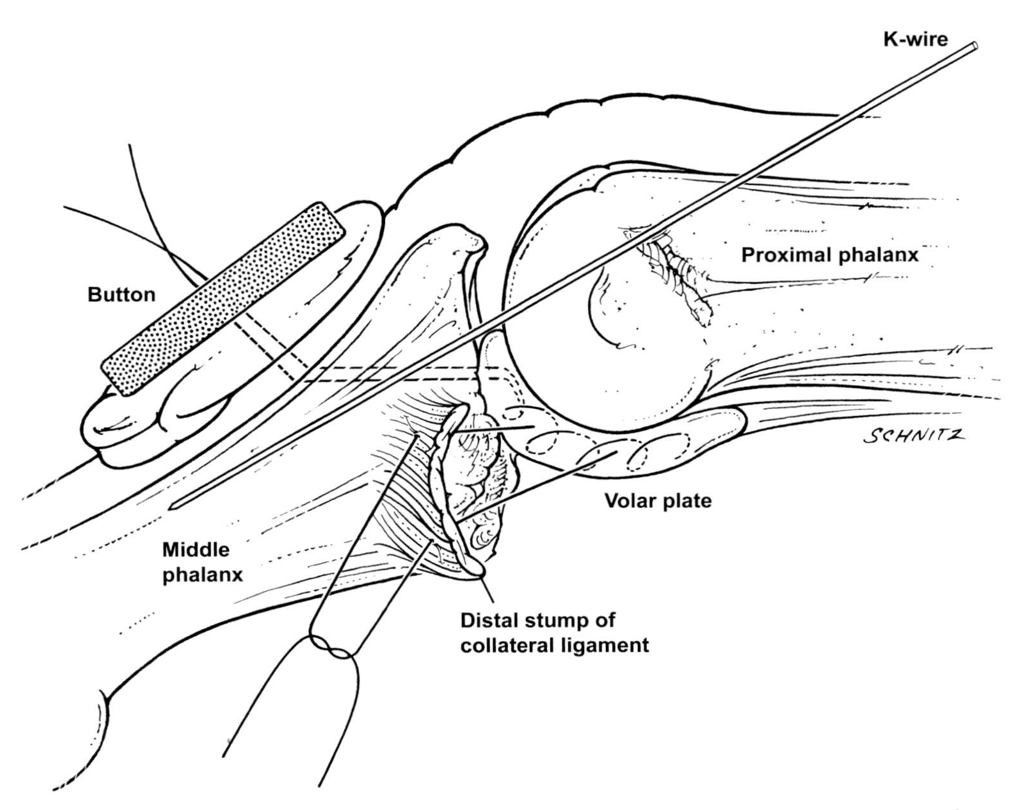

Figure 5.16. Sutures are tied over a padded button, drawing the volar plate into the defect and simultaneously reducing the PIP joint. A 4-0 nylon suture attaches the lateral margin of the volar plate to the distal stump of the collateral ligament.

COMPLICATIONS

Complications include redisplacement, PIP angular deformity, PIP flexion contracture, and DIP joint stiffness. If redisplacement occurs soon after the K-wire or pull-out sutures are removed, a closed reduction and pinning for 4 additional weeks should be performed. If it occurs later during the patient's rehabilitation but the patient is regaining acceptable painless motion, then the situation can be accepted. Angular deformity results if a symmetrical trough is not created. PIP flexion contracture or joint stiffness occurs if the collateral ligaments are not excised and full passive range of motion is achieved at the time of operation. DIP joint stiffness (loss of flexion) occurs in patients operated on late secondary to extensor mechanism (lateral band) contracture or adhesions. If recognized at surgery, I will pin the DIP joint in flexion. If it is a problem postoperatively, a distal Fowler release of the lateral bands can be performed.

Of course, accelerated arthrosis at the PIP joint may accompany any significant trauma. Although VPA provides a serviceable joint and can enhance the function and increase the longevity of the joint, later salvage procedures are sometimes necessary.

RESULTS

Ninety to 95 degrees of PIP joint motion (Fig. 5.2) can be achieved under ideal conditions in acute cases, as we originally reported in 1980. In malunion or reconstructive cases (Figs. 5.3 and 5.4), usually 4 or more months after injury 75 to 80 degrees of PIP joint motion can be expected, because a more extensive joint release is usually necessary.

In cases of osteoarthritis after this injury, gratifying results may be achieved usually after a year or more (Figs. 5.5–5.7). Some of our patients have been followed up for 30 years. One interesting finding is that joints can remodel as bone fills in distal to the volar plate (Fig. 5.2).

RECOMMENDED READING

1. Agee J. Unstable fracture dislocations of the proximal interphalangeal joint of the fingers: a preliminary report of a new technique. *J Hand Surg* 3:386–389, 1978.
2. Eaton RG. *Joint Injuries of the Hand*. Springfield, IL: Charles C. Thomas, 1972:3–34.
3. Eaton RG, Malerich MM. Volar plate arthroplasty for the proximal interphalangeal joint: a ten year review. *J Hand Surg* 5:260–268, 1980.
4. Malerich MM, Eaton RG. The volar plate reconstruction for fracture-dislocation of the proximal interphalangeal joint. *Hand Clinics* 10:251–260, 1994.
5. Schenck RR. Dynamic traction and early passive movement for fractures of the proximal interphalangeal joint. *J Hand Surg* 11A:850–858, 1986.
6. Stark HH. Use of internal fixation for closed fracture of phalanges and metacarpals. *J Bone Joint Surg* 48A:493–502, 1966.
7. Williams RMM, Stern P, Kiefhaber TR, et al. Treatment of unstable PIP fracture-dislocations using a hemi-hamate autograft. Paper presented at: 57th Annual Meeting of the American Society for Surgery of the Hand, Phoenix, Arizona, October 3–5, 2002.
8. Zemel NP, Start HH, Ashworth CR, et al. Chronic fracture dislocation of the proximal interphalangeal joint: treatment by osteotomy and bone graft. *J Hand Surg* 6:477–455, 1981.

6

Malunion and Nonunion of the Phalanges and Metacarpals

Jesse B. Jupiter

MALUNION

Indications/Contraindications

One of the most common complications following metacarpal and phalangeal fractures is angular and/or rotational deformity of the osteoarticular column. For the subset of patients in whom symptomatic malunion results after fracture or its treatment, corrective osteotomy may be necessary. Osteotomies are also indicated for congenital malformations, growth disturbances, fixed flexion contractures, nonunion with deformity, and paralysis.

As a general rule, the indications for operative correction are based upon a number of factors, including the functional deficit, any associated pathology lesions, and the location and affect of the malunion. More often than not, deformity involving the middle or distal phalanges and thumb will offer less functional impairment than more proximal lesions involving the proximal phalanges or metacarpals.

Etiology

The majority of fractures of the phalanges and metacarpals heal without deformity, provided that appropriate indications for treatment are followed, techniques of immobilization are observed, and patient compliance is exercised. Associated soft-tissue injury, open fractures, and inadequate skeletal fixation may result in deformity.

Extra-articular malunion can produce "scissoring" of adjacent digits, disturbance of musculotendinous balance, pain, and reduction of strength (Fig. 6.1). The extra-articular malunion associated with open fractures or after initial operative treatment of the fracture

Jesse B. Jupiter, M.D.: Orthopaedic Surgery, Harvard Medical School, Boston, MA, and Orthopaedic Hand Surgery, Massachusetts General Hospital, Boston, MA

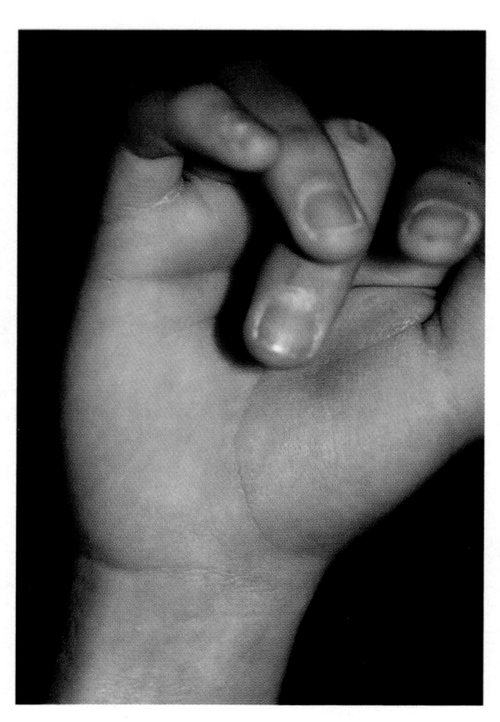

Figure 6.1. Rotational malunion of the ring ray manifests as "scissoring" or overlap when the digit is flexed (From: Buchler U, Gupta A, Ruf S. Corrective osteotomy for post-traumatic malunion of the phalanges in the hand. *J Hand Surg* 21B:33–42, 1996.)

may also be associated with tendon adhesions, trophic changes, or joint stiffness. Intra-articular malunion may cause stiffness, pain, arthritis, or instability.

Evaluation and Classification

It is essential to obtain a thorough history regarding the original injury, treatment, hand dominance, occupation, avocational pursuits, and patient compliance.

Radiographic examination should include anteroposterior (AP), lateral, and oblique projections, with similar films of the contralateral digit for comparison. More complex deformities require a true AP and lateral x-ray proximal and distal to the malunion site to use for preoperative planning and to superimpose on a tracing of the contralateral skeletal unit.

Deformity involving a joint is best evaluated by computed tomography (CT) or three-dimensional reconstructed CT scans (Table 6.1).

Indications and Timing of Corrective Osteotomy

The timing of intervention is intellectually divided into three periods. The first is relatively acute, when manipulative reduction is still possible. This may in reality be considered redisplacement rather than malunion, even when fracture callous is present.

The second is up to about 10 weeks after injury, when the fracture callous is still malleable, articular fragments can be defined, and the original fracture line in the diaphysis is still apparent.

The third stage is associated with trophic conditions or when extreme swelling would preclude operative intervention. When an intra-articular malunion presents beyond 6 months after injury, late osteotomy through the original fracture line is not typically feasible.

Preoperative Planning

In addition to the skeletal elements, careful assessment should include the status of the soft-tissue envelope, gliding capacity of the flexor and extensor tendons, joint mobility, and neurovascular status.

Table 6.1. *Malunions Are Classified as Follows*

1. Location	extra-articular intra-articular combined proximal or distal metaphysis diaphysis
2. Direction	flexion/extension deformity radial/ulnar deviation rotation shortening offset combinations
3. Associated soft-tissue lesions	contracture adhesions deficiency neurovascular deficit
4. Skeletal maturity	growing mature
5. Time frame	developing established
6. Isolated versus combined	only bone involved combined with tendon, joint, or other structures trophic conditions

The outlines of the proximal and distal fragments are traced onto separate sheets of paper. These are lined up onto a tracing of the opposite normal bone, and the type of correction, required bone graft, location, and type of fixation can be determined. This type of preoperative planning will facilitate the intraoperative execution of the osteotomy. Appreciating the three-dimensional characteristics of the rotational deformity, and the influence and geometry of the osteotomy, is critical to successful reconstruction (Fig. 6.2).

Complex malunions involving structures other than just the skeletal deformity may require concomitant capsulotomy, tenolysis, or soft-tissue reconstruction.

Location

For the most part, corrective osteotomy is best performed at or adjacent to the site of the deformity. While it is feasible to correct some modest rotational deformities of the pha-

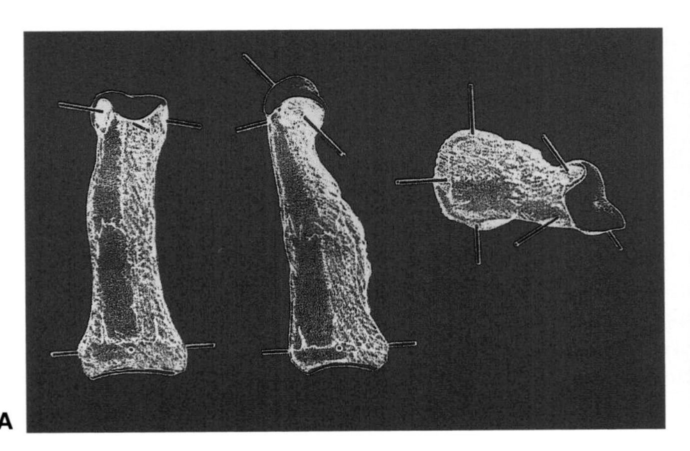

A

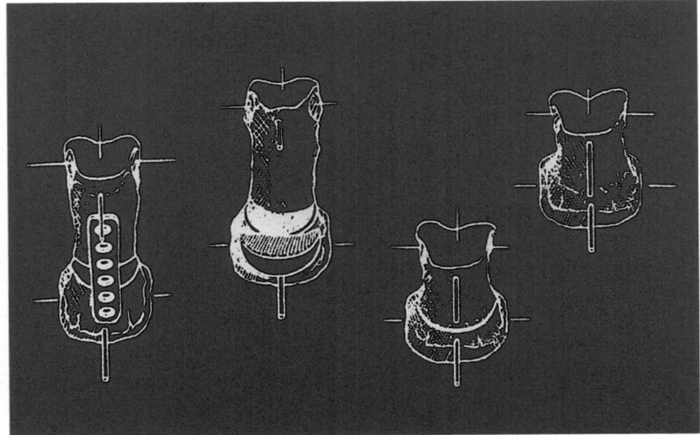

B

Figure 6.2. A: Imaging and preoperative planning are critical tools to assist the surgeon in appreciating the key relationships between the region of maximum deformity, the axis of the osteoarticular column, and the adjacent joint relationships. Orientation pins (later explained in greater detail) are the intraoperative key to alignment and derotation. **B:** Three-dimensional planning leads to successful restoration of the phalangeal (or metacarpal) anatomy.

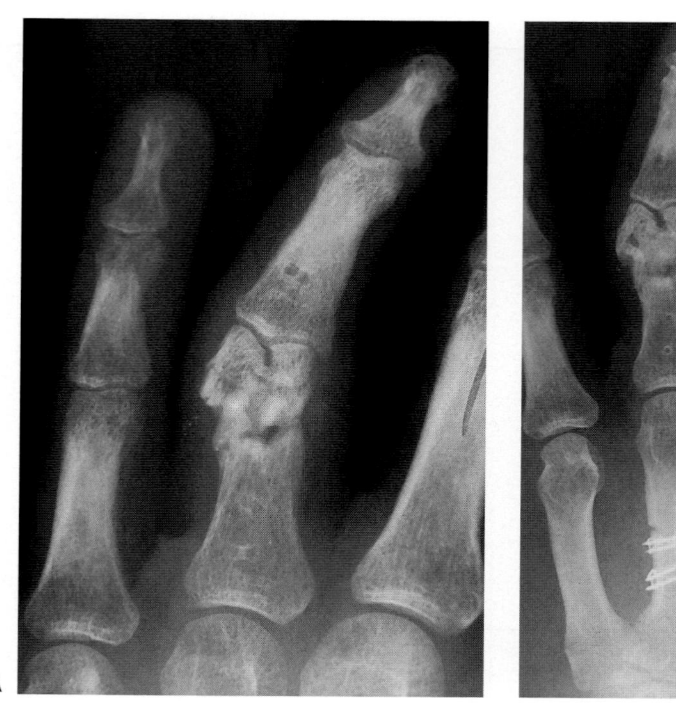

Figure 6.3. A: The location of the fracture and resulting deformity causing the greatest functional limitation involving the PIP joint. In selected cases, it is unrealistic to operate at the site of the original injury. **B:** A basilar osteotomy of the metacarpal affects the rotation needed to avoid overlap with the adjacent digit, while the tenuous PIP joint relationships are left undisturbed. (From: Faierman E, Jupiter JB. Deformity and nonunion following fractures. In: Tubiana R, Gilbert A, eds. *Bone and Skin Disorders*. London: Martin Dunitz, 153–170, 2002.)

langes with a rotational osteotomy at the metacarpal level, this has the potential of creating further deformity and impingement of an adjacent digit. Osteotomy at the metacarpal base level (Weckesser) is logical in some cases when extensive dissection and skeletal work would not be well accommodated at the phalangeal level (Fig. 6.3).

Surgery

Axillary or supraclavicular block anesthesia is preferred. After sterile preparation of the entire extremity, the arm is exsanguinated and a brachial tourniquet inflated to a pressure of 250 mm Hg. The arm is positioned on a hand table with an image intensifier readily available.

The type of osteotomy and the method of internal fixation will depend upon both the direction of the deformity and the need for associated soft-tissue or joint procedures.

The surgical exposure to diaphyseal or metaphyseal malunion is generally through a midaxial skin incision. This will permit excellent exposure of both the skeletal deformity and the flexor and extensor tendons and adjacent articulations.

In contrast, articular deformity correction will require a dorsal approach, permitting capsulotomy and a more proximal extension if needed.

Proximal phalangeal angular deformity may be best suited for an incomplete opening-wedge osteotomy. This type of osteotomy is relatively uncomplicated to perform, restores length, rebalances the extension tendon tension, and is stable due to complete bone contact. As a result, the requirement for internal fixation is diminished, and often a tension wire is sufficient for fixation.

Angular deformity in a volar direction can also be corrected with a transverse opening-wedge osteotomy. Because of the deforming forces that tend to recreate the deformity, a stronger plate and screw implant will be required.

An isolated rotational malunion of the proximal phalanx is corrected with a complete transverse osteotomy with low-profile plate fixation. Metacarpal rotational osteotomies can be performed in a similar manner or alternatively with a step-cut osteotomy.

Intraoperative evaluation of the planned correction can be accomplished by placing two small Kirschner wires perpendicular to the diaphysis in two places, one proximal and one distal to the site of deformity. Correction can be judged when both sets of Kirschner wires become parallel.

Complex deformity, which is a combination of vectors, is treated best by a single oblique cut combined with an interpositional bone graft and stable plate fixation. This stable fixation is particularly important when associated tenolysis and/or capsulectomies, requiring early mobilization, are performed.

The implant selected will depend upon the size of the bone to be corrected, the need for an interpositional bone graft, and the associated soft-tissue procedure required. Osteotomies in the metaphyseal regions are preferentially stabilized with condylar plates. It is my preference to use a slightly larger size implant for osteotomy correction than for acute fracture fixation; thus, a 2.0-mm condylar plate is used for proximal phalangeal correction and a 2.4-mm plate is used for metacarpal osteotomy fixation in most average-sized patients (Fig. 6.4).

Postoperative Management

Kirschner Wire or Tension Wire Fixation. The initial operative dressing is removed at 10 days, at which time sutures are removed. A low-profile removable Orthoplast splint can be used and gentle motion initiated. Upon removal of the wire, usually at 3 weeks postoperatively, active range-of-motion exercises are accelerated and the splint is discontinued. Buddy straps to adjacent digits may be useful to promote comfortable motion.

Plate Fixation. The postoperative dressing is removed at 48 hours, and active range-of-motion exercises under the supervision of a hand therapist are begun. Coban wraps and

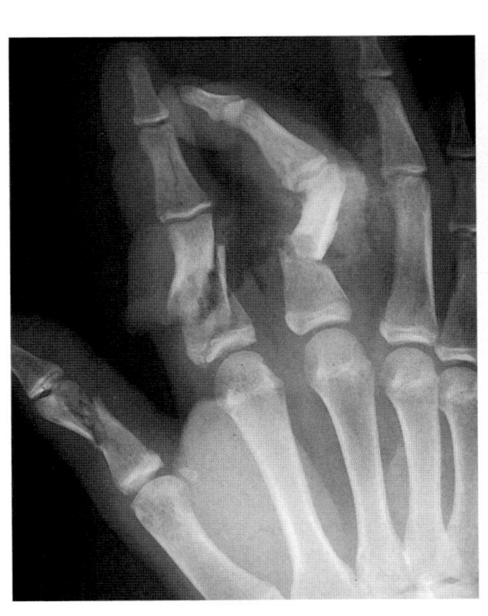

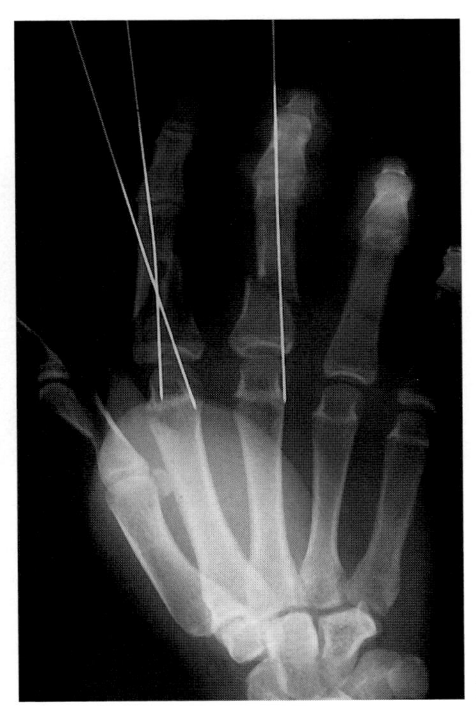

Figure 6.4. A: A young male sustained a crush injury involving the index, long, and thumb rays with associated soft-tissue injuries. **B:** Initial fixation was inadequate to maintain stability.

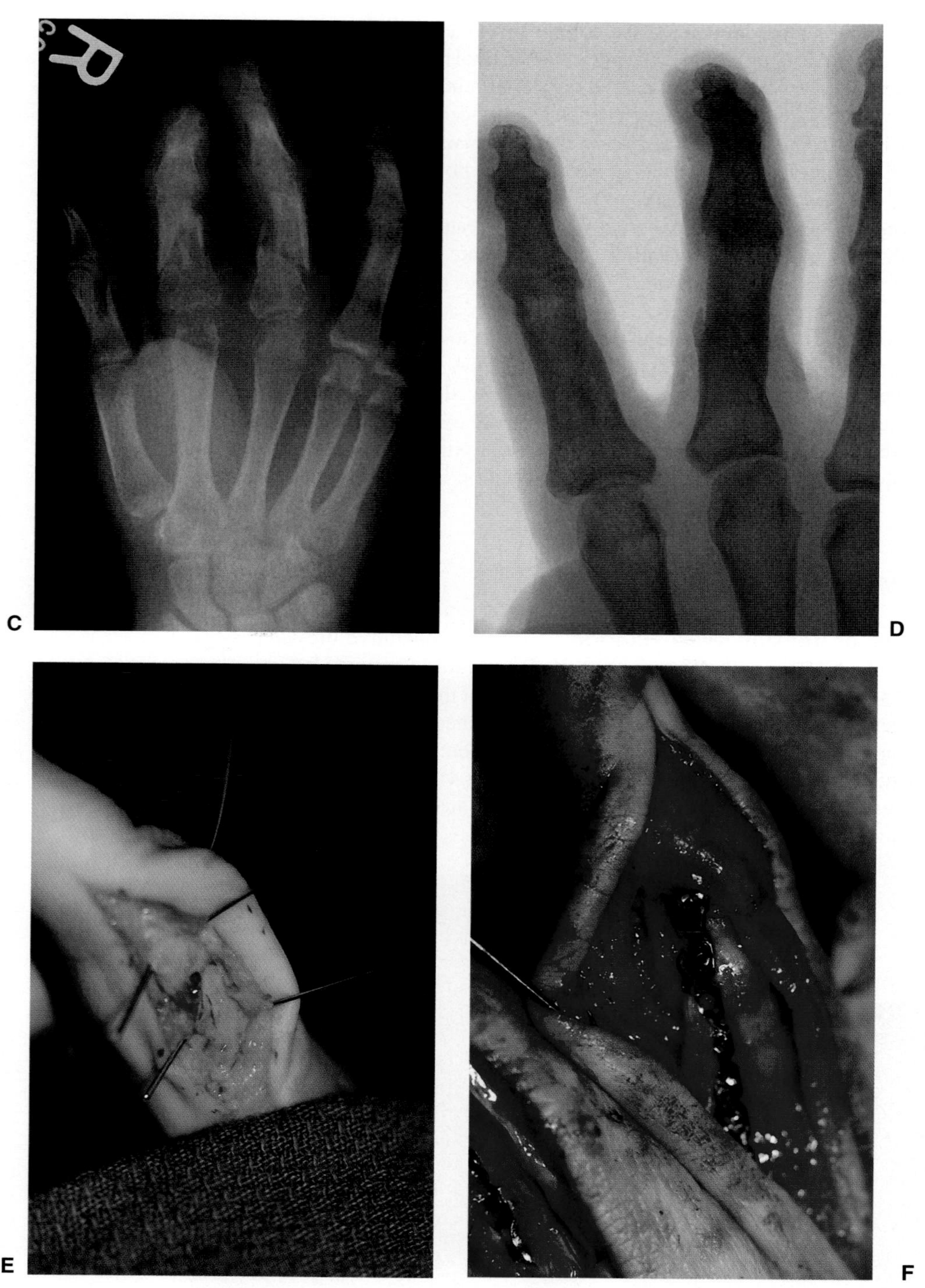

Figure 6.4. *Continued.* **C:** Early in the postinjury course, the pins were removed and the adjacent rays rotated in a way that resulted in dysfunctional positioning. **D:** The phalangeal fractures healed, but the malangulation and malrotation persisted. **E:** After extensive preoperative planning, the osteotomies were conducted through midaxial incisions. Orientation pins were placed prior to bone cuts and eventually aligned according to plan. **F:** In both the long ray and the index ray (foreground), condylar blade plates were chosen for their stability and fragment-control capability.

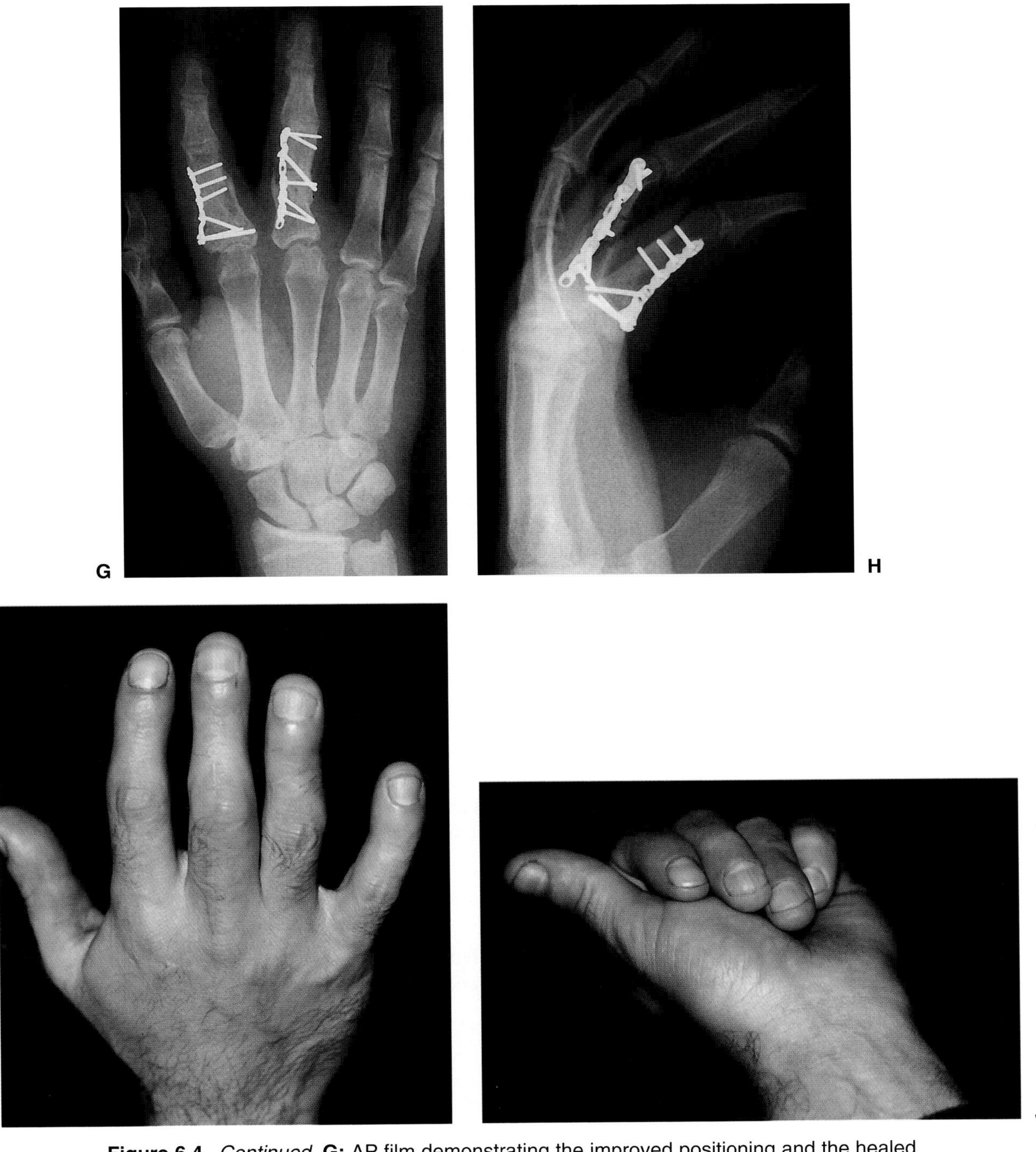

Figure 6.4. *Continued.* **G:** AP film demonstrating the improved positioning and the healed osteotomies. **H:** The lateral projection demonstrates excellent PIP joint alignment. Meticulous scrutiny of that relationship is necessary to verify that diaphyseal or metaphyseal osteotomy has the desired result at the joint level. **I, J:** Clinical alignment in extension and elimination of scissoring or overlap were accomplished. (From: Faierman E, Jupiter JB. Deformity and nonunion following fractures. In: Tubiana R, Gilbert A, eds. *Bone and Skin Disorders*. London: Martin Dunitz, 153–170, 2002.)

buddy straps should be the only support. In those instances in which tenolyses or capsulotomies were performed, dynamic splinting may be required within 10 to 14 days.

It will not be uncommon, especially with the phalangeal osteotomy, to have some deficit of full proximal interphalangeal joint extension. Plate removal and extensor tenolysis may be considered, but not before 4 to 6 months after osteotomy.

Complications

Stiffness. As with any operative intervention of the digits, residual tendon adhesions or articular stiffness can result. When a plate is used for stability, the osteotomy implant itself may interfere with tendon gliding and will require removal when associated tenolysis is performed.

Loss of Reduction. Inadequate internal fixation can result in loss of fixation and subsequent loss of correction. As a general rule, one should consider using implants one size larger than would be required for an acute fracture at the same level. Thus, in the proximal phalanx, where a 1.5-mm plate would be sufficient for fracture fixation, a 2.0-mm implant might be best for corrective osteotomy fixation, especially when soft-tissue releases are needed.

Inadequate Correction. Poor preoperative evaluation of the deformity or inadequate preoperative planning can result in insufficient correction of the deformity. Integrated assessment both clinically and radiologically is mandatory to judge the accuracy of the realignment.

NONUNION

Indications/Contraindications

Failure of a phalangeal or metacarpal fracture to heal will result in a functional deficit. If recognized early, operative intervention will minimize late functional impairment. Asymptomatic nonunions such as might be seen with comminuted tuft fractures of the distal phalanx should not require intervention.

Etiologies

Nonunion of fractures of tubular bones result from loss of bone substance, inadequate immobilization, fracture distraction due to inadequate Kirschner wires, or infection.

Classifications

A nonunion can be classified as either atrophic (lacking intrinsic biological capacity to heal) or hypertrophic (biologically active but lacking stability). The former are the sequelae of open fractures, infections, or bone loss, whereas the latter can be found after unstable fixation with longitudinal or crossed Kirschner wires or unstable plate fixation. When an atrophic nonunion exists, nonunion debridement, autogenous bone graft, skeletal realignment, and stable internal fixation will be required. In contrast, our experience has shown that well-aligned hypertrophic nonunions require only stable internal fixation to achieve union.

Preoperative Planning

A thorough history of the original injury is important to rule out the potential of infection if an open injury or prior surgery has occurred. The clinical alignment, mobility of adjacent joints, neurovascular status, and quality of soft-tissue coverage must all be evaluated, and deficiency of any one of these components will influence operative decision-making.

Adequate radiographic evaluation will include AP, lateral, and oblique radiographs of the involved bone and intact opposite digit.

On the basis of clinical and radiologic evaluation, one can generally determine the type and alignment of the nonunion and plan surgical exposure, internal fixation, and the potential need for autogenous bone graft.

Surgery

Anesthesia. Brachial plexus block is preferred, as an adequate amount of autogenous bone graft, if required, can be obtained from the distal radius. A pneumatic tourniquet is used and, after exsanguination of the limb, applied to 250 mm Hg. A C-arm should be available.

Hypertrophic Nonunions. Diaphyseal hypertrophic nonunions of either phalanges or metacarpals will respond to stable internal fixation, preferably with plate and screws. When associated with an angular deformity, the implant, if surgically possible, is applied on the tension side and functions as a tension-bond plate.

Reduction and compression can be achieved using the implant on the tension side. The implant must be strong enough to withstand this load; therefore, a 2.4-mm dynamic compression plate in the proximal phalanx is preferred.

Atrophic Nonunion. In the absence of active infection, the management of an atrophic nonunion consists of debridement of the fibrous interposition material to create vascular bone ends, interposition bone graft, skeletal realignment, and stable plate fixation.

Unless a major skeletal deficit is present, we prefer to use cancellous autograft compacted in a small syringe whose diameter is equal to that of the involved skeletal structure. The plunger is removed and the cancellous graft is placed into the barrel of the syringe. The plunger is reinserted and the graft is compacted and pushed out the top of the syringe with the blunt end of a Kirschner wire. The graft can be shaped at the ends to precisely fit into the two bony ends and rapidly incorporates in the presence of stable plate fixation.

Infected atrophic nonunions are treated with debridement, realignment, external fixation, and secondary bone grafting with or without internal fixation. Prolonged courses of antibiotics are not as necessary as with long bone infections. We give a 2-week course of culture-specific antibiotics after debridement and wound closure.

Postoperative Management

The postoperative management is similar to that described for corrective osteotomy for malunion.

RECOMMENDED READINGS

1. Buchler U, Gupta A, Ruf S. Corrective osteotomy for post-traumatic malunion of the phalanges in the hand. *J Hand Surg* 21B:33–42, 1996.
2. Duncan KLT, Jupiter JB. Intraarticular osteotomy for malunion of metacarpal head fractures. *J Hand Surg* 14A:888–893, 1989.
3. Faierman E, Jupiter JB. Deformity and nonunion following fractures. In: Tubiana R, Gilbert A, eds. *Bone and Skin Disorders*. London: Martin Dunitz, 2002:153–170.
4. Froimson A. Osteotomy for digital deformity. *J Hand Surg* 6A:585–589, 1981.
5. Jupiter JB, Koniuch M, Smith RJ. The management of delayed union, and nonunion of the metacarpals and phalanges. *J Hand Surg* 10A:357–366, 1985.
6. Manktelow RT, Mahoney JL. Step osteotomy: a precise rotation osteotomy to correct scissoring deformities of the fingers. *Plast Reconstr Surg* 68:571–576, 1981.

usually with some element of a rotational displacement. The spectrum of injuries that may result ranges from a mild sprain of the collateral ligaments to significantly comminuted intra-articlar fracture-dislocations.

In the most common fracture-dislocation pattern, the volar margin of the base of the middle phalanx, is fractured by a sheer-impaction mechanism or avulsion (Fig. 7.2A). If the volar articular involvement is more than 40% of the cartilage surface, dorsal subluxation or frank dislocation usually occurs. Injuries of greater magnitude, and slightly different force application, can lead to central impaction of the base of the middle phalanx. These are also known as pilon fractures (Fig. 7.2B).

Preoperative Planning

Clinical Evaluation. The examination of the PIP joint begins with inspection of the soft-tissue envelope. The surgeon must note whether the injury is open or closed, the extent of joint swelling, and the location of any abrasions. A detailed neurovascular examination is also performed. The axial and rotational alignment of the digit should be assessed. Both the active and passive range of motion is documented. Tendon and neurovascular function are assessed before and after preliminary reduction.

Radiographic Evaluation. Patients with injuries to the PIP joint require radiographs in the anteroposterior (AP) and lateral planes (Figs. 7.3A, B). Lateral views in varying degrees of flexion may be helpful to determine the reducibility of volar fragments of the P2 phalanx. The ability to assess the behavior of the fracture-dislocation under image intensification (biplanar fluoroscopy) is advantageous. Oblique radiographs are sometimes beneficial as they allow the surgeon to accurately assess the fracture and degree of comminution. Radiographs of the metacarpophalangeal joint and distal interphalangeal joint should be performed to rule out associated injuries. Traction radiographs can aid in determining reducibility of the joint

The advent of the small fluoroscopy unit aids significantly in the assessment of the PIP-level injury. In addition to static assessment of the joint, stability and fragment behavior through the arc of motion can be assessed in "real time."

A

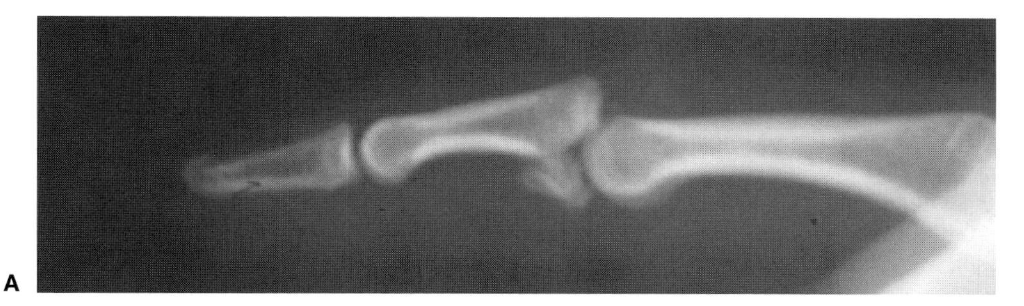

B

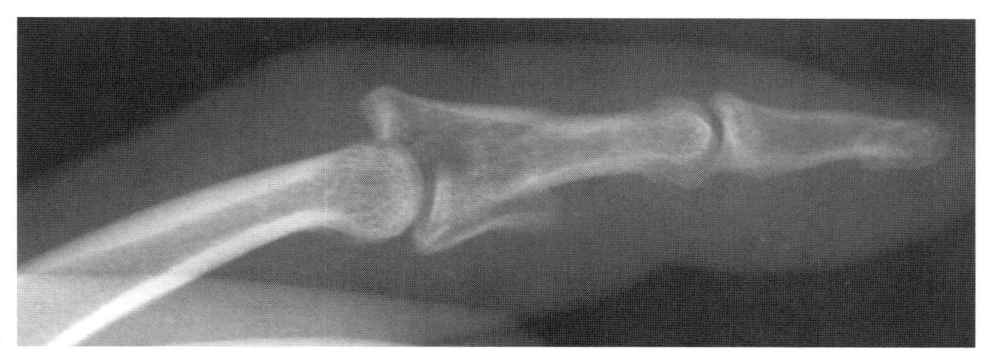

Figure 7.2. A: Lateral radiograph demonstrating volar injury to base of P2. **B:** Lateral radiograph demonstrating pilon injury to base of P2.

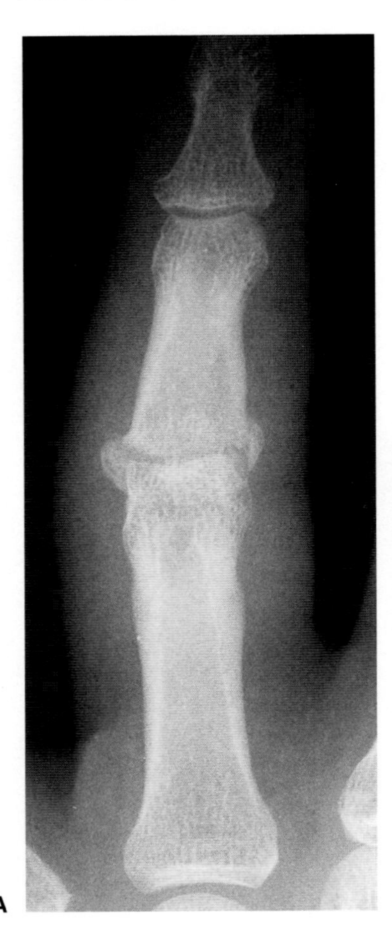

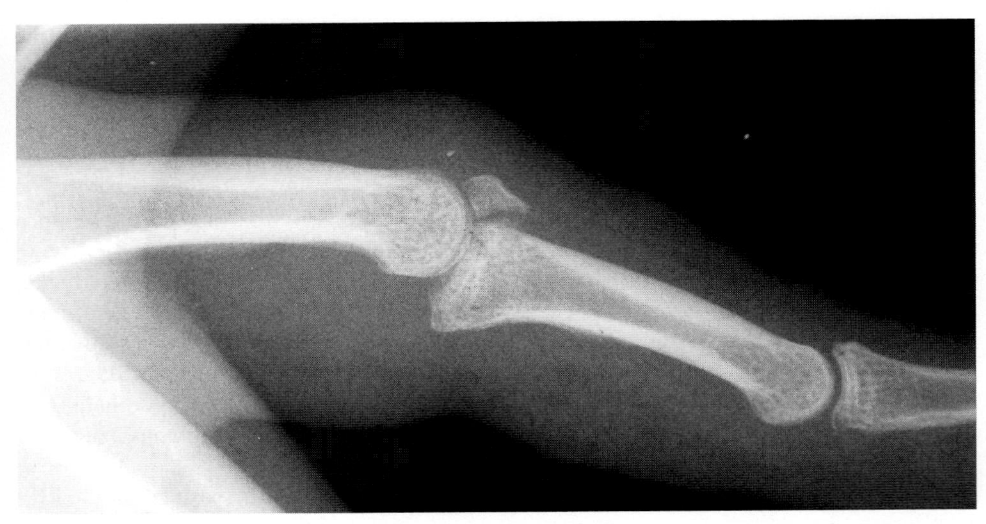

Figure 7.3. **A:** AP radiograph of injury to PIP joint. **B:** Lateral radiograph of injury to PIP joint.

Decision to Apply a Dynamic External Fixator. It cannot be emphasized enough that the dynamic external fixator is a neutralization device. Its application is reserved for fractures and fracture-dislocations that are challenging, not straightforward PIP dislocations without bony injury that are easily reduced and maintain an anatomic reduction through the majority of the motion arc.

The decision to apply the fixator is an important one because it introduces potential morbidity, increases surgical time and complication rates, and can make the postoperative course more difficult for some patients. However, when tenuous fixation needs to be protected while a motion program initiates, or minimal dissection and ligamentotaxis is preferable to extensive exposure of comminuted fracture, then the dynamic fixator is invaluable. Regardless, the external fixator does not replace sound fracture principles; it is almost always an adjunctive procedure, not a primary one.

Surgery

The patient is placed supine on the operating room table and positioned such that the arm can be placed in the center of the hand table. The surgery may be performed under any type of regional anesthesia, including local or axillary blocks. In the more cooperative patient, a wrist block may be utilized. After the administration of anesthesia, a well-padded tourniquet is placed around the brachium. The arm is subsequently prepared and draped, and exsanguinated before tourniquet inflation.

Choice of Fixator

There are multiple factors that must be considered when deciding upon an external fixator for the PIP joint. Some of the variables include: surgeon experience, availability, performance, and cost. In general, unilateral fixators do not provide adequate stability or control to handle the types of complex fracture-dislocations for which the surgeon would need to apply a frame. Asymmetric impaction and extensive soft-tissue disruption typically require the "control" afforded by bilateral frames.

Despite this, we believe that it is important to develop familiarity with several frame designs and their application. Intra-operative flexibility may need to be maintained, as placement of fixation or technical challenges may require the surgeon to revert to an alternative choice of "homemade" or commercially available frame.

We have extensive experience with all frames, and prefer the Biosymmetric Fixator™ (Biomet, Warsaw, IN, U.S.A.) because it is easy to apply, it permits ultimate control of the most unstable PIP or DIP joint problems, it can be used as a static or dynamic frame, it allows for variable distraction, and the box configuration is biomechanically strong.

This device has a radiolucent frame that does not obscure the PIP joint (Fig. 7.4). This allows for easy visualization of the joint reduction at the time of surgery and during follow-up. It can be placed in a static fashion or a dynamic mode and easily converted, so it can even be used as a mini-external fixator for complex fracture, but then be converted to a dynamic distraction frame to allow early motion.

The other commercially available frame, the Compass Hinge™ (Smith-Nephew Richards, Memphis, TN, U.S.A.) allows for very facile conversion from static to dynamic modes. However, elements of the frame and the worm gear are not radiolucent, and often obscure visualization of the joint. We have used this device successfully, but its ability to control the extremely complex fracture-dislocations is limited because it is unilateral and anchored to the phalanges only with smooth wires, which tend to deform or loosen. The passive motion advancement feature is unique and clever, but can be duplicated by cooperative patients who pursue a supervised rehabilitation regimen.

Bent wire fixators are of lower cost and are made from readily available materials. These are a good option if cost is a factor or a commercial fixator is not available. Having some facility with the application of one or more of these frames is essential for any surgeon treating complex hand trauma.

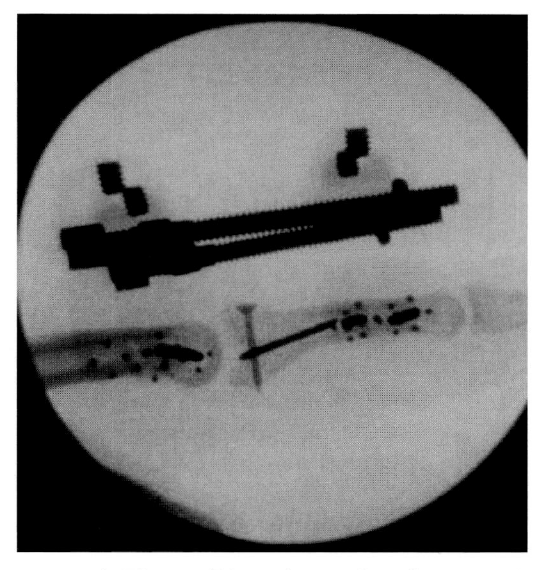

Figure 7.4. The Biosymmetric Fixator (Biomet) seen in a flouroscopic lateral image. The device has a radiolucent frame that does not obscure the PIP joint.

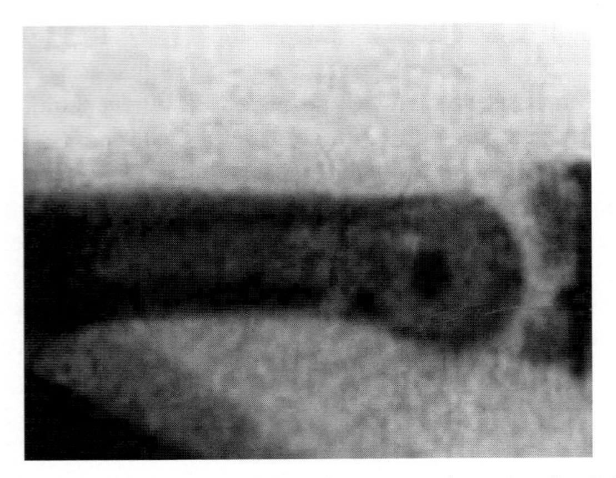

Figure 7.5. Placement of the pin across the axis of rotation.

Application of the BioSymMetRic™ PIP External Fixator

Step 1: Placement of the Axis of Rotation Pin. Regardless of fixator-model choice, the most integral step in the application is the identification and instrumentation of the PIP axis of rotation. The axis of rotation for the PIP joint is a single point that is equidistant from the distal, palmar, and dorsal surfaces of the head of the proximal phalanx.

Under fluoroscopic guidance, obtain a lateral of the proximal phalanx. In this view, the head of the proximal phalanx appears as a single circle. Care must be exercised to obtain a lateral view where the P1 condyles completely overlap; it is easy to accept slight rotation, which may result in suboptimal performance of the frame. Place the tip of one of the external fixator pins in the center of this circle. Bring your hand into the plane of the fluoroscopy beam and drive the pin across the axis. If the pin is placed correctly, it appears as a single dot on a perfect lateral of the proximal phalanx (Fig. 7.5).

We have developed a trick that allows accurate localization of the axis of rotation using basic dermoglyphics. By flexing the PIP joint maximally the flexion crease points to the axis. Despite swelling, which may be excessive in some cases, the axis can then be determined by inferring the midaxis of the bone and locating the point of intersection between the flexion crease line carried dorsally and the midaxial line. This technique is surprisingly accurate and saves time and potential morbidity of multiple pinning attempts (Fig. 7.6).

Step 2: Placement of the Distal Pins in the Middle Phalanx. The frame of the external fixator has radiographic markers that can be used as a guide to pin placement. Prior

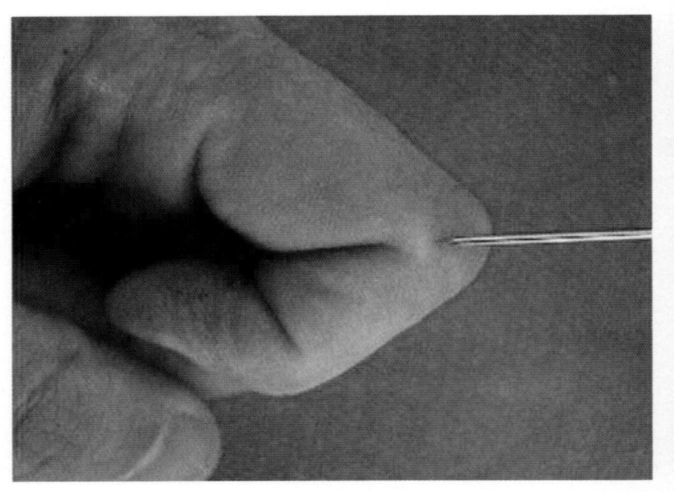

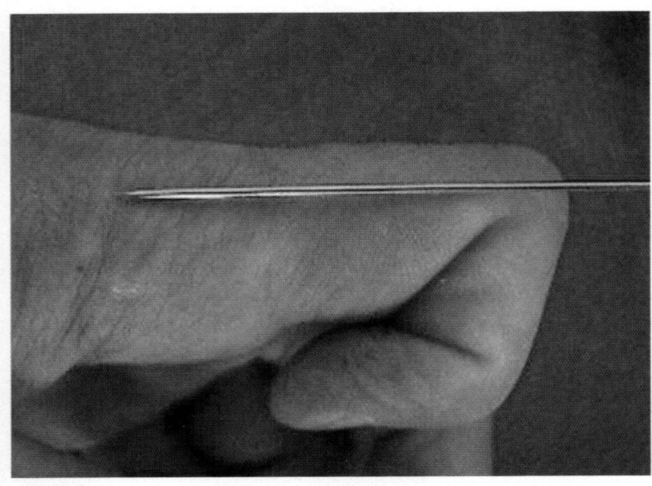

Figure 7.6. A, B: The pin is localizing the P1 axis of rotation base on the topographic anatomy. The axis located at the midway point between the dorsal limit of the PIP flexion crease and the dorsum of the PIP joint.

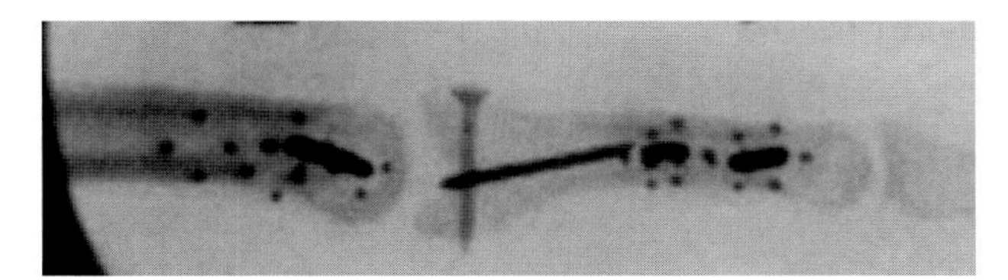

Figure 7.7. Placement of the distal pins in P2.

to pin insertion through the frame, ensure that room has been left for eventual distraction, if that feature is to be employed. The two pins in the middle phalanx should pass transversely through the axis in a parallel orientation to each other. By doing so, the proximal and middle phalanges will be held in a linear relationship when the frame is applied. Place the two pins in the middle phalanx in the aforementioned position under fluoroscopic guidance.

First, place the distal pin. Although both the P1 and P2 phalanges are instrumented, the unstable joint can still be positioned with flexibility. One of the greatest advantages of the bilateral frame designs is that the ultimate position of the fixator is not determined until the second P2 pin is placed, thus establishing the axial alignment of the P1 and P2 phalanges, and therefore the joint reduction (Fig.7.7).

It can be difficult to visualize this important concept, but consider the flexibility in positioning that still exists when the P1 axis pin and the distal-most P2 transverse pin are inserted. The PIP joint can still be positioned in space to align or be distracted. When the alignment is verified, the second, or more proximal, of the P2 pins then establishes the linear or coaxial alignment of the joint in an anatomic position.

Step 3: Application of the Frame. The frame is quadrangular in shape, controlling the PIP joint from both sides, and actually affording the potential to differentially distract the joint on the side of asymmetrical depression (Figs.7.8A, B). The protruding radial and ulnar pins are slid into the appropriate holes of the frame's body, if they were not already directed to those positions by using the frame as the pinning guide.

The radial and ulnar sides of the fixator are connected and stabilized dorsally by two transverse rails. Use an Allen wrench to loose the rails. Adjust the width of the frame. Leave room between the skin and the frame to allow for swelling and prevent irritation. Tighten the dorsal screws with the Allen wrench. Cut the pins flush against the frame. Place the pin caps in the inserter and slide the cap over the cut end of the pin. The caps have a machined break-off point. Stabilize the frame in one hand and twist the inserter with the other hand. The cap will break off and sit flush over the pins within the frame.

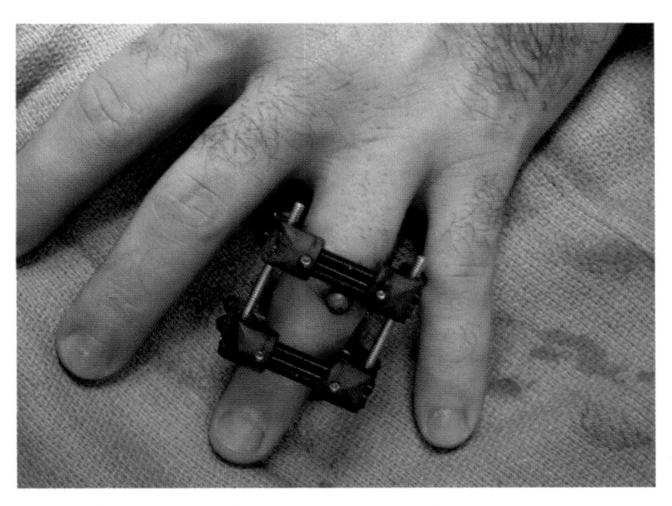

A

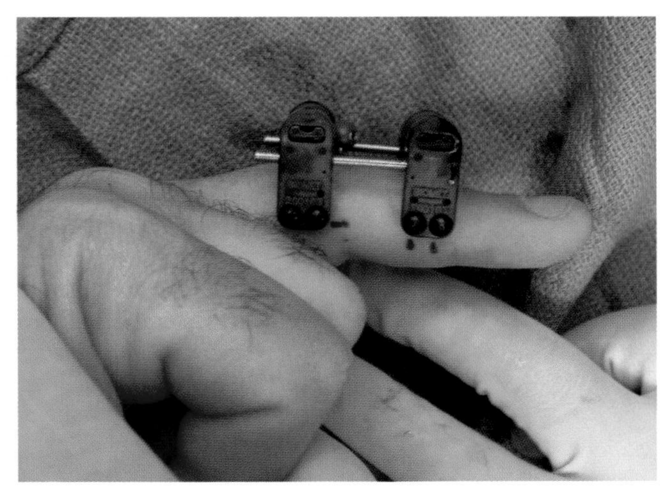

B

Figure 7.8. A: PA clinical view of the Biomet Biosymmetric Fixator **B:** Lateral clinical view of the Biomet Biosymmetric Fixator.

Step 4: Applying Distraction. The screw mechanism for distraction is located at the distal aspect of the frame so it can be accessed for later adjustment in an office setting. Both the radial and ulnar sides of the frame have a distraction mechanism. This allows for differential distraction and correction of radial/ulnar deviation that may be an issue in more comminuted pilon fractures or for protection of tenuous fixation or incompetent soft tissues.

Place the Allen wrench in either the radial or ulnar distractor, and under fluoroscopic guidance turn the wrench clockwise; this will apply distraction. This step should be performed on each side of the frame until joint congruity is achieved. The surgeon may find the ligamentotaxis applied to the frame to be beneficial for specific fragment reduction, particularly of those peripheral fragments attached to the collateral ligaments and volar plate.

Step 5: Application of dressing. Apply a nonadhesive dressing around the pins, followed by a light compressive dressing. Plaster immobilization is typically not needed, since the frame is most often utilized in situations where the surgeon wishes to promote early motion. Eventual transfer to a removable orthosis or dressing that permits active motion is made. We advocate initiating a program when swelling starts to diminish, typically two to five days postoperative.

Step 6: Final Radiographs. Obtain final AP, lateral, and oblique radiographs to document joint reduction and pin placement (Fig. 7.4). Observing the affect of differential distraction on the PIP joint is one of the many benefits of employing intra-operative image intensification.

Step 7: Locking the frame in static mode/Converting the Frame to Dynamic Mode. In certain situations, such as an avulsion of the central slip insertion, it may be beneficial to initially hold the patient in extension until the dorsal fragment has healed back to the P2 phalanx. This may also be beneficial when comminuted fractures are treated with the frame in a statis mode like a mini-external fixator.

To make the frame a static fixator, place the most proximal pin in the fixator. Visualize the radiographic markers in the frame under fluoroscopy. Drive the pin across the proximal phalanx. Cut the pin and apply the cap as in Step 3.

When the surgeon is ready to allow the patient to begin motion, the fixator can be converted from the static to dynamic mode in the office. Loosen the dorsal screws with the Allen wrench. Collapse the width of the frame. Cut one end of the most proximal pin flush with the skin. Prep this side of the skin with betadine. From the opposite side, remove this pin with a needle holder. Restore the original width of the frame. Tighten the dorsal screws with the Allen wrench. In this manner, the degree of traction is not disturbed.

Bent Wire Fixator

There has been substantial interest in developing "homemade" bent wire fixators in the last half decade. Agee, Slade, and others have reported their innovative designs for these devices. We will review here a frame of less sophistication that could be engineered by almost any surgeon without extensive knowledge of these more elaborate designs. This frame requires no special tools, rubber bands, or pins of differing size or composition (threaded vs. unthreaded). It can be thought of as an almost universal "bailout" when a frame is needed and resources or experience dictate an external fixator of less complexity or expense than the myriad of other designs.

Step 1: Placement of the Axis of Rotation Pin. Under fluoroscopic guidance, obtain a lateral of the proximal phalanx. In this view, the head of the proximal phalanx appears as a circle. Place the tip of a long 0.045-inch Kirschner wire in the center of this circle. Bring your hand into the plane of the fluoroscopy beam and drive the pin across the proximal phalanx. If the pin is placed correctly, it appears as a single dot on a perfect lateral of the proximal phalanx.

Step 2: Placement of the Middle Phalanx Pin. Under fluoroscopic guidance, place a second 0.045-inch Kirschner wire of standard length in the middle phalanx distal to the injury and bisecting the dorsal and volar cortices (Fig. 7.9).

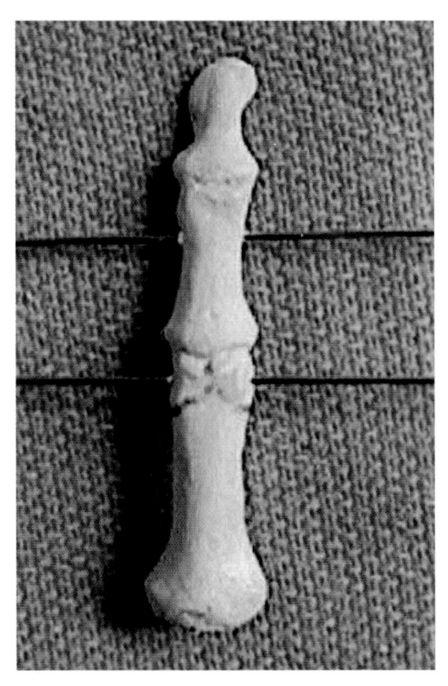

Figure 7.9. Sawbone depiction of the proximal and distal pin placement for a bent wire fixator.

Step 3: Bending the Pins. On each side of the digit, bend the axis of rotation pin 90 degrees in the direction of the fingertip. Make sure the wire extends past the fingertip (Fig. 7.10). Bend the distal most aspect of the pin into an "S" configuration (Fig. 7.11). Bend the middle phalanx pin into a "U" configuration (Fig. 7.12A).

Step 4: Linkage of the Bent Wires. Link the vertical aspect of the proximal pin "S" proximally around the distal pin "U" (Fig. 7.12B).

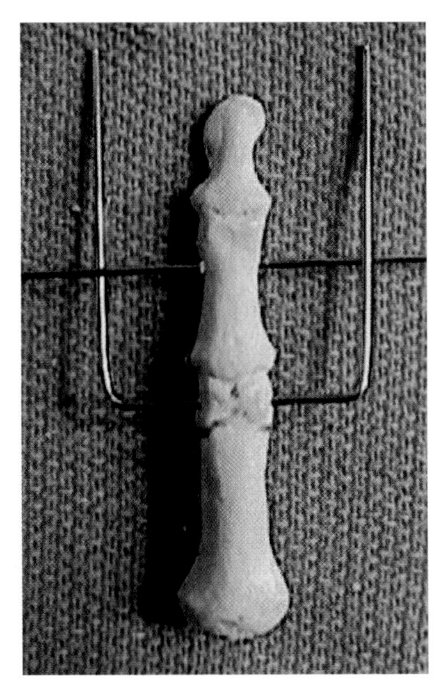

Figure 7.10. The proximal pin is bent 90º in the direction of the fingertip.

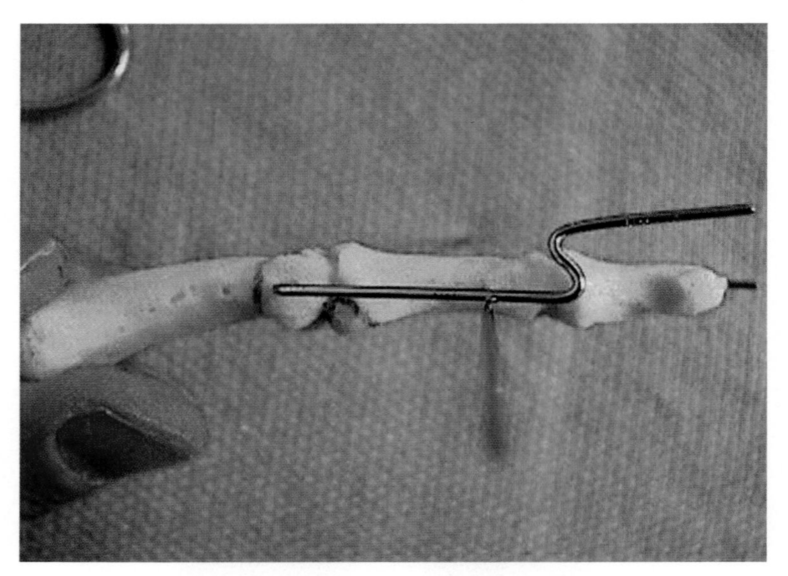

Figure 7.11. The proximal pin is bent into an "S" configuration.

Step 5: Check the Reduction Under Fluoroscopy. The wires should not obscure the visualization of the reduced joint.

Step 6: Placement of the Reduction Pin. Hold the joint reduced. Place a third 0.045-inch Kirschner wire of standard length just distal to the zone of injury at the base of the middle phalanx. If the middle phalanx dorsally subluxates, place the third wire just below the bent axis pin. The axis pin suppresses the reduction pin and reduces the joint. If the middle phalanx volarly subluxates, place the reduction pin just dorsal to the bent axis pin.

Step 7: Application of Dressing. Apply a nonadhesive dressing around the pins, followed by a light compressive dressing.

Step 8: Final Radiographs. Obtain final AP, lateral, and oblique radiographs to document joint reduction and pin placement.

POSTOPERATIVE MANAGEMENT

Remove the initial operative dressing within three to five days. Active range-of-motion exercises and edema control are begun under the guidance of a hand therapist. Radiographs should be checked at two-week intervals. Remove the frame in the office at four weeks

A

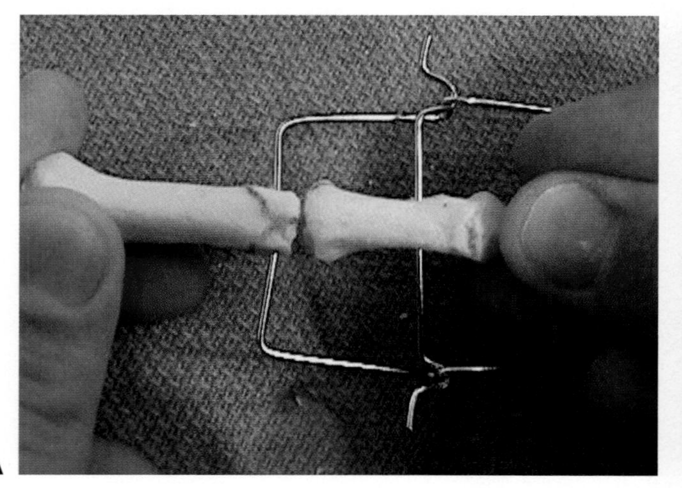

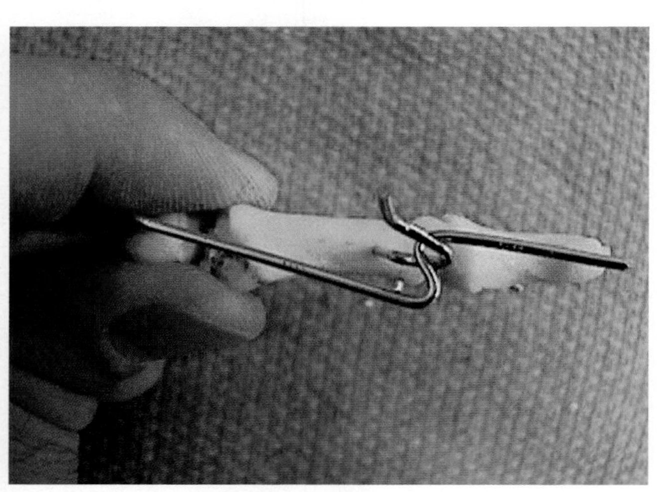

B

Figure 7.12. A: The distal pin is bent into a "U" configuation. **B:** Lateral view of bent wire fixator demonstrating linkage of the proximal and distal wires.

or when radiographs show fracture healing. The patient continues active and passive range-of-motion exercises and starts a progressive strengthening program.

Rehabilitation

The external fixator is used for force neutralization in PIP joint surgery. Although the frame can be utilized alone, it is most often employed with primary joint fixation designed to reconstruct or salvage the articular relationships. Since that fixation is often tenuous, and the proclivity of the PIP joint to become stiff is significant, some mechanism is needed to protect the construct while promoting motion.

Rehabilitation plans vary depending on whether the fixator is locked or allows PIP motion. When the fixator is used for arthrodesis or primary tubular bone fixation, the protocols that apply to those entities should be followed. This chapter focuses on those pathologies and surgical situations in which we sought to establish a conventional PIP joint relationship and pursue the ultimate goal of functional motion.

With this appreciation of the basic philosophy behind using an external fixator in mind, individualize the immediate postoperative and medium-term plan for motion recovery. This plan includes a brief period (3 to 5 days) of bulky immobilization to allow swelling to dissipate. During this period, any active motion can commence. During the entire course, adjacent joint mobilization (presumably MCP and DIP in the majority of cases) should be aggressively pursued.

PIP motion can be initiated when it has been demonstrated that digital swelling will not create problems at the pin interfaces or with the frame body. The patient is encouraged to pursue an active and active-assisted program as often as is comfortable. This maximizes motion and minimizes tendon adhesions and arthrofibrosis. Again, it is assumed that the distraction is protecting any fixation construct that may have been used to support the juxta-articular skeleton.

In about half of the patients we have treated with the frame, some early DIP lag occurs. We suggest a program of specific work on active terminal extension and night splinting of that joint alone to combat that byproduct of slightly limited extensor excursion.

Although each program is patient-specific, we have typically instituted a gentle passive-motion program when the swelling has diminished to an extent that permits this to be done with relative ease and comfort. A general rule would be when the patient has active excursion exceeding about 60 to 75 degrees, then the passive program can commence. As with all rehabilitation, the level of comfort and amount of swelling are important guides. Anticipate that the patient will have episodes of progression and regression, and set realistic expectations for short- and long-term goals.

We have not advocated anesthetic blocks or PIP manipulations to "jump start" a motion program. Search for the root reason for retarded progress before introducing another invasive variable or potentially causing further inflammation or injury to the traumatized system.

The frame is usually discontinued at around postoperative week four or five in the majority of our patients, when the basic osseous and soft-tissue work no longer needs the protection of the fixator. At this time an even more aggressive blocking and passive program can be added to the rehabilitation program. Dynamic splinting may be of benefit in certain circumstances.

We advocate the glove rubber band, a simple, inexpensive technique for use when recovery of the terminal degrees of PIP and DIP joint motion is sought (Fig. 7.13). This has been one of the best ways for the patient to recover terminal composite flexion, but limits to the longevity of wear (usually less than five to seven minutes per session) must be appreciated. Make sure patients refrain from falling asleep when the band is on in case of untoward effects from slippage around the neurovascular bundles.

It is rare that we actually design a true strengthening program for patients with single-digit injuries. The deconditioning they have experienced from the infirmity should usually reverse with more normal hand-use patterns. For those with more specific hand-intensive demands, perhaps a strengthening program would be beneficial.

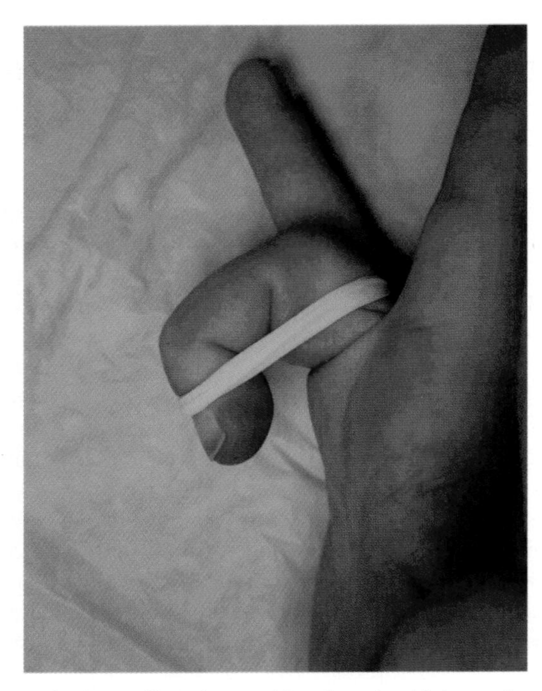

Figure 7.13. Photograph shows the glove rubber band, which can be effective for recovery of terminal composite flexion when motion at the PIP and DIP joint permit. Use is limited to less than five to seven minutes per session.

RESULTS

For use of the external fixator, the injury and reconstructive challenge must be significant enough to warrant additional intervention, morbidity, potential complication, and arduous rehabilitation.

These are the reasons we utilize only bilateral fixator options. If the problem was bad enough to need a fixator, then it needs optimal levels of control and flexibility in positioning and distraction. Usually, the joint has been significantly compromised, and simple unilateral control is inadequate, as we need to combat drift into malangulation and malrotation.

We have selected only the most challenging PIP joint fractures and fracture-dislocations for which we bring out the external fixator. We sense a trend toward a refocusing on the use of frames. As in the use of other technologies, the pendulum swing may have favored more liberal use of the devices a half decade ago, and now more experience and communication has lead to greater appreciation of the indications and expected outcomes.

Although problems may accompany the use of the frame, we have experienced reasonably pleasing results as compared with outcomes with other salvage procedures for these most injured joints. Despite our modest expectations, we have been able to restore what we consider a functional outcome to a majority of patients.

Our definition of success is based on recovery of 75° or more of PIP motion, stability, comfort, and ability to resume tasks of vocation and avocation. Recognizing that this population is mixed, and the severity and character of injuries is likewise, we have been successful in this pursuit in over 50 cases we have followed. Over half of the patients recover greater than 90 degrees of motion, and no patients have had to change jobs due to the PIP joint sequelae. With these criteria as a base, we have had good or excellent results in 82% of our reviewed cases.

Persistent instability is almost never a problem. The difficulty is stiffness. In only two patients of our index group was some type of progressive deformity due to lack of stability considered the germinal problem. Both of those patients had largely a failure of the bony elements of the reconstruction.

We have never encountered a septic arthritis, and we have not had to return any patient to a formal operating room setting for an infectious complication. The use of oral antibiotics or the discontinuation of a pin earlier than desired has been seen in about 20% and 5% of cases, respectively. We have never experienced a frame breakage since abandoning unilateral fixators, none of which are included in the cases we are recounting.

A persistent extensor lag at both the PIP and DIP joints (defined as greater than 5 degrees different from the contralateral comparison digit) has been seen in over 40% of patients. Interestingly, patients complain less of this limitation at the PIP joint than they do with the DIP outcome. Most say this is for cosmetic, rather than functional, reasons.

It is difficult to normalize data regarding functional parameters, even objective ones like grip strength, because of the variability in the patient population. However, grip strength is seldom affected to a significant extent. Only when the small finger ray is involved does it appear to impact with a modest diminution. Without premorbid or reliable contralateral comparisons due to hand dominance, it is not adequate to project true limitations based on the treatment course selected.

An external frame is indicated in those cases that are distinctly advanced on the scale of combination trauma and technical challenge. The outcome will be most determined by timely primary intervention, but the use of a frame as an adjunct may have positive influence as it promotes early protection and accelerated rehabilitation in this subset of challenging injuries.

COMPLICATIONS

Loss of Reduction

Loss of reduction can occur due to inadequate tightening of the frame. To avoid this, the surgeon needs to check all aspects of the frame prior to leaving the operating room and upon each return visit in the office. In addition, loss of reduction can occur secondary to inappropriately placing a fracture in immediate dynamic mode. Fractures with a dorsal fragment at the base of P2 to which the central slip inserts should have that fragment protected in the static mode for three weeks and with the frame then converted to a dynamic mode.

Pin-Tract Infection

Early pin-tract cellulitis is treated with oral antibiotics and digital splinting to decrease joint motion. Infections occurring two weeks after surgery may need the fixator removed and the digit immobilized with a splint. Motion can be restarted when the soft tissues have improved and radiographs show evidence of healing. Failure to recognize the pin-tract infection early can lead to osteomyelitis or a septic joint. We have not yet seen this happen.

Stiffness/Flexion Contracture

Flexion contractures can be prevented with an early postoperative therapy program monitored by a certified hand therapist. Active extension exercises with the MCP joint blocked in flexion helps to concentrate the extensor force on the PIP joint. Static night splinting of the PIP joint can also be instituted.

Articular Incongruity

Articular incongruity results from inadequate interpretation of the reduction at the time of surgery. The surgeon must not leave the operating room without perfect AP and lateral views of the PIP joint. Oblique views also help in judging the reduction. Sometimes, despite an excellent reduction, post-traumatic osteoarthritis develops. This is a result of the initial trauma.

RECOMMENDED READING

1. Agee JM. Unstable Fracture Dislocations of the Proximal Interphalangeal Joint. Treatment with the Force Couple Splint. *Clin Orthop* 214:101–112, 1987.
2. Bain GI, Mehta JA, Heptinstall RJ, et al. Dynamic External Fixation for Injuries of the Proximal Interphalangeal Joint. *JBJS* 80B:1014–1019, 1998.
3. Hastings H II, Ernst JM. Dynamic External Fixation for Fractures of the Proximal Interphalangeal Joint. *Hand Clinics* 4:659–674, 1993.
4. Kiefhaber TR, Stern PJ. Fracture Dislocations of the Proximal Interphalangeal Joint. *JHS* 23A:368–378,1998.
5. Krakauer JD, Stern PJ. Hinged Device for Fractures Involving the Proximal Interphalangeal Joint. *Clin Orthop* 327:29–37, 1996.
6. Salter RB. The Physiologic Basis of Continuous Passive Motion for Articular Cartilage Healing and Regeneration. *Hand Clin* 10:211–219, 1994.
7. Schenck RR. Dynamic Traction and Early Passive Movement for Fractures of the Proximal Interphalangeal Joint. *JHS* 11A:850–858, 1986.
8. Seno N, Hashizume H, Inoue H, et al. Fractures of the Base of the Middle Phalanx of the Finger. *JBJS* 79B:758–763, 1997.
9. Stern PJ, Roman RJ, Kiefhaber TR, et al. Pilon Fractures of the Proximal Interphalangeal Joint. *JHS* 16A:844–850, 1991.
10. Suzuki Y, Matasunaga T, Sato S, et al. The Pins and Rubber Traction System for Treatment of Comminuted Intraarticular Fractures and Fracture-Dislocations in the Hand. *JBJS* 19B:98–107, 1994.
11. Wolfe SW, Swigart CR, Grauer J, et al. Augmented external fixation of distal radius fractures: a biomechanical analysis. *J Hand Surg* 23A:127–134, 1998.

PART II

Fractures and Dislocations: The Thumb

8

Surgical Treatment of Acute and Chronic Incompetence of the Thumb Metacarpophalangeal Joint Stabilizers

Steven Z. Glickel

INDICATIONS/CONTRAINDICATIONS

The indication for repair of an acute tear of the ulnar collateral ligament (UCL) of the metacarpophalangeal (MP) joint of the thumb is a complete tear. Stener described the lesion that bears his name, in which the proximal end of the torn collateral ligament lies superficial to the proximal margin of the adductor aponeurosis. The distal end of the ligament, or the bony insertion of the proximal stump on the ulnar base of the proximal phalanx, lies deep to the adductor aponeurosis. The ligament cannot heal with tissue interposed, so this represents an absolute indication for surgical repair. A complete tear without a Stener lesion is a strong relative indication for repair. It is certainly the case that some complete tears will heal adequately with cast or splint immobilization. However, several authors have recommended early repair for all complete tears, noting that some patients with complete tears may have displacement of the torn ends of the ligament even without a Stener lesion, resulting in chronic laxity and/or pain. I agree with this recommendation for most patients except those who are conspicuously low demand. The indication for surgery for acute radial collateral ligament (RCL) tears is not quite as clear. Some authors recommend nonoperative treatment with immobilization for complete tears. Others make a strong case for repair

Steven Z. Glickel, M.D.: Orthopaedic Surgery, Columbia University, New York, NY, and Orthopaedic Surgery, St. Luke's-Roosevelt Hospital Center, New York, NY

if the tear is complete. Dray and Eaton recommend repair if a complete tear is accompanied by volar subluxation of the MP joint.

Campbell described the lesion known as the "gamekeeper's thumb," in which the ulnar collateral ligaments of Scottish gamekeepers became attenuated by repetitive radially directed force against the ulnar side of the thumb when used to fracture the necks of rabbits. The gamekeeper's thumb is a form of chronic instability, which may also be the result of failure of recognition of an acute tear, an untreated acute tear, or failure of an acute repair. Patients with chronic instability of either the UCL or RCL deserve a trial of conservative treatment. The MP joint should be splinted with a customized hand-based thermoplastic splint including only the MP joint (thumb cone or short opponens splint). Nonsteroidal antiinflammatory medication may improve the synovitis and pain resulting from instability. The indications for UCL reconstruction are failure of conservative treatment with persistent pain and instability of the MP joint. Rarely is instability alone a sufficient indication for surgery. Typically, patients complain of exacerbation of pain by activities such as writing, turning keys in locks, and unscrewing jar tops. They sometimes have difficulty holding large objects, such as a half-gallon container of milk, because they do not have a stable post against which to support the object. Kessler and Heller suggested that chronic instability of the RCL is rarely symptomatic. I have not found that to be the case. Patients complain of pain and weakness when doing torsional motions, such as turning doorknobs and unscrewing jar tops, and with axial compression on the thumb tip.

Contraindications to reconstruction of UCL or RCL tears include osteoarthritis, "multidirectional" instability, or fixed subluxation of the joint. Mild chondromalacia may be tolerated, but established osteoarthritis is a contraindication to reconstruction and an indication for MP arthrodesis. If an arthritic joint is reconstructed, pain is likely to persist and increase over time, necessitating conversion to arthrodesis. Very rarely, a patient may have gross instability of both collateral ligaments or one collateral ligament and the volar plate, which is a relative contraindication to reconstruction since reconstruction of one collateral ligament alone might not be adequate to stabilize the joint. An equally rare circumstance is a joint in which the collateral ligament is so unstable that it becomes fixed in an angulated position at the MP joint. The intact collateral ligament shortens because of the chronic deviation toward that side. In order to reconstruct the incompetent ligament, the intact ligament would have to be released, creating the "multidirectional" instability mentioned previously.

PREOPERATIVE PLANNING

The assessment of instability of the thumb MP collateral ligaments is primarily clinical with radiographic correlation. Special studies are usually not necessary. Clinical examination begins with observation. If there is a significant ligament injury, there is usually swelling, and, in the acute setting, there may be ecchymosis on the injured side of the joint. The resting posture of the thumb at the MP joint is occasionally indicative of pathology. In rare instances, the joint is angulated at rest if the collateral ligament is grossly incompetent and the instability is chronic. Thumbs with RCL instability often have a dorsal prominence of the radial side of the metacarpal head. This is less common with UCL instability.

Joint tenderness is usually discretely localized to the area of pathology. Palpation of a fullness on the ulnar side of the metacarpal head is strongly suggestive of a Stener lesion. Stability of the collateral ligaments is tested in extension and 30 degrees of flexion. There is no consensus in the literature concerning the degree of instability that is diagnostic of a complete tear. The criteria that are probably most accurate were described by Heyman et al. and include 35 degrees of laxity of the ulnar side of the MP joint when stressed in extension and 15 degrees more laxity than the contralateral thumb when stressed in 30 degrees of flexion. Laxity in extension suggests that the accessory and proper collateral ligaments are both torn. A more subtle finding is the presence or absence of a discrete endpoint to the joint opening with stress. Absence of an endpoint is strongly suggestive of a complete ligament tear (Fig. 8.1). Mildly increased joint opening compared to the contralateral side with a discrete endpoint may be indicative of a partial or grade 2 tear.

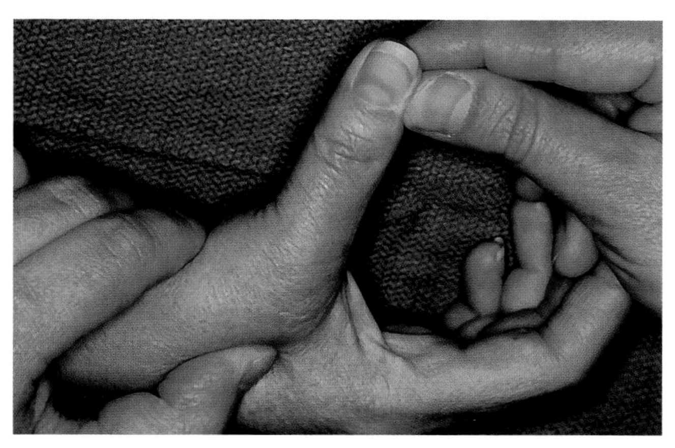

Figure 8.1. The ulnar joint opens approximately 35 degrees with radially directed stress. Lack of a clear endpoint is strongly suggestive of a complete tear of the UCL.

Obtain plain PA, lateral, and oblique radiographs to rule out a fracture. On the ulnar side, fractures are usually avulsions from the ulnar base of the proximal phalanx since the site of the ligament injury is generally distal. On the radial side, avulsions may either be from the base of the proximal phalanx or the radial side of the metacarpal head if the avulsion is proximal. The lateral X-ray may show volar subluxation of the MP joint, which is fairly common as result of extension of the collateral ligament tear to involve the dorsal capsule. This may occur with UCL or RCL tears. It is rare to have an isolated tear of the dorsal capsule causing volar subluxation without an associated collateral ligament injury. Stress views of the MP joint have been recommended to radiographically demonstrate instability. My personal approach is to rely almost exclusively on physical examination and plain x-rays to make the diagnosis; I generally do not get stress views. There have been numerous studies looking at the efficacy of special radiographic studies, including arthrograms of the MP joint, ultrasonography, and magnetic resonance imaging. My feeling is that none of these studies is necessary. Most surgeons will repair a complete ulnar collateral ligament tear with or without a Stener lesion, so it becomes somewhat of a moot point if the Stener lesion is present or not. Arthrograms are invasive, uncomfortable, and add relatively little information to a good physical examination.

REPAIR FOR ACUTE INJURIES

The involved limb is anesthetized with a regional block, either axillary or supraclavicular. A forearm or brachial tourniquet is used. Prep and drape the extremity with a stockingette and an impervious extremity drape. Expose the UCL using a "lazy S"-shaped incision with the vertical limb of the "S" overlying the ulnar side of the MP joint. Elevate skin flaps. Identify, mobilize, and gently retract the invariably present branch of the dorsal sensory branch of the radial nerve. Examine the proximal margin of the abductor aponeurosis for the presence of a Stener lesion. Incise the abductor aponeurosis longitudinally, parallel and approximately 3 mm volar to the EPL tendon. Reflect the flaps of the aponeurosis dorsally and volarly, exposing the underlying ligament and joint. Assess the location of the tear within the ligament. Most commonly, it is torn distally from its insertion on the base of the proximal phalanx or within the substance of the ligament. Deviate the proximal phalanx radially and explore the joint for chondral injuries or other pathology.

If the ligament is torn within its substance, reapproximate the torn ends directly using several figure-of-eight braided synthetic sutures like 3-0 and/or 4-0 Ethibond (Ethicon, Cincinnati, OH, U.S.A.). Do not tie the sutures until all have been placed. It is easiest to place the volar sutures first. It can be difficult to manipulate a large needle around the volar aspect of the joint. For this reason, Ethicon made a customized "UCL" needle with a short radius of curvature that facilitates placement of sutures at the base of the ligament. Repair the dorsal capsule of the MP joint if the ligament tear propogated into the capsule. Once all sutures have been placed, reduce the joint, correct any volar subluxation, and tie the sutures from volar to dorsal. In the past, I transfixed the MP joint with a Kirschner wire, but have not done that for several years with no apparent deterioration in results.

Most often the ligament is avulsed from its insertion on the ulnar base of the proximal phalanx. In that case, the ligament needs to be reattached to bone. This may be done with a pullout suture or, as is currently my preference, using bone anchors. Mobilize the avulsed ligament and retract it proximally. Usually two anchors are sufficient to reattach the ligament. My preference is to use the mini Mitek bone anchor, to which is attached a 2-0 Ethibond suture. Drill holes for the anchor with the drill bit that comes with the set. This can be done by hand using a T-wrench with a Jacob's chuck to hold the drill bit. Place one hole dorsally and the other volarly in the base of the proximal phalanx approximately 5 mm distal to the articular surface. Insert anchors in each of these holes using the introducer on which the anchor and suture are mounted. Minimally decorticate the bone proximal to the drill holes to enhance reattachment of the ligament. Advance the ligament to as nearly an anatomic position as possible and suture it volarly and the capsule dorsally with the 2-0 Ethibond sutures. Place additional figure-of-eight sutures of 3-0 Ethibond to reinforce the repair, assuming that there is any intact periosteum remaining at the base of the proximal phalanx. Repair the abductor aponeurosis with 4-0 Vicryl (Ethicon, Cincinnati, OH, U.S.A.) interrupted sutures and close the skin with absorbable sutures like 5-0 Vicryl rapide (Ethicon, Cincinnati, OH, U.S.A.). Dress the wound with a moist gauze, fluffed gauze sponges, and a Kling wrap. Apply a short-arm thumb spica cast.

Repair of the radial collateral ligament is similar to that for the UCL with a few notable exceptions. There is no equivalent to the Stener lesion on the radial side of the MP joint, so both ends of the torn RCL will be deep to the abductor aponeurosis. The incidence of proximal and distal tears of the RCL is approximately equal, in contrast to the UCL, where distal tears are much more common than proximal. Repair tears in the substance of the RCL in a manner similar to that described above for the UCL using multiple 3-0 or 4-0 Ethibond sutures. If the ligament is avulsed from its insertion on the base of the proximal phalanx or from its origin on the radial side of the metacarpal head, reattach it using two mini Mitek bone anchors. Since the normal origin of the RCL is relatively dorsal on the metacarpal head, place the anchors in approximately that position. Repair the abductor aponeurosis with interrupted sutures of 4-0 Vicryl, and the skin with 5-0 Vicryl rapide. A short-arm thumb spica cast is worn for six weeks.

There are relatively few pitfalls in repair of the collateral ligaments as long as the procedure is done in a timely manner avoiding fibrosis and shortening of the torn ligament. A scarred ligament may not be able to be brought out to its physiologic resting length, resulting in a repair that is too tight, which limits range of motion of the joint. My experience has also been that if a subacutely torn ligament is repaired, the repair may not hold up over time, resulting in some recurrent laxity. This is presumably because the connective tissue has been permanently altered by the chronicity of the injury and resultant fibrosis. It is also possible to simply make the repair too tight or too loose if the sutures are not placed with the ligament at its physiologic length. This may occur with direct repair of an intrasubstance tear where the ends of the ligament are overlapped too much in the interest of creating a "snug" repair. When a torn ligament is reattached to bone, the site of reattachment may be either too close to or too far from the joint, making the repair too loose or too tight respectively.

RECONSTRUCTION FOR CHRONIC INSTABILITY

The procedure is usually performed under regional anesthetic, which may be either an axillary block or a supraclavicular block depending on the preference of the anesthesiologist. Position the patient supine on the operating room table. Sterilely prep the extremity. Place a tourniquet on the brachium. A forearm tourniquet is not used because of the necessity to harvest a forearm tendon for use in the reconstruction. Drape the extremity with a stockingette and prefabricated extremity drape. Exsanguinate the limb and inflate the tourniquet to 80 to 100 mm of mercury greater than systolic pressure. The ulnar aspect of the MP joint may be exposed using one of several skin incisions. My preference is a "lazy S"-shaped incision with the proximal limb parallel to the ulnar side of the thumb metacarpal; the transverse limb extends slightly obliquely from dorsal to volar at the level of the joint, and the distal, longitudinal limb volar to the mid-axial line (Fig. 8.2). Alternative incisions include a straight mid-axial or a chevron-shaped incision with its apex slightly volar to the mid-axial line and the longitudinal limbs extending just dorsal to the mid-axial line. Elevate the skin flaps and retract them with a 4-0 silk suture. A branch of the dorsal sensory branch of the radial nerve invariably crosses the operative field. Retract it gently to avoid a neurapraxia postoperatively. The need to dissect out the branch of the nerve is particularly compelling in procedures in which there is scarring either from the initial injury or a failed primary operative procedure. Advise the patient in advance of the procedure of the possibility of having numbness on the dorsum of the thumb distal to the incision, and that although this numbness is usually temporary, it may be permanent.

As the procedure was originally described, the next step involves mobilization of a flap of abductor aponeurosis distal to the vertical fibers or the sagittal band. Try to preserve the sagittal fibers as long as they are not densely adherent to the underlying torn ligament. Outline a triangular flap of abductor aponeurosis with the longitudinal limb approximately 2 to 3 mm volar to the EPL tendon and extending from the level of the vertical fibers distally. Make a vertical limb of the incision along the distal edge of the sagittal fibers. The flap is reflected volarly and distally, exposing the ulnar side of the base of the proximal phalanx. If the aponeurosis is adherent and unable to be separated from the underlying ligament, incise it longitudinally and repair the vertical fibers at the end of the procedure (Fig. 8.3). Expose the joint by retracting the intact vertical fibers and examine the articular cartilage. Degeneration of the articular cartilage, particularly with ebernation, is a clear indication to abort the planned reconstruction and proceed with MP arthrodesis.

To proceed with reconstruction, excise any remaining ligament (Fig. 8.4). Three gouge holes are needed through which to pass the tendon graft used for the reconstruction. Plan for two gouge holes on the ulnar side of the phalangeal base, one dorsal and one volar. Make the dorsal hole at the "1 o'clock" position and the volar hole at the "5 o'clock" position. Start the holes so that the proximal extent of the cortical opening is approximately 7–8 mm distal to the joint. This prevents inadvertently enlarging the hole too close to the articular surface. Separate the holes sufficiently far from each other to avoid inadvertently breaking the bridge between them. Make the holes with three hand-held gouges of increas-

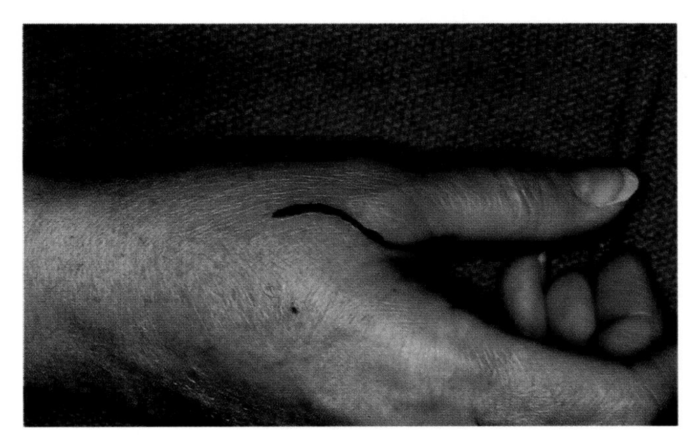

Figure 8.2. Use a "lazy S"-shaped incision to expose the ulnar side of the thumb MP joint.

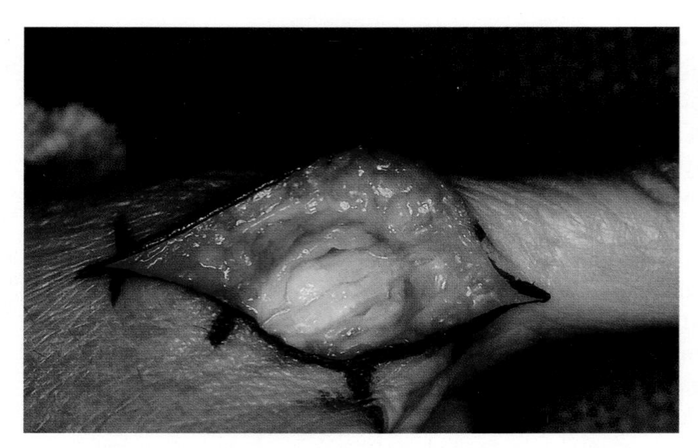

Figure 8.3. Incise the adductor aponeurosis to expose the ulnar side of the MP joint, including the torn UCL.

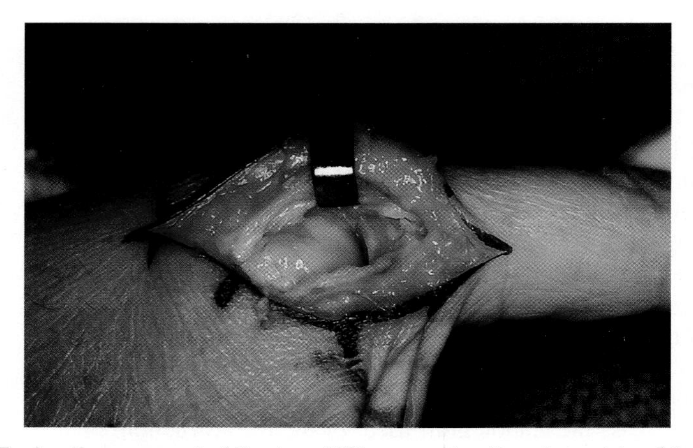

Figure 8.4. Excise the remnant of the torn UCL, exposing the ulnar side of the MP joint and base of the proximal phalanx. Inspect the joint for the presence or absence of degenerative disease.

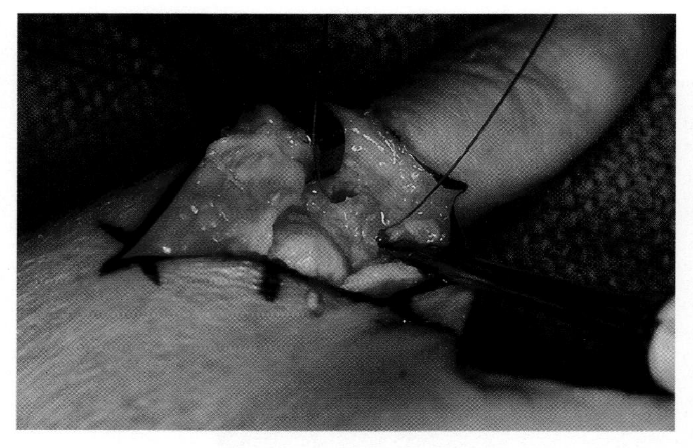

Figure 8.5. Make holes in the base of the proximal phalanx using hand-held gouges of increasing size. Connect the holes within the medullary canal. A 28-gauge stainless steel wire is passed through the hole for later use to pass the tendon graft.

ing diameter (Walter Lorenz, Jacksonville, FL). Direct the proximal phalangeal gouge holes toward each other within the medullary canal so that they connect (Fig. 8.5). Place a 28-gauge stainless steel wire through the gouge hole to be used for later passage of the tendon graft. This can be more difficult than it seems. Bend the end of the wire into a gentle curve simulating the radius of curvature of the hole in the medullary canal. Introduce the wire into one of the holes and retrieve the end through the other using a hemostat with a fine tip. Secure the ends of the wire with a clamp to avoid inadvertently pulling it out of the hole as the procedure progresses.

Make another hole in the metacarpal neck. Begin the hole with the small gouge on the ulnar side of the metacarpal neck in the area of the origin of the collateral ligament, slightly dorsal to the longitudinal axis of the bone. Direct the hole radially and slightly proximally across the medullary canal, emerging on the radial side. Enlarge the hole with the medium and large gouges. Make a 1-cm incision over the tip of the gouge, emerging on the radial side of the metacarpal. Place another 28-gauge stainless steel wire through this gouge track using the concavity of the gouge as a guide to its passage. Clamp the ends of this wire as well.

Harvest a tendon graft. The preferred donor is the palmaris longus tendon, if available. Expose the distal end of the tendon through a 1-cm transverse incision at the level of the distal wrist crease. Mobilize the tendon. Identify and protect the median nerve to avoid inadvertent injury. The palmaris longus can be removed with a tendon stripper. Alternatively, my preference is to make a second, proximal incision. Identify the musculotendinous junction by applying traction to the distal end of the tendon. Make an incision measuring approximately 1.5 cm over the musculotendinous junction; divide the tendon. Withdraw the palmaris into the distal incision with firm traction. If the patient does not have a palmaris longus tendon, alternative donors include the plantaris, a toe extensor, or a strip of the FCR tendon. My preference is the FCR since it obviates the need for a second surgical field. The fact that the surface of the tendon is not perfectly smooth is of little concern since it is not required to glide through a fibrosseous sheath.

Place a 0.045-inch Kirschner wire from distal to proximal in the center of the metacarpal head, emerging on the radial side of the metacarpal shaft. Withdraw it from proximally into the medullary canal, so that the end of the pin is just proximal to the level of the subchondral bone of the metacarpal head for later use to transfix the MP joint. Tie the wire in the proximal phalanx around one end of the tendon graft (Fig. 8.6). Moisten the graft with saline and carefully draw it through the hole in the medullary canal at the base of the proximal phalanx. Pull the tendon with a twisting motion to avoid excessive force that might crack the bony bridge between the two holes. It is generally easier to place the tendon in the volar hole and withdraw it through the more dorsal hole. Pull the tendon far enough that

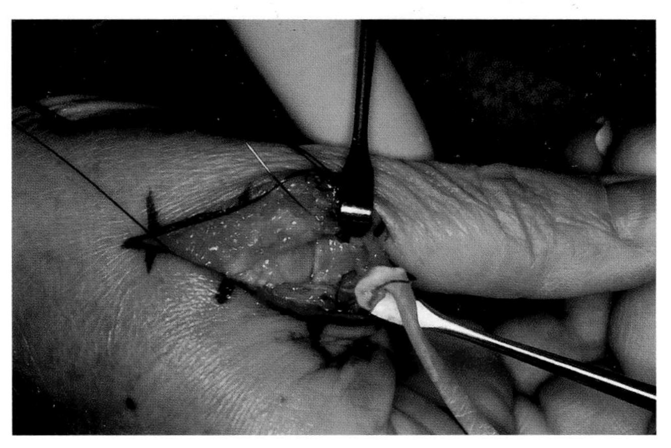

Figure 8.6. Tie the end of the stainless steel wire emerging from the volar gouge in the base of the proximal phalanx around one end of the tendon graft.

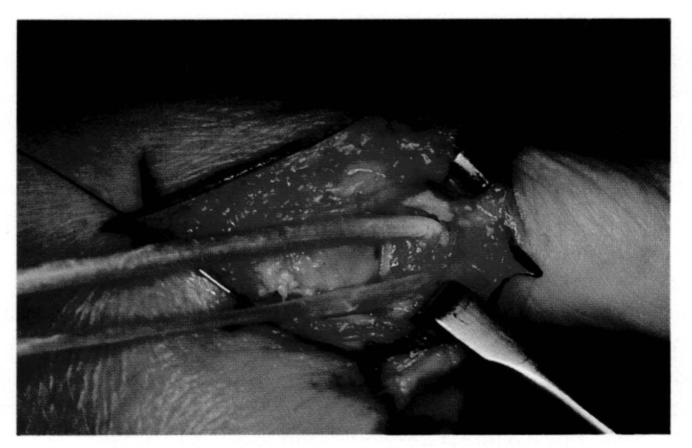

Figure 8.7. Pull the tendon graft through the hole in the medullary canal using the wire as a guide; equal length limbs emerge from the proximal phalanx dorsally and volarly.

the two limbs of the graft are of equal length (Fig. 8.7). Remove the wire from the end of the tendon. If the sagittal fibers are intact, pass both limbs of the tendon beneath it. Tie the wire on the ulnar side of the thumb metacarpal around both ends of the tendon graft simultaneously. Draw the wire through the medullary canal of the metacarpal from ulnar to radial, delivering the two equal lengths of tendon graft through the hole and into the radial incision (Fig. 8.8). Place the MP joint in neutral flexion and slightly overreduce the joint by radially deviating the proximal phalanx on the metacarpal head. Tension the graft by applying traction to both limbs simultaneously (Fig. 8.9). Tie the ends of the graft in a knot (Fig. 8.10). Suture the knot to the adjacent periosteum with two mattress sutures of 3-0 braided synthetic suture material like Ethibond (Fig. 8.11). An alternative to this part of the procedure is the way that the procedure was initially described (Figs. 8.12, 8.13, 8.14). Pull the tendon ends through a stab wound on the radial side of the thumb and place the ends of the graft through either the holes of a button or rubber catheter. Tie the ends in a knot and suture them (Fig. 8.15). In either case, test the tension on the graft by ulnarly deviating the proximal phalanx. The joint should open no more than 5 to 10 degrees. It should also be possible to flex the joint through a nearly full range of motion without excessive force. If the tension is felt to be appropriate, transfix the joint with the previously placed 0.045-inch Kirschner wire.

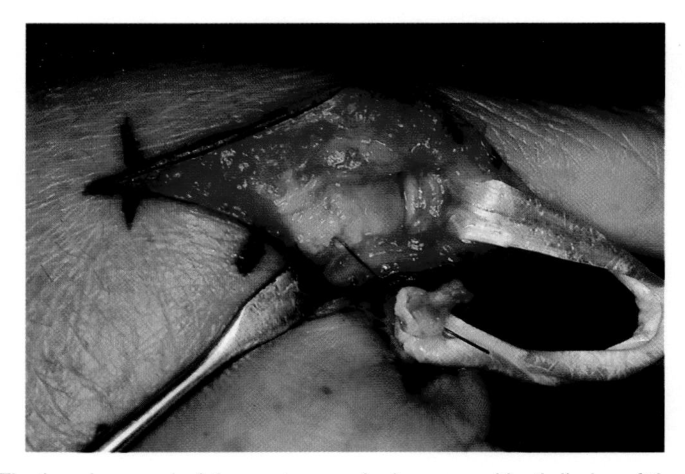

Figure 8.8. Tie the ulnar end of the metacarpal wire around both limbs of the graft and pull them through the metacarpal hole, emerging on the radial side.

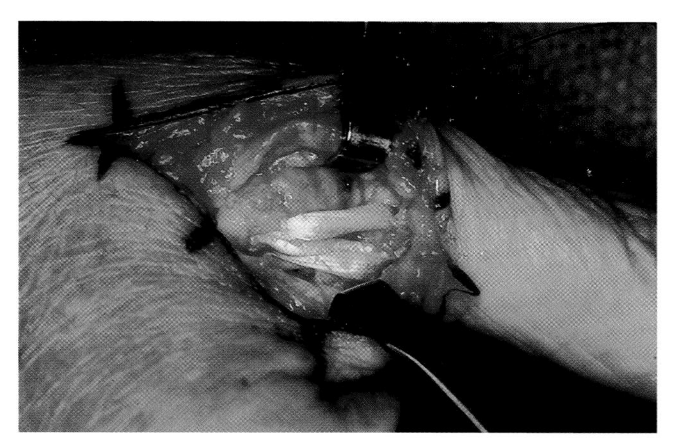

Figure 8.9. The two limbs of the graft are seen crossing the ulnar side of the joint in a configuration that closely resembles that of the normal UCL.

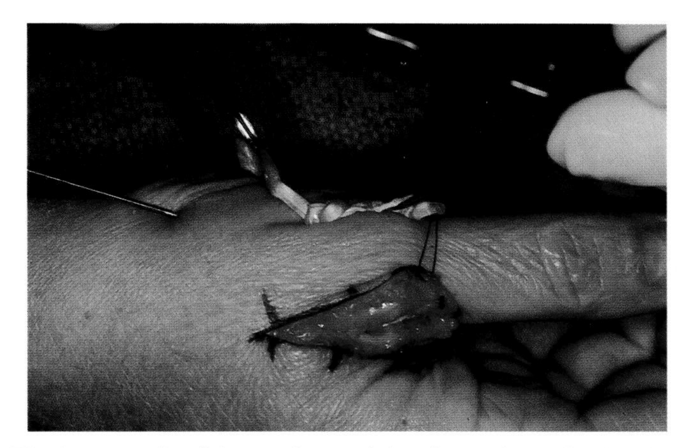

Figure 8.10. Tie the two tails of the tendon graft in a knot after adjusting the tension of the reconstruction.

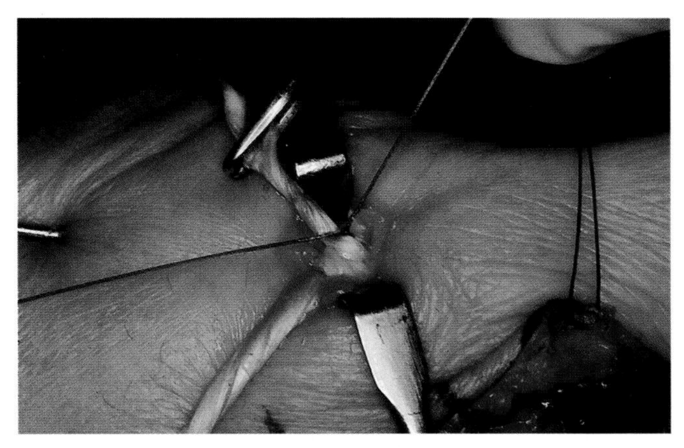

Figure 8.11. The knot is sutured with two 3-0 Ethibond horizontal mattress sutures.

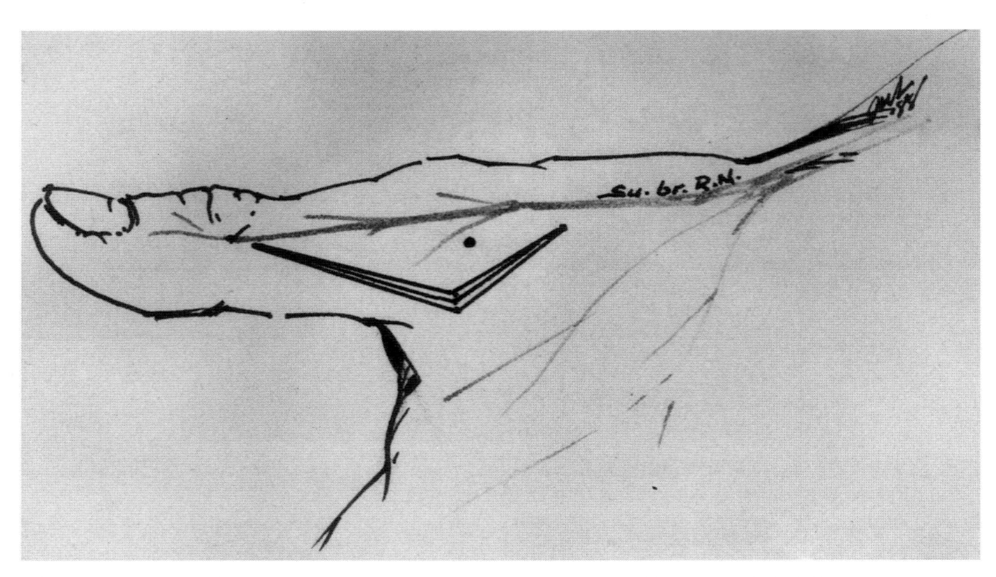

Figure 8.12. An alternative incision to expose the ulnar side of the MP joint is a chevron-shaped incision with its apex just volar to the midaxial line. (From Glickel S, Malerich M, Pearce S, et al. Ligament replacement for chronic instability of the ulnar collateral ligament of the metacarpophalangeal joint of the thumb. *J Hand Surg* 18A:930, 1993, with permission.)

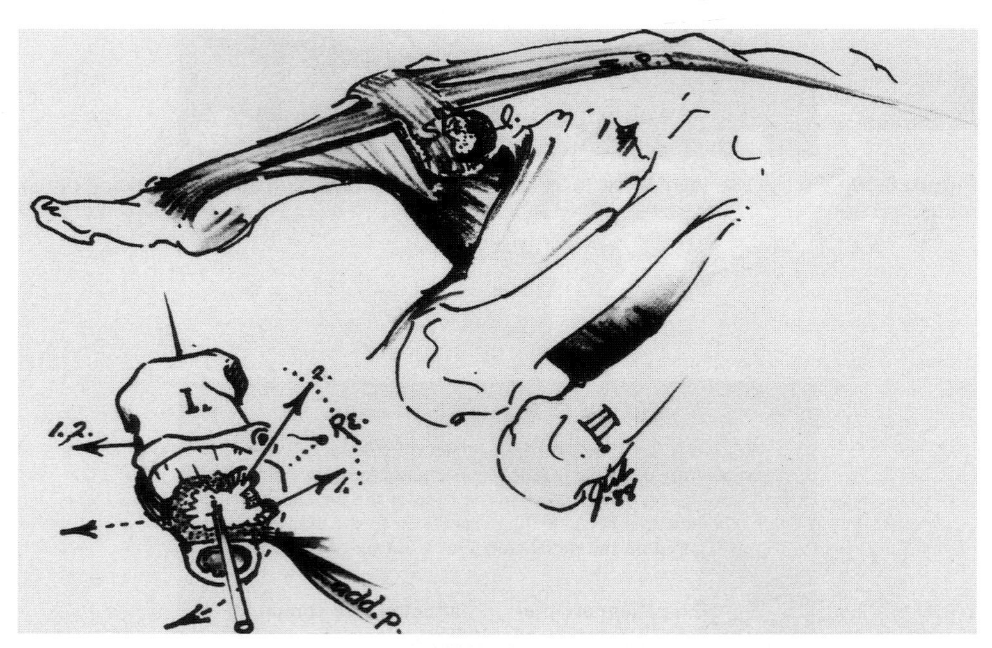

Figure 8.13. Create a flap of the adductor aponeurosis by making an "L"-shaped incision with the transverse limb distal and parallel to the sagittal band and the longitudinal limb parallel and just volar to the EPL tendon. If the sagittal band is too scarred to be dissected free of the underlying ligament, it may be incised parallel to the EPL tendon, as well. (From: Glickel S, Malerich M, Pearce S, Littler JW. Ligament replacement for chronic instability of the ulnar collateral ligament of the metacarpophalangeal joint of the thumb. *J Hand Surg* 18A:930, 1993, with permission.)

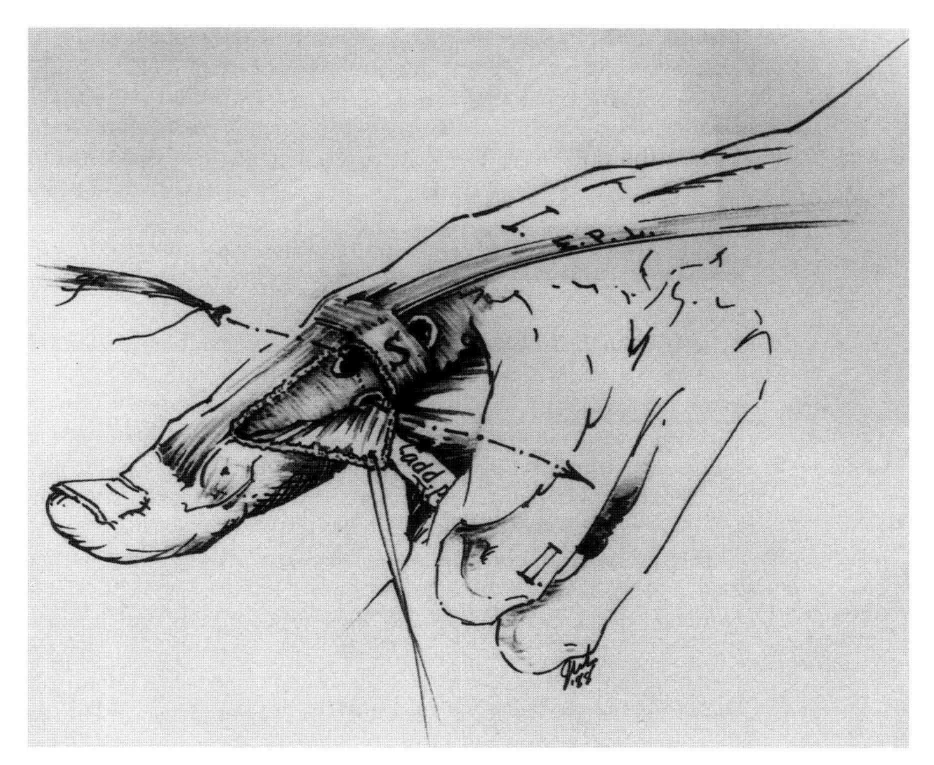

Figure 8.14. Use a 28-gauge stainless steel wire to pull the tendon graft through the holes in the phalangeal base. (From: Glickel S, Malerich M, Pearce S, et al. Ligament replacement for chronic instability of the ulnar collateral ligament of the metacarpophalangeal joint of the thumb. *J Hand Surg* 18A:930, 1993, with permission.)

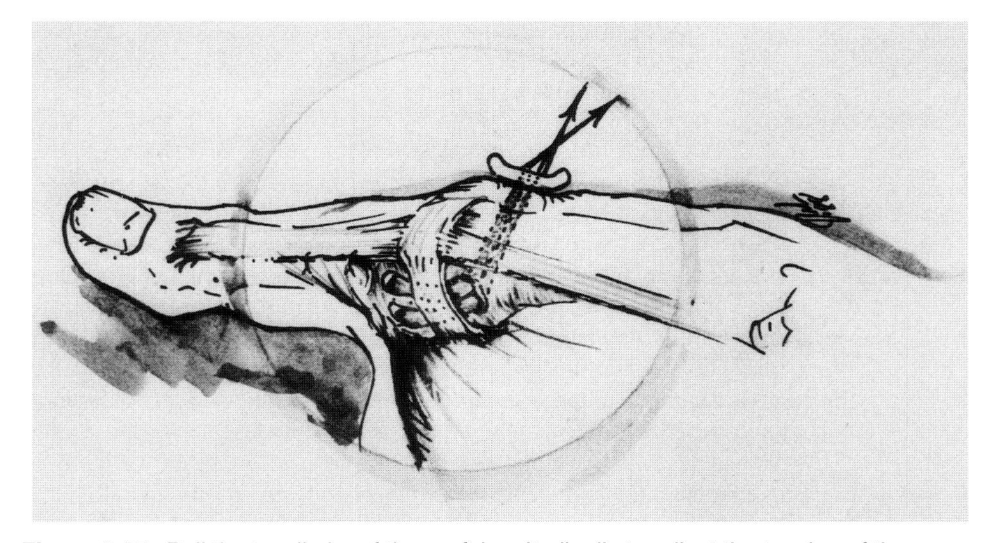

Figure 8.15. Pull the two limbs of the graft longitudinally to adjust the tension of the reconstruction. Tie the ends of the graft in a knot where they emerge from the hole in the metacarpal neck. Suture the knot with 3-0 Ethibond. (From: Glickel S, Malerich M, Pearce S, et al. Ligament replacement for chronic instability of the ulnar collateral ligament of the metacarpophalangeal joint of the thumb. *J Hand Surg* 18A:930, 1993, with permission)

Suture the adductor aponeurosis with simple interrupted sutures of 4-0 Vicryl. Close the skin incision with simple or mattress sutures of a rapidly absorbable suture like 5-0 Vicryl rapide (Ethicon, Cincinnati, OH, U.S.A.) or 5-0 plain catgut so the cast does not have to be changed to remove sutures. Alternatively, the skin can be closed with a running subcuticular suture of 4-0 Prolene (Ethicon, Cincinnati, OH, U.S.A.) Dress the wound with a moist gauze, fluff sponges, and Kling gauze. Apply a short-arm thumb spica cast, which is worn for six weeks.

Reconstruction of chronic instability of the radial collateral ligament of the thumb MP joint is essentially the mirror image of the procedure for ulnar collateral laxity. My experience has been that the sagittal band on the radial side can rarely be easily separated from the underlying torn, fibrotic RCL, so incise the vertical fibers of the sagittal band along with the more distal part of the abductor aponeurosis, the entirety of which is carefully dissected from the underlying tissue. Explore the joint. Degenerative disease is a contraindication to reconstruction and should be treated with arthrodesis. Intact articular cartilage portends well for a successful reconstruction. Excise the remnants of the torn RCL. Make holes in the radial base of the proximal phalanx in the "7 o'clock" and "11 o'clock" positions. The remainder of the procedure is essentially the same as for the UCL reconstruction.

There are potential pitfalls to this technique. If the bridge of bone between the gouge holes at the base of the proximal phalanx is too narrow, it can fracture, which would be a significant problem since it would leave a gaping hole in the bone. Therefore, the holes should be started as far dorsally and volarly as possible in order to widen the bridge. If the hole is made with a hand-held gouge, the cutting edge of the instrument should be turned away from the bony bridge so that the hole is enlarged toward the dorsal and volar aspects of the bone rather than toward the midline. Bringing the ends of the tendon graft through the skin and tying them over a button causes dimpling of the skin in one-third of patients. This is aesthetically unappealing to some patients, who also do not like seeing their tendon exposed. Therefore, I have abandoned this technique.

It is very uncommon for this reconstruction to be too tight. When the tension of the reconstruction is set, the two ends of the graft should be pulled as firmly as possible and then a little tension relaxed from the maximally tight point. It is my impression that the reconstruction loosens slightly during the healing and rehabilitation process. The reconstruction can certainly be made too loose, so the surgeon must check the tightness of the joint prior to transfixing it with the K-wire. Another potential pitfall is to ignore or underestimate the degree of degeneration of the joint either preoperatively or during the procedure. A corollary of this is that the surgeon should resist being "talked into" reconstructing an osteoarthritic joint by an imploring patient who wants to retain motion. The likelihood is that the joint will deteriorate over time.

POSTOPERATIVE MANAGEMENT

The surgeon's expectations of the results of repair or reconstruction of the collateral ligaments of the thumb MP joint vary somewhat depending upon the chronicity of injury relative to the surgery. Most patients who have radial or ulnar collateral ligament repairs do quite well. It is uncommon for the ligament to not be rendered permanently stable. Instances of persistent or recurrent instability occur with extenuating circumstances like systemic ligament laxity, re-injury, or temporal relationship to the hormone changes of pregnancy. Patients occasionally have mild to moderate stiffness of the MP joint. The expectations for collateral ligament reconstruction are only slightly less optimistic. The likelihood of the joint being stable postoperatively is very high. Recurrent laxity is uncommon and tends to occur in unusual circumstances, such as those noted for repair. The joint may be slightly stiffer after repair and pinch strength slightly lower.

Patients are advised that the operation is moderately painful for the first two or three days postoperatively. They will be in a cast that ties up the thumb but allows motion of the digits. When the cast is removed they will have significant stiffness of their operated thumbs. They will need to work with a hand or occupational therapist to regain motion, and that is likely to be an arduous process. Patients undergoing either repair or reconstruction are advised that the procedure should render their injured thumb stable. On average, they regain three-quarters of the range of motion of the thumb MP joint and nearly full motion of the interphalangeal (IP) joint. Their grip strength should return to nearly normal and pinch strength should be within 85 to 90% of normal. The skin incision heals well with a faint, flat scar.

REHABILITATION

Continue cast immobilization for 4 weeks for acute UCL repairs, 5 weeks for acute RCL repairs, and 6 weeks for reconstruction of either ligament. When the cast is removed, remove the K-wire from the reconstructed thumbs. Refer both repair and reconstruction patients to the hand therapist for a thumb cone splint immobilizing only the MP joint; the IP joint is free. Begin active and gentle active-assisted range of motion. In addition to therapy sessions, advise the patient to work on active range-of-motion exercise 4 times per day, doing 10 to 12 repetitions of extension and flexion each time. Instruct UCL patients to avoid radially directed force on the tip of the thumb. Conversely, instruct RCL patients to avoid ulnarly directed force on the tip of the thumb. Eliminate the splint after 2 weeks. Patients continue to work on range-of-motion exercise and begin strengthening the hand with therapeutic putty and light gripping activities. They avoid torque and forceful resisted strengthening of the thumb until 3 months after the surgery, and then do progressive pinch and grip strengthening and light free weights. Unrestricted activity is allowed at 4 months postoperatively.

RESULTS

The results of repair of the radial and ulnar collateral ligaments of the thumb MP joint have been consistently quite good in my experience. The joint is stabilized by the procedure, and that stability holds up over time with rare exceptions. Range of motion of the MP joint is usually 85% to 90% or more of the contralateral side. Pinch and grip strength are usually very close to the contralateral, normal hand. Patients are generally able to use their thumb normally for strenuous activity requiring forceful pinch and grasp, including contact sports. The integrity of the articular cartilage also is maintained over time unless there was a significant chondral injury at the time of the initial repair.

Reconstruction of the collateral ligaments using the technique described in this chapter produces results only slightly less favorable than repair. Range of motion of the MP joint averages approximately 80% of the uninjured side. Motion of the IP joint is often limited initially postoperatively, but tends to normalize during the first month or two out of the cast. Grip strength gradually improves to close to the contralateral thumb, and pinch strength averages about 90% of the normal thumb. Patients are able to use their thumbs in an unrestricted way for all activities, including forceful pinch and grasp. None of the reconstructions that had normal or minimally degenerated cartilage required revision due to development or progression of degenerative disease.

COMPLICATIONS

Many patients develop transient hypesthesia on the dorsoulnar or dorsoradial aspects of the thumb distal to the surgical site, due to traction on the respective digital branch of the dorsal sensory branch of the radial sensory nerve. That is almost always self-limiting, resolving within a few weeks. The few patients who had persistent or recurrent instability after repair or reconstruction had specific etiologies. These included laxity soon after pregnancy, which presumably was related to peripartum hormonal changes. The oldest patient to have a UCL reconstruction also had the most severe instability preoperatively. She had significant stiffness of the MP joint postoperatively. The reconstruction was probably made too tight in an overenthusiastic effort to stabilize the grossly lax joint. The initial description of the technique involved bringing the ends of the tendon graft through a stab wound on the side of the metacarpal, tying them over a button or catheter. One-third of those patients developed a dimple where the graft penetrated the skin. In the current iteration of that part of the procedure, the tendon is tied beneath the skin. Somewhat surprisingly, this does not cause a perceptible bump beneath the skin. These patients do not develop dimpling of the skin, but do have a longer scar on the side of the thumb opposite the tear.

RECOMMENDED READINGS

1. Abrahamsson S, Sollerman C, Lundborg G, et al. Diagnosis of displaced ulnar collateral ligament of the metacarpophalangeal joint of the thumb. *J Hand Surg* 15A:457, 1990.
2. Alldred AJ. Rupture of the collateral ligament of the metacarpophalangeal joint of the thumb. *J Bone Joint Surg* 37B:443, 1955.
3. Bowers WH, Hurst LC. Gamekeepers thumb: evaluation by arthrography and stress roentgenography. *J Bone Joint Surg* 59A:519, 1977.
4. Camp RA, Weatherwax RJ, Miller EB. Chronic post-traumatic radial instability of the thumb metacarpophalangel joint. *J Hand Surg* 51:221, 1980.
5. Campbell CS. Gamekeeper's thumb. *J Bone Joint Surg* 37B:148, 1955.
6. Coonrad RW, Goldner JL. A study of the pathological findings and treatment in soft-tissue injury of the thumb metacarpophalangeal joint. *J Bone Joint Surg* 50A:439, 1968.
7. Dray GJ, Eaton RG. Dislocations and ligament injuries in the digits. In: Green DP, ed. *Operative Hand Surgery*, 2nd ed. New York: Churchill Livingstone, 1988:777–811.
8. Eaton RG. *Joint Injuries of the Hand.* Springfield, IL: Charles C. Thomas, 1971.
9. Engel J, Ganel A, Ditzian R, et al. Arthrography as a method of diagnosing tear of the ulnar collateral ligament of the metacarpophlangeal joint of the thumb (gamekeeper's thumb). *J Trauma* 19:106, 1979.
10. Frank WE, Dobyns J. Surgical pathology of collateral ligamentous injuries of the thumb. *Clin Orthop* 83:102, 1972.
11. Glickel SZ, Malerich M, Pearce SM, et al. Ligament replacement for chronic instability of the ulnar collateral ligament of the metacarpophalangeal joint of the thumb. *J Hand Surg* 18A:930, 1993.
12. Hergan K, Mittler C, Oser W. Ulnar collateral ligament: Differentiation of displaced and nondisplaced tears with ultrasound and MR imaging. *Radiology* 194:65–71, 1995.
13. Heyman P, Gelberman RH, Duncan K, et al. Injuries of the ulnar collateral ligament of the thumb metacarpophalangeal joint-biomechanical and prospective clinical studies on the usefulness of valgus stress testing. *Clin Orthop* 292:165, 1993.
14. Hoglund M, Tordai P, Muren C. Diagnosis by ultrasound of dislocated ulnar collateral ligament of the thumb. *Acta Radiologica* 36:620–625, 1995.
15. Kessler I. Complete avulsion of the ulnar collateral ligament of the metacarpophalangeal joint of the thumb. *Clin Orthop* 29:196, 1961.
16. Kessler I, Heller J. Complete avulsion of the ligamentous apparatus of the metacarpophalangeal joint of the thumb. *Surg Gynecol Obstet* 116:95, 1963.
17. Kohut G, O'Callaghan B. Gamekeeper's thumb ligament localization by echography. *Ann Chir Main* 12:252–262, 1993.
18. Neviaser RJ, Wilson JN, Lievano A. Rupture of the ulnar collateral ligament of the thumb (Gamekeeper's thumb): correction by dynamic repair. *J Bone Joint Surg* 53A:1357, 1971.
19. Osterman AL, Hayken GD, Bora FW Jr. A quantitative evaluation of thumb function after ulnar collateral repair and reconstruction. *J Trauma* 21:854, 1981.
20. Palmer AK, Louis DS. Assessing ulnar instability of the metacarpophalangeal joint of the thumb. *J Hand Surg* 3A:542, 1978.
21. Resnick D, Danzig LA. Arthrographic evaluation of injuries of the first metacarpophalangeal joint: Gamekeeper's thumb. *Am J Roentgenol* 126:1046, 1976.
22. Smith RJ. Post-traumatic instability of the metacarpal joint of the thumb. *J Bone Joint Surg* 59A:12, 1977.
23. Spaeth HJ, Abrams RA, Bock GW, et al. Gamekeeper's thumb: Differentiation of nondisplaced and displaced tears of the ulnar collateral ligament with MR imaging. *Radiology* 188:533, 1993.
24. Stener B. Displacement of the ruptured ulnar collateral ligament of the metacarpophalangeal joint of the thumb: a clinical and anatomical study. *J Bone Joint Surg* 44B:869, 1962.
25. Strandell G. Total rupture of the ulnar collateral ligament of the metcarpophalangeal joint of the thumb. *Acta Chir Scand* 118:72, 1959.

9

Surgical Treatment of Fractures of the Thumb Metacarpal Base: Bennett's and Rolando's Fractures

Keith B. Raskin and Steven S. Shin

INDICATIONS/CONTRAINDICATIONS

The thumb ray is susceptible to various injuries, which can result in unstable fracture dislocations of the carpometacarpal (CMC) joint. Two common fracture patterns of the thumb metacarpal accompanied by intra-articular extension into the CMC joint are the single fractures (Bennett's fracture) and more complex T- or Y-type fractures (Rolando's fracture). The main indication for surgical intervention of Bennett's and Rolando's fractures are grossly displaced, unstable, or irreducible fracture-subluxations of the first CMC joint.

Although there were original suggestions that these fractures may be well-suited for treatment by early unrestricted motion, without fracture reduction, there is a growing trend to follow the principles of general fracture management for articular injuries, in which accurate reduction diminishes the potential for late complications. There are several reports detailing the direct relationship between the accuracy of the articular reduction and the potential for development of posttraumatic arthritis.

Due to the multiple deforming forces at the first CMC joint, these fractures are likely to displace if left untreated. Even with accurate reduction and cast immobilization, it is essential to closely monitor these fractures during the healing phase, due to potential secondary displacement, caused by the influence of the musculotendinous forces about the thumb. Concomitant soft-tissue injuries or fractures of adjacent bones can also contribute to the need for surgical stabilization of these fractures.

Keith B. Raskin, M.D.: Department of Orthopaedic Surgery, New York University School of Medicine, New York, NY

Steven S. Shin, M.D.: Orthopaedic Surgery, New York University School of Medicine, New York, NY

In the Bennett's fracture, the thumb metacarpal shaft is displaced by the force of the abductor pollicis longus (APL) and the adductor pollicis (AP), and to a less degree by the more distally inserting extensor pollicis longus (EPL), while the volar-ulnar basilar fragment is held in its anatomic position by the anterior oblique ligament (AOL). The APL, AP, and EPL muscles tend to pull the metacarpal shaft dorsally, proximally, and radially. The same muscles are responsible for the tendency for displacement in Rolando's fractures, except the APL can also displace the dorsal-radial basilar fragment. Due to the potential for posttraumatic arthritis, accurate reduction and stable fixation are recommended.

As can be inferred, the relative contraindications for surgical treatment of these fractures are nondisplaced or stable fractures that are well-maintained with cast immobilization with less than 1 mm of displacement. Closed reduction and cast immobilization of these fractures have achieved good results, provided that there is no further displacement over time.

PREOPERATIVE PLANNING

The initial preoperative planning begins with a thorough history and physical examination. Commonly, the patient describes direct trauma to the thumb tip, either in a sports-related injury or fall. It is important to determine in the mature patient whether there is a preexisting arthritic condition so commonly identified at the basal joint. This may be described by the patient as a chronic, progressive weakness or pain with specific daily activities.

Ecchymosis surrounding the CMC region of the thumb is often present, along with an associated loss of motion and creitus on attempted movement (Fig. 9.1). In the more significantly displaced fractures, a prominence or a "shelf" deformity may be present at the base of the thumb metacarpal, due to the metacarpal shaft displacement. An open injury is uncommon. The thumb, hand, and wrist should be carefully assessed for concomitant injuries. A complete neurovascular examination is performed prior to surgical consideration. Suspicion of evolving compartment syndrome in severe injuries should be maintained.

Postero-anterior, lateral, and oblique radiographic views of the thumb are mandatory for evaluation of the fracture. Contralateral radiographs aid in determining the normal appearance of the basal joint in each patient. A traction radiograph may also be helpful in evaluating the effect of ligamentotaxis on the fracture reduction. This is best-suited for intraoperative assessment under regional or general anesthesia.

A preoperative determination for timing of the surgery is based upon the amount of associated edema. If significant soft-tissue edema is present, closed manipulation and accurate articular reduction may be compromised. I prefer to provide patients with protective thumb spica splints and instruct them on strict limb elevation. Usually, within 24 to 48

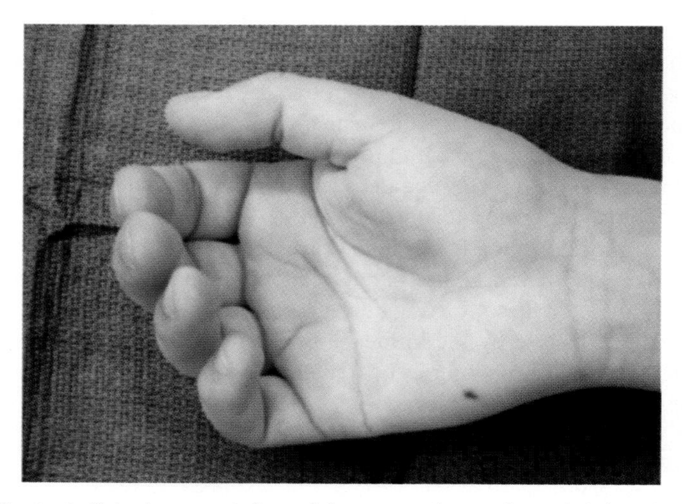

Figure 9.1. Typical clinical presentation of thenar ecchymosis and deformity at the carpometacarpal joint.

hours the edema has substantially reduced, and we can then safely proceed with the definitive reduction and fixation.

In both the Bennett's and Rolando's fracture, the goals of treatment are to restore the articular congruity at the CMC joint of the thumb, while regaining the relative position of the metacarpal shaft and articular surface with the trapezium. These goals are to be achieved with the least invasive methods. Several treatment options are currently available for Bennett's fractures, including closed reduction and percutaneous pinning; oblique pin traction and casting; open reduction and internal fixation (ORIF) with pins; ORIF with screws, and external fixation. Similar treatment options have also been described for Rolando fractures.

The least invasive surgical treatment of these fractures is closed reduction with percutaneous smooth-wire fixation. Open reduction and internal fixation should be reserved for those cases in which closed reduction is unsuccessful; a relative indication to proceed with ORIF is a fracture fragment of greater than 25–30% of the articular surface.

SURGERY

The patient is placed in a supine position and receives regional anesthesia with either general anesthesia, a proximal block (axillary, superclavicular, infraclavicular), or a wrist block (Fig. 9.2) (with or without thumb CMC infiltration) (Fig. 9.3). Intravenous sedation assists in muscular relaxation. The involved extremity is then prepped and draped in the usual sterile fashion. The arm is positioned at 90 degrees from the body on an armboard extension. Intraoperative fluoroscopy is helpful for real-time assessment of fracture reduction and fixation.

Closed Reduction with Percutaneous Pinning of Bennett's and Rolando's Fracture

Bennett's Fracture. The authors prefer closed reduction and percutaneous pinning in the majority of the Bennett's fracture during the acute phase when the fracture fragment is less than 25–30% of the articular surface. This method requires gentle longitudinal traction, abduction, and pronation of the thumb while applying direct pressure over the dorsal-radial portion of the metacarpal base (Fig. 9.4 A–C). Once the reduction has been obtained, intraoperative fluoroscopy is utilized while maintaining traction to confirm restoration of articular congruity (Fig. 9.5 A–D). A 0.045-inch smooth Kirschner wire is then inserted with power instrumentation, usually starting at the dorso-radial metacarpal shaft, in one of several configurations.

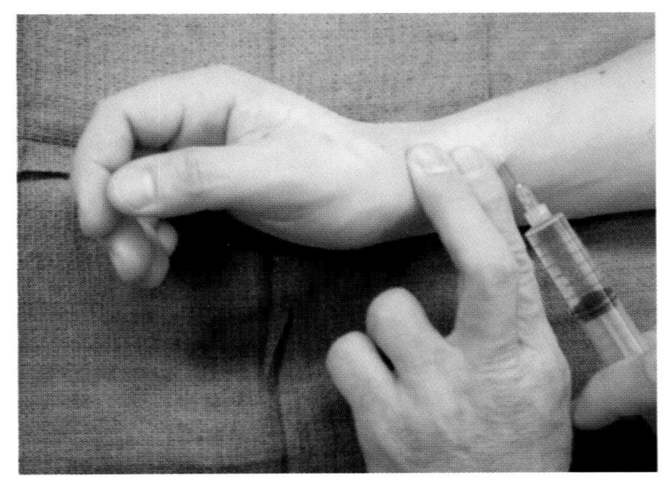

Figure 9.2. Subcutaneous local anesthesia injected for the radial nerve distribution safely performed at two fingerbreadths proximal to the radial styloid.

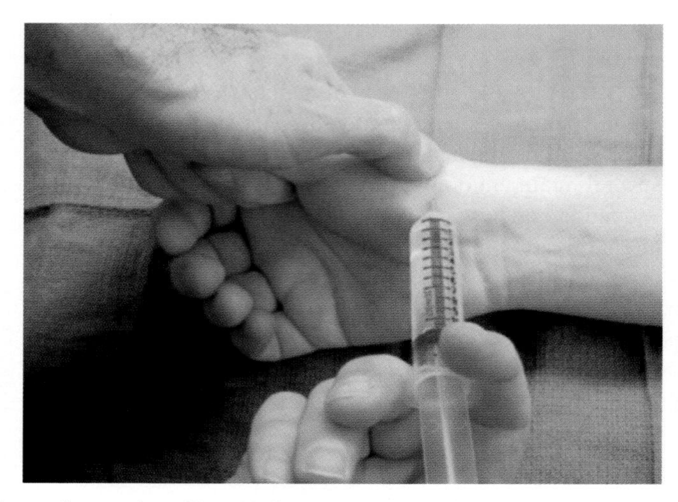

Figure 9.3. A small quantity of local infiltration into the CMC joint improves the quality of the block.

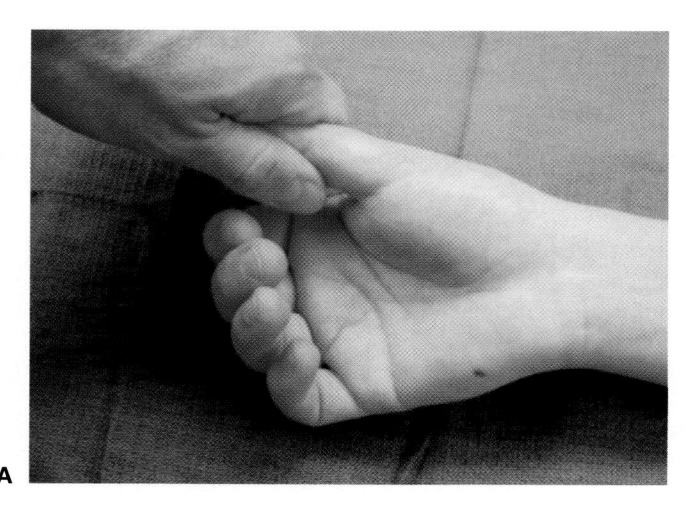

A

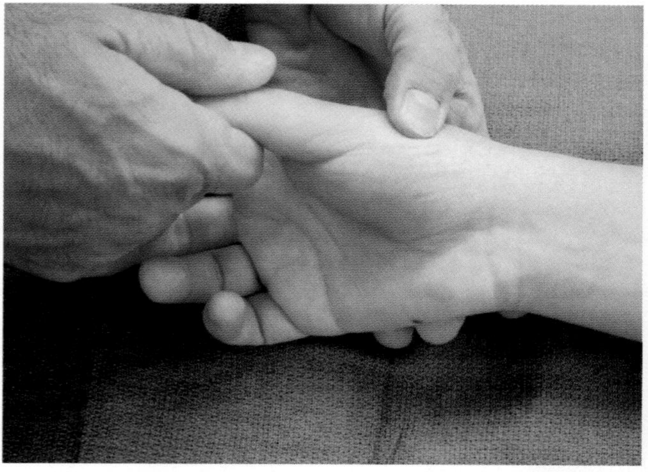

B

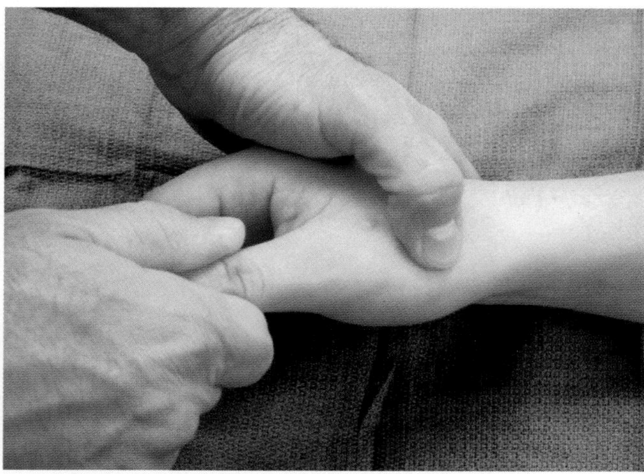

C

Figure 9.4. A: Direct longitudinal traction at the distal phalangeal level is initially preformed, followed by **(B, C)** gentle abduction and manual reduction at the fracture site.

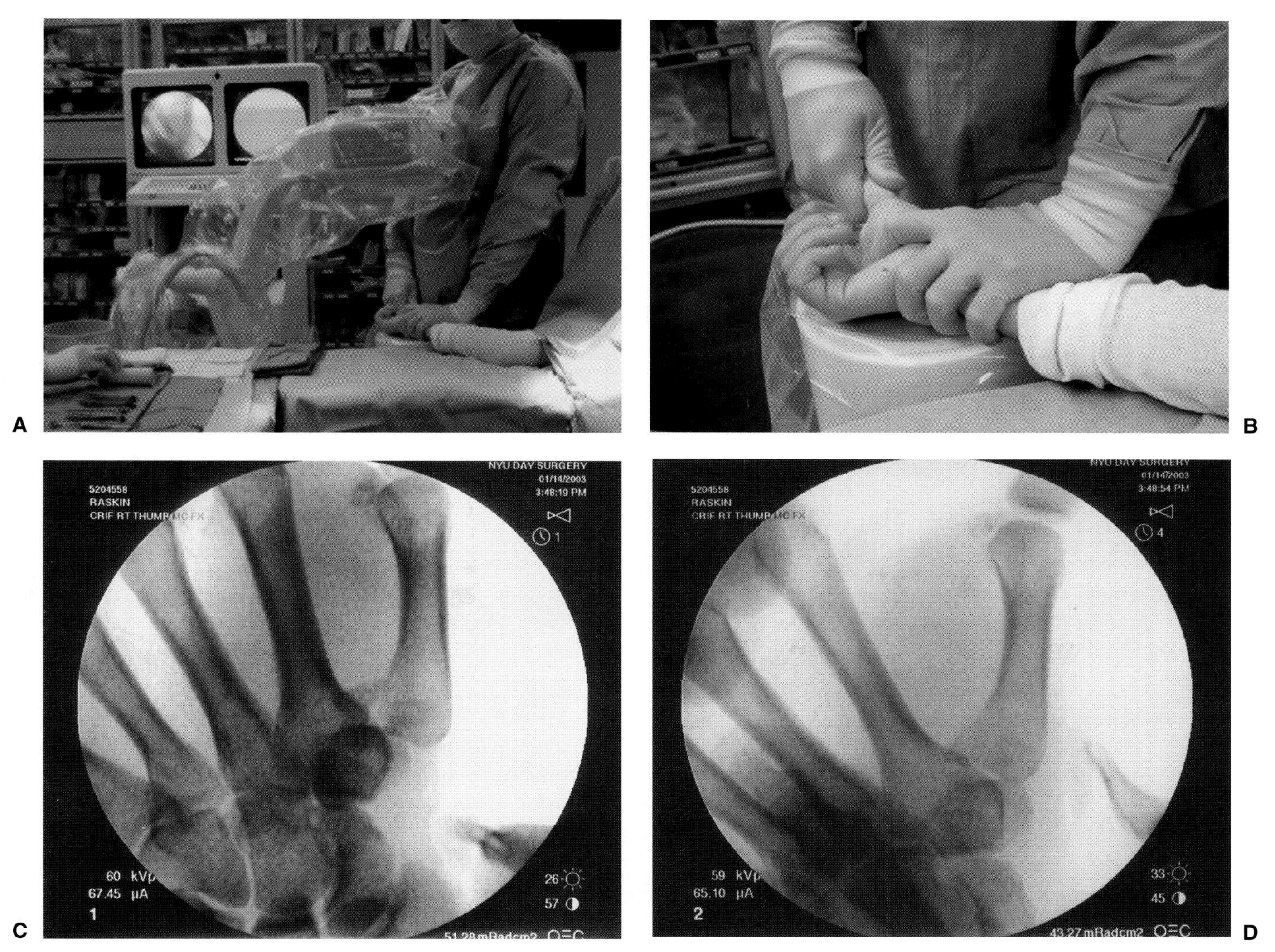

Figure 9.5. **A:** The thumb is positioned over the fluoroscopy unit with the arm positioned at 90 degrees from the body. **B:** The longitudinal traction and reduction position is maintained for fluoroscopic imaging. **C, D:** Pre and postreduction imaging at the fracture site.

The wire does not need to cross the fracture site, but should gain stability into the adjacent carpal bones and/or the index metacarpal. A second and possibly third Kirschner wire is drilled in a diverging manner to gain fracture stability in three planes (Fig 9.6 A,B). The hand is once again positioned over the fluoroscopy unit to verify reduction and fixation wire placement (Fig. 9.7 A,B). Final radiographs are assessed to determine articular alignment along with reduction of the CMC subluxation and appropriate placement of the percutaneous wires (Fig. 9.8).

If incomplete reduction of the fracture is identified, then a secondary closed reduction should be attempted prior to considering an open reduction and internal fixation of the fracture. Once successful closed reduction has been accomplished, the wires are then bent and cut outside of the skin (Fig. 9.9 A,B). An alternative method of cutting the pins beneath the skin has not been necessary due to the relatively short period of time to union in the majority of these fractures.

A well-padded thumb spica plaster splint is applied and the hand elevated in a postoperative foam pillow until the soft-tissue edema resolves. The patient is encouraged to begin active digit range-of-motion exercises during the early postoperative period (Fig. 9.10 A,B). This is followed by thumb spica cast immobilization until fracture union, usually

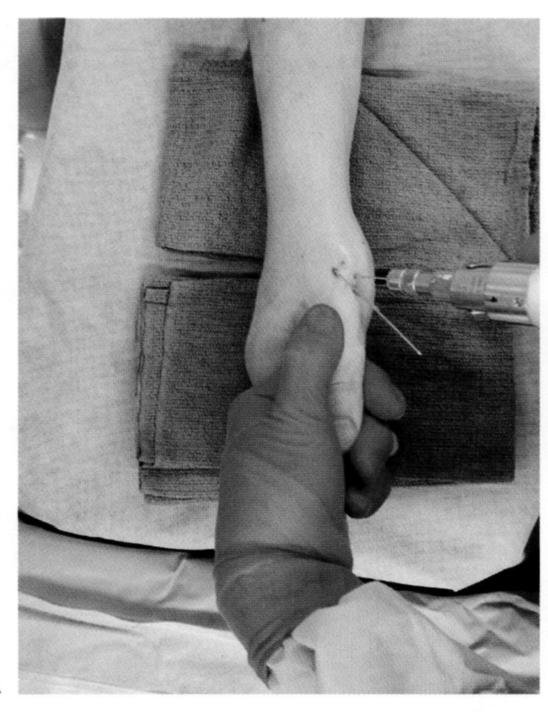

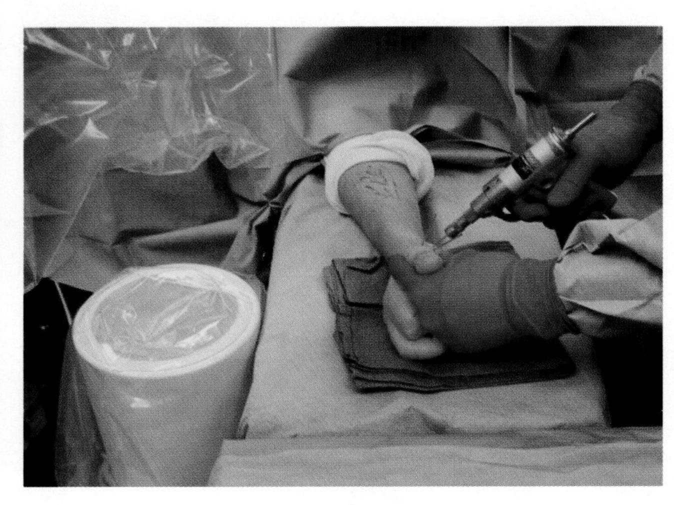

A B

Figure 9.6. A: The reduction is maintained during the wire insertion. **B:** Multiple wires are inserted in a diverting configuration.

within four to five weeks. If the fracture does not reduce adequately, of course, open reduction and internal fixation is performed.

Rolando's Fracture. If a successful closed reduction of the Rolando's fracture can be achieved under fluoroscopic guidance, percutaneous pinning is an equally accepted form of fixation. The classic T- or Y-type fractures, with larger fragments, are more amenable to closed reduction and pinning. Similar maneuvers to closed reduction of the Bennett's fracture are used in the reduction of this fracture. One or two Kirschner wires are then placed through the basilar fragments to restore the articular surface. The reduced metacarpal base can then be secured to the metacarpal shaft with additional Kirschner wires placed in a similar manner to that described for Bennett's fractures. After confirmation of adequate reduction and internal fixation of the fracture, a similar postoperative thumb spica splint is applied.

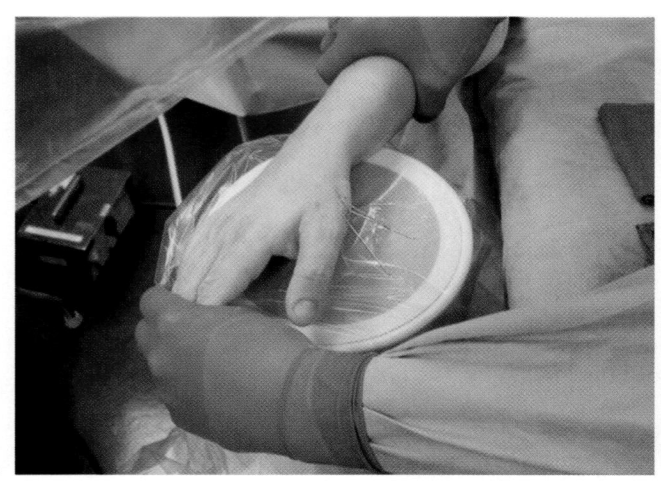

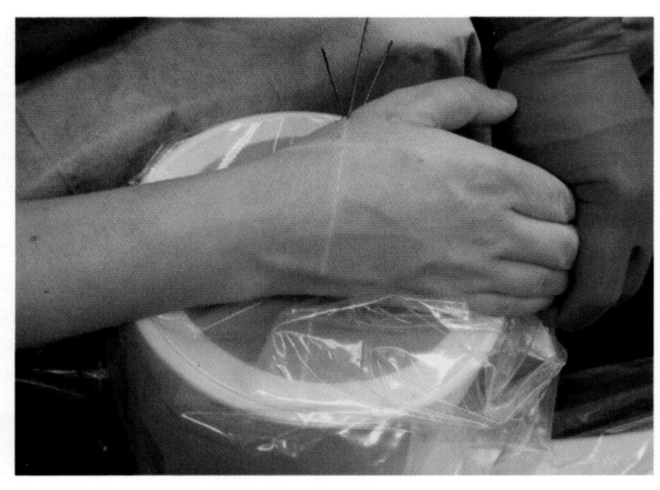

A B

Figure 9.7. A, B: The hand is once again positioned over the fluoroscopy unit for P/A, lateral, and oblique views.

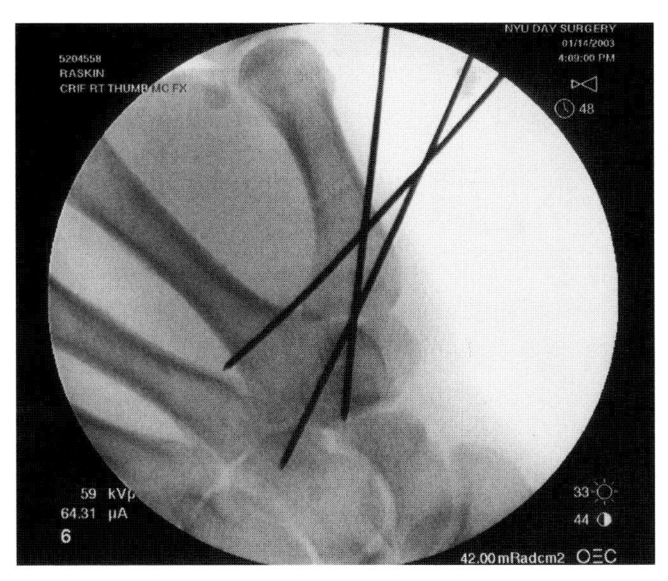

Figure 9.8. Final lateral radiograph demonstrating restored articular congruity with reduction of CMC subluxation, along with appropriate wire placement.

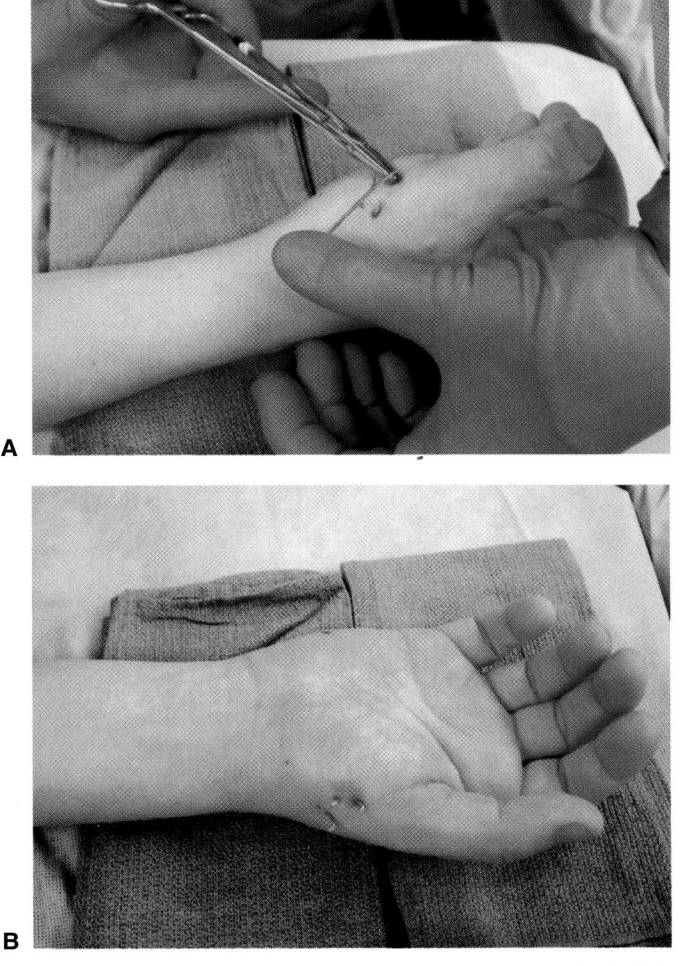

Figure 9.9. **A:** The wires are bent and cut outside the skin. **B:** The final clinical appearance.

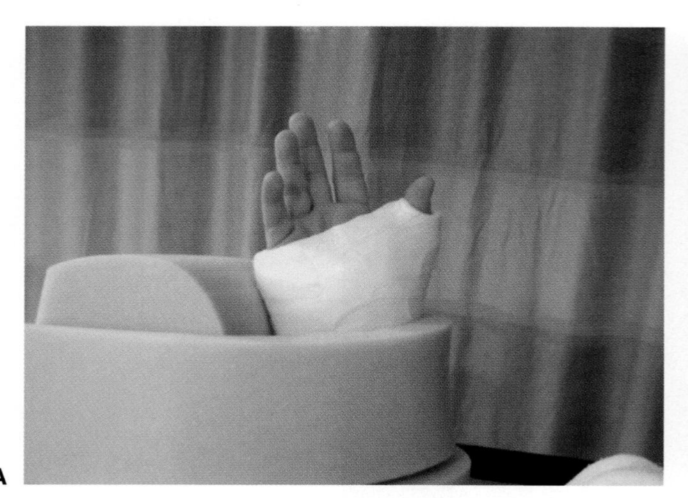

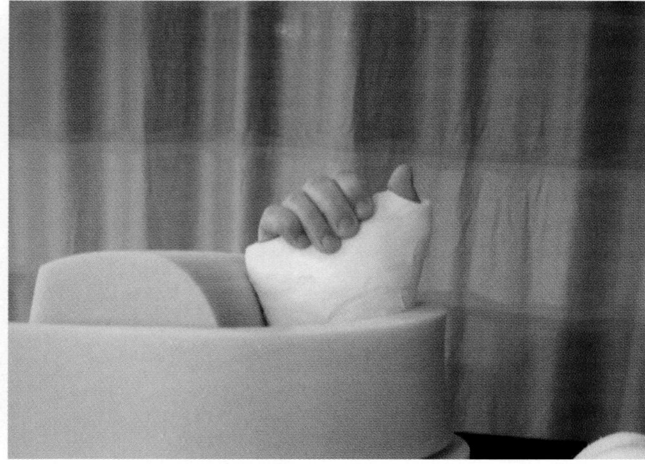

Figure 9.10. A, B: The immediate postoperative elevated position of the hand, with active digit range of motion.

Open Reduction and Internal Fixation of Bennett's and Rolando's Fracture

Bennett's Fracture. The authors recommend ORIF of the Bennett's fracture when the fracture fragment is larger than 25–30% of the articular surface or if unreducible by closed methods. A Wagner approach is used through an incision on the dorsal-radial aspect about the glaborous border over the CMC joint and curved volarly to the distal wrist crease up to the flexor carpi radialis tendon. Care is taken to avoid injury to the palmar cutaneous branch of the median nerve. The thenar muscles are carefully reflected extraperiosteally from the volar aspect of the trapezium and proximal metacarpal. A longitudinal capsulotomy is then made to expose the CMC joint. All soft-tissue attachments to the fragments should be preserved.

A tenaculum or dental pick may be used to reduce the fracture, and K-wires are placed in a dorsal to volar direction to maintain the reduction. A small 1.5- to 2.7-mm compression screw can be used in lag configuration for fracture fixation if the fragments are large enough (Fig. 9.11 A,B). The incision is then repaired with absorbable deep sutures

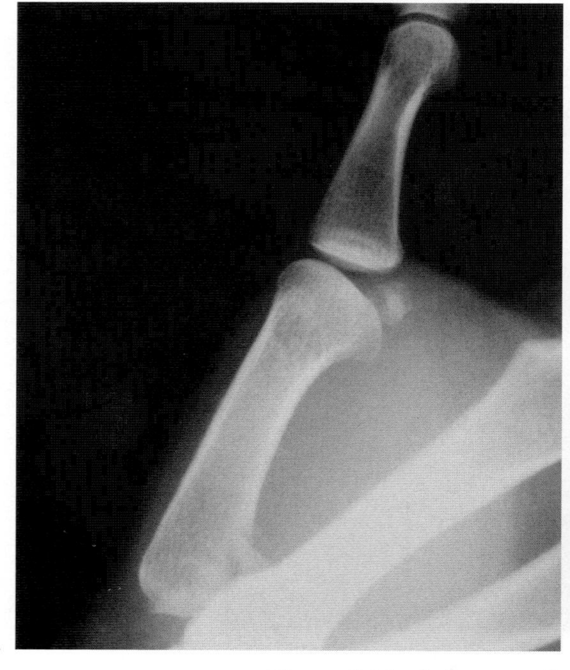

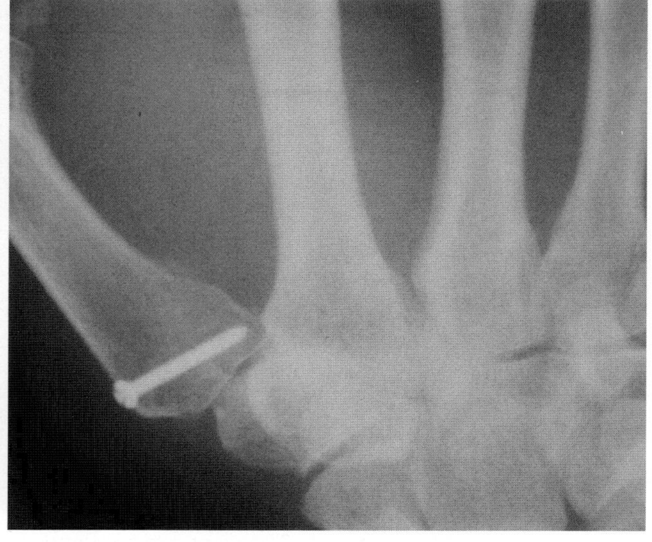

Figure 9.11. A: Preoperative radiograph of a displaced Bennett's fracture involving 25% of the articular surface. **B:** Long-term postoperative radiograph of the Bennett's fracture healed with restored congruity and intact lag compression screw.

and 5-0 nylon sutures for the skin layer. A postoperative thumb spica splint is then applied.

Special consideration is made for those complex fractures associated with concomitant trapezial body fractures. The articular surface of the trapezium should be reduced and stabilized prior to reduction and fixation of the metacarpal articular fracture. These fractures are often well-suited for intrafragmentary compression screw fixation (Fig. 9.12 A–E).

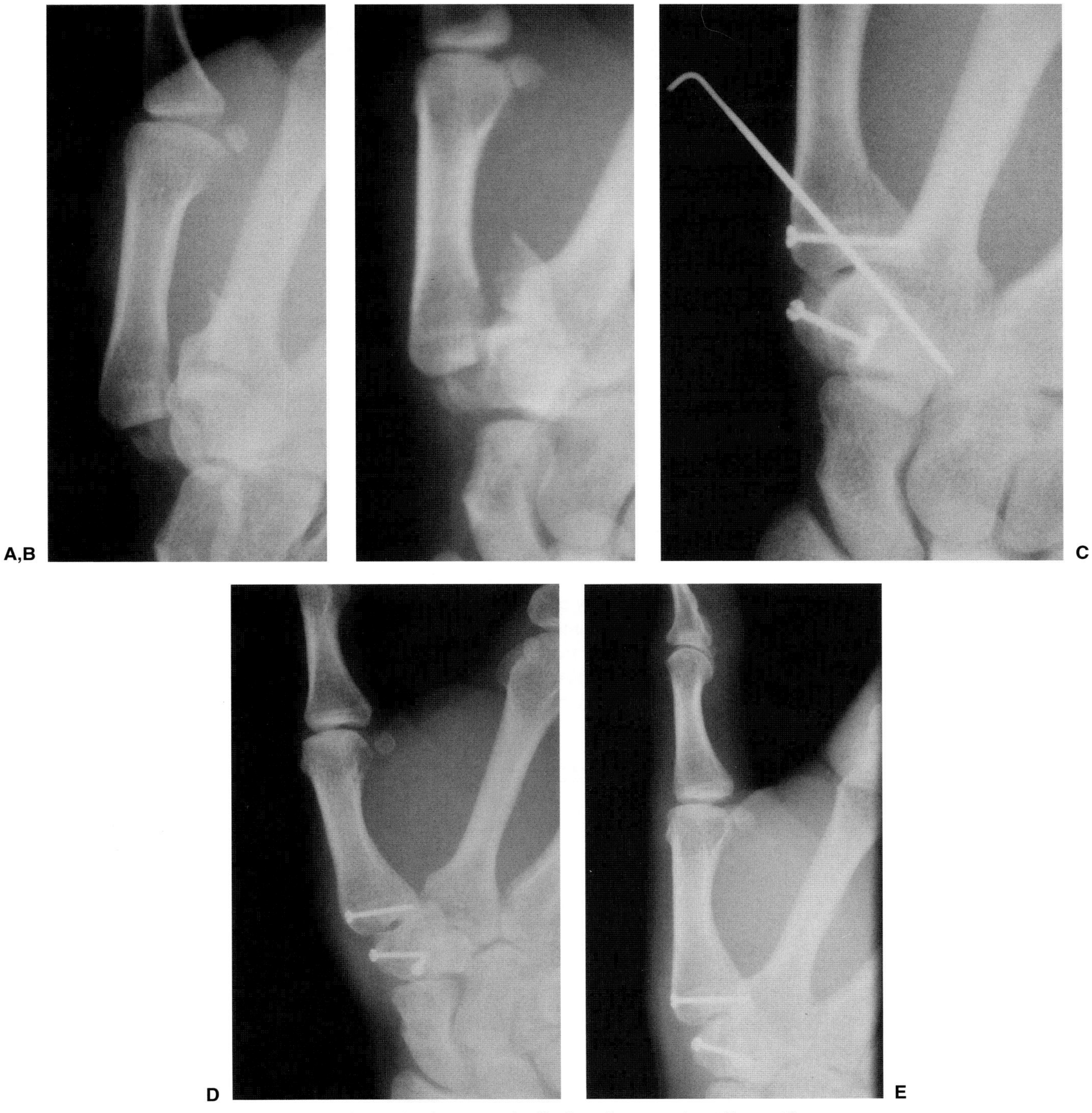

Figure 9.12. A, B: Preoperative radiograph of a severely displaced concomitant Bennett's fracture and trapezial body fracture. **C:** Immediate postoperative and **D, E:** Long-term follow-up radiograph demonstrating restored alignment without post-traumatic arthritis.

Rolando's Fracture. A similar approach as described above for the Bennett's fracture is used for Rolando's fractures. The radial end of the incision may be extended distally along the thumb metacarpal shaft. Sensory branches of the radial nerve should be protected. Open reduction and Kirschner wire fixation alone may be sufficient to achieve and maintain an anatomic reduction. However, plate fixation may be preferable if two large basilar fragments are present. The fracture is reduced and provisionally fixed with a Kirschner wire. Then a small 2.0- to 2.7-mm T- or L-plate can be placed along the thumb metacarpal, with the transverse portion of the plate on the basilar fragments. Lag screws can then be inserted through the holes of the transverse portion of the plate and offset laterally in the holes to provide for fragmentary compression. The fracture pattern may require a lag screw placed outside of the plate. The stabilized articular fragments can now be reduced and secure through the plate to the intact portion of the metacarpal shaft. The incision site is repaired and thumb spica splint immobilization applied.

POSTOPERATIVE MANAGEMENT

Bennett's Fracture

The splint is removed for pin site inspection at one week and is replaced with a thumb spica cast until fracture union, commonly identified at four to six weeks postoperatively. The pins can then be removed and hand therapy instituted along with intermittent protective immobilization in a removable thumb spica splint for two to four more weeks. If screw fixation is used, active range of motion and intermittent splinting can be initiated at one to two weeks in a compliant patient.

Rolando's Fracture

For fractures treated with closed reduction and percutaneous pinning, the thumb spica splint may be removed at one week for pin inspection. The splint is then replaced with a thumb spica cast and worn for three to five more weeks, at which point the pins may be removed if there is radiographic evidence of healing. A removable splint is intermittently worn outdoors for two to four more weeks, during which time active range of motion is advanced as tolerated.

For fractures treated with stable plate fixation, a removable splint is worn for four to six weeks and active range of motion begun within the first or second week.

REHABILITATION

After completion of healing of the CMC fracture dislocation, a removable orthoplast thumb spica splint is worn for comfort as a therapy program is followed. The thumb range of motion is restored through a progressive program of opposition to the digits along with retropulsion exercises. As the motion is recovered, strengthening exercises are performed. The patient is weaned from the splint over a period of several weeks.

RESULTS

The majority of patients with Bennett's and Rolando's fractures experience a successful recovery after surgical intervention. It is uncommon for patients to require further surgery for a malunion, residual stiffness, instability, or post-traumatic arthritis after the recommended management. The predictable outcome from appropriate treatment of this injury in an otherwise healthy patient is a full functional recovery. If there is an underlying history of pre-existing basal joint osteoarthritis, there is an increased risk of progression requiring reconstructive surgery in the future.

COMPLICATIONS OF BENNETT'S AND ROLANDO'S FRACTURES

If the intra-articular fracture is not adequately reduced, the resulting malunion, if associated with a persistent subluxation, may progress to arthritis of the first CMC joint. A corrective osteotomy of the thumb metacarpal has been described to correct the malunion, assuming it is recognized before degenerative changes of the joint are observed. Once degenerative arthritis has developed, arthrodesis or arthroplasty of the first CMC joint may be necessary. Nonunion of the thumb metacarpal base is extremely rare.

RECOMMENDED READING

1. Blum L. The treatment of Bennett's fracture-dislocation of the first metacarpal bone. *J Bone Joint Surg* 23: 578–580, 1941.
2. Breen TF, Gelberman RH, Jupiter JB. Intra-articular fractures of the basilar joint of the thumb. *Hand Clin* 4: 491–501, 1988
3. Foster RJ, Hastings H II. Treatment of Bennett, Rolando, and vertical intra-articular trapezial fractures. *Clin Orthop* 214:121–129, 1987
4. Gedda KO. Studies on Bennett's fracture: anatomy, roentgenology, and therapy. *Acta Chir Scand Suppl* 193, 1954.
5. Gedda KO, Moberg E. Open reduction and osteosynthesis of the so-called Bennett's fracture in the carpometacarpal joint of the thumb. *Acta Orthop Scand* 22:249–257, 1953.
6. Gelberman RH, Vance RM, Zakaib GS. Fracture of the base of the thumb: treatment with oblique traction. *J Bone Joint Surg* 61A:260–262, 1979.
7. Giachino AA. A surgical technique to treat a malunited symptomatic Bennett's fracture. *J Hand Surg* 21A: 149, 1996.
8. Griffiths JC. Fractures of the base of the first metacarpal bone. *J Bone Joint Surg* 46B:712–719, 1964
9. Heim U, Pfeiffer KM. Small Fragment Set Manual. *Internal Fixation of Small Fractures*. 2nd ed. New York: Springer-Verlag, 1982.
10. Hughes AW. Bennett's fractures fixed using the Herbert scaphoid screw. *J R Coll Surg Edinb* 30:231–233, 1985.
11. Johnson EC. Fractures of the base of the thumb: a new method of fixation. *JAMA* 126:27–28, 1944.
12. Kjaar-Petersen K, Langhoff O, Andersen K. Bennett's fracture. *J Hand Surg* 15B:58–61, 1990.
13. Livesley PJ. The conservative management of Bennett's fracture-dislocation: a 26-year follow-up. *J Hand Surg* 3B:291–294, 1990.
14. Oosterbos CJM, De Beor HH. Nonoperative treatment of Bennett's fracture: a 13-year follow-up. *J Orthop Trauma* 9:23–27, 1995.
15. Pollen AG. The conservative treatment of Bennett's fracture-subluxation of the thumb metacarpal. *J Bone Joint Surg* 50B:90–101, 1968.
16. Proubasta, IR. Rolando's fracture of the first metacarpal. *J Bone Joint Surg* 74B:416–417, 1992.
17. Ruedi TP, Burri C, Pfeiffer KM. Stable internal fixation of fractures of the hand. *J Trauma* 11:381–389, 1971.
18. Salgeback S, Eiken O, Carsam N, et al. A study of Bennett's fracture. *Scand J Plast Reconstr Surg* 5: 142–148, 1971.
19. Segmuller G. *Surgical Stabilization of the Skeleton of the Hand*. Baltimore: Williams & Wilkins, 1977.
20. Spanberg O, Thoren L. Bennett's fracture. A new method of treatment with oblique traction. *J Bone Joint Surg* 45B:732–736, 1963.
21. Stern PJ. Fractures of the Metacarpals and Phalanges. In: Green DP, ed. *The Operative Hand Surgery*. Philadelphia: Harcourt Health Sciences, 1999.
22. Thoren L. A new method of extension treatment in Bennett's fracture. *Acta Chir Scand* 110:485–492, 1955.
23. Thurston AJ, Dempsey SM. Bennett's fracture. A medium- to long-term review. *Aust N Z J Surg* 63:120–123, 1993.
24. Van Niekerk JLM, Ouwens R. Fractures of the base of the first metacarpal bone: results of surgical treatment. *Injury* 20:359–362, 1989.
25. Wagner CJ. Methods of treatment of Bennett's fracture-dislocation. *Am J Surg* 80:230–231, 1950.
26. Wagner CJ. Trans-articular fixation of fracture-dislocation of the first metacarpal-carpal joint. *West J Surg Obstet Gynecol* 59:362–365, 1951.
27. Wiggins HE, Bundens WD Jr, Park BJ. A method of treatment of fracture dislocations of the first metacarpal bone. *J Bone Joint Surg* 36A:810–819, 1954.

PART III

The Pediatric Hand

10

Fixation of Fractures in the Child's Hand

Donald S. Bae and Peter M. Waters

INTRODUCTION

Children use their hands to explore their environment and participate in play and sports activities. For these reasons, fractures of the hand are common in skeletally immature patients. While most children's hand fractures can be treated nonoperatively, a small percentage of hand injuries account for the majority of unfavorable outcomes. These fractures require careful surgical treatment to promote optimal healing, improved appearance, and prevent long-term functional compromise.

Several principles germinal to the care of skeletally immature patients should be followed. First, unique characteristics of the physis, or growth plate, must be understood. Physeal fractures constitute approximately one-third of pediatric hand fractures. Although children have the advantage of bony remodeling with growth, maximal remodeling occurs in the plane of joint motion. Furthermore, the remodeling potential is greater in younger patients and in fractures located adjacent to the physis.

Conversely, epiphyseal injuries and coronal or rotational deformities have little remodeling potential. Surgical approaches and fracture fixation, when possible, should not violate the physis to avoid the complications of growth disturbance. This is typically accomplished with periosteal sutures or fine, smooth wires that do not cross the growth plate.

The small size of structures in the child's hand presents another challenge. Given the generous amount of subcutaneous soft tissue, deformity may be more subtle and palpation and reduction maneuvers less precise. Furthermore, the tissue available for fixation or repair is more tenuous than in adults.

Finally, postoperative mobilization must be more restrictive in children, who may not comply with postoperative activity restrictions. Casts are more frequently utilized, with in-

Donald S. Bae, M.D.: Orthopaedic Surgery, Harvard Medical School, Boston, MA, and Department of Orthopaedic Surgery, Children's Hospital Boston, Boston, MA
Peter M. Waters, M.D.: Orthopaedic Surgery, Children's Hospital, Boston, MA

corporation of adjacent fingers, the whole hand, and/or the elbow to prevent the loss of immobilization and/or secondary displacement. Postoperative stiffness is not as prevalent as in adults, and with proper surgical techniques, fracture nonunion is rare.

Rather than provide a comprehensive review of pediatric hand fractures, this chapter will focus on three specific injuries in the skeletally immature hand requiring surgical treatment. Emphasis will be placed on surgical technique, postoperative care, and the avoidance of complications. Throughout the discussion, underlying principles of fracture care in the pediatric patient population will be highlighted.

SALTER-HARRIS III FRACTURE OF THE PROXIMAL PHALANX OF THE THUMB

Indications/Contraindications

Salter-Harris III fractures are intra-articular and usually not amenable to closed reduction (Fig. 10.1). Salter-Harris III fractures of the proximal phalanx of the thumb represent the pediatric equivalent of the adult "gamekeeper's thumb." Given the strength of the ulnar collateral ligament relative to the physis, a radially directed force to the metacarpophalangeal (MCP) joint will typically result in an avulsion fracture of the proximal phalangeal epiphysis. Displaced Salter-Harris III fractures of the proximal phalanx of the thumb require open reduction and internal fixation to restore articular congruity, joint stability, and physeal alignment.

Preoperative Planning

Patients and/or parents will describe a radially directed force imparted to the thumb, typically during sports participation or a fall. Physical examination reveals tenderness and swelling at the ulnar base of the proximal phalanx. Laxity with radial stress may be elicited. Gentle examination techniques are required in the acute setting, particularly in the younger, anxious child. Plain anteroposterior (AP) and lateral radiographs of the thumb will confirm the diagnosis. In cases in which there is laxity with radial stress and negative radiographs, one can conclude that there has been an injury to the ulnar collateral ligament of the thumb MCP joint.

Surgery

Patients are positioned supine with the affected extremity placed on a radiolucent hand table (Fig. 10.2). A well-padded tourniquet is placed on the upper brachium, and the entire extremity is prepped and draped after the induction of general anesthesia. The limb is exsanguinated with an Esmark bandage and the tourniquet is raised to 250 mm Hg.

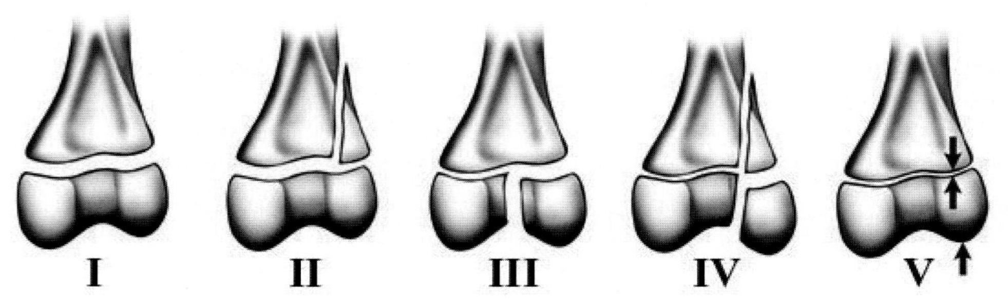

Figure 10.1. Salter-Harris classification of physeal fractures.

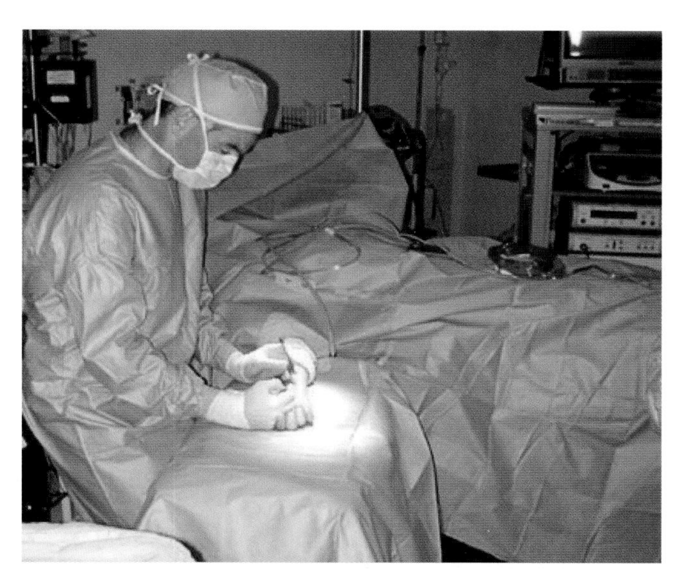

Figure 10.2. Intraoperative positioning of the patient. The entire upper extremity is prepped and draped after application of an upper extremity pneumatic tourniquet. A radiolucent arm table is utilized; alternatively, the collecting plate of a fluoroscopy unit may be used to support the limb in very young patients.

An incision is made over the dorsal-ulnar aspect of the thumb MCP joint (Fig. 10.3). Subcutaneous dissection is performed in line with the skin incision, protecting the radial sensory nerve. The adductor pollicis fascia is released from its insertion on the extensor tendon. As the ulnar collateral ligament is usually intact, the MCP joint should be exposed through the fracture site. The ligament should not be divided. If better visualization of the articular surface is necessary, the dorsal capsule may be incised.

A 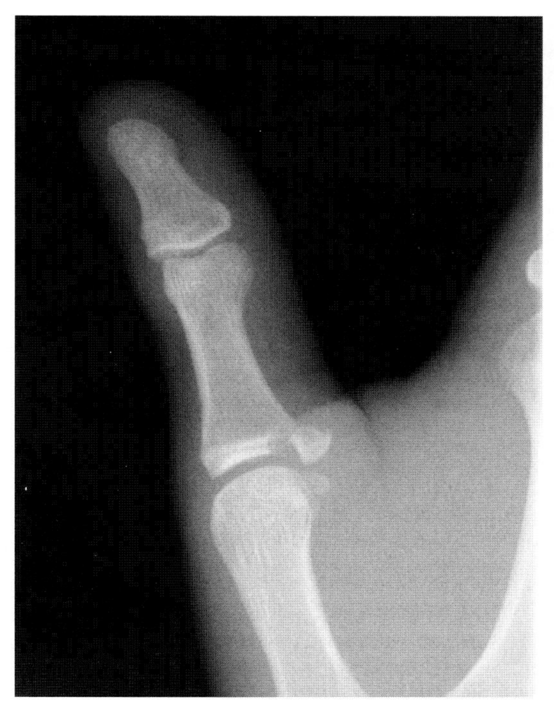

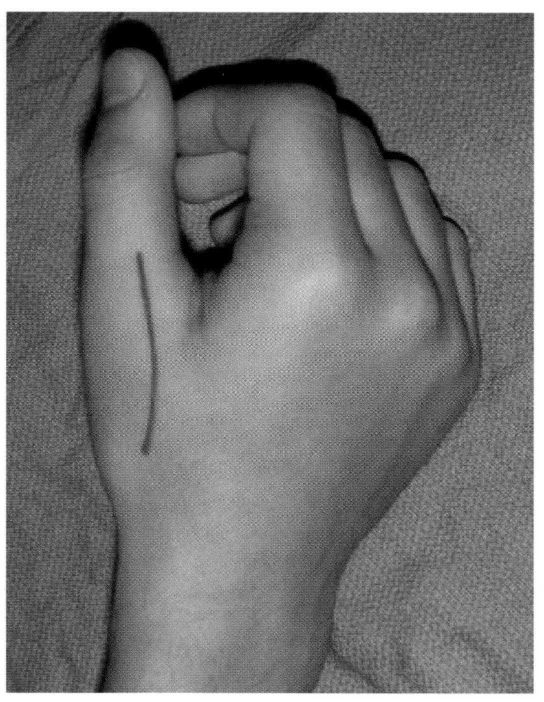 B

Figure 10.3. Salter-Harris III fracture of the proximal phalanx of the thumb. **A:** Preoperative radiograph demonstrating a displaced Salter-Harris III fracture of the proximal phalanx of the thumb. **B:** Planned surgical incision over the dorsoulnar aspect of the thumb MCP joint.

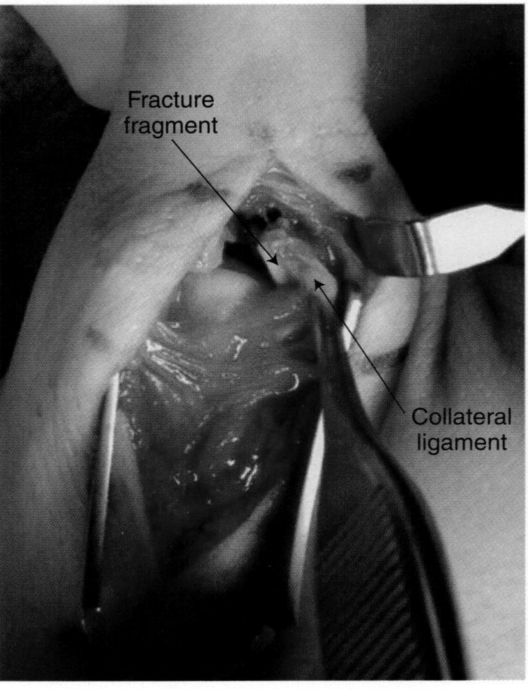

C,D

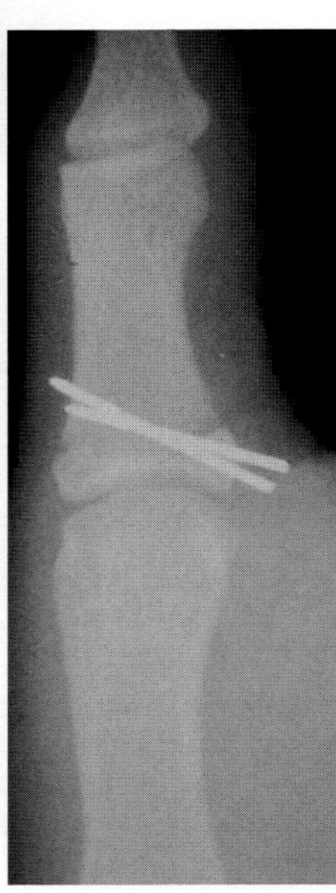

E

Figure 10.3. *Continued.* **C:** Superficial exposure of the adductor fascia, held in forceps, and the extensor mechanism, exposed by a retractor. **D:** Displaced fracture fragment. Note the intact ulnar collateral ligament, held by forceps. The fracture fragment is indicated by the arrow. **E:** Postoperative radiographs demonstrating anatomic reduction and pin fixation.

After cleaning and irrigating the fracture site, carefully reduce the avulsed epiphyseal fracture fragment. Place two parallel or slightly divergent smooth Kirschner (K-) wires into the reduced epiphyseal fragment, across the fracture site, and into the opposite radial cortex. Intraoperative fluoroscopy is helpful to confirm anatomic reduction and appropriate placement of the wires (Fig. 10.3). If the ulnar collateral ligament is noted to be lax or avulsed, its insertion may be advanced or repaired with fine absorbable sutures to the underlying periosteum. The tourniquet is released and adequate hemostasis achieved. We prefer to bend and cut the wires superficial to the skin. Perform a layered closure, carefully reapproximating the adductor pollicis fascia. Care must be made to avoid suturing the extensor mechanism to the underlying joint capsule, which may interfere with thumb flexion. The skin is closed with 4-0 absorbable suture in a subcuticular fashion. A bulky dressing and thumb spica cast is then applied.

Postoperative Management and Rehabilitation

Patients remain in the thumb spica cast for 4 to 6 weeks until radiographic evidence of fracture healing. After this time, the cast is discontinued and the smooth wires are removed, usually in the office setting without the need for anesthesia. Range-of-motion and strengthening exercises are begun with a home program. A protective splint for potential traumatic activities is utilized until full motion and strength are achieved, which almost always occurs by 8 to 12 weeks postoperatively. At that time, unrestricted activities are performed.

Results

With prompt diagnosis and appropriate treatment, using the techniques described here, patients may expect full recovery of thumb MCP range of motion and stability. To our knowledge, there have been no peer-reviewed publications reporting the results of surgical treatment of Salter-Harris III fractures of the proximal phalanx of the thumb. However, our experience with this technique has been universally successful, with patients returning to activities as tolerated.

Complications

Failure of diagnosis or inadequate treatment may result in an incongruent or unstable joint, both of which may lead to pain and limitations of strength, motion, and function. Nonunion, MCP joint instability, and/or posttraumatic arthrosis are the risks of nonoperative treatment of a displaced fracture. In the absence of MCP joint arthrosis, nonunions may be treated with open reduction, bone grafting, and internal fixation. Small fracture fragments may be excised with ulnar collateral ligament advancement and repair. Persistent instability secondary to ligamentous injury is treated with ulnar collateral ligament reconstruction. In the setting of arthrosis, MCP joint arthrodesis may be used as a salvage procedure.

PHALANGEAL NECK FRACTURE

Indications/Contraindications

Also known as subcapital or subcondylar, phalangeal neck fractures almost exclusively occur in children, usually due to crush injury of the digit in a closing door or swing. The distal fragment is often rotated and displaced in extension as the patient attempts to draw the hand away. The middle phalanx is involved more frequently than the proximal phalanx, and the border digits are most affected. As the phalangeal condyles are not completely ossified in younger patients, these injuries often present with innocuous-appearing radiographs, sometimes characterized as only a small fleck or "cap" of bone. For this reason, a high index of suspicion must be maintained and radiographs carefully reviewed to prevent missed diagnoses.

Al-Qattan has recently classified these fractures into three types: type I are nondisplaced; type II are displaced with some bone-to-bone contact; and type III are completely displaced without any bony apposition. Type II and III fractures have little remodeling potential, are prone to nonunion, and are at high risk for secondary displacement after closed reduction alone. These fractures should be treated with closed or open reduction and pin fixation.

Preoperative Planning

Patients with phalangeal neck fractures present with pain and limited motion after a crush and withdrawal injury. AP radiographs of the hand may demonstrate subtle findings, and a true lateral radiograph of the affected digit is critical to make the correct diagnosis and assess for rotational deformity (Fig. 10.4). Oblique radiographs may be the most helpful views to demonstrate or characterize this pattern of injury.

Surgery

Patients are positioned, prepped, and draped as previously described. Closed reduction is performed with longitudinal distraction, followed by hyperflexion of the interphalangeal (IP) joint and volar-directed pressure on the distal fracture fragment. Radial-ulnar angulation and malrotation are corrected at the same time. With fluoroscopic guidance maintaining the involved IP joint in flexion, crossed K-wires (usually 0.035) are inserted at the

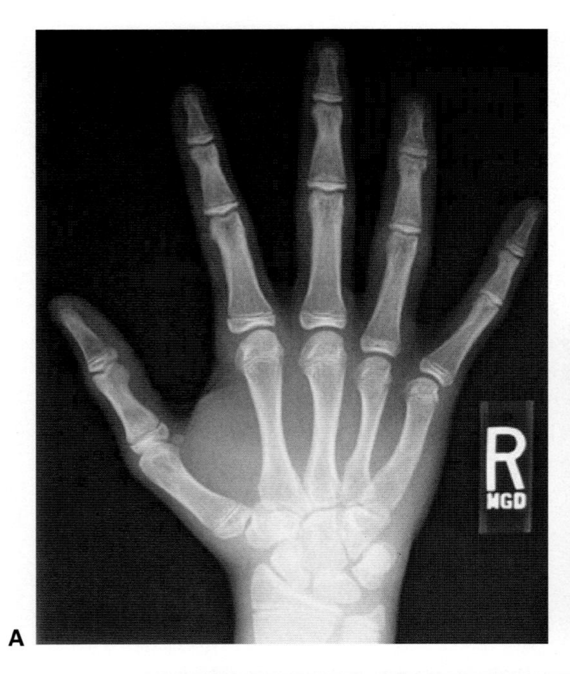

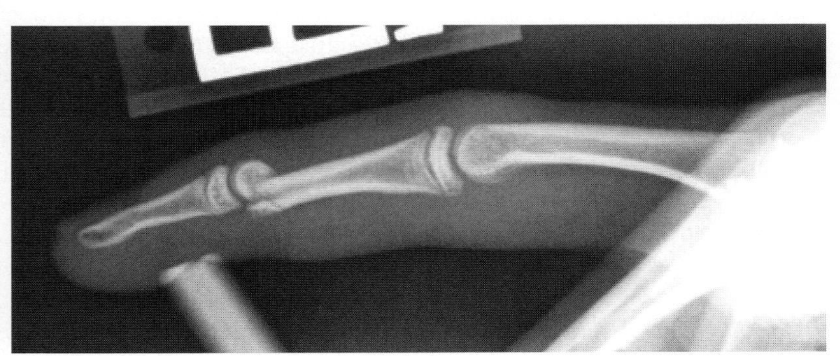

A

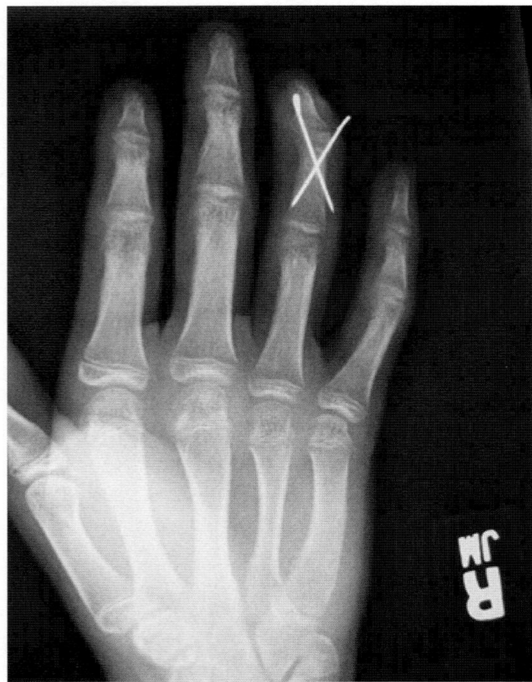

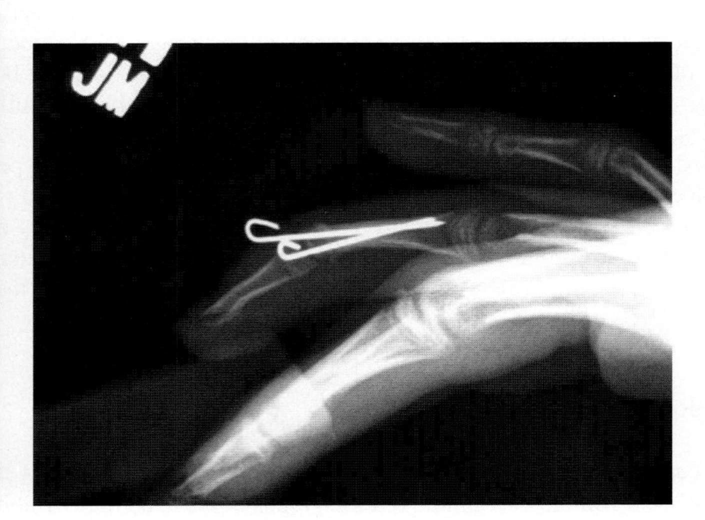

B

Figure 10.4. Phalangeal neck fracture. **A:** Preoperative AP and lateral radiographs demonstrating a displaced phalangeal neck fracture of the ring finger middle phalanx. **B:** Intraoperative AP and lateral radiographs demonstrating anatomic reduction and percutaneous pin fixation.

collateral recesses and passed across the fracture site, engaging the opposite cortex. K-wires should not cross at the fracture site (Fig. 10.4). Careful attention is made not to pass wires through the proximal articular surface or physis. Wire placement and fracture stability are confirmed fluoroscopically. If adequate reduction and fixation are achieved, the wires are left protruding through the skin and the hand is immobilized in a cast extending to the fingertips.

If adequate reduction cannot be achieved by closed manipulation, open reduction should be performed. We prefer a dorsal approach, mobilizing the lateral bands volarly and the extensor mechanism dorsally, to gain access to the phalangeal neck. Alternatively, a midaxial incision may be utilized. Soft-tissue attachments to the fracture fragment are preserved to prevent disruption of the vascular supply and subsequent osteonecrosis. Once the reduction is performed, percutaneous pinning and cast immobilization may be performed as described above.

Postoperative Management

Patients are casted until 4 weeks postoperatively, at which time the K-wires are removed and gentle range-of-motion exercises are begun. It is important to maintain fixation for 4 weeks, as premature K-wire removal may predispose to secondary displacement.

Results

With prompt diagnosis and appropriate treatment, patients may expect almost universal fracture healing and good to excellent functional results. Our results are consistent with those reported by Al-Qattan and others. Timely treatment, anatomic reduction of fracture fragments, and secure fixation and cast immobilization for 4 weeks are the keys to achieving good functional results.

Complications

Loss of motion is a common complication of phalangeal neck fractures in the skeletally immature patient. This is usually secondary to late presentation with either an incipient or established dorsal malunion and bony formation within the subcondylar fossa (Fig. 10.5). If detected before the fracture has completely united in a malrotated or displaced position, percutaneous pin osteoclasis may be performed. A smooth wire is inserted percutaneously into the fracture site through the fracture callus under fluoroscopic guidance. If malunion has occurred, patients may require a subcondylar fossa reconstruction to regain IP flexion (Fig. 10.5). Loss of extension may also occur, particularly with dorsal approaches, if the extensor mechanism is not carefully handled and preserved.

Osteonecrosis of the phalangeal head is another potential complication. The distal fracture fragment is small, can be predominantly cartilaginous, and has a tenuous blood supply. For this reason, it is critical to maintain ligamentous attachments, avoid excessive manipulation, and minimize trauma to the articular fragment during the reduction and passage of K-wires.

EXTRAPHYSEAL PHALANGEAL FRACTURE

Indications/Contraindications

Extraphyseal fractures of the phalanges are not as common as physeal fractures. The fracture pattern and forces imparted by the adjacent musculotendinous units dictate the subsequent deformity and displacement. In general, up to 20 degrees of angulation in the plane of digital motion may remodel with growth, although this is dependent upon patient age and fracture location. Coronal and rotational displacements, however, have poor remodeling potential. Furthermore, small fracture fragment size and interposed periosteum and/or soft tissue may preclude closed reduction. For these reasons, extraphyseal phalangeal fractures with greater than 20 degrees of sagittal angulation or any coronal or rotational displacement should be reduced and internally stabilized. Extreme care

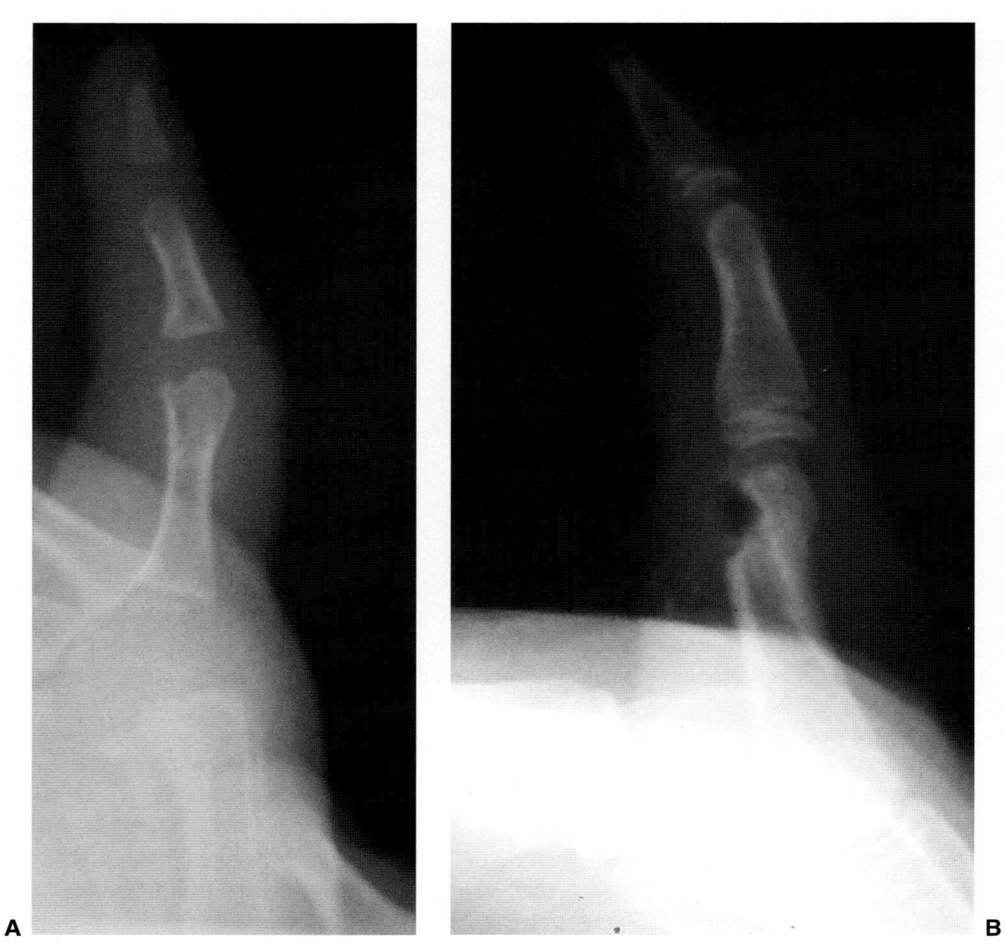

Figure 10.5. Phalangeal neck fracture malunion. **A:** Lateral radiograph demonstrating a proximal phalangeal neck fracture malunion with significant bony formation within the subcondylar fossa. **B:** Lateral radiograph after subcondylar fossa reconstruction.

and meticulous technique must be exercised, as these fractures are predisposed to poor functional outcomes.

Preoperative Planning

Patients will typically present with pain, swelling, ecchymosis, and limited motion. Careful examination of the plane of the fingernails or cascade with digital flexion or wrist tenodesis may reveal malrotation. Plain AP and lateral radiographs will confirm the diagnosis and provide further information regarding displacement, angulation, and/or rotation (Fig. 10.6). Spiral-oblique fractures are particularly prone to coronal and rotational malalignment. Oblique radiographs of the affected digits are often helpful in subtle injuries.

Surgery

After the induction of adequate anesthesia, patients are positioned, prepped, and draped as described above. Closed reduction is performed with longitudinal traction and exaggeration of the deformity, followed by correction of the angular and/or rotational deformity. In proximal phalangeal injuries, flexion of the MCP joint will aid in reduction by stabilizing the proximal fracture fragment and relaxing the deforming force of the intrinsic

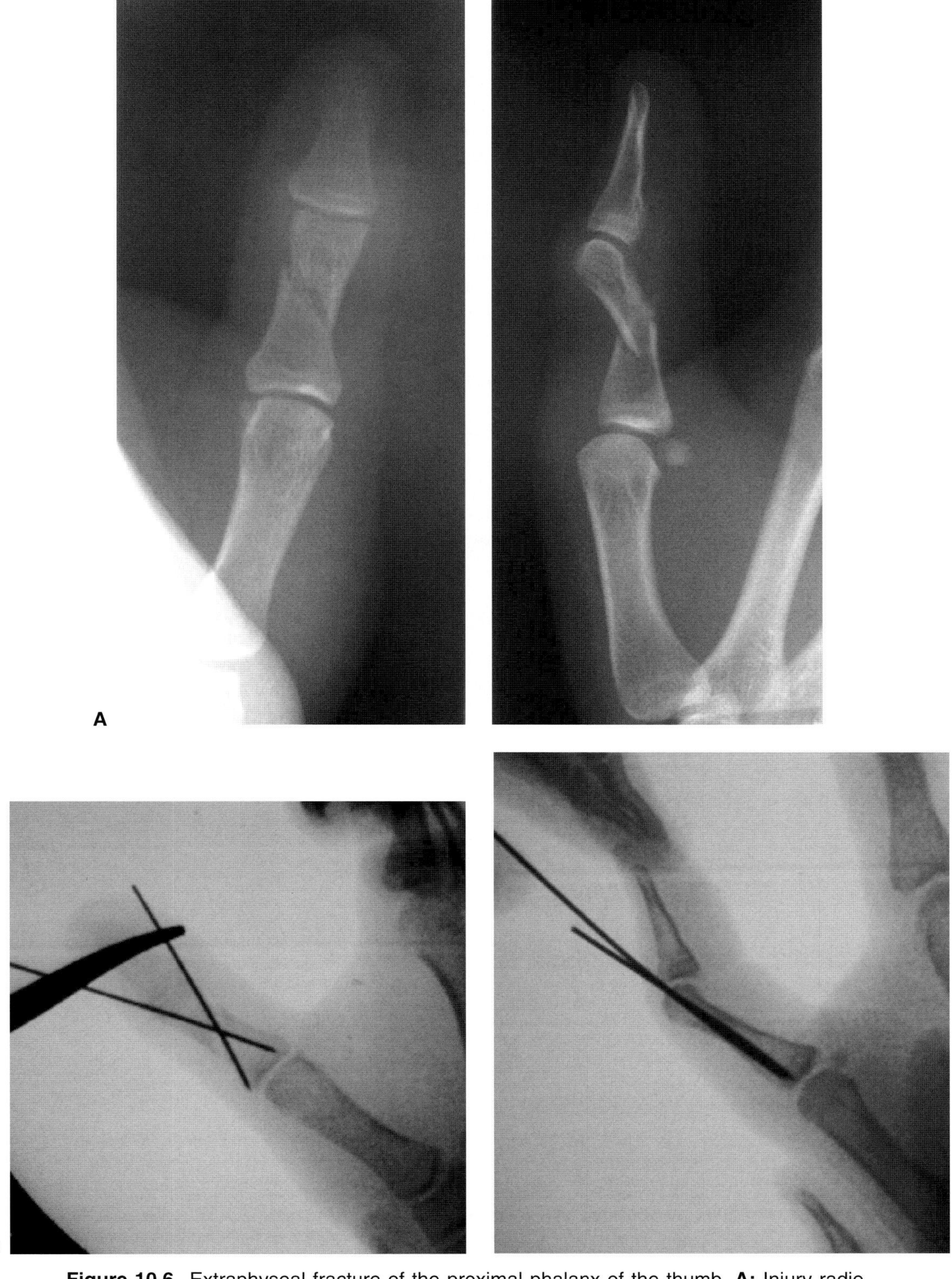

Figure 10.6. Extraphyseal fracture of the proximal phalanx of the thumb. **A:** Injury radiographs demonstrating a proximal phalangeal fracture of the thumb with apex volar angulation. Despite attempted closed reduction, there was persistent fracture instability and unacceptable angulation in the sagittal plane. **B:** Intraoperative radiographs demonstrating anatomic reduction with fixation using percutaneous K-wires.

musculature. The reduction is confirmed by clinical inspection and fluoroscopy. Fracture stabilization is then achieved with percutaneous K-wires placed in the midaxial line (Fig. 10.6). Ideally, K-wires are placed orthogonal to the fracture line. Crossed K-wire fixation may be required in predominantly transverse fracture patterns. K-wires are left superficial to the skin, and the hand is immobilized in a cast extending beyond the fingertips.

Open reduction is performed when closed reduction is unsuccessful, as may occur with soft-tissue or periosteal interposition. For fractures involving the proximal two-thirds of the phalanx, a dorsal tendon-splitting approach is preferred. In fractures of the distal one-third, open reduction may be performed by elevating the lateral bands and/or mobilizing the extensor mechanism to gain access to the zone of injury. The fracture is reduced and checked with fluoroscopy. Smooth K-wire fixation is then performed as previously described. In older patients with large fracture fragments, internal fixation using interfragmentary compression screws with or without neutralization plates may be considered.

Postoperative Management

Casts are discontinued at 3 to 4 weeks postoperatively and K-wires are removed. Gentle range-of-motion exercises are initiated at this time. Injuries of the proximal interphalangeal joint are particularly at risk for permanent stiffness, emphasizing the need for early motion. Patients are allowed to return to full activities at 6 to 8 weeks postoperatively. Formal physical or occupational therapy is rarely required.

Results/Complications

With prompt diagnosis and timely surgery, patients may expect almost universal fracture healing and restoration of full function. Complications of redisplacement, stiffness, and persistent deformity may be avoided by expeditious treatment with meticulous surgery and appropriate postoperative immobilization. In rare instances of malunion with persistent deformity and/or functional compromise, corrective osteotomy may be performed. Typically, this may be performed at the basilar metaphysis, which is technically less challenging and provides for adequate correction.

RECOMMENDED READING

1. Al-Qattan MM. Phalangeal neck fractures in children: classification and outcome in 66 cases. *J Hand Surg* 26B:112–121, 2001.
2. Al-Qattan MM, Cardoso E, Hassanain J, et al. Nonunion following subcapital (neck) fractures of the proximal phalanx of the thumb in children. *J Hand Surg* 4B:693–698, 1999.
3. Barton NJ. Fractures of the phalanges of the hand in children. *Hand* 11:134–143, 1979.
4. Bhende MS, Dandrea LA, Davis HW. Hand injuries in children presenting to a pediatric emergency department. *Ann Emerg Med* 22:1519–1523, 1993.
5. Davies MB, Wright JE, Edwards MS. True skier's thumb in childhood. *Injury* 33:186–187, 2002.
6. DeJonge JS, Kingma J, Van Der Lei B, et al. Phalangeal fractures of the hand: an analysis of gender and age related incidence and aetiology. *J Hand Surg* 19B:168–170, 1994.
7. Fisher MD, McElfresh EC. Physeal and periphyseal injuries of the hand. *Hand Clinics* 10:287–301, 1994.
8. Gabuzda G, Mara J. Bony gamekeeper's thumb in a skeletally immature girl. *Orthopedics* 14:792–793, 1991.
9. Hastings H, Simmons BP. Hand fractures in children: a statistical analysis. *Clin Orthop* 188:120–130, 1984.
10. Leonard MH, Dubravcik P. Management of fractured fingers in the child. *Clin Orthop* 73:160–168, 1970.
11. Salter RB, Harris WR. Injuries involving the epiphyseal plate. *J Bone Joint Surg* 45A:587–622, 1963.
12. Simmons BP, Peters TT. Subcondylar fossa reconstruction for malunion of fractures of the proximal phalanx in children. *J Hand Surg* 12A:1079–1082, 1987.
13. Stein F. Skeletal injuries of the hand in children. *Clin Plast Surg* 8:65–81, 1981.

11

Index Pollicization for Congenital Absence and Hypoplasia of the Thumb

Joseph Upton

INTRODUCTION

During the past five decades, no area of hand surgery has changed as much as thumb reconstruction. Techniques for reconstruction following traumatic total or subtotal loss with the transposition of an index or other digit were introduced and refined after the World War II era. Many ingenious methods of pollicization were introduced as basic principles evolved. The introduction of microvascular techniques have made the reattachment of amputated parts the procedure of choice following most traumatic injuries and, as such, have greatly reduced the need for post-traumatic pollicization.

Despite our enthusiasm for microvascular applications in hand surgery and a plethora of new techniques, index pollicization remains the procedure of choice for congenital absence and severe hypoplasia of the first ray. The early contributions of Gosset, Hilgenfeld, and Bunnell in the treatment of traumatic loss were later refined for the child with congenital differences by Littler and Buck-Gramcko. Over the past 25 years, we have built upon this foundation and added further adaptations in a series of 270 pollicization procedures.

INDICATIONS

Thumb Hypoplasia and Absence Deformities

Any child with severe bilateral absence or hypoplasia of the thumb (Types IIIB, IV, and V) is an excellent candidate for pollicization, barring any accompanying major neurologic, cardiovascular, or hematologic deficiency that would prevent the child from using the

Joseph Upton M.D.: Division of Plastic Surgery, Harvard Medical School, Boston, MA, and Department of Surgery, Children's Hospital, Beth Israel Deaconess Medical Center, Boston, MA

upper extremity effectively. Most experienced surgeons would recommend this procedure for unilateral absence or hypoplasia as well. Those with severe mental retardation or proximal limb deficiencies, such as shoulder-to-hand phocomelia, may not be good candidates. Important initial considerations in these patients include the motion status of the shoulder and elbow, as well as the arm and forearm length, all of which determine the position of the hand and arm in space. The child must be able to use her/his new thumb effectively to justify this procedure. Additional indications include the rare mirror hand, five-fingered hand, and other unique malformations.

Aesthetic Indications

The importance of appearance has been long overlooked by authors of congenital hand texts. Older children, and particularly teenagers, prefer a one-thumb, three-fingered hand to the four-fingered hand with or without the abducted and slightly pronated index finger. When the normal or slightly stiff index finger has been repositioned as a thumb early in life, all children will adapt and use this ray effectively as a thumb. Creation of a deep, broad first web space, and the size of the intrinsic muscles on the radial side of the thumb, are key variables that impact the final appearance of the new thumb, which, distally, will always be thinner than the normal thumb.

Type IIIB Thumb

The decision to ablate a good-looking thumb with large phalangeal components and a deficient metacarpal with no carpometacarpal (CMC) joint is difficult for parents in most cultures. In our experience, these families are usually members of strict religious groups and believe that God put it there for a reason. However, many of these patients have bilateral, asymmetrical malformations. It is best to pollicize the most normal index digit first so that the parents may become encouraged by the early outcome and agree to have the same procedure on the opposite hand (Fig. 11.1). However, it is not always possible to convince some parents, who will doctor shop until they find a surgeon willing to build upon the existing hypoplastic thumb. Stabilization of the deficient thumb metacarpal with bone or tendon grafts followed by tendon transfers can be completed in multiple stages. Microvascular transfer of the second toe metacarpal (MP) joint with overlying soft tissue to reconstruct the new thumb CMC joint has also been performed in these thumbs. The long-term outcomes have been less satisfactory than a well-performed index pollicization. All experienced pediatric hand surgeons prefer the index pollicization to microvascular alternatives for these indications.

CONTRAINDICATIONS

Children with severe associated malformations, especially neurological, with little chance of function should not be subjected to this additional operation. However, these bed-ridden patients should be distinguished from those ambulatory children with mild retardation who use their arms and hands adroitly in their activities of daily living. All cases must be individualized, as there are very few absolute contraindications for this procedure.

Those with radial deficiencies have a smaller, stiff, often-contracted index ray and are not good candidates for a formal index pollicization. Judicious rotation-recession osteotomy of the index ray with and without joint arthrodeses is often preferred.

In some cases of thumb hypoplasia, the remaining elements are severed enough to initiate augmentation instead of pollicization. Despite the intellectual appeal of maintaining a five-digit hand, reconstruction of some of their Type IIIA thumbs is demanding, and results are often inferior to pollicization.

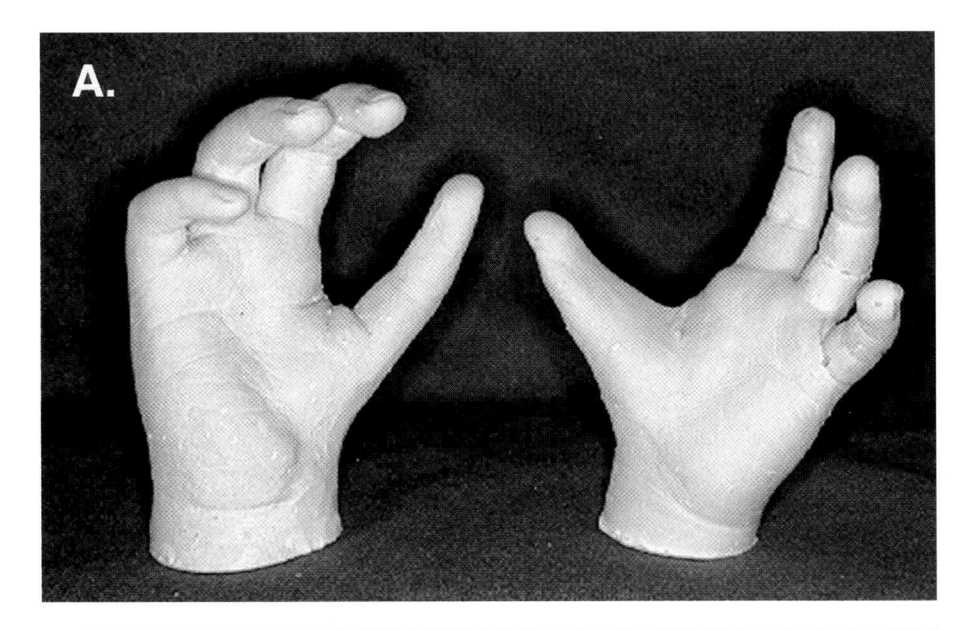

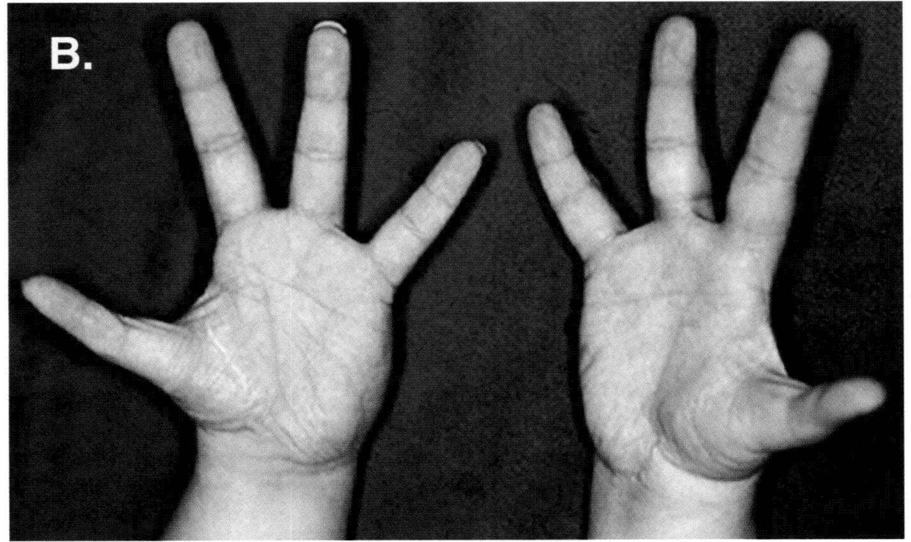

Figure 11.1. Top: Postoperative mold of two patients show the difference between a thumb with a deep webspace on the left and one with a balanced and more natural web on the right. Both had normal index fingers preoperatively. The hand on the right had more tissue advanced from the ulnar side of the thumb into the webspace. **Bottom:** The hands of a 25-year-old accountant are seen 24 years following a pollicization of the right hand and 21 years following the same procedure on the left side. Because she had a Type III B hypoplastic thumb on the left side, it took almost 3 years to convince the parents that this was the appropriate procedure for the left hand.

PREOPERATIVE PLANNING

Physical Examination

A careful physical examination is often all that is necessary to adequately assess these hands. These patients usually fall into two major groups: those with a normal index finger and good thenar muscles, and those with radial dysplasias, previous centralizations, and stiff index rays. A detailed documentation of active and passive range of motion, the presence and strength of intrinsic muscles, and flexion contractures of the index and/or other digits should be carefully recorded. Videotapes provided by occupational therapists are very helpful for evaluations of older children and all postoperative patients.

Radiology

Routine anteroposterior (AP) and lateral radiographs are obtained. Angiograms are obtained only on limbs with unusual anomalies, such as the mirror hand or other bizarre malformations in which the arterial blood supply to the index digit may be in question.

Parents and Family

Often the surgeon's hardest job is to counsel discriminating parents who have carefully watched their child adapt to every task presented. The use of pre and postoperative hand molds, photographs of other patients, and actually meeting other patients who use their new thumbs is quite useful. It is very important to give the parents of these children an accurate expectation of the postoperative outcome and to emphasize the diminished pinch and grasping ability of these new thumbs. These new thumbs will never be normal, but the final outcome will be better than those achieved with alternative reconstructions.

Timing of Pollicization

Some controversy will always exist regarding the optimal time for an index pollicization. Although some experienced surgeons such as Dieter Buck-Gamcko and Guy Fouchet have performed these operations on children less than 4 months of age, most wait until the child is between 12 and 24 months of age. Pollicization in a 12-month-old toddler is much easier than that in a 2- to 3-month-old baby. I have found that the size of the hand and not the chronological age of the child is the primary consideration. Other advantages of waiting include improved cooperation of the child and increased likelihood of performing a much more precise operation on a larger hand. The 1- to 2-year age range is also preferable with our limited knowledge of neuromuscular maturation and central conditioning and plasticity of the cerebral cortex.

SURGERY

Incisions

In contrast to post-traumatic thumb reconstructions, adequate skin cover is present in congenital cases, and the need for skin grafts is usually a reflection of poor incision planning. A racquet-shaped incision is made across the base of the thumb 1.0 to 2.0 mm proximal to the digitopalmer flexion crease. The radial extension of this incision may extend either toward the palm or directly along the radial border of the hand (Figs. 11.2, 11.3). Once this incision is made through the dermal layer, upward traction of the skin will enhance the decompression of the fibrous septae, anchoring the skin to the palmar aponeurosis. If this dissection is kept above the palmer fascia, there is no danger of neurovascular injury. The palmer aponeurosis should not be elevated with the flap (Fig. 11.4, bottom).

The dorsal incision extends over the index finger at the MP joint level. In most children, two large dorsal veins can be located on either side of the dorsal midline. Once the tight dermal layer has been penetrated, upward traction of the skin flap will enable both sharp and blunt scissor dissection between the two layers of fat on the dorsal surface of the hand. The important dorsal veins and nerves are located between these two layers, which may not be anatomically distinct but which are easily separated with proper retraction (Fig. 11.4, top). If the surgeon retains a generous layer of fat on the dorsal flap, the blood supply to

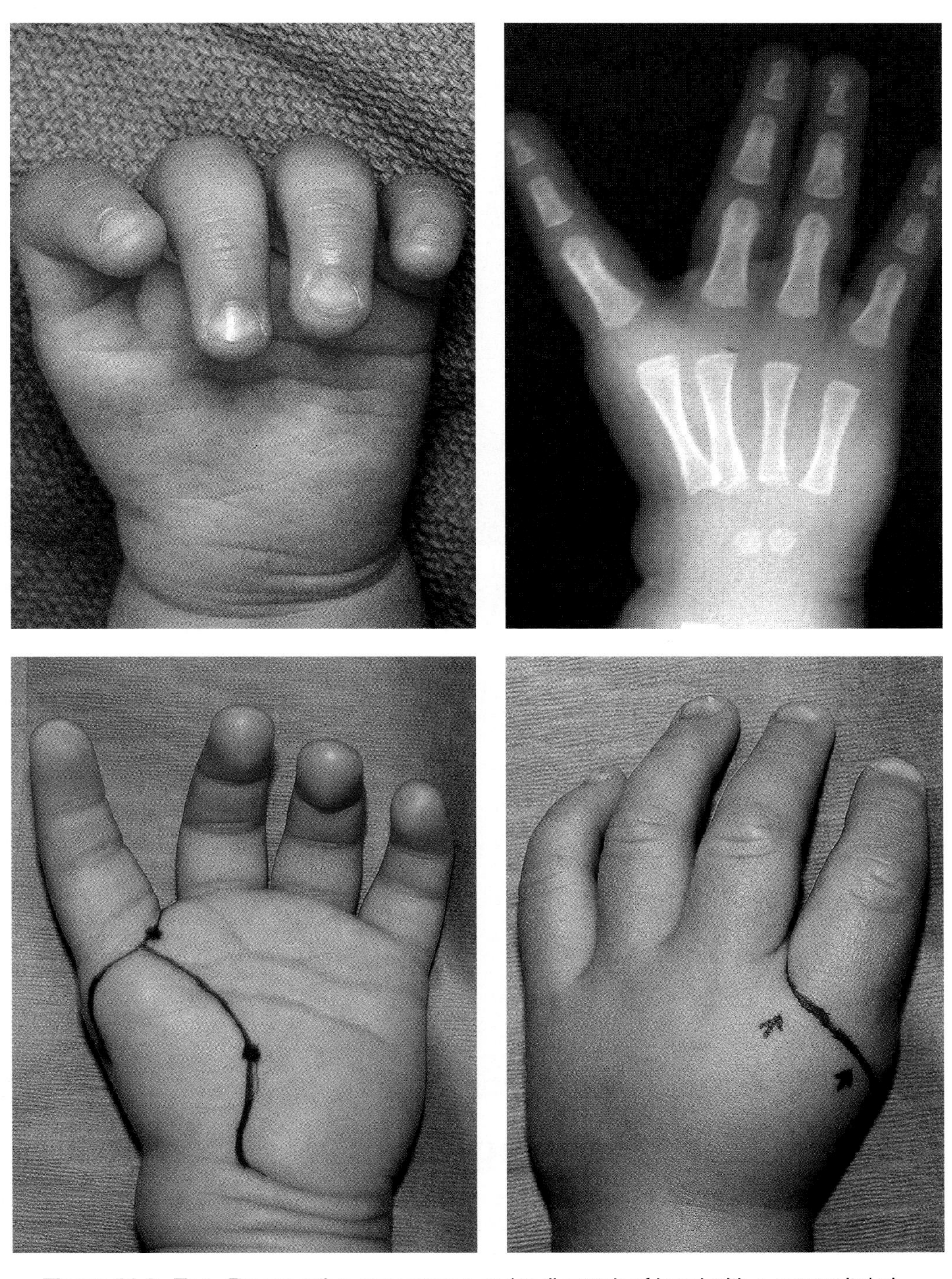

Figure 11.2. Top: Preoperative appearance and radiograph of hand with a congenital absence of the thumb (Type V). Abduction and autopronation of the most radial ray is common. Joint motion is normal. **Bottom:** The palmer incision marks the presence of the future thenar flexion crease, is made 2.0 to 3.0 mm proximal to the digitopalmer flexion crease, and extends toward the base of the index finger. The markings on the dorsal view indicate the most likely position of dorsal veins (*arrows*). The circle on the palmer surface indicates the planned change of position.

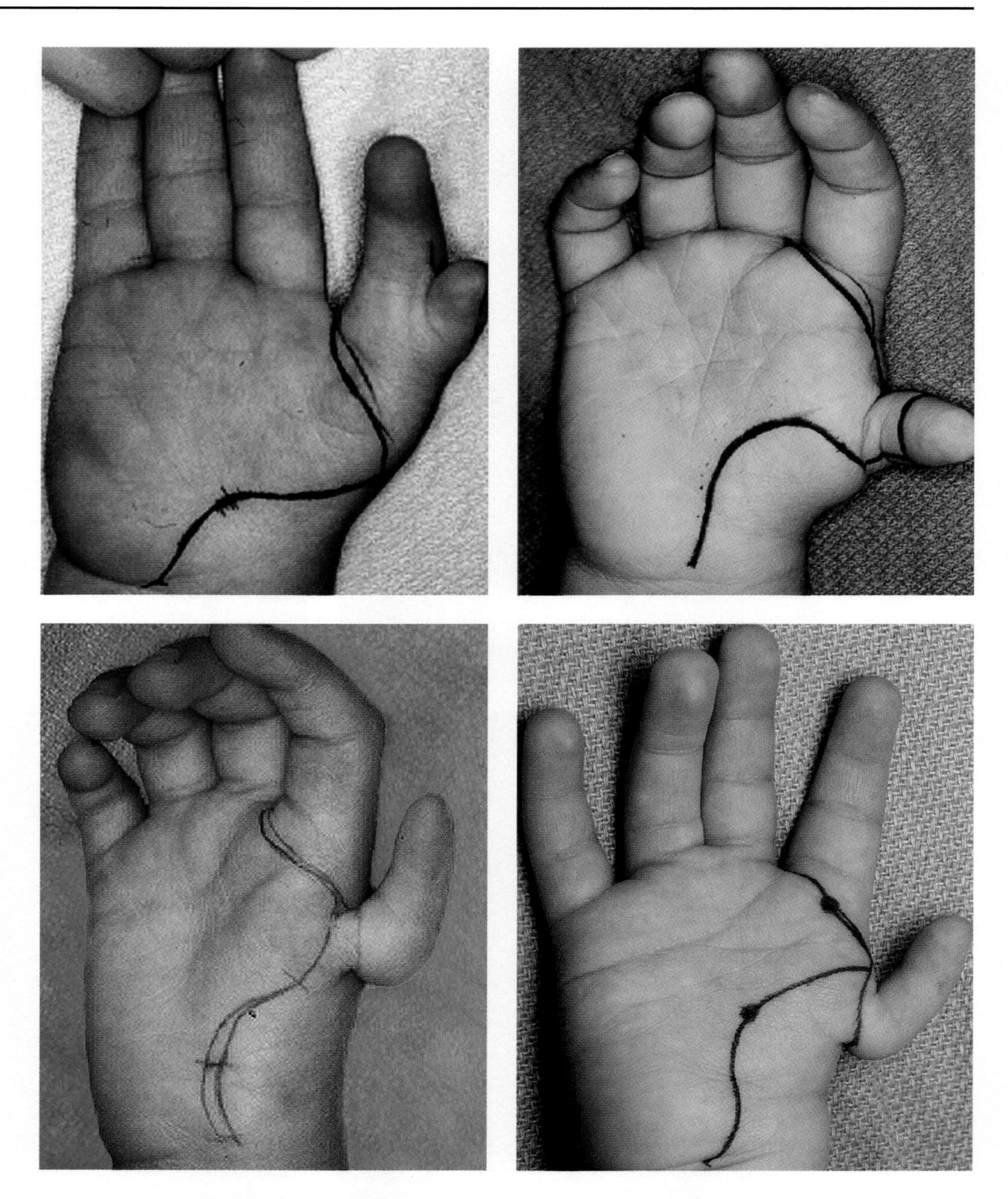

Floating thumb, pouce flotant

Figure 11.3. Alternative incisions have been used in the presence of hypoplastic thumbs. The most important and permanent landmark is the position of the new thenar flexion crease. Additional skin is not needed for index pollicization. One should save as much tissue as possible and discard extra flap after the thumb has been seated in full palmer abduction.

this region will not be compromised. The dorsal flap is raised three to four centimeters proximal for visualization of the venous drainage plexus and to allow ligation of branch(s) to the long finger, which, if left intact, will tether full proximal movement of the digits later in the procedure (Fig. 11.4).

One of the most important functions of these incisions is the creation of a normal-appearing first web space, which means extending the level of the web on the ulnar side of the new thumb to the MP joint, formerly the index proximal interphalangeal (PIP) joint.

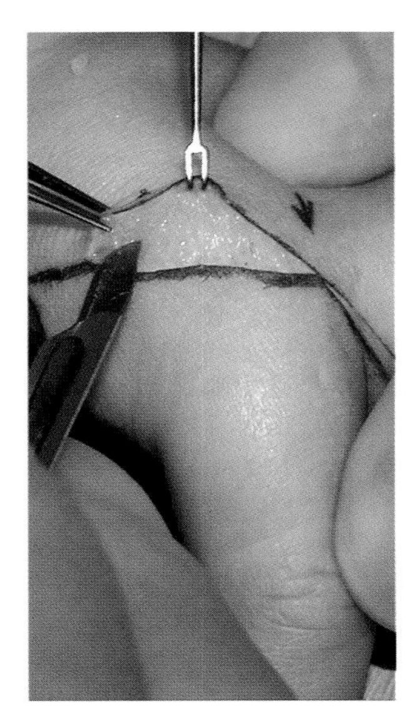
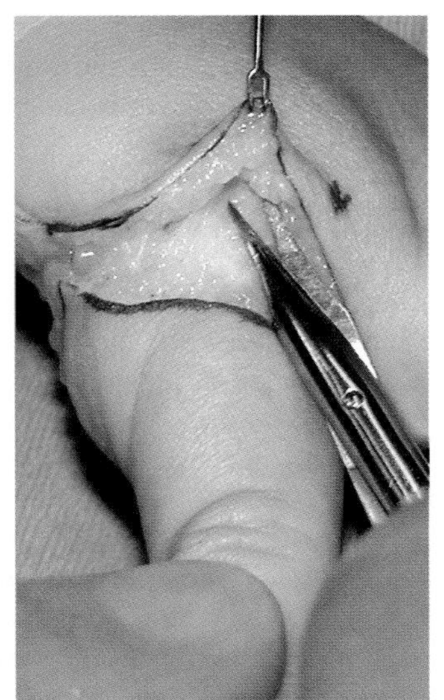
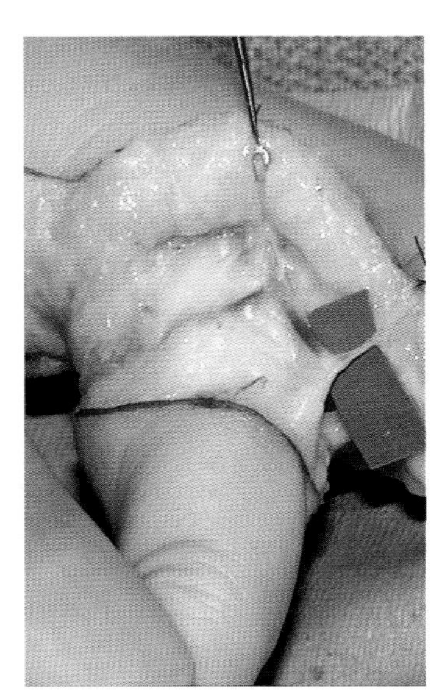

Dorsal flap elevation

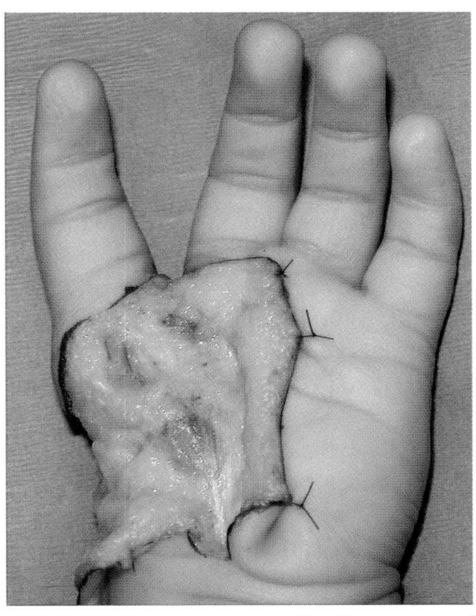
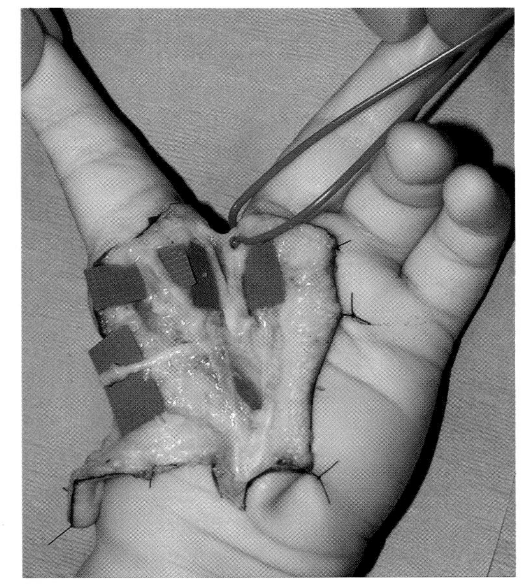

Palmar flap elevation

Figure 11.4. Top: The dorsal incision is made to the subdermal plane. Upward traction and scissor dissection separate the two layers of fat. The dorsal veins and nerves are in the deep layer. A connecting branch to the long finger (beneath green background) is ligated. **Bottom:** The palmer flap is raised above the palmer aponeurosis and extended ulnar only far enough to expose the neurovascular bundle. Note the asymptomatic neuroma that formed after removal of a hypoplastic thumb (Type IV) in the newborn nursery. Both bundles are exposed, with a red loop around the radial digital artery to the long finger.

This is accomplished by advancing tissue from the ulnar side of the new thumb into the new web space. The dorsal cutback incision, which permits this advancement and is delayed until the precise location of the incision, can be made later in the operation.

Incisions: Types IIB, IV

Small non-functional thumbs attached by diminutive soft-tissue pedicles should be ablated in the newborn nursery. The larger, hypoplastic thumb is usually saved until a later decision can be made in regard to its usefulness. There is no standard method for the introduction of this tissue. It is best to plan incisions first as though there were no thumb remnant, and then one can incorporate the extra tissue into the original design (Figs. 11.3 and 11.4).

In addition to the Types IIB and IIV thumb hypoplasias, a small thumb may be joined to the index ray by a simple or complete soft-tissue syndactyly, most commonly seen in the Holt Oram syndrome (congenital heart defect plus a radial dysplasia). Occasionally, a mitten hand will present with thumb absence and syndactyly between the index and long digits. There is no consensus upon whether to treat these soft-tissue connections prior to or at the same time as index pollicization. Twenty years ago, we performed these separately but now prefer to correct everything at the time of pollicization.

Soft-tissue Dissection

Neurovascular Structures. Following elevation, the dorsal and palmar flaps are secured with traction sutures. The palmer flap does not need to be elevated further than the longitudinal fibers of the palmar aponeurosis to the long finger. Removal of these fibers to the index finger exposes the palmar arch and common vessels to the index long web space. The distal bifurcation is identified and the ulnar arborization looped. Neural loops around either side of the vessels (artery and venae commitantes) are easily identified with traction on the common nerve (Fig. 11.5, top). Neural loops can be gently teased apart. The rarely encountered arterial loop around the nerve requires ligation of one limb without disturbance of the vascular continuity. The distal bifurcation to the radial side of the long finger is then ligated.

In contrast, the entire vascular bundle to the radial side of the index digit does not require much manipulation. These vessels are much smaller than the dominant vessels on the ulnar side of the index finger.

Connective Tissue. Following identification of both neurovascular bundles, the A-1 pulley is identified with midline scissor dissection. A full trigger release extending up into the A-2 pulley is performed. The transverse metacarpal ligament (inter volar plate ligament) within the index long web space is exposed and transected (Fig. 11.5, bottom). This affords an increased mobility of the index ray. Investing fascia of the palmer interosseous muscle, the dorsal interosseous muscle, and the dorsal fascia within the subcutaneous tissue planes are next released.

Intrinsic Muscles. The insertion of the intrinsic muscles to the index finger are then detached, and the individual muscles raised and mobilized. The insertions of the 1st dorsal interosseous are best identified with incision of the fascia over the lumbrical to the index finger (Fig. 11.6, top right) and following the muscle to its attachment to the extensor mechanism, where the insertions of the 1st dorsal interosseous muscle (abductor indicis muscle) are easily visualized (Fig. 11.7). At least 2.0 to 3.0 mm of distal aponeurosis is retained for suture fixation when these bone and tendon insertions are detached. The 1st dorsal interosseous muscle varies in size and bulk tremendously and with normal index rays often has two parts, an outer muscle to the extensor mechanism and a large inner muscle belly inserting into the base of the proximal phalanx. The distal one half of these intrinsic muscles are teased apart and their proximal periosteal and other soft-tissue origins not dissected.

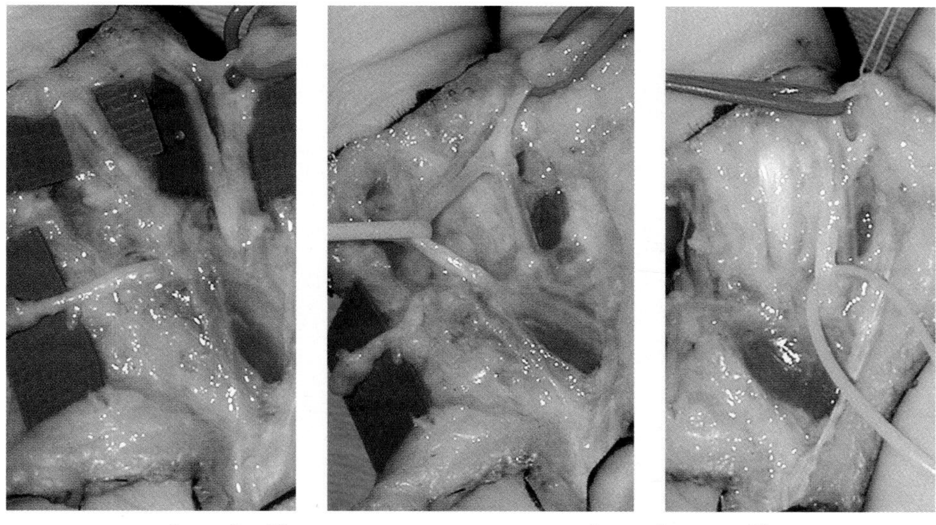

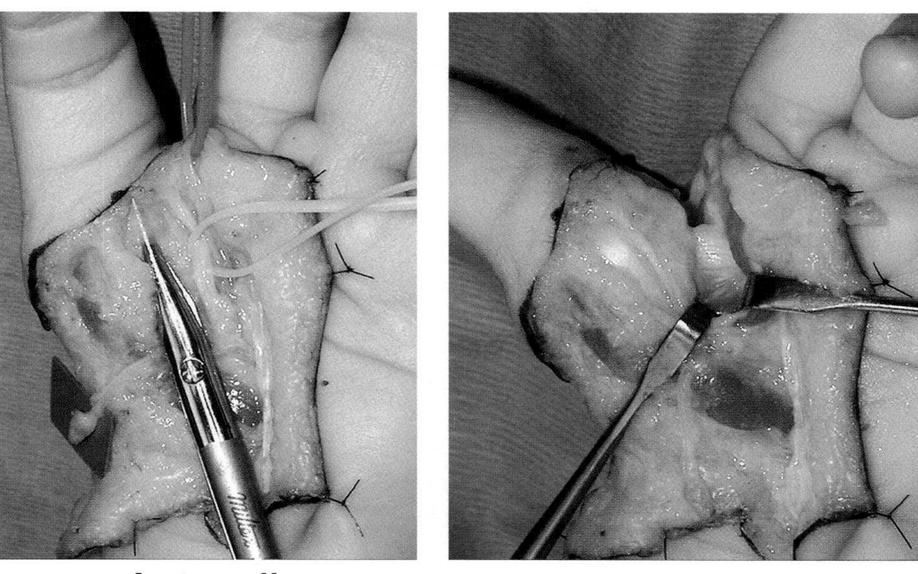

Figure 11.5. Top: The radial neurovascular bundle has been isolated. On the ulnar side careful scrutiny for the presence of arterial or neural loops must be done. **Bottom:** The first annular pulley is dissected in the midline and decompressed. Following ligation of the artery to the long finger, the transverse metacarpal ligament is easily identified before transection.

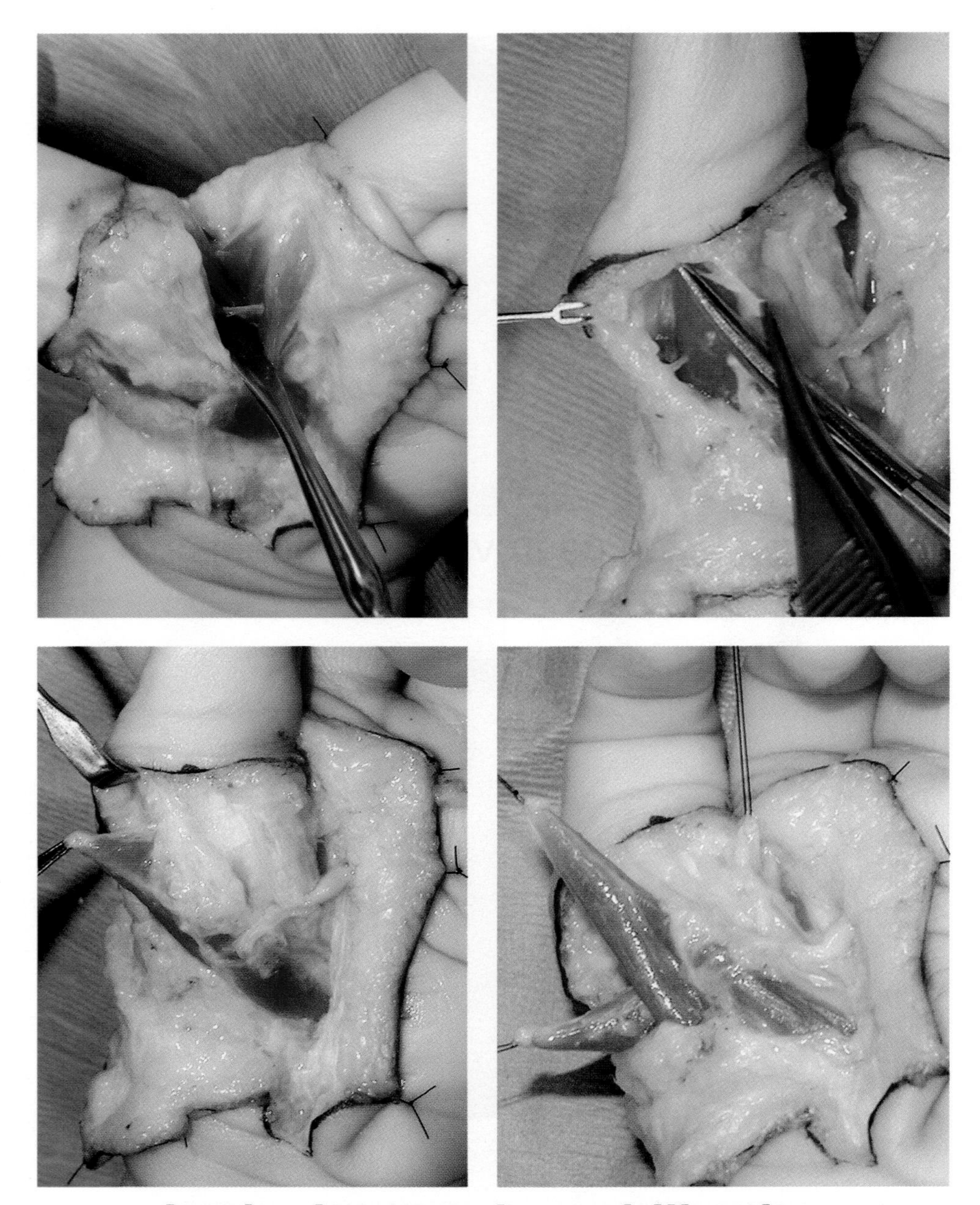

Intrinsic muscle mobilization

Figure 11.6. Top: Additional mobility of the index ray is obtained with release of fascial bands between intrinsic muscles. The distal aponeurosis and distal insertion of the radial intrinsic muscles are easily located with release of the investing fascia from proximal to distal. **Bottom:** At least 2.0 to 3.0 mm of aponeurosis should be kept for securing sutures. The 1st DI often has more than one muscle belly.

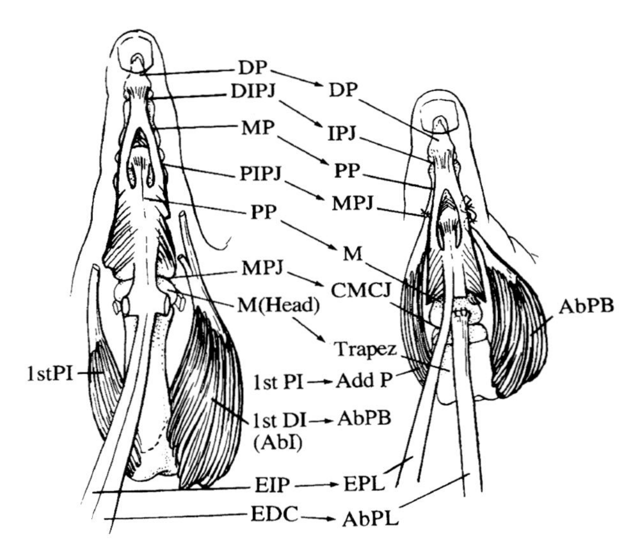

Figure 11.7. Rebalancing of the extrinsic and intrinsic muscles from a left index finger to the new left thumb (right). DP = distal phalanx, MP = middle phalanx, PP = proximal phalanx, M = metacarpal, DIPJ = distal interphalangeal joint, PIPJ = proximal interphalangeal joint, MP = metacarpophalangeal joint, CMCJ = carpometacarpal joint, EDC = extensor digitorum comminus tendon, EIP = extensor indicis proprius tendon, 1st PI = first palmer interosseous (ulnar interosseous) muscle, 1st DI = first dorsal interosseous muscle (radial interosseous, abductor indicis), AbPB = abductor pollicis brevis, AddP = adductor pollicis muscle, FPB = flexor pollicis brevis muscle, AbPL = abductor pollicis longus tendon.

Skeletal Shortening. Once the soft-tissue dissection has been completed, the index metacarpal is exposed, the extensor tendon and dorsal veins are retracted, and subperiosteal dissection is completed from the metacarpal base to the epiphyseal plate within the metacarpal head. The collateral ligaments and palmar plate stabilizers to the MP joint are preserved. The periosteum and fascia of the palmar (ulnar) interosseous muscle are usually the final fibers to be released during this part of the dissection. Two metacarpal osteotomies are done: a distal cut through the epiphysis (Fig. 11.8, top right) and an oblique proximal cut through the metaphysis.

The metacarpal head is then recessed (shortened) and rotated in 90 to 100 degrees of pronation, and fixed with one or more non-absorbable sutures anterior to the index metacarpal base with the index MP joint (now the thumb CMC joint) in a hyperextended position (Fig. 11.9). This joint positioning, as advocated by Buck-Gramcko, prevents hyperextension of the new thumb. Note that the index MP joint is a hyperextension joint, and the normal thumb CMC joint is not a hyperextension joint. This repositioned new thumb lies (1) with the metacarpal head pronated 100 degrees (relative to its former position), (2) flexed 35 to 40 degrees, and (3) abducted 20 to 30 degrees in a radial position.

This skeletal shortening and recession is one of the most critical steps in a pollicization procedure and usually occurs at the end of a normal tourniquet run of 90 minutes. Placement of the metacarpal head is often facilitated by the dissection of a space anterior to the base of the index metacarpal during the periosteal elevation.

Incision. The rotation-recession maneuver of the index finger invites a Y-to-V advancement of tissue from the radial side of the hand into the dorsal and/or radial surface of the new thumb. The exact placement of the incision is determined by the tissue availability. The thumb is first held in a position of full palmer abduction and the soft tissue draped over it. A longitudinal incision, usually dorsal but sometimes more radial, extends out to the new MP extension crease (Fig. 11.10). If performed before tourniquet release, the dorsal venous system is easier to identify and to dissect. This incision then provides excellent exposure of the entire extensor mechanism and releases tissue for advancement from the ulnar side of the thumb toward the radial side of the long finger. This movement provides a much more pleasing and normal-appearing first web space.

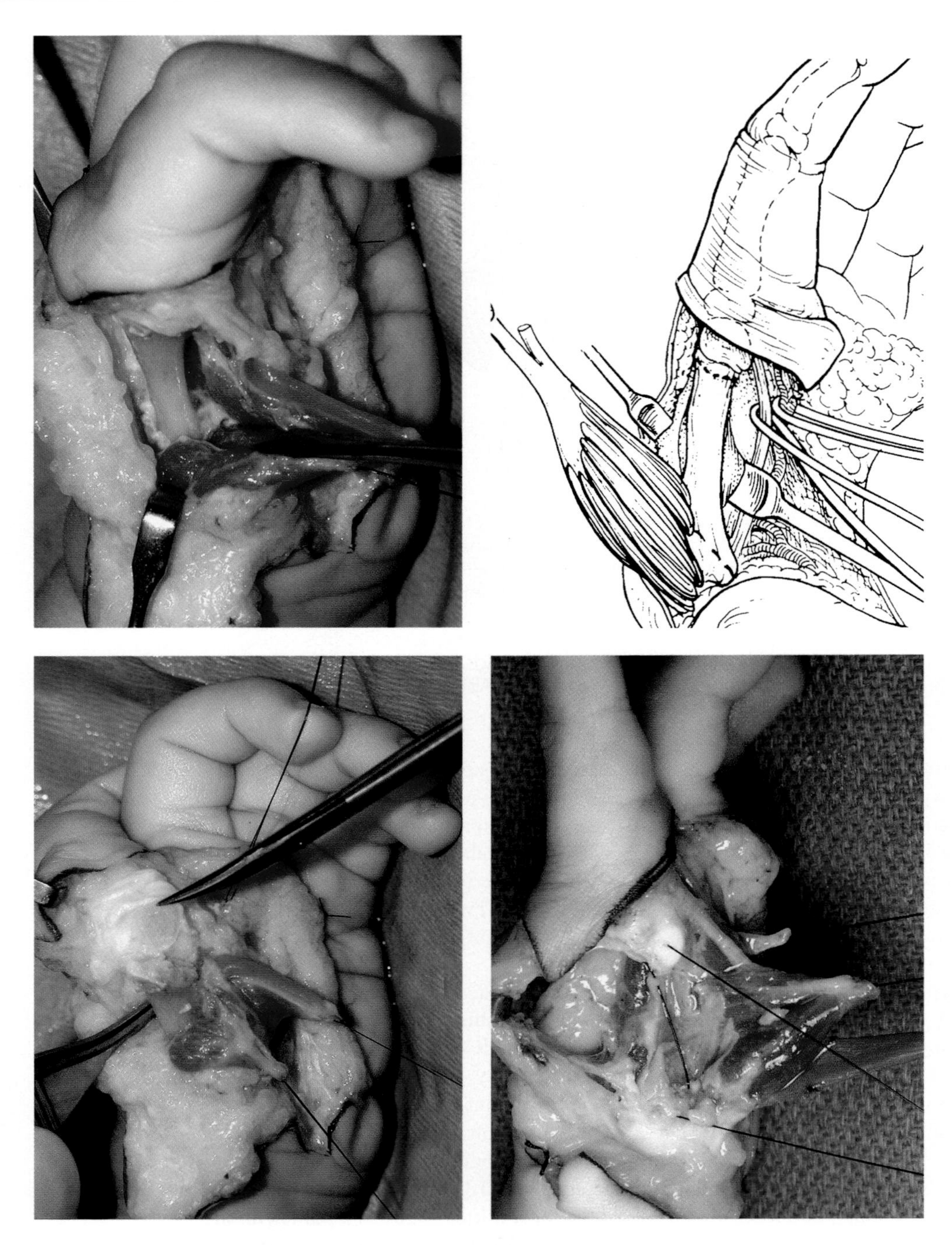

Skeletal shortening

Figure 11.8. Top: Periosteum is elevated over the entire metacarpal and the intrinsic muscles left attached to the periosteum. The illustration shows the placement and extent of metacarpal resection. **Bottom:** This distal osteotomy is through the epiphysis, which appears white and is easily distinguished from cancellous bone. An interosseus suture is used to fix the hyperextended metacarpal head anterior to the base of the index metacarpal. The schematic illustration shows the repositioning of the metacarpal head, which becomes the thumb trapezium.

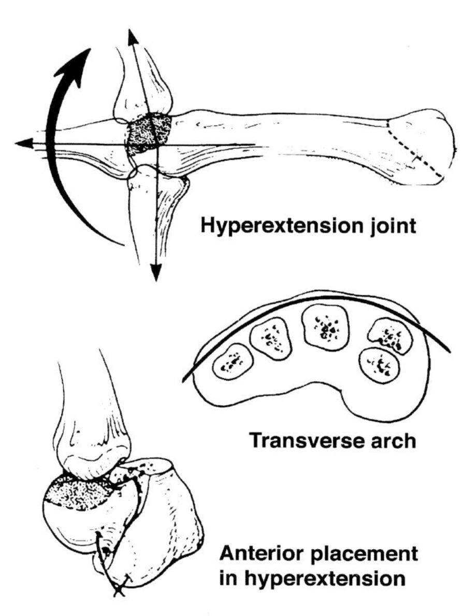

Figure 11.9. Top: A normal index metacarpophalangeal joint is a hyperextension joint. In some individuals, up to 90 degrees of hyperextension beyond neutral position is possible. **Middle:** The placement of the metacarpal head, which becomes the new thumb trapezium, anterior the base of the metacarpal creates a new transverse palmar arch and more effectively places the thumb in a more palmar position. **Bottom:** An oblique cut is made in the metacarpal base just above the CMC articulation.

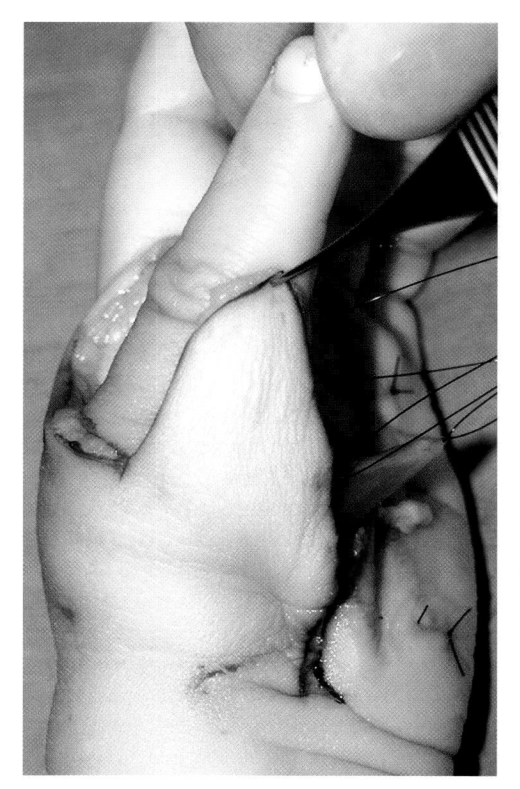

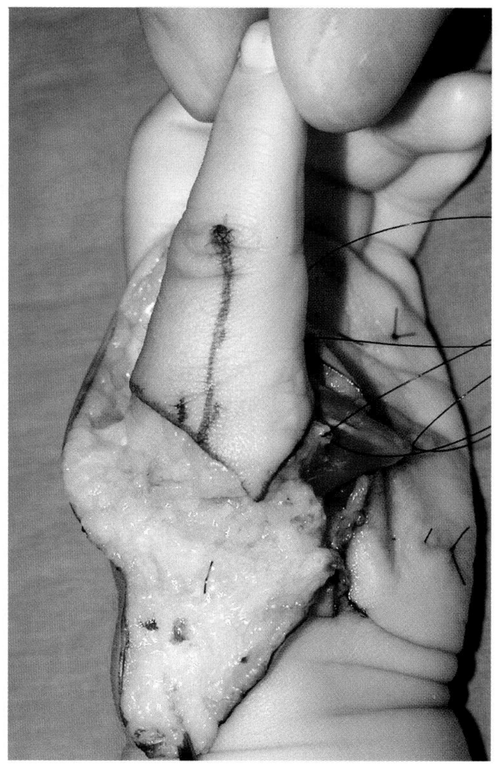

Figure 11.10. With the new thumb held in optimal palmer abduction, the available skin flap is then draped over the thumb. At this point the exact placement of the cutback incision can be determined. The soft tissue on the ulnar side is advanced into the new first web space, and that on the radial side is used to improve the bulk of the thenar region.

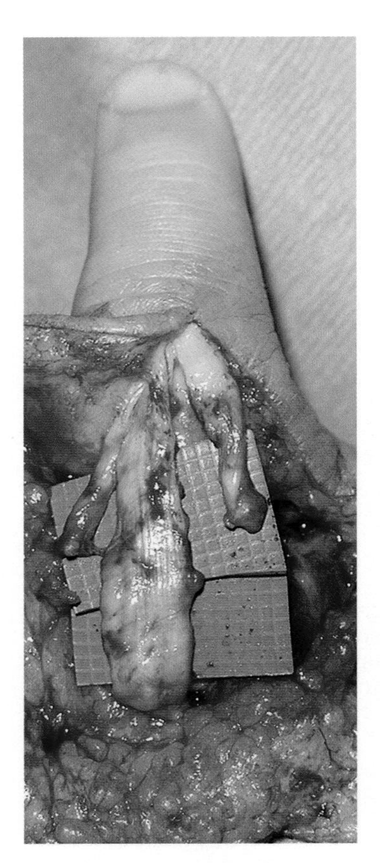

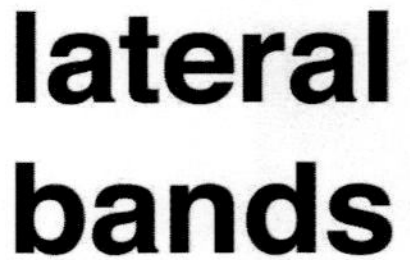

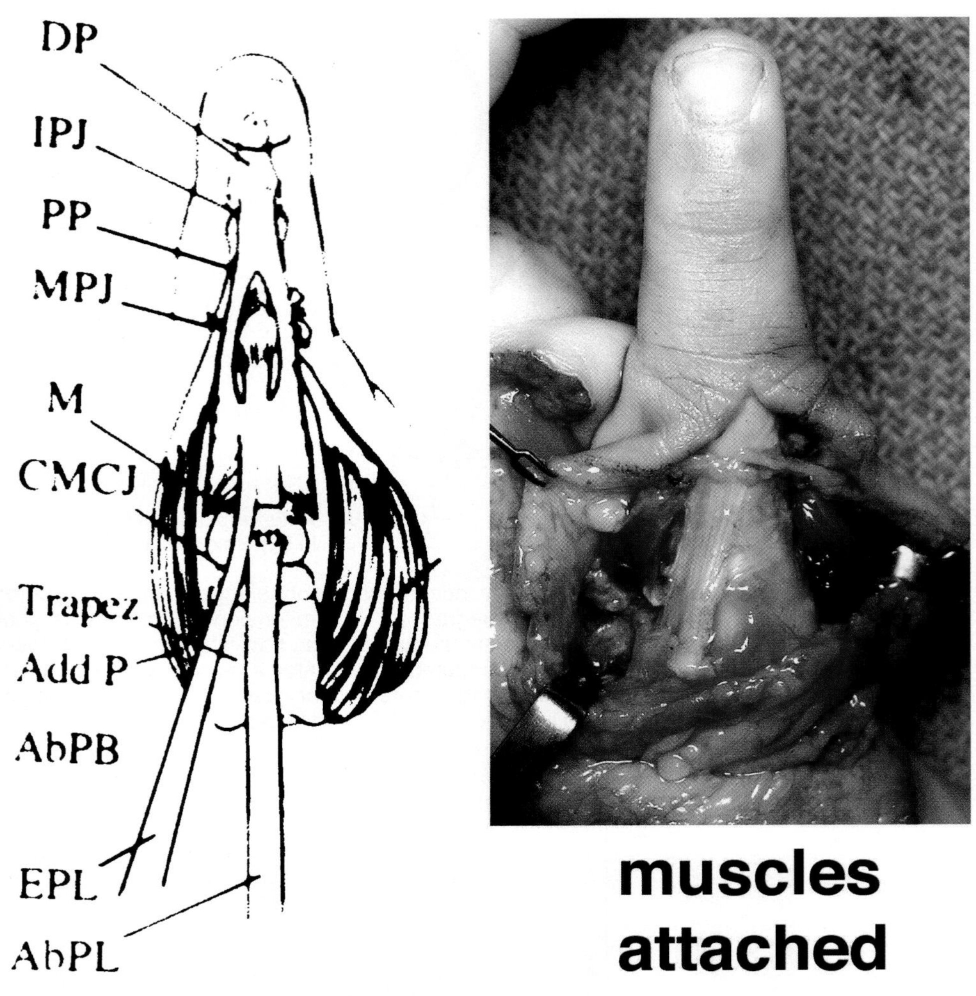

Figure 11.11. The lateral bands are separated from the central portion of the extensor mechanism. The index EDC is attached to the ulnar base of the new thumb metacarpal, and the EIP is shortened and attached to the central extensor of the index to become the new thumb EPL.

Extrinsic Tendon Rebalancing. The extrinsic flexor tendons are not altered, as they will shorten and adjust to proper tension with time and growth. Within 18 months, strong flexion is present. This is not true for the extensor muscle tendon units, which must be shortened (Fig. 11.11). Alteration of the flexor is helpful and indicated in the stiff index finger, where there are predictable changes in the flexor mechanism.

Distally, the lateral bands are separated from the central portion of the extensor, and proximally, the indicis proprius is separated from the more radial central extensor tendon. Both are incised. The common extensor is advanced to the base of the thumb metacarpal held in 40 degrees of extension. Insertion well to the ulnar side provides an additional amount of pronation to the thumb ray. The extensor indicis proprius is then shortened and reattached to the central portion of the extensor mechanism to become the extensor pollicis longus. End-to-end, simple overlap, or interweave suture techniques work equally well.

Intrinsic Muscle Reattachment. The intrinsic muscles are next reattached (Fig. 11.11). The 1st PI becomes the adductor pollicis and is attached to the ulnar side of the thumb proximal phalanx (formerly the index middle phalanx). Some surgeons prefer to interweave the lateral band through this muscle, which then makes it part of the extensor mechanism. This muscle is often small and has poor mechanical advantage as an adductor of the thumb. However, strength can be reinforced by transfer of a superficial flexor tendon at a later date.

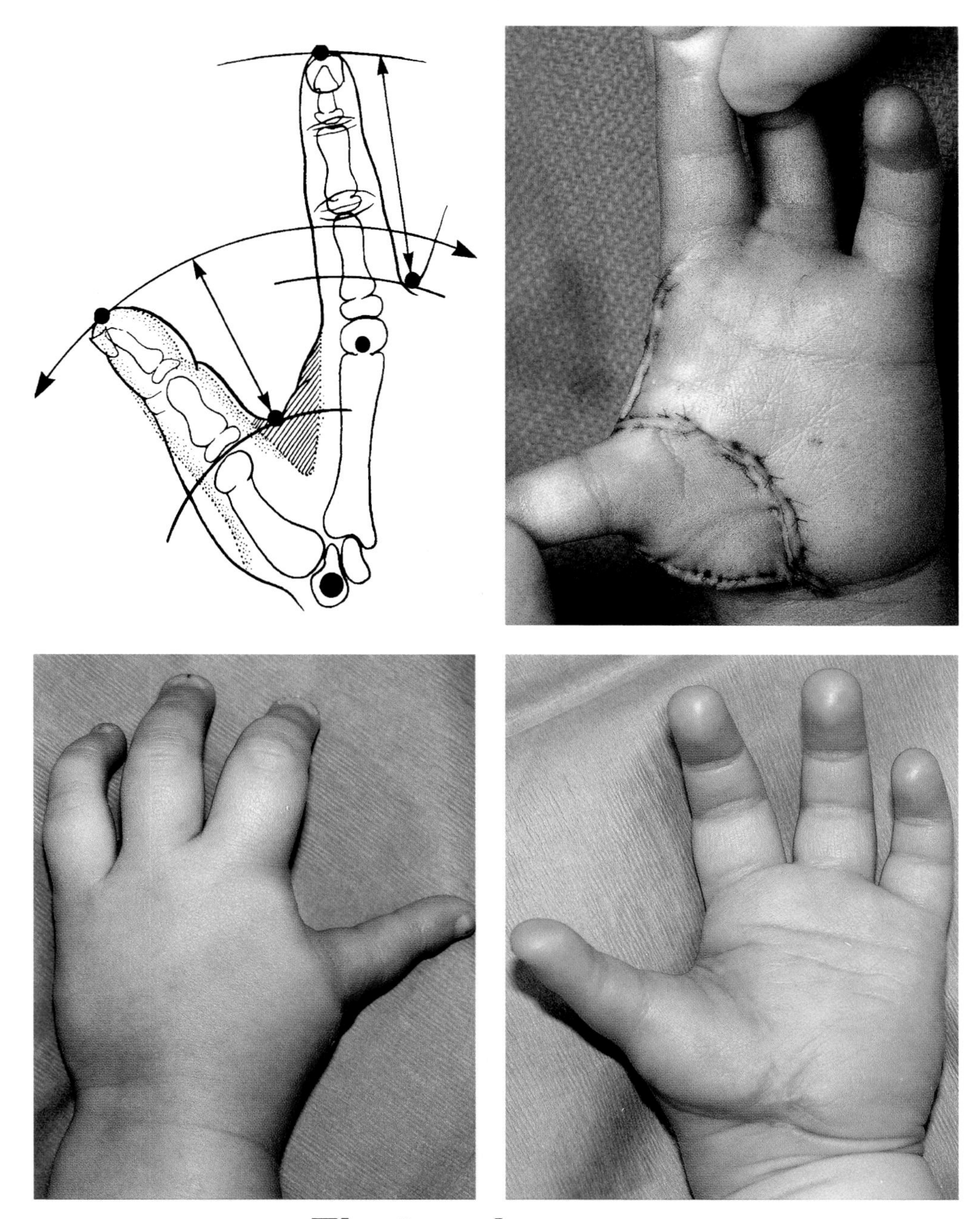

First web space

Figure 11.12. Top: The new 1st webspace extends gently between the MP joint of the thumb and index fingers. If the index ray were transposed without soft-tissue alteration, an unusually deep web space would result, and the transposed ray would appear more like a digit than a thumb. With advancement of the dorsal tissue from the index and advancement of the local tissues, a normal web can be achieved. **Bottom:** With proper positioning, the simulation of the normal web space as seen four months postoperatively is critical to the appearance of the new thumb.

The first DI (radial interosseous, abductor indicis) is attached to the radial side of the proximal phalanx (formerly the index middle phalanx). If two muscles are present, which is often the case, the more external part is interwoven into the extensor mechanism and the inner portion attached directly to the proximal phalanx to simulate the abductor pollicis brevis, thereby providing strong abduction and a strong resistance to hyperextension.

Skin Closure. Skin closure provides a remarkable amount of stability to the ultimate position of the new thumb in palmar abduction. The most proximal portion of the radial flap is first inset into the base of the new thenar eminence, which is then established and closed with absorbable 5-0 and 6-0 mild chromic sutures. The upper portion of the first web space at the base of the long finger is closed next. If the thenar flexion crease is in an optimal position, the tissue on the ulnar side of the thumb has been advanced into the new first web space. The flap from the dorsum of the hand is next advanced over the thumb and first web space. Necessary trimming is often needed to create a gentle web, which extends between the thumb and long finger at the MP joint level. If this web is excessively deep, the new thumb will retain its appearance as a digit (Fig. 11.12). The excessive fat that is often present in young children may be found on the dorsal surfaces. This should be gently dispersed beneath the skin flap and debulked at a later date.

Technical Caveat: Position of the Stiff Index Finger. Motion limitations at the interphalangeal joint levels of the index are not a contraindication to formal pollicization. Many children present with a normal, mobile index on one side and a stiff, contralateral index associated with a radial deficiency. It is wise to transpose the normal index first. On the opposite hand as much active and passive motion should be gained before pollicization. This often may involve a joint release with Z-plasty, a formal syndactyly separation, or an excision of a hypoplastic thumb. Once the metacarpal head is fixed anterior to the index metacarpal base, the new thumb should be placed in full palmer abduction with limited flexion. Because the thumb will function more as a mobile post than a thumb with full active range of motion, it should be positioned closer to the long finger and with enough pronation to make thumb-to-long-finger contact possible (Fig. 11.1 and Fig. 11.14). The extrinsic flexor is also shortened appropriately because the increases of muscle excursion and strength with growth are not as predictable when the entire muscle tendon unit is hypoplastic (Fig. 11.13).

POSTOPERATIVE MANAGEMENT

The incisions are covered with xeroform, one layer of wet gauze, and an additional layer of dry gauze. A bulky fluff dressing is then applied, and the entire upper extremity is immobilized with a well-padded long arm cast extending well proximal to the elbow flexed 90 degrees. This flexed position must be maintained during the application of the soft dressing, in order to avoid antecubital pressure, which can potentially occur when the extremity is wrapped in extension and then flexed at the elbow. The distal half of the thumb is exposed, and the parents are instructed to call if the thumb begins to disappear into the dressing, a sure sign that the child is beginning to wiggle out of the cast.

Three to four weeks later this cast is removed under sedation and a thumb spica splint made for wear at night. An active range-of-motion program is started, and no restraints are placed on the child during preschool or at play.

RESULTS

The new thumb will never be normal because the skeletal foundation, including an intact CMC joint stabilized by a normal cone thenar muscle, is absent. Nail width, pulp volume, phalangeal lengths, joint relationships, thenar and web space contours will not precisely mimic the normal thumb (Fig. 11.15).

A review of the literature over the past 50 years shows that although more parameters for measurement have been developed, the basic conclusions have not changed: Those with a

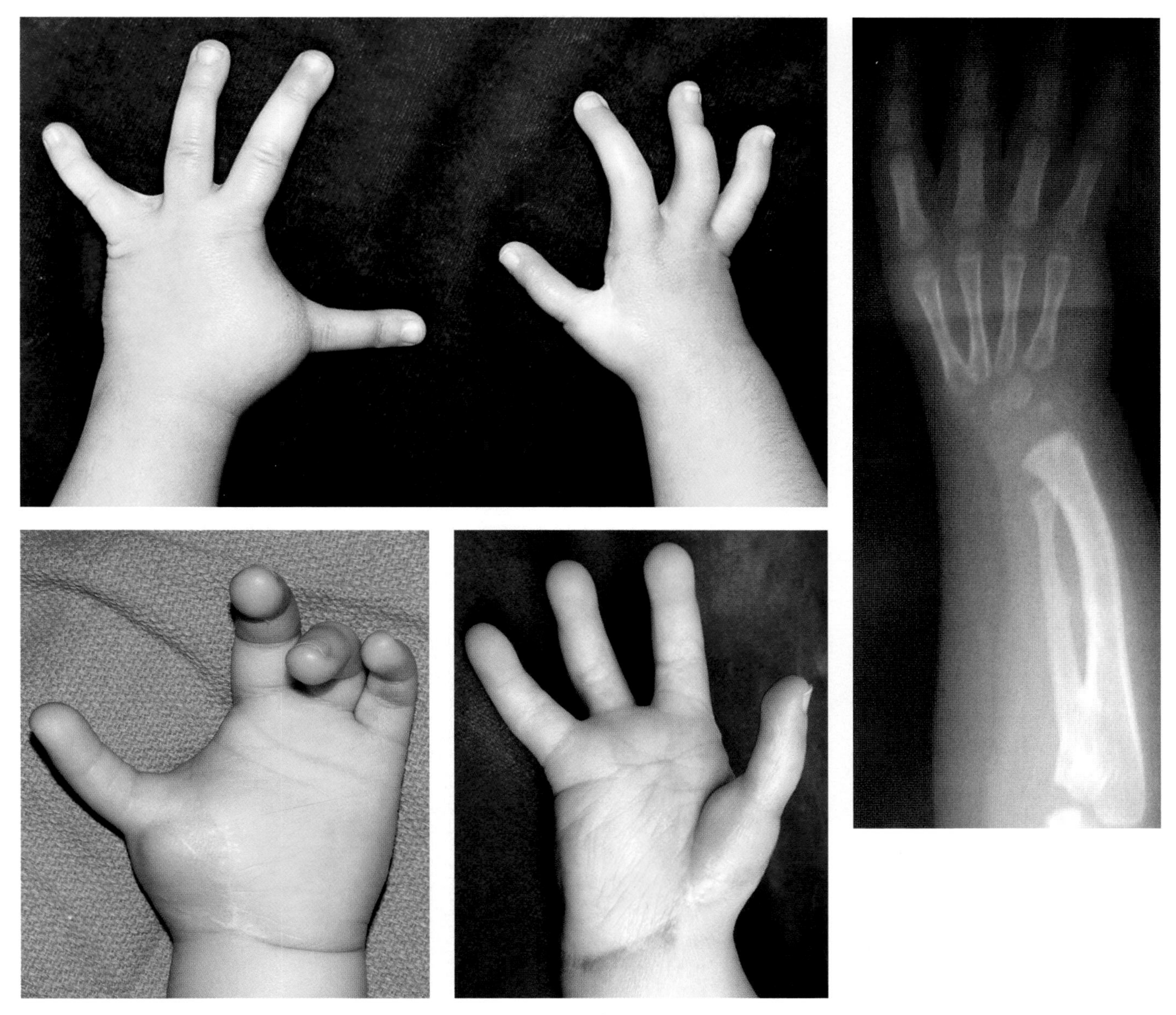

Figure 11.13. Top: This patient with the Holt-Oram syndrome has a hypoplastic thumb syndactylized to the index ray with a complete syndactyly. In one operation the hypoplastic thumb was removed prior to a formal index pollicization. Because this digit is stiff, it is positioned closer to the long finger in less palmer abduction. **Bottom:** Eighteen months later, he has maintained an excellent pinch and grasp between the less-than-normal thumb and the best ray of the hand, the fifth digit.

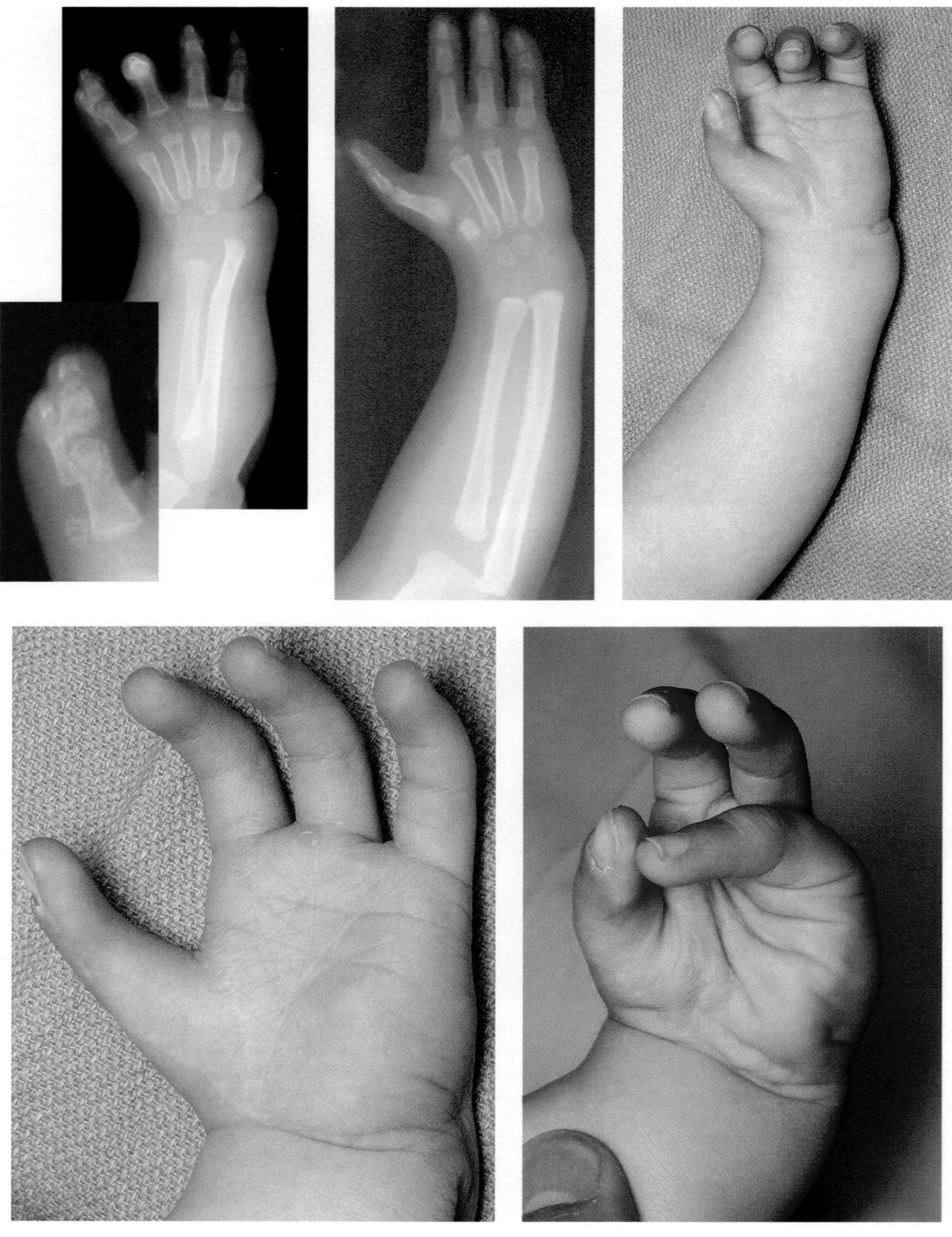

Figure 11.14. This child had a normal index finger on the left hand and a stiff index association with a radial club hand on the right hand. During the formal pollicization, the left side was placed in greater palmer abduction and extension with a larger first web space than the right side, where limited mobility of the thumb is predictable.

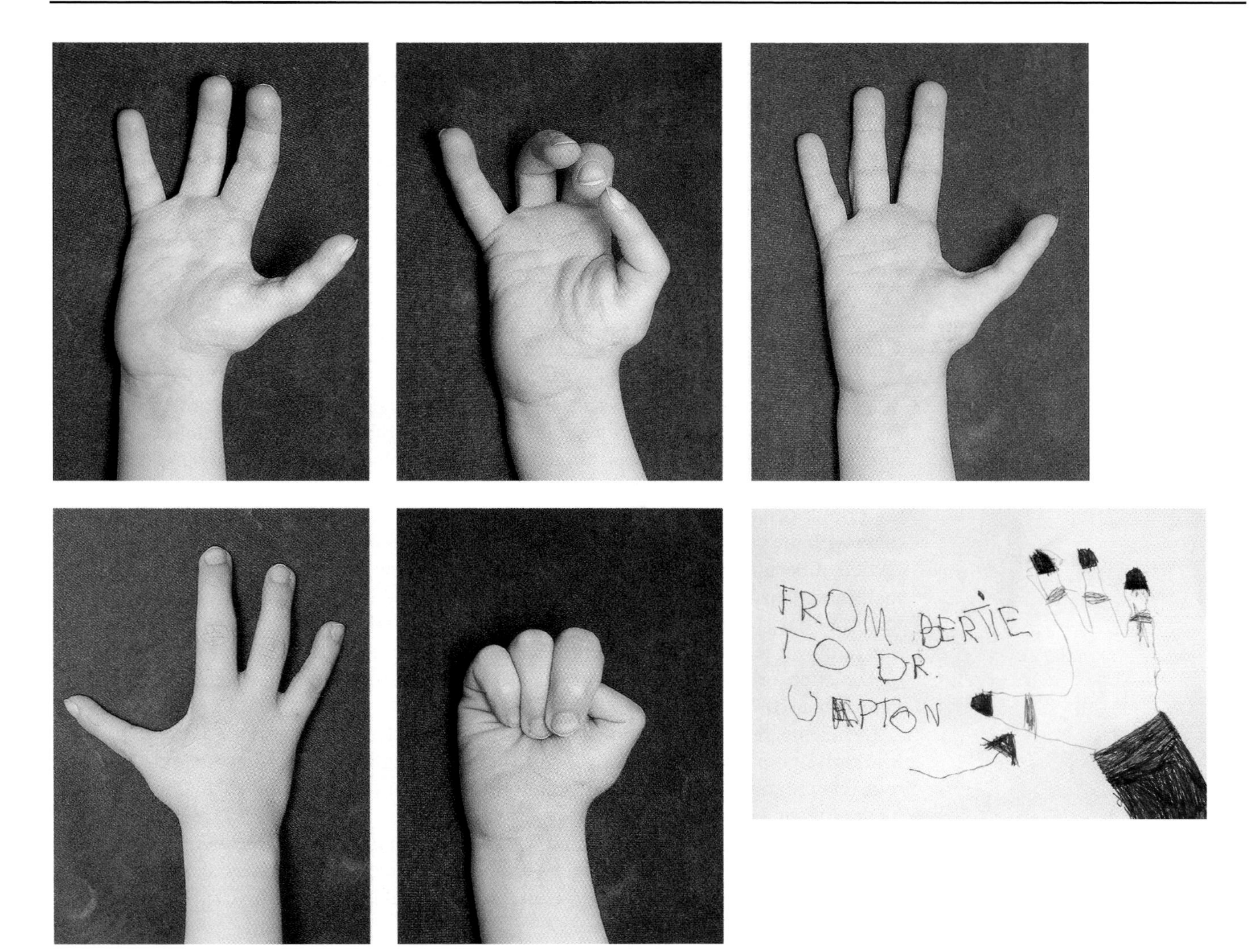

Figure 11.15. Top: Four years after pollicization of an index finger with normal range of motion and complement of intrinsic muscles, good flexion and full extension of the thumb is demonstrated. The thumb to long finger pinch is approximately 60% of normal for his age and sex. Palmar abduction through the AbPB (formerly the 1st DI) is present but weak. **Bottom:** Despite the slender distal contour, the gentle curve of the first web space makes this digit appear more like a thumb than a transposed index finger.

normal index ray prior to pollicization had much better outcomes than those with associated conditions such as the radial club hand, a mirror hand, a five-fingered hand, or following a previous syndactyly release. An ongoing study of our outcomes greater than 10 years postoperatively definitely reveals these two general groups of patients.

Any assessment of the aesthetic and functional outcomes following pollicization is difficult at best. Manske's careful follow-up of 52 patients included range of motion, strength (pinch and grip), hand usage, and a timed-activity test. This study of two case reports confirmed the observation that following pollicization of a normal index finger, there was a marked reduction in strength in comparison to a normal thumb. However, these new thumbs did function significantly better than a pollicized index finger associated with radial club hand, mirror hand, five-fingered hand, or a syndactyly. However, the diminished function does not mean that these children do not use their hands. To the contrary, they adapt quite effectively, and their primary deficit is the manipulation of small objects. Secondary procedures such as opposition transfers and arthrodeses were more commonly performed in the latter group.

The appearance of a pollicized digit is much more difficult to determine because of the subjective interpretation required. Some have tried to quantify by measuring the length of the digit relative to the PIP flexion crease, the resting posture of the new thumb, and the rotation relative to the other digits. Others have emphasized the creation of a web across the first web space, which avoids the appearance of a finger positioned on the side of the hand. We have observed that the parents and grandparents are almost uniformly pleased with the postoperative appearance and that the patients do not have much of an opinion until they are teenagers, at which time many will let you know whether they like their thumbs or not. Just ask!

COMPLICATIONS

Most problems occur as a result of inexperience and/or a hastily performed operation. Although we have never seen vascular compromise following index to thumb transposition, this catastrophe can occur. Infection and hematomas are rare, but wound dehiscence and maceration, often interpreted as infection, may result from inadequate immobilization, the primary cause of complication in pediatric hand surgery. Failure to ablate the growth plate with the metacarpal osteotomy will enable the new thumb to grow at the metacarpal level and become too long. Hyperextension of the new thumb will occur when the index metacarpal head, which becomes the thumb trapezium, is not seated in hyperextension. Islands of bone spicules will develop within periosteum left attached to intrinsic muscles, but this rarely affects function. Adherence of the extrinsic tendons will occur more commonly on the extensor side than the flexor side. However, these potential problems have occurred in less than 10% of our cases.

Deficient strength in both pinch and grasping should not be interpreted as complications. Similarly, poor abduction power or adduction strength necessitating secondary tendon transfers are more a function of the malformation than complications related to poor judgment or technical errors on the part of the surgeon.

Undeniably, experience is essential with the index pollicization procedure, which is perhaps the most elegant in hand surgery. Both improvement of outcomes and refinement of one's technique can only be gained with a very critical appraisal of individual results!

RECOMMENDED READING

1. Barton N, Buck-Gramcko D, Evans DM, et al. Mirror hand treated by true pollicization. *J Hand Surg* 11B:320–336, 1986.
2. Bayne LG. Long-term review of the surgical treatment of radial deficiencies. *J Hand Surg* 12A:169–179, 1987.
3. Buck-Gramcko D. Pollicization of the index finger: methods annd results in aplasia and hypoplasia of the thumb. *J Bone Joint Surg* 53A:1605–1617, 1971.
4. Buck-Gramcko D. Complications and bad results in pollicization of the index finger (in congenital cases). *Ann Chir Main Membr Suppl* 10:506–512, 1991.
5. Buck-Gramcko D. Pollicization in congenital malformations of the hand and forearm. *Congenital Malformations of the Hand and Forearm.* London: Churchill-Livingstone 1988:379–402.
6. Dijkstra-Zwollw R. Functional results of thumb reconstruction. *Hand* 14:120–128, 1982.
7. Eaton C, Lister GD. Syndactyly. *Hand Clinics* 6:555–575, 1990.
8. Egloff D, Verdan CL. Pollicization of the index finger for reconstruction of the congenitally hypoplstic or absent thumb. *J Hand Surg* 8:839–848, 1990.
9. Erhardt R. Sequential levels in the development of prehension. *Am J Occup Ther* 592–596, 1974.
10. Flatt A. *The absent thumb in congenital hand anomalies*. St. Louis: Quality Medical Publ, 1994.
11. Harrison H. Upper limb anomalies: pollicization for congenital deformities of the hand. *Proc Roy Soc Med* 66:634–638, 1973.
12. Harrison S. Pollicisation in cases of radial club hand. *Br J Plast Surg* 3:192–200, 1970.
13. Hentz VR. The surgical management of congenital hand anomalies. In: Littler J, ed. *Reconstructive Plastic Surgery. 6. The Hand and Upper Extremity*. Philadelphia: WB Saunders, 1977:3306–3349.
14. Hentz VR. Traditional techniques for thumb reconstruction: guidelines for indications. In: Landi: A, ed. *Reconstruction of the Thumb.* London: Chapman Hall Ltd, 1990:170–186.
15. Kaplan EB. *Functional and Surgical Anatomy of the Hand*. Philadelphia: Lippincott, 1984.
16. Lister G. The choice of procedure following thumb amputations. *Clin Orthop* 195:45–51, 1985.
17. Littler J. Neurovascular pedicle method of transposition for reconstruction of the hand. *Plast Reconstr Surg* 12:303–319, 1953.

18. Manske P. Reconstruction of the congenitally deficient thumb. *Hand Clin* 8:177–196, 1992.
19. Manske P, Rotman MB, Dailey LA. Long-term functional results after pollciization for the congenitally deficient thumb. *J Hand Surg* 17A:1064–1073, 1992.
20. Michon J, Merle J, Bouchon Y, et al. Functional comparison between pollicization and toe-to-hand transfer for thumb reconstruction. *J Reconstr Microsurg* 1:103–112, 1984.
21. Percival NJ, Chandraprakasam T. A method of assessment of pollicisation. *J Hand Surg* 16B:141–143, 1991.
22. Roper B, Turnbull TJ. Functional assessment after pollicisation. *J Hand Surg* 11B:399–403, 1986.
23. Sekiguchi J, Ohmori K, Kobayashi S, et al. Functional results after pollicization in congenital cases. *J Jpn Soc Surg Hand* 10:890–894, 1994.
24. Sherik SK, Flatt AE. Functional evaluation of congenital hand anomalies. *Am J Occup Ther* 25:98–104, 1971.
25. Sykes PJ, Percival NJ. Pollicization of the index finger in congenital anomalies. *J Hand Surg* 16B:144–147, 1991.
26. Taylor N, Jebsen RH. Evaluation of hand function in children. *Arch Phys Med Rehabil* 54:129–135, 1973.
27. Upton J. Pollicization for the aplastic thumb. *Current Therapy in Plastic and Reconstructive Surgery: Trunk and extremities.* In: Marsh J, ed. Toronto: BC Decker 1989:232–237, 1989.
28. Ward J, Pensler JM, Parry SW. Pollicization for thumb reconstruction in severe pediatgric hand burns. *Plast Reconstr Surg* 76:927–932, 1985.

12

Release and Reconstruction of Digital Syndactyly

Michelle A. James

INDICATIONS/CONTRAINDICATIONS

Syndactyly, or failure of the separation of digits, is the most common congenital hand malformation, with an occurrence of approximately 1 in 2,500 births. It may be inherited as an autosomal dominant trait; whether genetic or not, it frequently occurs as an isolated anomaly. It may also occur in both fingers and toes, and it may occur together with polydactyly of the hand or feet or as part of a syndrome such as Poland syndrome or Apert syndrome. Syndactyly also occurs in ulnar deficiency and central deficiency. Webbed digits seen in congenital constriction ring syndrome (CCRS; also called Streeter's dysplasia or amniotic band syndrome) occur because previously separated digits fuse together prenatally; thus, in CCRS, acrosyndactyly (fused tips with sinuses in the webs) and nonadjacent syndactyly may occur.

Syndactyly occurs most commonly between the long and ring fingers (Fig. 12.1, A and B), followed by the ring-small, index-long, and least commonly thumb-index web spaces.

Release of thumb-index syndactyly improves hand function as it enables cylindrical grasp. Release of syndactyly involving border digits (thumb-index or ring-small) is indicated because the differential length and growth patterns of adjacent digits can induce an angular or longitudinal growth deformity, most often of the longer digit. Release of long-ring and index-long syndactyly is performed to improve appearance, increase grasp span, provide independent mobility of the involved digits, and enable ring and glove wear.

Release of complicated syndactyly (Table 12.1) may be contraindicated if one or both of the fingers is so hypoplastic that it could not function on its own. This can be difficult to discern before release.

Michelle A. James, M.D.: Orthopaedic Surgery, University of California, Davis School of Medicine, Sacramento, CA, and Orthopaedic Surgery, Shriners Hospital for Children Northern California, Sacramento, CA

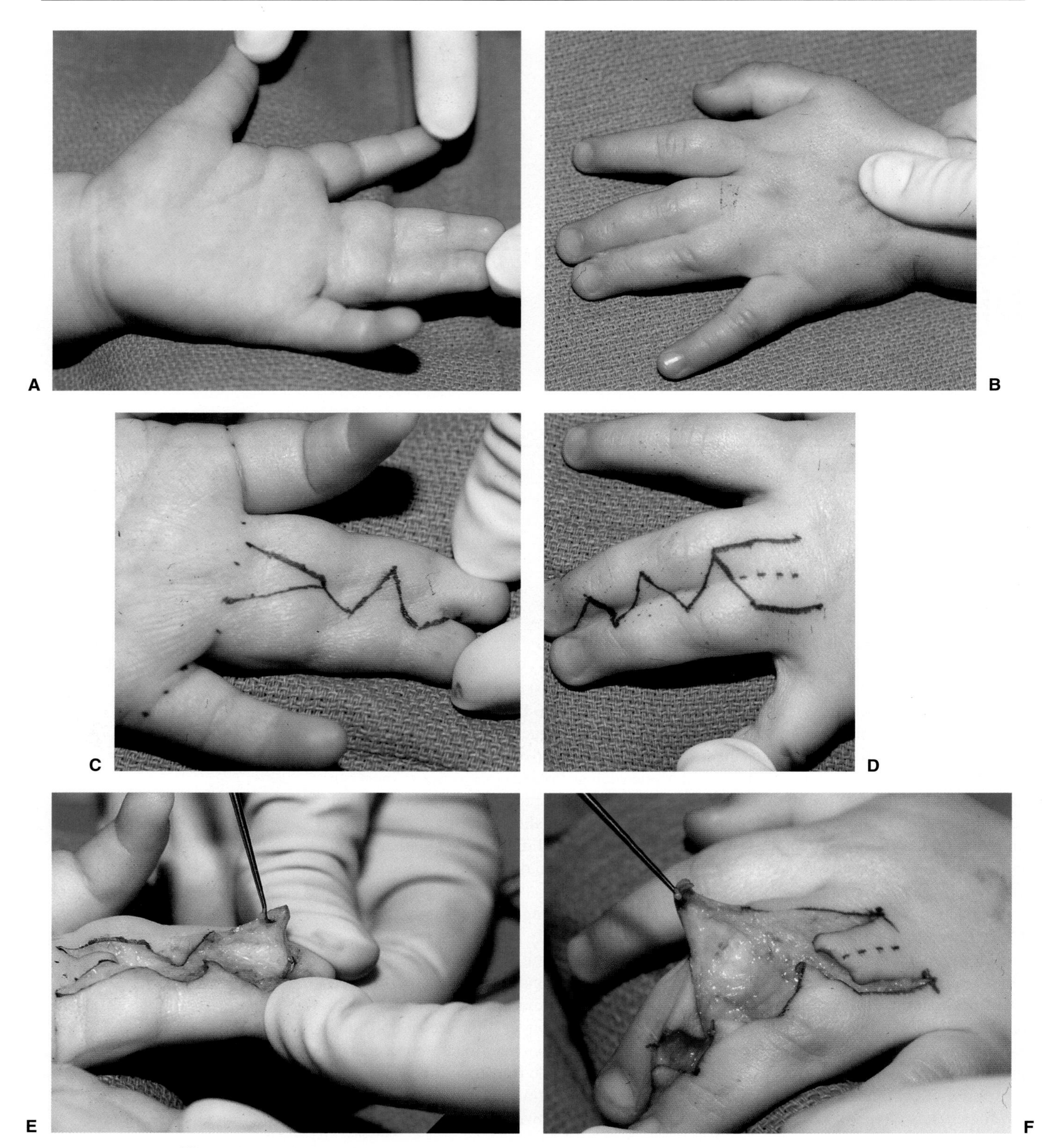

Figure 12.1. A: Palmar view of simple complete long-ring syndactyly. **B:** Dorsal view of simple complete long-ring syndactyly. **C:** Palmar incisions for simple complete long-ring syndactyly. **D:** Dorsal incisions for simple complete long-ring syndactyly. **E:** Elevation of flaps from the palmar aspect. **F:** Elevation of flaps from the dorsal aspect.

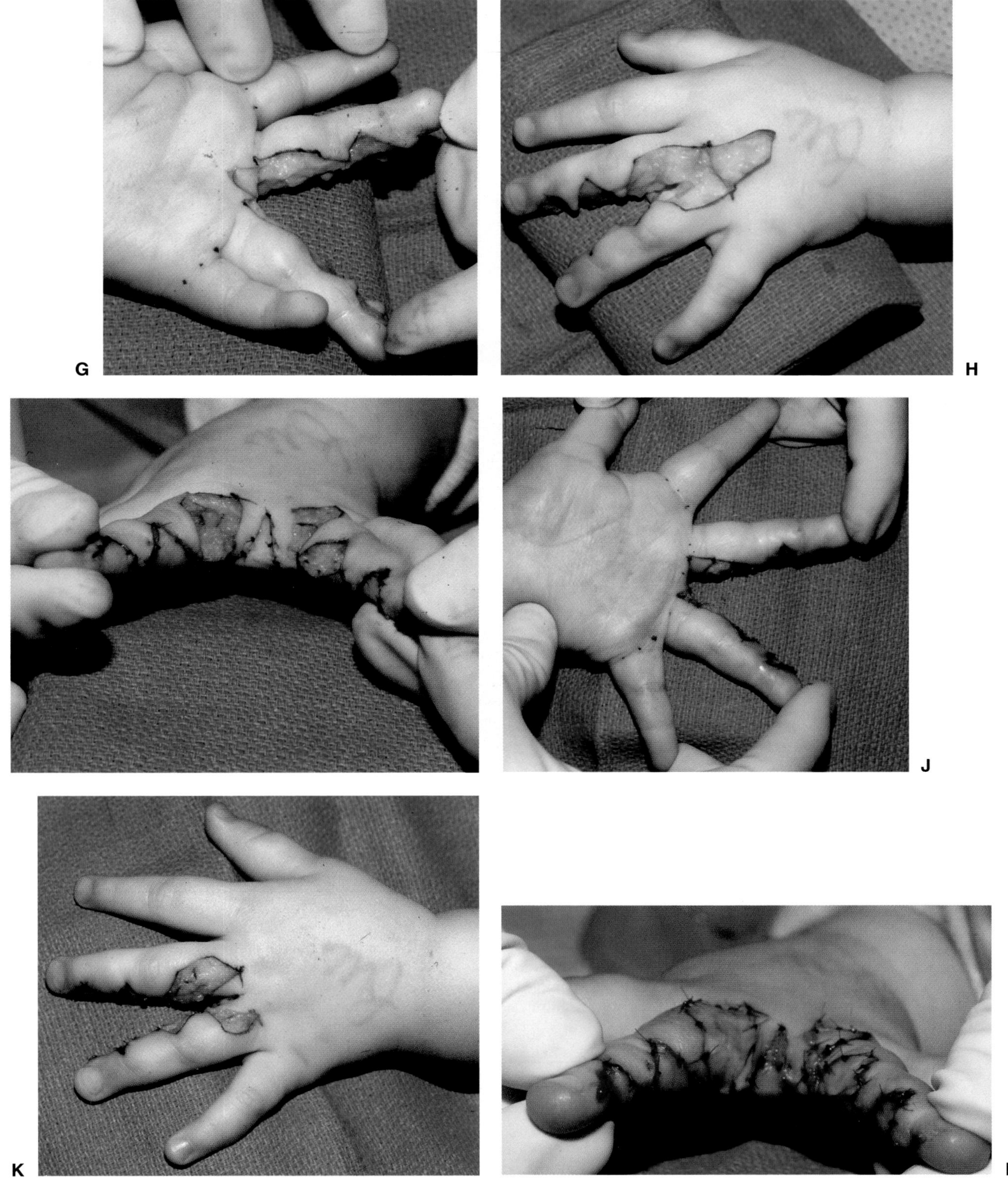

Figure 12.1. *Continued.* **G:** Separation of digits from the palmar aspect. **H:** Separation of digits from the dorsal aspect. **I:** Web with interdigitated local flaps sutured in place. Note that the dorsal trapezoidal flap has been split longitudinally, with the palmar triangle inserted into the split. **J:** Flaps sutured in place from the palmar aspect. **K:** Flaps sutured in place from the dorsal aspect. **L:** Web with local flaps and grafts sutured in place.

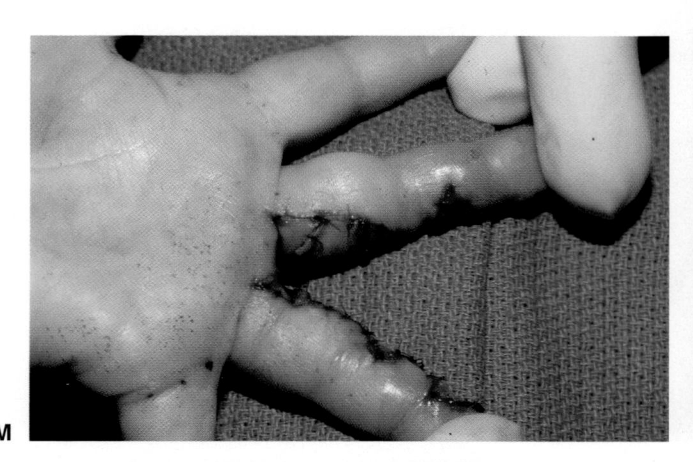

M

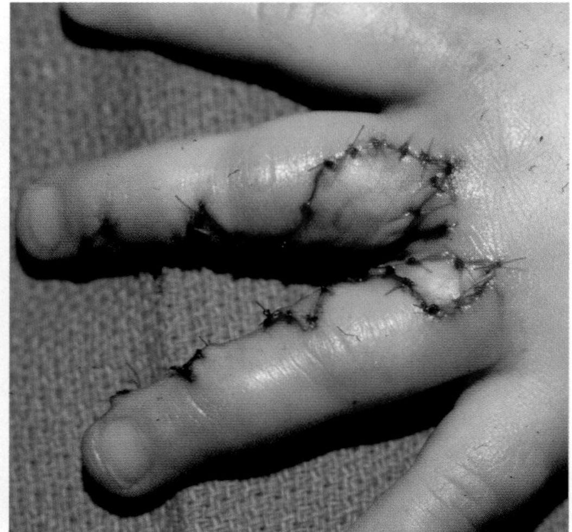

N

O

Figure 12.1. *Continued.* **M:** Flaps and grafts sutured in place from the palmar aspect. **N:** Flaps and grafts sutured in place from the dorsal aspect. **O:** Fiberglass shell covering bulky compressive dressing. See Figure 12.8 for 6-month follow-up of the same patient.

Table 12.1. *Classification of Syndactyly*

Extent of webbing	Incomplete	Syndactyly does not extend to fingertips
	Complete	Syndactyly extends to fingertips
	Synonychia	Affected digits share a common nail
Presence of bony abnormalities	Simple	Soft-tissue connection only
	Complex	Synostosis
	Complicated	Bony malformation (polydactyly, dislocation, longitudinal epiphyseal bracket)

PREOPERATIVE PLANNING

Syndactyly is classified on the basis of clinical and radiographic findings, by both the degree of webbing and the presence of bony fusion or other bony anomalies (Table 12.1). Radiographs of both hands (and feet, if toe syndactyly is present) help the surgeon classify the syndactyly.

The skin of the normal web space between the triphalangeal digits gently deepens from dorsal to volar halfway between the metacarpophalangeal and proximal interphalangeal joints (MPJ and PIPJ). In the mildest forms of syndactyly, the web is proximal to the PIPJ; this minimal anatomic variant can be adequately deepened without using a skin graft. Release of syndactyly distal to the PIPJ almost always requires additional skin.

Syndactyly-release incisions are planned so that the new web is composed of local flaps of native skin as opposed to skin grafts (Fig. 12.1, C and D), and the incisions on the sides of the fingers are angled to minimize the effects of graft and scar contraction during growth. Full-thickness skin grafts are almost always used because they are more durable and contract less than split-thickness grafts. However, even full-thickness grafts can contract and are slightly more likely to become hyperpigmented than split-thickness grafts.

Graft should be harvested from an inconspicuous location such as the upper groin (the surgeon should avoid harvesting from areas that will bear pubic hair at a later date, or the graft will bear hair in its new location) or the antecubital fossa. The groin provides more skin than the antecubital fossa, but because groin skin tends to be darker, the antecubital fossa is preferred by some surgeons because of its color match to the skin of the hand. Skin from the antecubital fossa has additional advantages: it is in the same surgical field as the hand, so that prepping and draping an additional surgical field is not necessary, and the graft can be harvested under tourniquet.

If the child has other congenital differences that may require ablation or amputation of tissues, including skin, the surgeon should plan syndactyly release at the same surgical sitting to harvest skin that would otherwise be discarded (Fig. 12.2, A and B).

Although most hand surgeons use full-thickness grafts in syndactyly reconstruction, there are reports of methods that decrease or eliminate the need for a graft. Special circumstances may be encountered in which avoiding graft harvest may be attractive, but it must be remembered that syndactyly is a problem of skin insufficiency. Therefore, these alternative techniques to spare the child a graft harvest are not yet widely accepted.

Neurovascular anomalies commonly accompany syndactyly. The common digital arteries may branch more distal than in normal, separated digits, and one branch may require ligation at the time of release. A distally branching common digital nerve can be separated by incising the epineurium and isolating the fascicles supplying each finger.

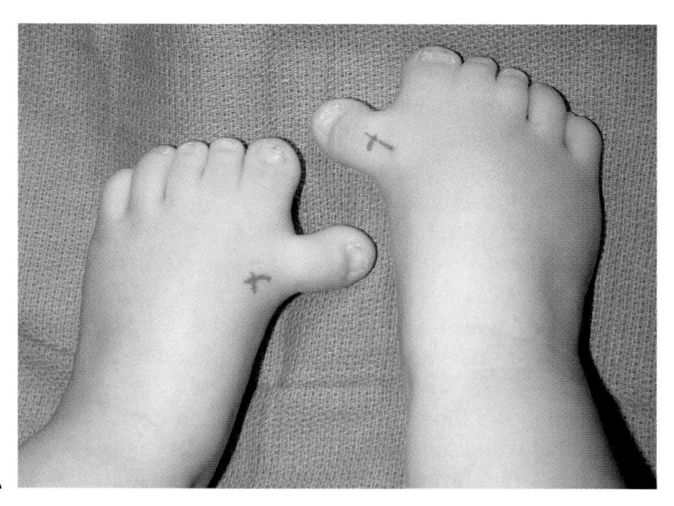

A

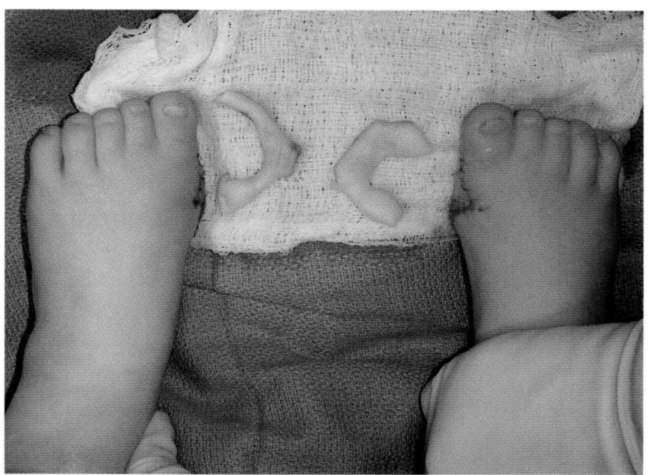

B

Figure 12.2. A: Toe polydactyly in a child with long-ring syndactyly. **B:** Skin harvested from ablated toes.

These are some of the reasons why creation of adjacent web spaces (i.e., operating on both sides of a single digit) at the same operation is never advocated. The chance of encountering an atypical vascular or nerve supply, coupled with the skin management challenges, make this practice far too risky for elective syndactyly release. Before performing the second release of a syndactyly involving a previously operated finger, careful scrutiny of the operative notes will hopefully reveal the status of the nerve and vessel on the initial operated side. Despite this relative assurance, a quick intraoperative pressure occlusion test of the digital vessels to ensure contralateral flow should be performed.

Several factors influence the timing of surgery. These include the digits involved (central versus border), the severity of the syndactyly (simple, complex), the influence of adjacent digits on growth (longitudinal, angular, or rotational malpositioning), and the general health status of the child.

Release of syndactyly involving the border digits can be contemplated at around 6 to 12 months of age, because pathologic influences of tethered growth may cause the longer digit to develop a flexion contracture and angulate toward the shorter one. While there is typically no such urgency to release long-ring or index-long syndactyly, parents may request earlier surgery. As long as the anesthetic risk is not increased by airway, pulmonary, or cardiac anomalies, the experienced hand surgeon can consider this preference without compromising the long-term result. However, there should never be an adverse decision made as a result of parental pressure; syndactyly release is almost always a completely elective procedure, and the safety and outcome must be maximized by respecting basic surgical tenets.

SURGERY

Complete Syndactyly Release (Fig. 12.1, A–O)

Position the patient in the supine position. For small children, place the child's head and ipsilateral shoulder on the securely attached hand table to allow the hand to reach the center of the proposed field. Perform the operation under general anesthesia and tourniquet control, using loupe magnification. Prepare and drape the full-thickness graft donor site (Fig. 12.3A), applying a sterile tourniquet if the antecubital fossa is used. Carefully plan and mark all flaps before inflating the tourniquet.

Place the base of the palmar "V" at the normal level of the proximal digital flexion crease (Fig. 12.1C). Place the base of the dorsal "rectangle" or trapezoid several millimeters proximal to this to create the normal dorsal-palmar slope of the web (Fig. 12.1D). The lengths of the palmar V and the dorsal rectangle should each be slightly longer than the depth of the palm. The sides of the dorsal rectangle should not extend beyond the midline of either digit.

The dorsal flap is fashioned as a trapezoid with the edge on the longer digit extending further distally than the edge on the shorter digit, creating an angulated distal margin (Fig. 12.1D). This prevents the most proximal dorsal triangle flap from being too acute. (If the syndactyly is complicated and there is no redundant soft tissue between the digits, consider using crossed triangles instead of the dorsal rectangle-palmar V technique described here.) Plan and mark the palmar and dorsal triangular flaps on the fingers to interdigitate with each other after the fingers are separated (Fig. 12.1, C and D), adjusting their lengths according to the amount of redundancy of skin between the digits. If a synostosis is present, plan the local flaps to cover the bony surfaces exposed by transecting the bony connection.

After exsanguinating the arm and elevating the tourniquet, use a single-prong skin hook and a sharp blade to elevate all flaps with a thin layer of subdermal fat to preserve the subdermal vascular plexus (Fig. 12.1, E and F).

Separate the digits carefully, protecting the flaps and searching for the neurovascular bundles. Avoid straying from the midline while separating the digits. Excise excess fat at the bases of the digits carefully, leaving a thin layer of subcutaneous fat as a graft bed. If the common digital artery and nerve bifurcate distal to the new web margin, separate the fascicles of the common digital nerve into the two proper digital nerves and ligate the

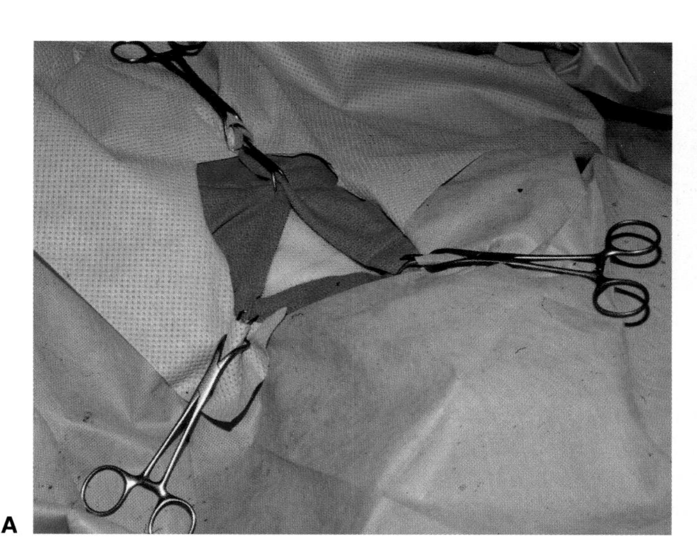

A

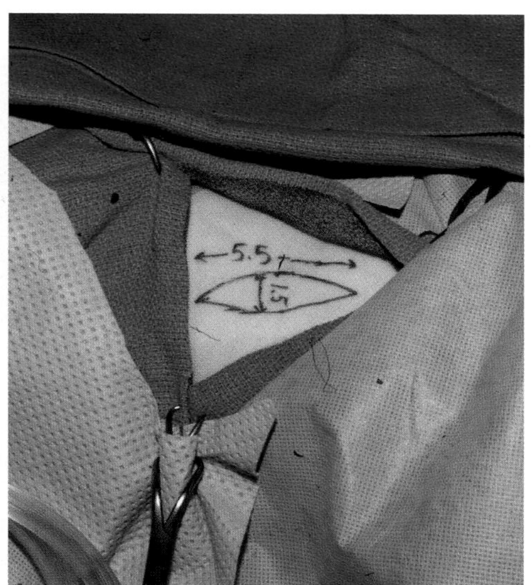

B

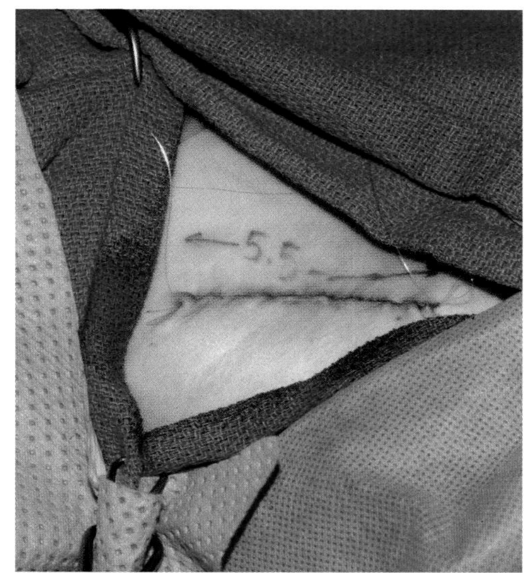

C

Figure 12.3. **A:** Groin full-thickness skin graft donor site, prepared and draped. **B:** Groin full-thickness skin graft donor site with incisions marked for harvesting skin, based on measurements of hand defects. **C:** Groin donor site after closure.

smaller of the two digital arteries or the artery that does not supply a border digit (e.g., preserve the radial digital artery to the small finger, since the ulnar digital artery to the small finger is often hypoplastic) (Fig. 12.1, G and H).

Split the dorsal rectangular flap longitudinally, almost to its base. Wrap half around each finger, suturing the corner closest to the midline of the flap in the triangular defect adjacent to the palmar triangular flap (Fig. 12.1I). Start suturing at the web and work distally, suturing the interdigitated flaps in place with 5-0 chromic or similarly sized absorbable suture (Fig. 12.1, J and K).

Synonychia, or shared nail elements, is encountered in most complete syndactylies regardless of whether they are simple or complex. If present, the surgeon can fashion nail folds to accommodate the newly transected nail by raising two long, narrow flaps across the fingertips, one based on each fingertip (Fig. 12.4). Each flap is the length of the nail. Raise these flaps carefully, dividing the nail, nail bed, and any synostosis of the distal phalanges, using a small bone cutter to transect the synostosis. Fold each flap down alongside the divided side of the nail to create the nail fold. In the smallest of fingers, this exercise may be almost impossible; in those cases in which the flap size is clearly insufficient to create two adjacent folds, maximize the reconstruction of the radial side nail fold of the ulnar digit.

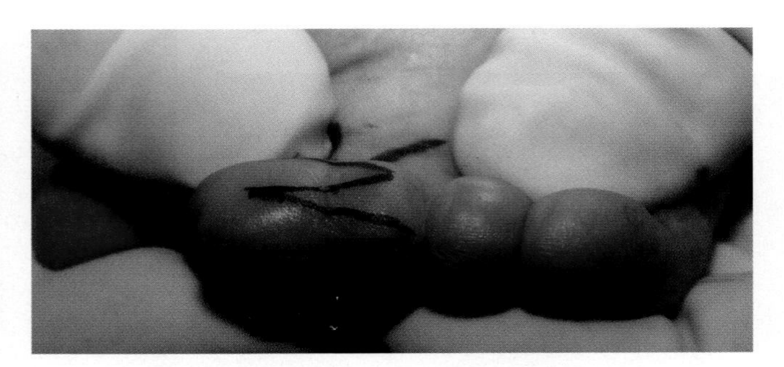

Figure 12.4. Synonychia flaps.

Use grafts for coverage on the proximal-dorsal aspect of each finger. Usually, one finger can be closed without any additional graft, and the remaining finger needs one to three grafts to fill in defects not covered by flaps. Measure the defects requiring grafts, adding the lengths of their longest sides together. The graft harvested will need to be as long as the sum of the lengths of the defects and as wide in the center as the widest defect. For example, if three grafts measuring 2 × 1 cm, 1.5 × 1.5 cm, and 2 × 0.5 cm are needed, the harvested graft should be an ellipse measuring 5.5 cm long and 1.5 cm across at its widest center point (Fig. 12.3B). Before obtaining graft from the groin, deflate and remove the tourniquet and achieve hemostasis. If graft is to be harvested from the antecubital fossa, leave the tourniquet inflated while the graft is harvested.

After anesthetizing the donor area with a local agent containing epinephrine, harvest full-thickness graft while stretching the skin. The epinephrine assists in hemostasis during and after the graft harvest, making it easier to raise the graft without the field being obscured with blood. The goal is to raise the flap with a minimum of subcutaneous fat on the graft; the depth of dissection should be closely monitored during the harvest. Remove any remaining dermis from the donor wound, achieve hemostasis, and close the wound cosmetically, in layers (Fig. 12.3C).

Suture the graft to the defects, usually with an absorbable suture material such as 5-0 chromic gut, starting at the corner of a smaller defect so that all excess graft ends up on one side of the defect. Stretch the graft snugly across the defect, insetting it, and trim the excess. Repeat with each defect, using the trimmed graft. Use graft from the middle of the ellipse to cover the largest defect (Fig. 12.1, L–N.)

Dress the hand wounds with nonadherent gauze, such as Xeroform or Adaptic, and moistened cotton balls to provide a bolster. Then apply a bulky compressive dressing and cover with a long-arm fiberglass cast shell with the elbow fixed at 90 degrees flexion (Fig. 12.1O). Leave the tip of the thumb exposed, and tell parents that if the thumb disappears the child is wiggling out of the cast and they should return for cast reapplication.

Partial Syndactyly Release (Fig. 12.5, A–F)

If the web does not need to be deepened more than the thickness of the palm, separation may be accomplished without the need for skin grafting. Different flap techniques have been described to close the deepened web. The three-square flap method works well if the dorsal, palmar, and distal aspects of the web are flat and approximately equal in size. In most cases of congenital syndactyly, a butterfly flap works best.

The dorsal aspect of the butterfly flap is a rectangle, based at the initiation of the web slope. On the palmar side, the flaps can either be a "Z" (Fig. 12.5C) or a squared-off "S," with the horizontal bottom of the Z or S at the level of the proximal digital flexion crease and the horizontal top along the web margin. After elevating the flaps, suture the distal margin of the dorsal flap to the palm at the level of the distal palmar flexion crease and wrap the two palmar flaps around the digits, filling the defects created by moving the dorsal rectangle (Fig. 12.5, E and F).

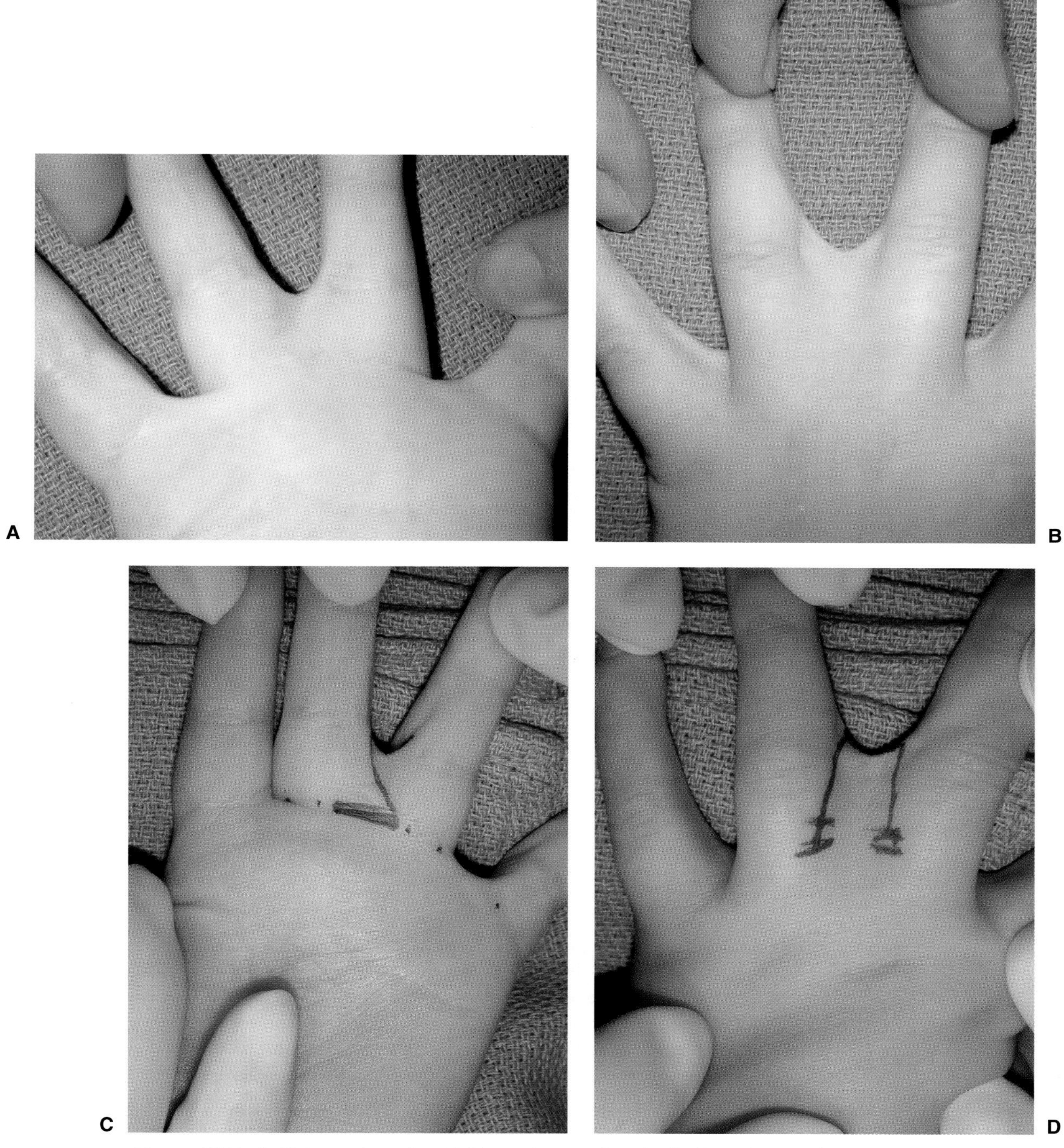

Figure 12.5. **A:** Palmar view of partial long-ring syndactyly. **B:** Dorsal view of partial long-ring syndactyly. **C:** Palmar incisions for butterfly flap. **D:** Dorsal incisions for butterfly flap.

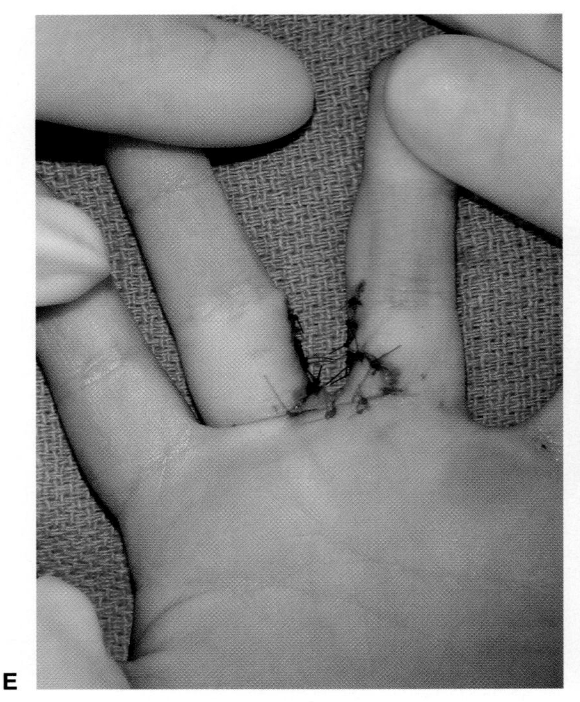
E

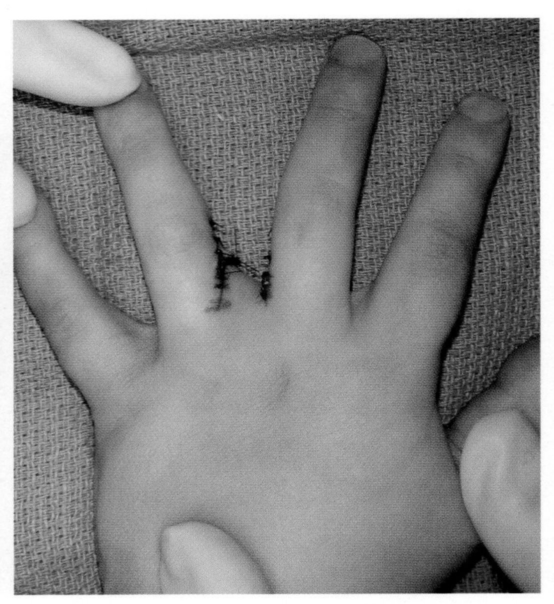
F

Figure 12.5. *Continued.* **E:** Flaps sutured in place from the palmar aspect. **F:** Flaps sutured in place from the dorsal aspect.

Thumb-Index Syndactyly Release (Dorsal Rotation Advancement Flap) (Fig. 12.6, A–H)

The thumb web should extend from the index MPJ to the thumb MPJ and should be lax enough to allow free palmar and radial abduction. For partial syndactyly, a simple or four-fold Z-plasty may be adequate. For complete syndactyly, the technique described above for fingers may suffice, but a dorsal rotation flap is often preferable.

Plan a large radially-based dorsal flap (Fig. 12.6, D and E). When measured from its point of rotation, the flap should be long enough to reach the middle of the thenar eminence to avoid contracture. Plan one or more zigzags on the palmar surface to avoid a longitudinal scar and to interdigitate if possible. Release the fascia of the first dorsal interosseous muscle in line with its raphe; in some cases, the adductor fascia may need to be incised. Protect the radial digital nerve to the index finger, as it is superficial and crosses the incision. When suturing the flaps in place, close the dorsal defect by bringing the skin edges together (Fig. 12.6G). Skin graft is not usually necessary. The scar will probably widen, but the appearance of a wide scar is less unsightly than the appearance of graft on the dorsum of the hand. The hand pictured in Figure 12.7 has a healed dorsal rotation advancement flap (note Fig. 12.7C).

Symbrachydactyly Release (Fig. 12.7, A–H)

The technique described for complete syndactyly is used, but resist the temptation to make the fingers appear longer by setting the web proximal to the normal level. This "phalangizes" the metacarpal and looks unattractive.

Separation of Syndactyly in Apert Syndrome

The treatment of this condition is as complex as the syndactyly and is beyond the scope of this chapter. Although many of the basic concepts are offered here, the planning of a

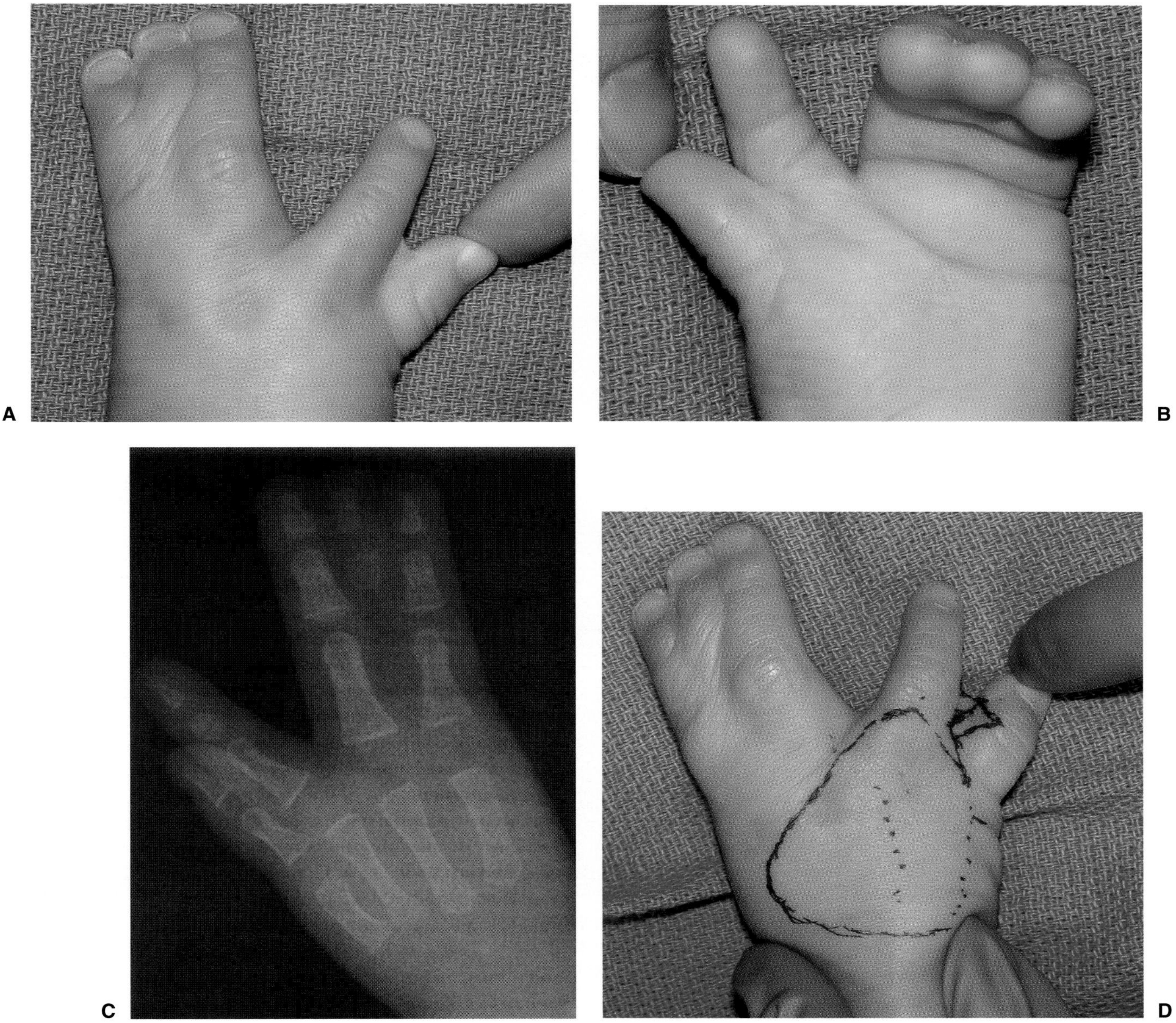

A B C D

Figure 12.6. A: Dorsal view of partial thumb-index syndactyly (with complete, complicated finger syndactyly). **B:** Palmar view of partial thumb-index syndactyly. **C:** x-ray of thumb-index syndactyly and complicated finger syndactyly. **D:** Dorsal incisions for dorsal rotation advancement flap.

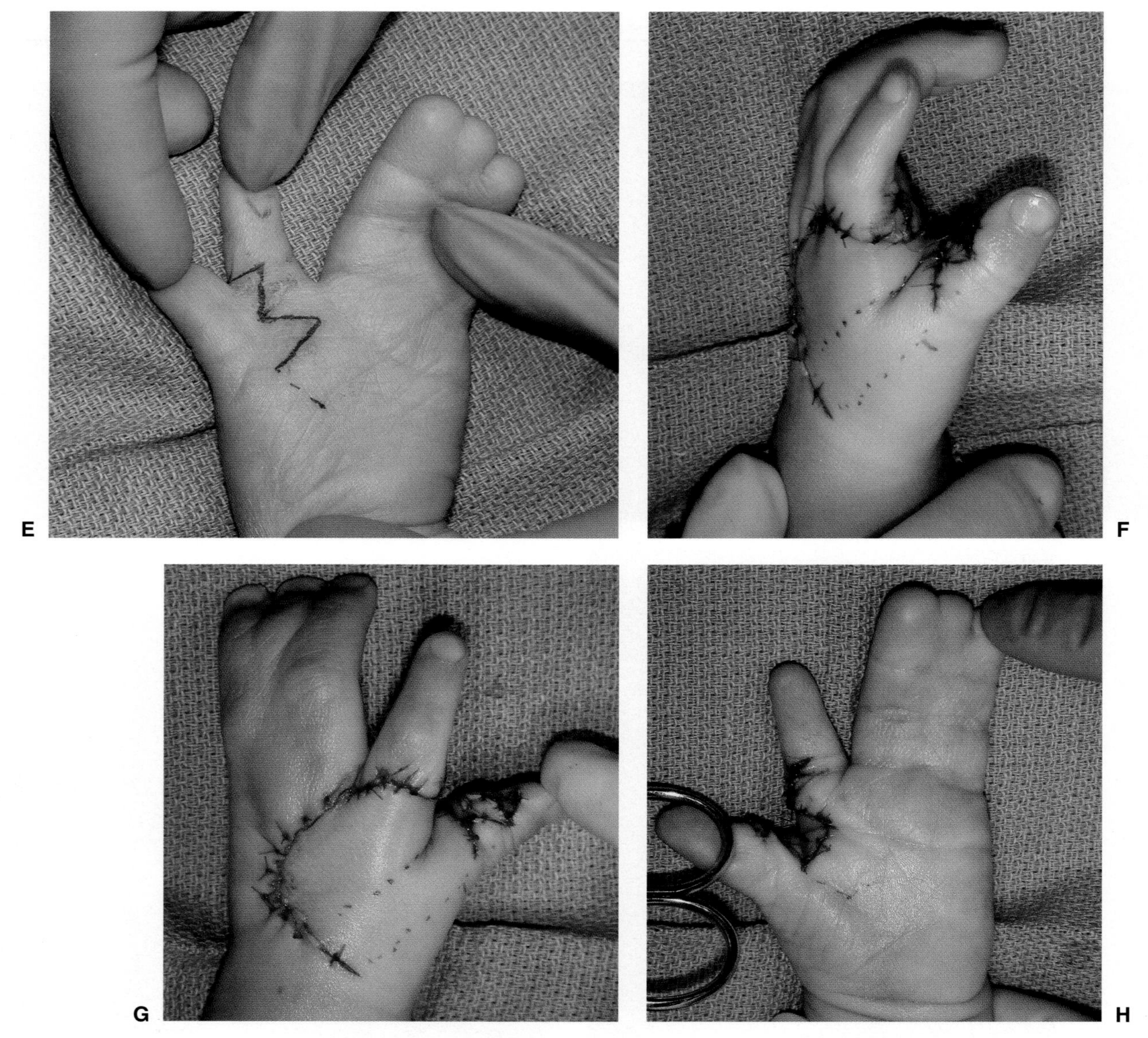

Figure 12.6. *Continued.* **E:** Palmar incisions for dorsal rotation advancement flap. **F:** Postoperative view of a web created by dorsal rotation advancement flap. **G:** Flaps sutured in place from the dorsal aspect. **H:** Flaps sutured in place from the palmar aspect.

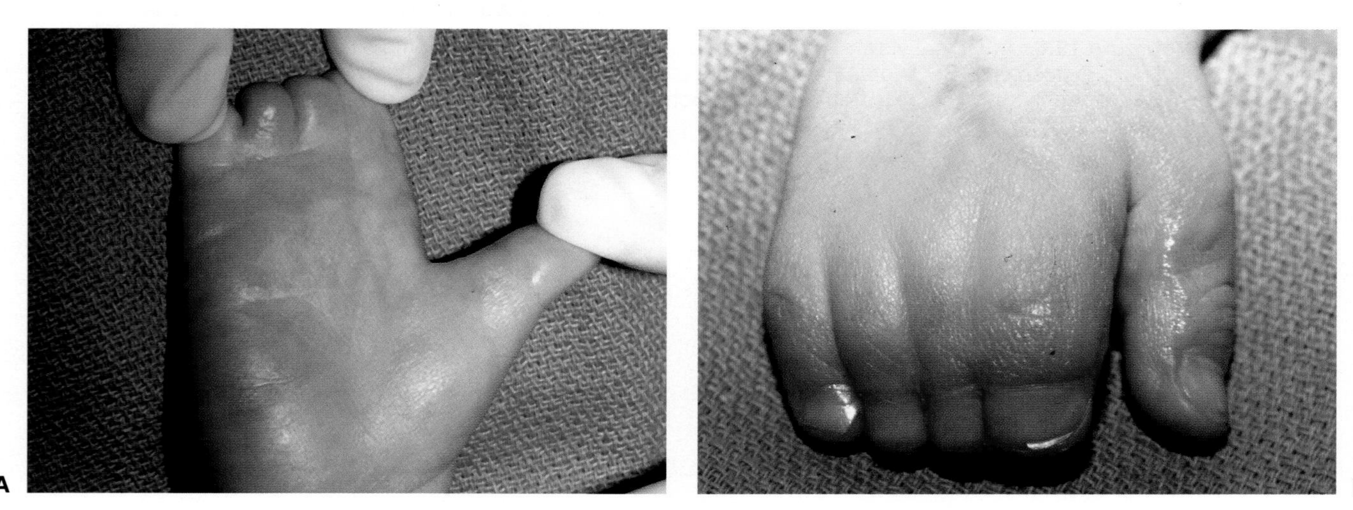

Figure 12.7. **A:** Palmar view of symbrachydactyly. **B:** Dorsal view of symbrachydactyly.

C D E F G H

Figure 12.7. *Continued.* **C:** First web (previous dorsal rotation advancement flap). **D:** Palmar incisions for index-long and ring-small syndactyly releases. **E:** Dorsal incisions for index-long and ring-small syndactyly releases. **F:** Flaps and grafts sutured in place from the palmar aspect. **G:** Flaps and grafts sutured in place from the dorsal aspect. **H:** Flaps and grafts sutured in place from the distal aspect.

multistep reconstruction is needed for this complex congenital difference. It is rare that a five-digit hand can be created in the setting of acrosyndactyly accompanying Apert's syndrome. See the work of Fereshetian, Upton, Van Heest, Al-Qattan, and Chang for details.

POSTOPERATIVE MANAGEMENT

Instruct the parents to keep the cast dry at all times and to return immediately for a cast change if it becomes wet or if the exposed tip of the thumb disappears (indicating that the child is slipping out of the cast). Leave the cast and bulky dressing in place for 3 to 4 weeks, then remove it and allow the child to use the hand without restrictions; no splinting or therapy is necessary.

RESULTS

The slope of the web created with a split dorsal rectangle and palmar V is very close to normal. Webs reconstructed with crossed triangle flaps appear less contoured or more "squared off." The skin graft scars are usually minimal, especially if the grafts are attached under slight tension, and are inset into the defects. Six-month postoperative results of complete syndactyly release are shown in Figure 12.8.

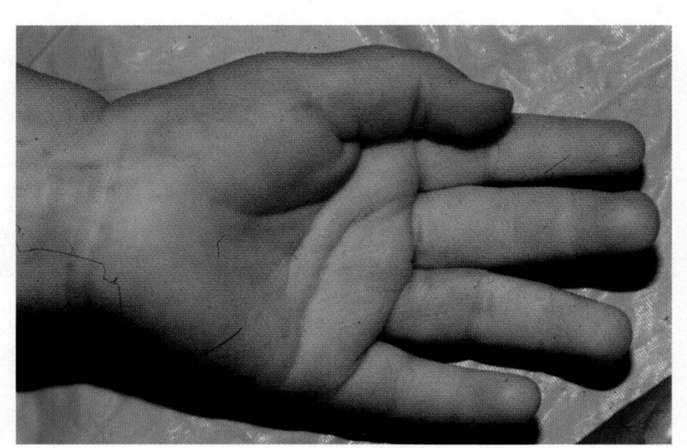
A

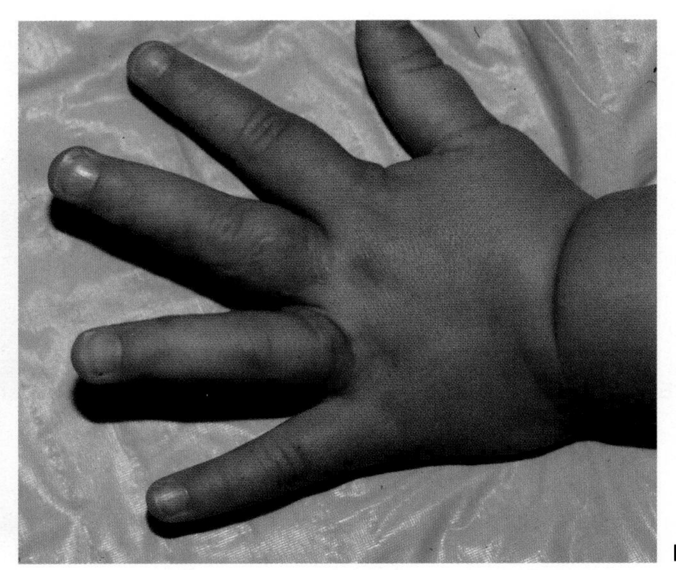
B

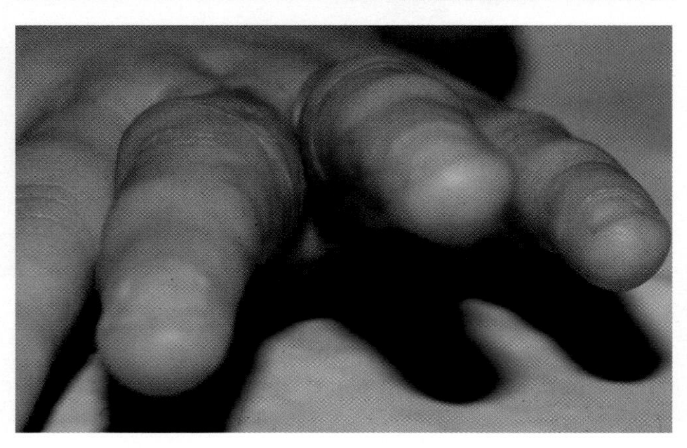
C

Figure 12.8. Six-month follow-up photographs of complete syndactyly release (same patient as in Fig. 12.1). **A:** Palmar view, 6 months after complete long-ring syndactyly release. **B:** Dorsal view, 6 months after complete long-ring syndactyly release. **C:** Long-ring web, 6 months after complete long-ring syndactyly release.

After separation, fingers with simple syndactyly usually function normally. Those with complex or complicated syndactyly may remain stiff and may develop deformity with growth. Parents should be informed of these facts from the outset, and periodic follow-up is suggested.

This operation is not simple. Like many hand operations, if it is not done well the first time it is very difficult to redo well. Operating through scarred beds, especially asymmetric webs, is challenging. The difficulty in managing the neurovascular bundles in a return operation is multiplied.

COMPLICATIONS

Hypertrophic scarring in the web and "web creep" (a web margin that ends up more distal because of excessive scarring or the influence of growth) may not be avoidable. However, these "complications" are often the result of too much tension in the web space closure. Pedicle flaps must be carefully planned so they cover the base of the web, as graft at the base will contract and narrow the web. Graft may be used generously, but each individual graft should not be too large for its space or the contour will not be smooth. When hypertrophic scarring occurs, it can be successfully treated with a custom-made compression glove or odoform petroleum spacers, as used by burn surgeons for the treatment of hand burns.

The pitfall of separating short fingers (symbrachydactyly) has already been described. The surgeon should avoid the temptation to make the webs deeper than normal level to make the fingers appear longer. These children will be just as functional, if not more so, with a web space that matches the architecture of their hand.

Groin donor graft tends to become hyperpigmented over time. Because this is especially noticeable in darker-skinned individuals, antecubital skin may be preferable.

ACKNOWLEDGEMENTS

Thank you to Julia Serat and Matt Harrison, photographers, for the intraoperative images.

RECOMMENDED READING

1. Al-Qattan MM. Classification of hand anomalies in Poland's syndrome. *Br J Plast Surg* 54:132–136, 2001.
2. Al-Qattan MM. The use of split thickness skin grafts in the correction of Apert's syndactyly. *J Hand Surg* 26B:8–10, 2001.
3. Al-Qattan MM, Al-Husain MA. Classification of hand anomalies in Apert's syndrome. *J Hand Surg* 21B:266–268, 1996.
4. Bandoh Y, Yanai A, Seno H. The three-square-flap method for reconstruction of minor syndactyly. *J Hand Surg* 22A:680–684, 1997.
5. Chang J, Danton TK, Ladd AL, et al. Reconstruction of the hand in Apert syndrome: a simplified approach. *Plast Reconstr Surg* 109:465–470; discussion 471, 2002.
6. De Smet L. Classification for congenital anomalies of the hand: the IFSSH classification and the JSSH modification. *Genet Couns* 13:331–338, 2002.
7. Deunk J, Nicolai JP, Hamburg SM. Long-term results of syndactyly correction: full-thickness versus split-thickness skin grafts. *J Hand Surg* 28B:125–130, 2003.
8. Dobyns JH, Wood VE, Bayne LG. Congenital Hand Deformities. In: Green DP, Hotchkiss RN, eds. *Operative Hand Surgery*. New York: Churchill Livingstone, 1993:251–548.
9. Eaton CJ, Lister GD. Syndactyly. *Hand Clinics* 6:555–576, 1990.
10. Ekerot L. Syndactyly correction without skin-grafting. *J Hand Surg* 21B:330–337, 1996.
11. Fereshetian S, Upton J. The anatomy and management of the thumb in Apert syndrome. *Clin Plast Surg* 18:365–380, 1991.
12. Flatt AE. Webbed Fingers. In: Flatt AE, ed. *The Care of Congenital Hand Anomalies*. St. Louis: Quality Medical Publishing, 1994:228–275.
13. Goodman FR. Limb malformations and the human HOX genes. *Am J Med Genet* 112:256–265, 2002.
14. Gould JS. Syndactyly. In: Carter PR, ed. *Reconstruction of the Child's Hand*. Philadelphia: Lea & Febiger, 1991:127–152.
15. Ireland DC, Takayama N, Flatt AE. Poland's syndrome. *J Bone Joint Surg* 58A:52–58, 1976.
16. James MA. Congenital Hand Malformations. In: Chapman MW, ed. *Chapman's Operative Orthopaedics*. Philadelphia: Lippincott Williams and Wilkins, 2001:1871–1941.

17. Marble K, Fudem G. First web space release with the dorsal hand rotation flap: closing the donor site. *Ann Plast Surg* 35:83–85, 1995.
18. McCarroll HR. Congenital anomalies: a 25-year overview. *J Hand Surg* 25A:1007–1037, 2000.
19. McCarroll HR Jr, Manske PR. The windblown hand: correction of the complex clasped thumb deformity. *Hand Clinics* 8:147–159, 1992.
20. Moore MH. Nonadjacent syndactyly in the congenital constriction band syndrome. *J Hand Surg* 17A:21–23, 1992.
21. Sandzen SC. Thumb web reconstruction. *Clin Orthop* 195:66–82, 1985.
22. Sommerlad BC. The open finger technique for release of syndactyly. *J Hand Surg* 26B:499–500, 2001.
23. Temtamy SA, McKusick VA. Syndactyly as Part of Syndromes. In: Bergsma D, Mudge JR, Paul NW, et al. eds. *The Genetics of Hand Malformations*. New York: Alan R. Liss, 1978:323–361.
24. Upton J. Apert syndrome: classification and pathologic anatomy of limb anomalies. *Clin Plast Surg* 18:321–355, 1991.
25. Van Heest AE, House JH, Reckling WC. Two-stage reconstruction of Apert acrosyndactyly. *J Hand Surg* 22A:315–322, 1997.

13

Reconstruction of the Duplicated Thumb

Gary M. Lourie

INDICATIONS/CONTRAINDICATIONS

Since its first description in 1645 by Digby, the treatment of the duplicate thumb continues to evolve. Even since the first edition of Master Techniques in Orthopaedic Surgery: The Hand, important contributions have been made. The infant with a duplicate thumb usually represents, by its presence, an indication for surgical reconstruction. This condition, seen in approximately 0.08 per 1,000 births, is equally seen in blacks and whites, but is slightly more common in Native Americans and Asians. It falls into the category of duplication as recommended by the International Federation of Societies for Surgery of the Hand (IFSSH).

Classifications developed by Bayne, Wassel, and others have accurately described the presentation of the duplicate thumb. The Wassel IV classification involves a single but widened metacarpal with duplication of the phalanges distally, and represents nearly 50% of all cases. Rarer presentations exist, but overall surgical goals remain the same: to ablate the hypoplastic component but combine structures from both thumbs to create a stable metacarpophalangeal joint, align bony units and centralize tendinous structures to optimize motion, and confirm a healthy sensate pulp for pinch and prehensile activity.

The progression of prehensile activity dictates the timing of surgical reconstruction. At month 6 of age, gross grasp and grip develop, with thumb and index finger function at 12 months of age. Voluntary release usually occurs at about 18 months of age, with established patterns seen between 2 to 3 years of age. There is no reason to operate before 1 year, as respiratory maturation will progress during this time and with age lessen the anesthetic risk. Some support is found in the Japanese literature for preoperative splinting; however, this splinting is cumbersome and usually not beneficial.

Surgery is indicated in the second to third year of life. The larger hand allows for easier dissection of neurovascular and tendinous structures. Further, postoperative casting will be easier to apply and maintain.

Gary M. Lourie, M.D.: Department of Orthopaedics, Emory University School of Medicine, Atlanta, GA, and Department of Hand Surgery, Scottish-Rite Children's Medical Center, Atlanta, GA

There are contraindications to surgery, but usually are the result of generalized systemic abnormalities that can exist with the duplicate thumb itself. Though conditions such as Holt-Oram, Diamond-Blackfan, and Fanconi's anemia are mostly seen with hypoplastic thumbs, it is not unusual to encounter these conditions, especially if the duplicate thumb involves a triphalangeal component; and to avoid possible catastrophic intraoperative events, hematologic indices, along with pediatric consultation, should be sought.

PREOPERATIVE PLANNING

Duplication of the thumb usually occurs as a sporadic mutation; however, rarely an autosomal dominant inheritance pattern can be seen. Because of this, genetic counseling should be offered to the patient's parents. A complete blood count (CBC), platelet count, along with prothrombin time (PT) should be assessed to rule out thrombocytopenia and coagulopathies. It is important early to explain to the parents that the child with a duplicate thumb will never have a completely normal thumb after surgical reconstruction. Even removal of the hypoplastic component and reconstruction of the dominant thumb will still leave the child with a smaller and stiffer thumb. Ezaki recommends referring to the duplicate thumb as a "split thumb" to impress this point upon the parents. Long-term studies have shown that even after surgical reconstruction, interphalangeal motion will be limited, averaging 0 to 30 degrees. The possibility of postoperative sequelae, such as the zigzag deformity, should be discussed with the parents along with the 25% need for revision later as the child grows. If these factors are discussed preoperatively, it will avoid any misconceptions that may arise later.

It is important in the child's first year of life to perform frequent physical and radiographic examinations. Not only do these visits allow for refinement of a surgical plan, but also cement the important bond with the family. Simple ablation of one of the duplicate thumbs has been met with failure, with best results seen with ablation of the hypoplastic component, centralization of the flexor and extensor tendons, alignment of bony units with osteotomies, reconstruction of the metacarpal phalangeal collateral ligament, and, through judicious use of skin incisions, providing good sensate coverage. Examining the child at play or examining for skin creases will reveal the more radial component to be usually hypoplastic and better suited for ablation. Palpation of the flexor and extensor tendons can give information about their contribution to the angular deformity. Frequently, the tendons are displaced in a radial direction and will need centralization. Lister has described the pollex abductus, an abnormal insertion of the flexor tendon radial that potentiates the angular deformity.

Frequent radiographs yield information on the status of the bony units. Most commonly in the Wassel IV presentation, a widened metacarpal head is present that requires intraoperative reduction. Angulation of the metacarpal ulnar and phalangeal angulation radial can be evaluated, confirming the later need for reconstructive osteotomies. Collateral ligament stability should be assessed, as most commonly the radiocollateral ligament of the metaphalangeal joint is unstable and will require reconstruction. Thenar muscle function should be assessed, as its usual insertion radial will need to be transferred at the time of reconstruction.

Radiographs may reveal, as Bayne has described, a "mixed quality of duplication." This is important, as rarely reconstruction will require removal of the radial component at the level of the metacarpal with transfer of the ulnar component to the base of the more radial metacarpal. Preoperative planning does not usually call for the use of arteriography. The arterial pattern, however, has been studied by Kitayama, who found that more than 75% of the time there is a digital vessel to each component, and 5% of the time involving only one digital vessel to the ulnar component. This highlights the possible ischemic consequence if the radial component is saved; in actuality, however, almost always the radial component is removed. Different presentations of the duplicate thumb do exist and will require alteration in the treatment scheme. Overall goals, however, remain the same, and because the

Wassel IV presentation (single but widened metacarpal with duplication of the proximal and distal phalanx) is the most common presentation, its surgical repair will be described in detail. In the rarer Wassel II presentation (single proximal phalanx with duplicate distal phalanx), the Bilhaut-Cloquet procedure with central excision of bone has been recommended, and the reader is provided references, though long-term follow-up has shown problems with the growth plate, nail growth, and stiffness.

SURGICAL TECHNIQUE

The surgery is performed under general anesthesia in the supine position, with the upper extremity on a hand table. The tourniquet is placed high on the arm to prevent breakthrough interosseous bleeding and, after exsanguination, inflated to approximately 100 mm above systolic pressure.

An incision is made beginning just distal to the carpometacarpal joint and continued to the base of the radial hypoplastic thumb. This incision can be either longitudinal, later closed with a Z-plasty, or can be constructed in a zigzag fashion. A longitudinal scar will contract and can contribute to a postoperative angular deformity and thus should be avoided (Fig. 13.1). The initial dissection should identify and retain all structures until the actual anatomic orientation is confirmed. Aberrant tendons along with neurovascular structures need to be identified, and only after it is determined to remove the more hypoplastic thumb can then the vascular structures be ligated. Tendons both extensor and flexor need to dissected proximal, and it is prudent to retain all parts even if anamolous, as they may later be useful for augmentation of the reconstructed thumb.

The flaps are developed and tagged with suture to help in exposure. Next the thenar muscles are identified and followed to their insertion, which usually is into the radial hypoplastic thumb. The insertion is released and tagged for later transfer to the ulnar thumb (Fig. 13.2). By tagging the thenar muscle after its release and retracting it more proximal, better exposure is given to the widened metacarpal head.

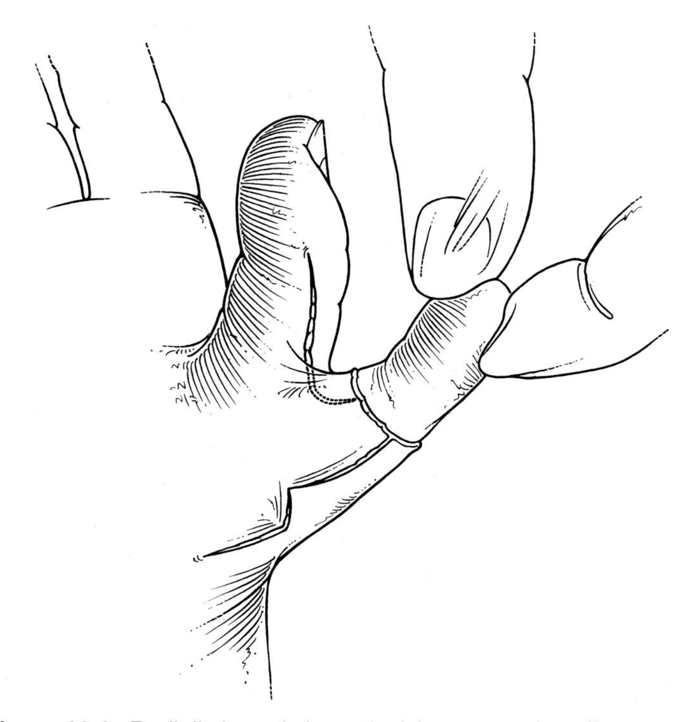

Figure 13.1. Radially based zigzag incision preserving all structures.

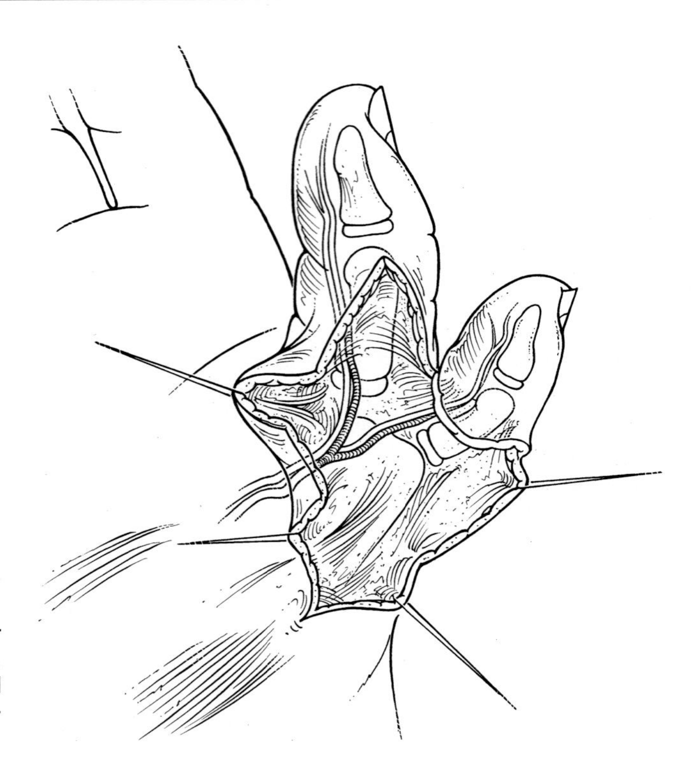

Figure 13.2. After the flaps are developed, the neurovascular bundles are identified and dissected out to their respective digits, the thenar muscles, usually attached radially, are detached and tagged and proximally retracted, giving exposure to the metacarpophalangeal joint.

A 10-mm-wide strip of tissue, including periosteum from P-1, capsule from the metacarpophalangeal joint, along with the proximally based periosteum of the metacarpal, is developed and tagged for later distal and volar advancement to reconstruct the radial collateral ligament of the MP joint (Fig. 13.3). With this strip developed, access to the MP joint is allowed and reveals a widened metacarpal head presenting as a dual-faceted structure (Fig. 13.4). The extra facet is removed with either a No. 15 blade or No. 69 Beaver blade. The metacarpal may also be angulated in an ulnar direction, and if present a closing wedge osteotomy-based radial is performed. Because the bony structures are delicate, the os-

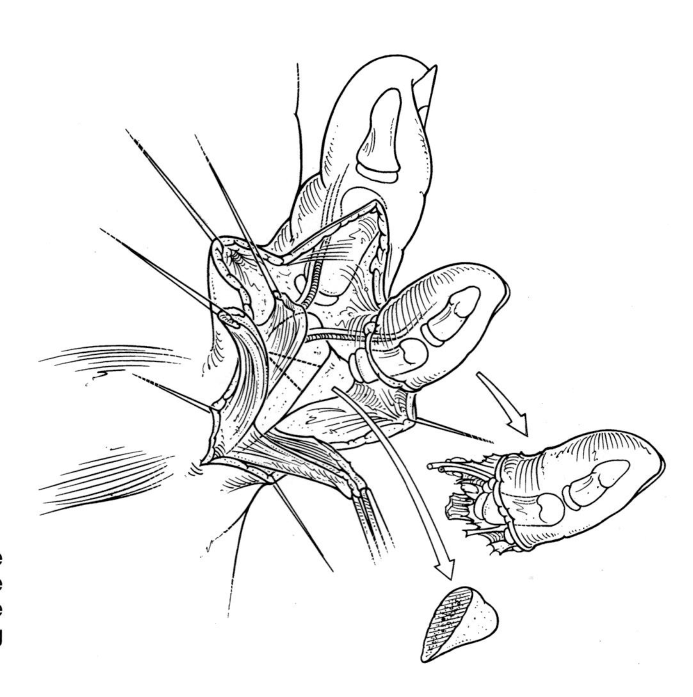

Figure 13.3. With the thenar muscles retracted, a 10-mm-wide periosteal capsular sleeve is raised for later reconstruction of the radial collateral ligament to the metacarpophalangeal joint. The widened metacarpal head is now visible, frequently presenting as a dual-faceted structure.

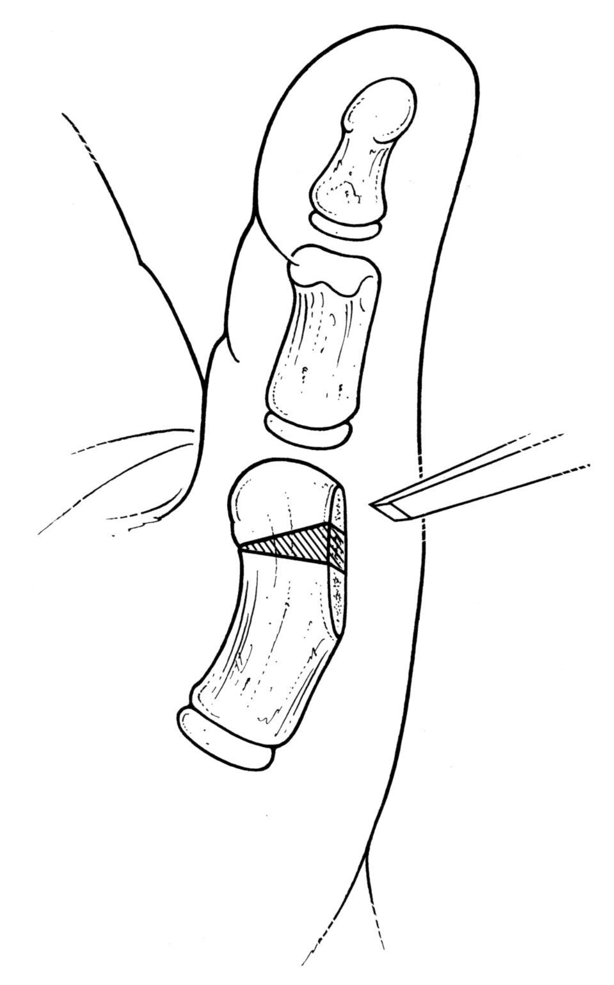

Figure 13.4. The combined reduction closing wedge osteotomy is illustrated.

teotomy is often performed with the use of a fine rongeur. By leaving the ulnar cortex intact, the osteotomy can be closed with manual pressure, correcting the angulation. Fixation is achieved with a Kirschner wire, usually 0.028 to 0.035/1000 of an inch in size (Fig. 13.5). Rarely the need for osteotomies at the level of the proximal phalanx will be necessary and must be performed to confirm that all joint surfaces are perpendicular to the longitudinal axis of the bone.

The reconstructed radial collateral ligament of the metacarpophalangeal joint is attached distal and volar to recreate its normal orientation (Fig. 13.5). The previously tagged thenar muscles are attached to the periosteum at the base of P-1 of the preserved thumb. The extensor pollicis longus and flexor pollicis longus tendons frequently need to be recentralized at this point. This is necessary to prevent potential angular deformity. Extra tendinous structures from the ablated thumb are used to augment the retained tendons. The incision is now closed, with particular attention to closing this in a zigzag fashion to avoid a longitudinal contracted scar.

Final trimming of the skin flaps is better done at the end of the procedure, though shortage of skin is rarely a problem. The pin is cut outside the skin, dressed, and the tourniquet released before final application of the dressing to confirm satisfactory capillary refill. Intraoperative radiographs confirm final position of the osteotomies. A long-arm splint is applied, incorporating all the digits, including the thumb, in a boxing-glove fashion to optimize the chance of the dressing remaining on for the entire postoperative period.

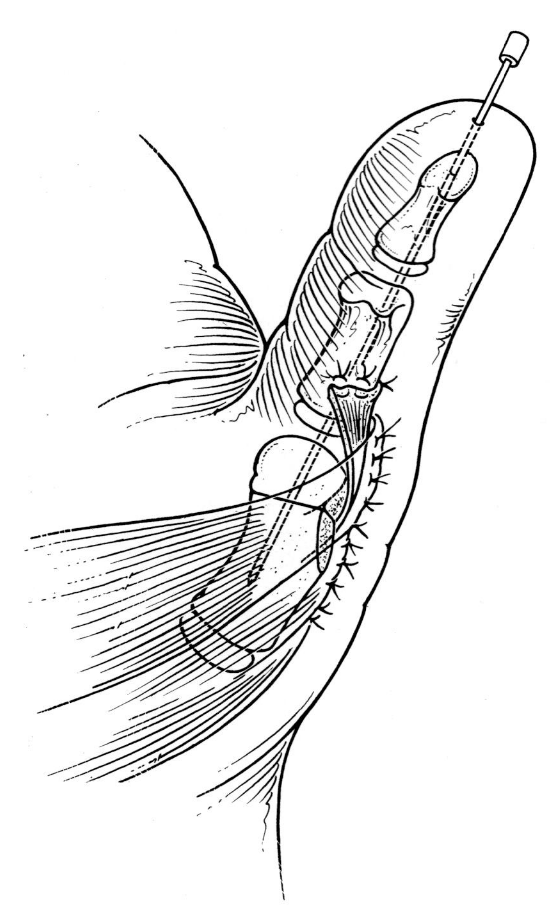

Figure 13.5. The reconstructed radial collateral ligament and advanced thenar muscles, along with longitudinal Kirschner wire aligning the osteotomies. The flaps are turned and closed in a zigzag fashion to prevent longitudinal linear contracture.

POSTOPERATIVE MANAGEMENT

The patient is usually admitted overnight, with the extremity elevated on one or two pillows. When the patient is discharged the next day, the extremity is immobilized in a sling or sling-and-swathe soft dressing.

If there are no postoperative problems, the patient is usually seen at 3 weeks, at which time radiographs are taken. If the osteotomies are healed, the pin is removed, and the patient is placed into a resting thumb-spica splint for an additional 3 weeks full time except for bathing and eating. During this time, initiation of active range of motion is performed. At the end of 6 weeks, the splint is usually reduced to nighttime and naptime wear, for an additional 6 months.

The early postoperative period is an optimum time to again discuss with the parents the long-term results of duplicate thumb reconstruction. Reaffirming that the final appearance of the reconstructed thumb will never retain the size of the contralateral is important. The interphalangeal motion will not increase greatly from preop measurements, usually maximizing in the 30-degree range. Continued growth of the thumb may result in an angular deformity known as the zigzag deformity, and parents must be reminded that there is up to a 25% need for revision surgery. Even though the reconstructed thumb will be slightly smaller and slightly stiffer, parents can expect their child to have excellent prehensile function and a thumb of satisfactory appearance if the surgeon adheres to the recommended principles.

COMPLICATIONS

The reconstruction of the duplicate thumb is difficult and can be fraught with complications. These include a longitudinal contracted scar, incomplete correction of the bony units, instability of the reconstructed metacarpophalangeal joint, and development of a characteristic angular deformity known as the zigzag deformity. Limited range of motion, especially at the interphalangeal joint, is not uncommon and averages less than 30 degrees. Repeat joint releases have not been successful; however, if pain develops an arthrodesis can be considered.

Instability at the metacarpophalangeal joint is the result of inadequate advancement of the periosteal capsular flap and often needs revision if the angular deformity becomes significant. Care must be taken in the initial operation in developing this flap, as retention of a bit of cartilage may later ossify and cause bony prominence and potentiate the instability. Reoperation can result in further joint stiffness and again if symptomatic, arthrodesis and chondrodesis can be done.

The most troublesome complication involves the zigzag deformity, which is manifested by ulnar deviation at the P-1 phalanx in combination with radial deviation at the P-2 phalanx. Many causes have been described, including incompetent radiocollateral ligament at the MP joint; a residual widened metacarpal head with undercorrection, both accentuated by a longitudinal scar and radial displacement of the extensor pollicis longus (EPL), and flexor pollicis longus (FPL). The pinch mechanism accentuates this collapse pattern, and the deformity can be aggravated by the rarely present pollex abductus, which involves the aberrant attachment of the FPL to the EPL radially. The deformity is unresponsive to splinting, and revision includes Z-plasty of the longitudinal scar, "slimming down" of the metacarpal head with osteotomy if needed, and removal of the radial half of the EPL tendon and reattachment of the FPL in a centralized position. Figure 13.6 shows the preoperative appearance of a 1-year-old infant with the characteristic deformity. The principles of reconstruction of the zigzag deformity are outlined in Figure 13.7, and the final postoperative appearance in Figure 13.8. Figures 13.9–13.12 demonstrate the scheme of treatment in a Wassel II thumb but highlight the important details similar to the Wassel IV reconstruction.

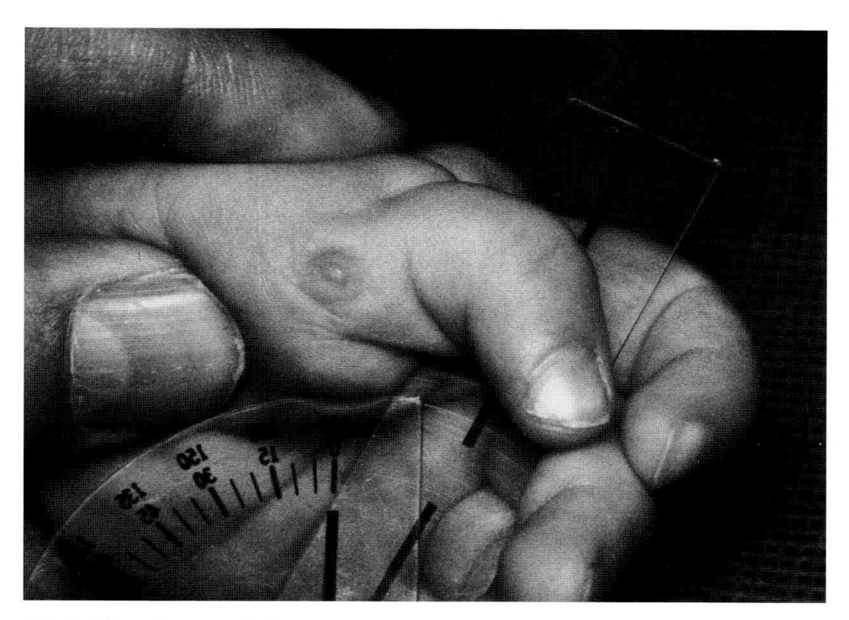

Figure 13.6. The characteristic zigzag deformity after simple ablation of the hypoplastic thumb.

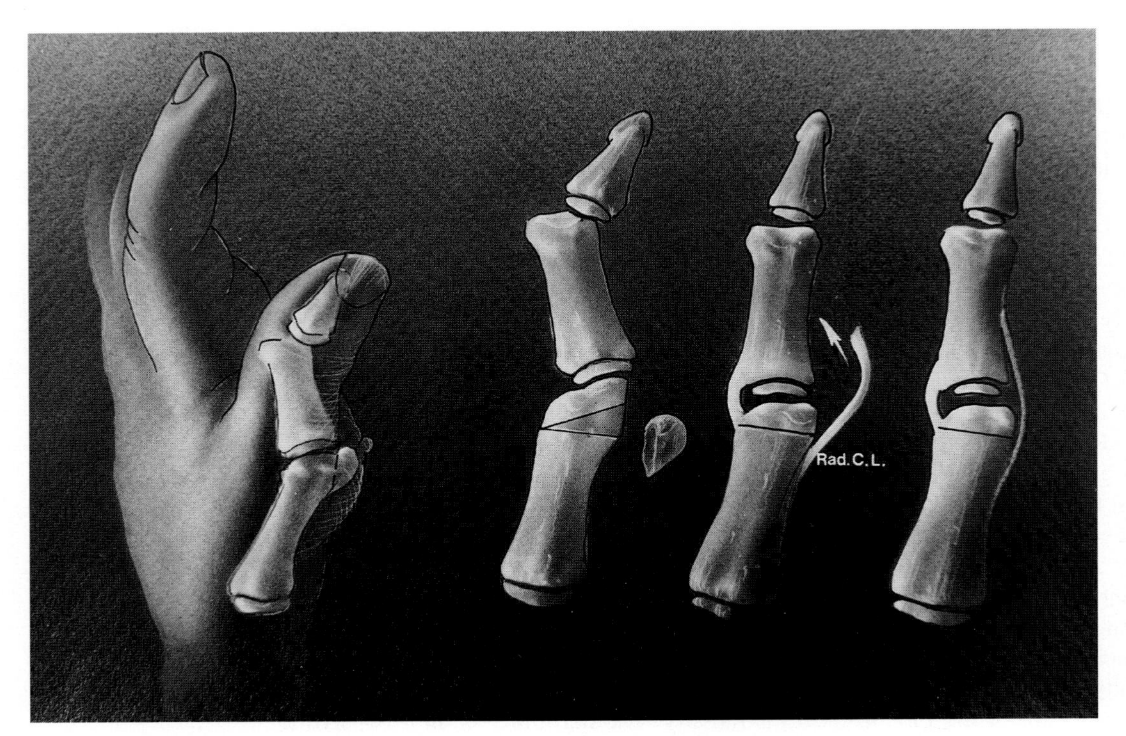

Figure 13.7. The proposed reconstruction of the zigzag deformity, with reconstruction of the radiocollateral ligament and reconstructive osteotomies to realign the bony units.

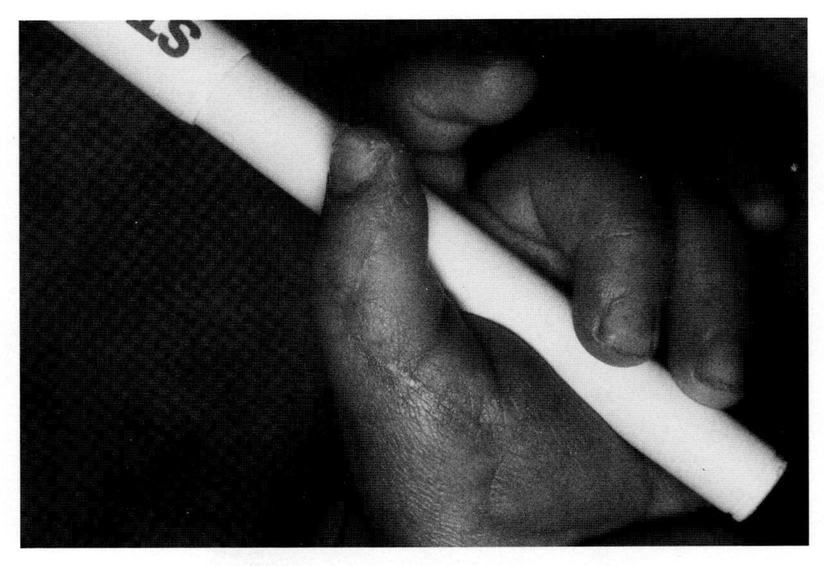

Figure 13.8. The postoperative correction.

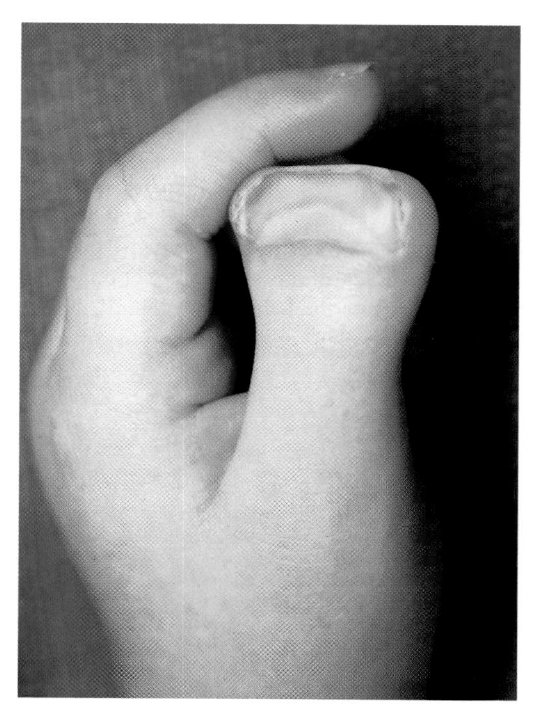

Figure 13.9. Preoperative appearance of a Wassel II thumb.

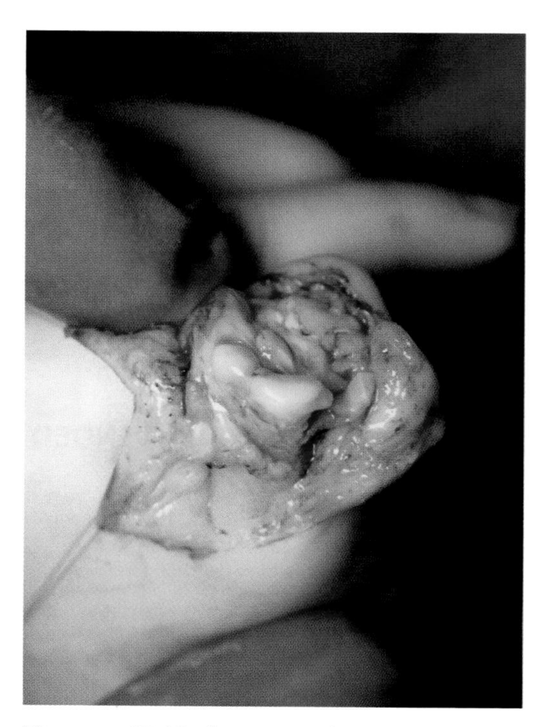

Figure 13.10. Intraoperative appearance demonstrating the dual facet of the proximal phalanx.

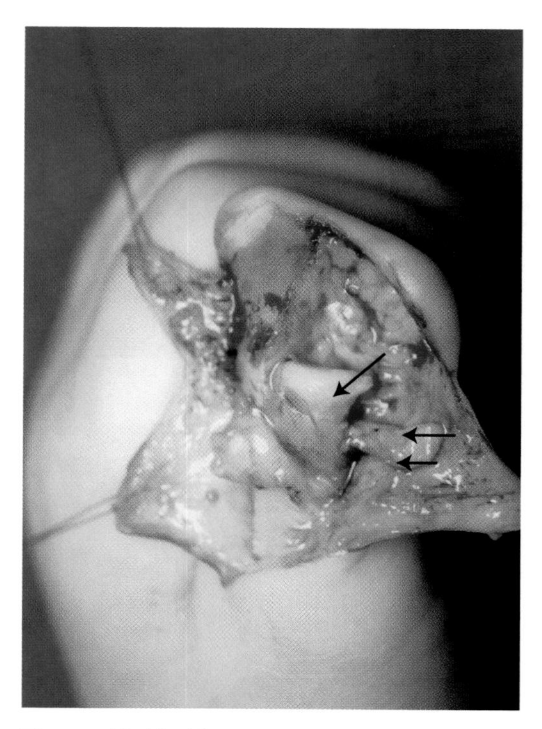

Figure 13.11. The reduction osteotomy has been completed (*single arrow*), and the developed peristeal capsular sleeve (*double arrow*) used to reconstruct the collateral ligament is shown.

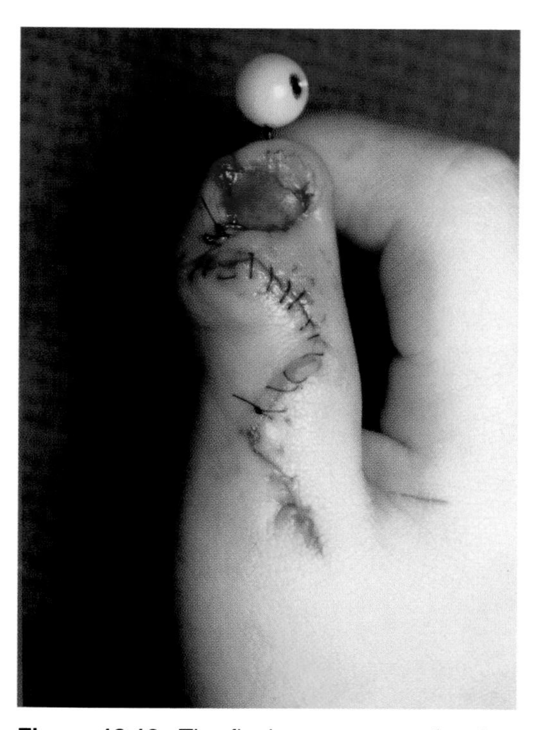

Figure 13.12. The final appearance after flap trimming and closure.

CONCLUSION

In conclusion, the successful treatment of the duplicate thumb requires adherence to established principles and recognition of detail to all aspects of the reconstruction. Preoperative discussion with the family is important to outline goals and possible pitfalls. The successful procedure includes: judicious use of skin incisions, reattachment of the thenar muscles, reconstruction of the metacarpophalangeal joint, osteotomies of the metacarpal and possibly the proximal phalanx to align bony units perpendicular to the longitudinal axis, and frequently redirection of tendinous structures. Though the reconstructed thumb may be somewhat smaller and stiffer than the contralateral, function should be satisfactory, and the infant should enjoy excellent prehensile activity.

RECOMMENDED READING

1. Dobyns JH, Lipscomb PR, Cooney WP. Management of thumb duplication. *Clin Orthop* 195:26–44, 1984.
2. Ezaki MB. Radial polydactyly. *Hand Clin* 6:577–588, 1990.
3. Goffin D, Gilbert A, Leclercq C. Thumb duplication: surgical treatment and analysis of sequels. *Annals of Hand and Upper Limb Surgery* 9:119–128, 1990.
4. Horii E, Nakamura R, Sakuna M, et al. Duplicated thumb bifurcation at the metacarpalphalangeal joint level: factors affecting surgical outcome. *J Hand Surg* 22A:671–679, 1997.
5. Kanavel AB. Congenital Malformations of the Hands. *Arch Surg* 25:308–316, 1932.
6. Kitayama Y, Tsukada S. Patterns of arterial distribution in the duplicated thumb. *Plast Reconstr Surg* 72(4):535–542, 1983.
7. Light TR. Treatment of preaxial polydactyly. *Hand Clin* 8:161–175, 1992.
8. Lister G. Pollex abductus in hypoplastic and duplication of the thumb. *J Hand Surg* 16A:626, 1991.
9. Marks TW, Bayne LG. Polydactyly of the thumb: abnormal anatomy and treatment. *J Hand Surg* 3:107–116, 1978.
10. Miura T. Duplicated thumb. *Plast Reconstr Surg* 6:470–479, 1982.
11. Miura T. An appropriate treatment for postoperative Z-formed deformity of the duplicated thumb. *J Hand Surg* 2:380–386, 1987.
12. Simmons BP. Polydactyly. *Hand Clin* 1:545–565, 1984.
13. Townsend DJ, Lipp EB Jr, Chun K, et al. Thumb duplication, 66 year's experience—a review of surgical complications. *J Hand Surg* 19A:973–976, 1994

PART IV

Nerve Disorders

14

Tendon Transfers for Radial Nerve Paralysis

Ioannis Sarris, Nickolaos A. Darlis, and
Dean G. Sotereanos

INDICATIONS/CONTRAINDICATIONS

The radial nerve is the most commonly injured nerve in the upper extremity. Denervation results in loss of wrist, thumb, and finger extension. Radial nerve dysfunction also affects the patient's ability to grasp and release objects, especially impairing power grasp.

Generally, once it is determined that the likelihood of recovery of the radial nerve is remote, tendon transfer procedures are indicated. In nerve palsies with progressive clinical or electrodiagnostic improvement, a reconstructive procedure is contraindicated. The etiologies associated with paralysis of the radial nerve can be divided into open or closed injuries. Open injuries with acute radial nerve palsy typically require primary exploration, whereas radial nerve dysfunction in the setting of closed injuries can usually be observed for up to 4 months.

The most common cause of radial nerve palsy is fracture of the humeral shaft, especially at the junction of the middle and distal third of the humerus (Holstein-Lewis fractures) (Fig. 14.1). At this point, the nerve penetrates the lateral intermuscular septum and is less mobile than in the spiral groove more proximal. Displaced oblique fractures at this level can directly damage the radial nerve. It is still controversial if Holstein-Lewis fractures with radial nerve deficits should be immediately explored. However, if initial nerve function exists that subsequently ceases, immediate exploration should be conducted. The radial nerve is also in danger from fractures of the middle third of the humeral shaft due to the close proximity to the bone in the spiral groove, where only a thin layer of the medial head of the triceps separates it from the bone.

Iatrogenic injuries may occur during fixation of humeral shaft fractures or other upper extremity procedures. When all reasonable precautions against nerve laceration were taken

Ioannis Sarris, M.D., Ph.D: Department of Orthopaedic Surgery, Allegheny General Hospital, Pittsburgh, PA

Nickolaos A. Darlis, M.D., Ph.D.: Department of Orthopaedic Surgery, Alleghany General Hospital, Pittsburgh, PA

Dean G. Sotereanos, M.D.: Department of Orthopaedic Surgery, Drexel University, College of Medicine, Philadelphia, PA, and Department of Orthopaedic Surgery, Allegheny General Hospital, Pittsburgh, PA

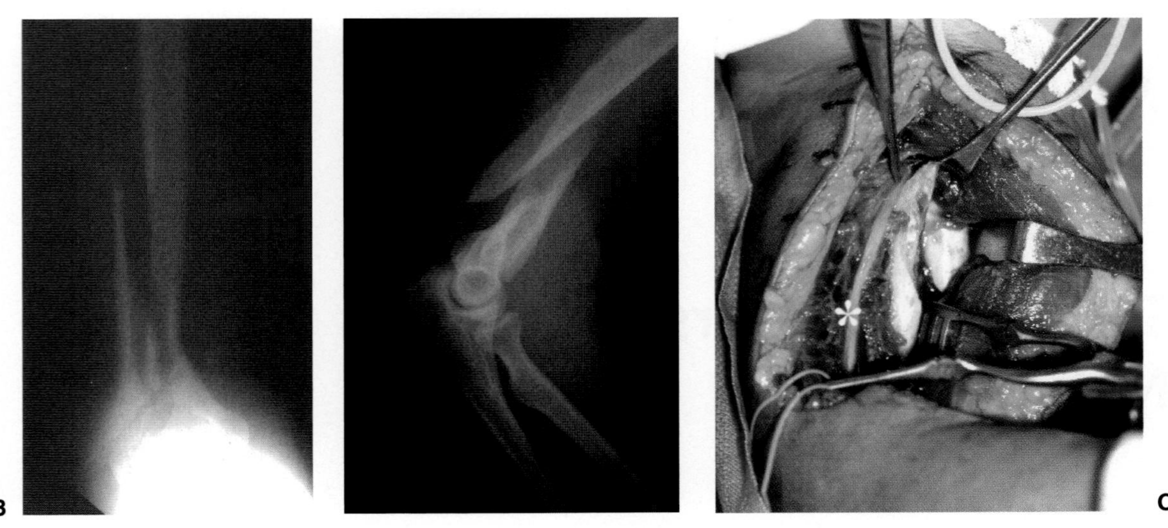

Figure 14.1. Posteroanterior **A:** and lateral **B:** radiographs of a Holstein-Lewis fracture of the distal third of the humerus. **C:** The close proximity of the radial nerve (star) to the fragments can be appreciated in this intraoperative photograph.

during the procedure, iatrogenic palsies can be observed for a 4-month period. This also applies to palsies after intramedullary nailing of the humerus.

Paralysis of the radial nerve can also occur from acute penetrating trauma (stab wounds, gunshot injuries, injections). Stab wounds often result in clean-cut radial nerve lacerations, and the nerve should be explored and primarily repaired. High-velocity gunshot injuries should undergo exploration and debridement, and the nerve should be tagged for secondary grafting. Nerve damage in these injuries is usually so extensive that primary repair cannot be undertaken. Low-velocity gunshot and shotgun injuries associated with radial nerve palsy can be observed for a 4-month period if there is no other indication for early exploration (e.g., suspected vascular injury).

Radial nerve paralysis without history of trauma usually occurs from tumors around the nerve or from progressive compression of the radial nerve at various levels and should be treated accordingly. Radial nerve palsies from prolonged external compression rarely cause long-term functional deficits. Alcohol- or drug-related palsies (Saturday night palsies) generally recover fairly quickly.

Diagnostic studies include plain radiographs in cases of fractures, dislocations, or suspected foreign body. Magnetic resonance imaging should be considered in the rare instance when a mass is suspected at any level along the course of the radial nerve. Electrodiagnostic studies are usually ordered 6 to 8 weeks after nerve injury and again at 4 to 5 months for comparison.

The indications for early exploration of the radial nerve include functional loss associated with penetrating trauma or instances in which the status of the nerve changed in subsequent examinations, especially a decrement after fracture manipulation. The nerve should also be explored when palsy occurs in association with a fracture pattern that per se warrants surgical treatment. In all other cases of radial nerve palsies, the patient should be closely observed for clinical or electrodiagnostic signs of reinnervation. If within 4 months after the injury there are no signs of reinnervation of the brachioradialis muscle, then surgical exploration is recommended. In cases in which immediate exploration is performed and the nerve is found to be contused or is lacerated and repaired, it is recommended to delay reconstruction with tendon transfers until recovery plateaus, typically about 6 to 8 months after injury. Nevertheless, a tendon transfer to restore wrist extension can be performed in conjunction with nerve repair in such patients (especially in delayed nerve grafting), as it provides dynamic stabilization of the wrist during the recovery period. Although results after radial nerve repair are generally good, it should be noted that fine, individual control of finger and thumb extension can be expected in less than half of the patients.

It is critical to maintain or restore joint suppleness before considering any tendon transfer. Consistent passive-motion programs, with or without other modalities, should be instituted immediately after injury. The use of a dynamic extension splint that keeps the wrist in 10 to 15 degrees of extension, and provides passive extension of the fingers and the thumb while allowing active flexion of the fingers under resistance, is generally recommended. A preoperative strengthening program of the unaffected muscles will lead to better results after surgical reconstruction, promoting faster rehabilitation. In cases of chronic radial nerve palsies with muscle fibrosis and joint contractures, tendon transfers are contraindicated.

PREOPERATIVE PLANNING

Preoperative planning is essential to any tendon transfer operation. It is important to discern the level of injury of the radial nerve. Loss of function of the triceps muscle usually reflects an injury at the brachial plexus. If the injury involves the proper radial nerve, at the level of the humerus the patient will lose function of the brachioradialis (BR), extensor carpi radialis longus (ECRL), and extensor carpi radialis brevis (ECRB) in addition to the muscles innervated by the posterior interosseous nerve (PIN). The term "high radial nerve palsy" is used for these cases. In "low radial nerve palsy," only the PIN-innervated muscles are affected and the patients are unable to extend their fingers at the metacarpophalangeal (MP) joints or the thumb. They also experience radial deviation of the wrist with dorsiflexion due to the preservation of the extensor carpi radialis longus, which inserts on the dorsoradial base of the index metacarpal. If the superficial radial nerve is preserved, the patients experience no sensory deficit, whereas in more proximal injuries, there is hypoesthesia of the dorsal aspect of the first web space. It should be noted that patients with radial nerve injury retain their ability to actively extend the fingers in the interphalangeal joints with the intrinsic muscles of the hand. The ability to extend the MP joints must be specifically examined to diagnose a radial nerve injury.

The presence of active contraction of the BR and wrist extensors allows for localization of the nerve injury to a point distal to the origin of the PIN. The importance of this distinction is the potential addition of two transferable muscles (BR and ECRL) and the synergistic action of wrist extension to the strength of finger flexion.

The soft-tissue coverage and potential tendon pathways of the transferred tendons should also be deemed to be "healthy" and adequate. Scars from previous incisions should be appreciated when planning the required incisions for the transfers. The strength of the donor-flexor muscles should also be examined. Supple joints are a prerequisite for tendon transfers; vigorous rehabilitation and even contracture releases can be used to maximize ultimate results. Any joint contractures, as previously mentioned, should first be released before proceeding to tendon transfers.

The decision of which functional muscle to use to substitute for a lost function is based on the well-established principles of tendon transfer:

- One "donor" musculotendinous unit must be chosen to substitute for one missing function.
- The donor tendon function must be of lesser importance than the function to be substituted (i.e., the donor tendon should be expendable).
- The muscle strength of the donor muscle must be adequate (typically at least M4), as it is expected to deteriorate (by at least one grade) after the transfer. The donor musculotendinous unit must have adequate length and excursion for its new function.
- A straight line of pull for the donor muscle must be established for the transfer.
- The new musculotendinous unit created with the tendon transfer must cross the minimum possible number of joints. If it is necessary to cross more than one joint and it is expected to exert its action at the most distal joint, the intermediate joints should be dynamically or statically stabilized.
- Tendon transfers between antagonist muscles should be avoided.

Radial nerve palsy distal to the innervation of the triceps usually requires tendon transfers to restore function. Muscles available for reconstruction are the extrinsic muscles of the volar forearm innervated by the median and ulnar nerves. Because of the numerous muscles available, several combinations of muscle transfers have been advocated in the literature.

Wrist Extension

For wrist extension, we prefer to transfer the pronator teres (PT) to the extensor carpi radialis brevis (ECRB) subcutaneously, over the fascia of the BR and the ECRL. A minor variation of this transfer includes PT insertion into both the ECRL and ECRB. However, transfer to the ECRL, or ECRL and ECRB, may result in radial wrist deviation and is generally not indicated.

Finger Extension

For finger extension, we prefer the use of the flexor carpi radialis (FCR), which is transferred to the extensor digitorum communis (EDC). Use of the flexor carpi ulnaris (FCU) for this transfer has fallen out of favor because it is a strong wrist flexor, an important wrist stabilizer, and may be an overly strong muscle to be used as a common finger extensor. Boyes has suggested the use of the flexor digitorum superficialis (FDS) of the long finger to the EDC and the FDS of the ring finger to the extensor indicis proprius to achieve more independent finger extension function; this combination may be too tedious.

Thumb Extension

For thumb extension, we prefer to transfer the palmaris longus (PL), when present, to the extensor pollicis longus (EPL). The EPL is rerouted out of the third dorsal compartment to accommodate a straighter line of pull and to provide some abduction in addition to extension. If the PL is not present, we usually use the FCR as the transferred muscle for both the EPL and the EDC, or if necessary, the FDS of the ring finger to the EPL. Boyes, to achieve a more anatomic reconstruction, suggested the use of the FDP of the ring finger to the EPL and the FCR to the abductor pollicis longus and the extensor pollicis brevis.

In summary (Fig. 14.2), our preferred tendon transfers for irreparable radial nerve palsy are (1) PT to ECRB, (2) FCR to EDC, and (3) PL to EPL.

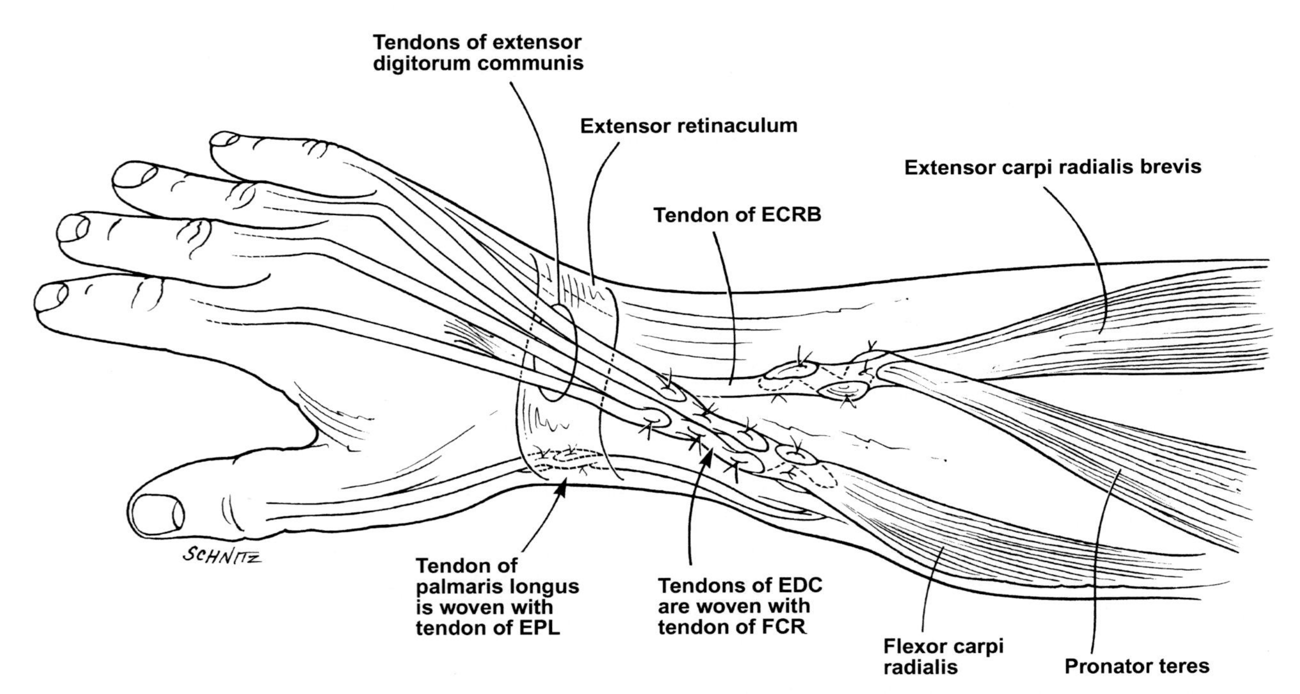

Figure 14.2. Diagrams of our preferred tendon transfers for irreparable radial nerve palsy: (**A**) PT to ECRB; (**B**) FCR to EDC; (**C**) PL to EPL. EPL = extensor pollicis longus; ECRL = extensor carpi radialis longus; ECRB = extensor carpi radialis brevis; PL = palmaris longus; FCR = flexor carpi radialis; PT = pronator teres; EDC = extensor digitorum communis; MC = metacarpal.

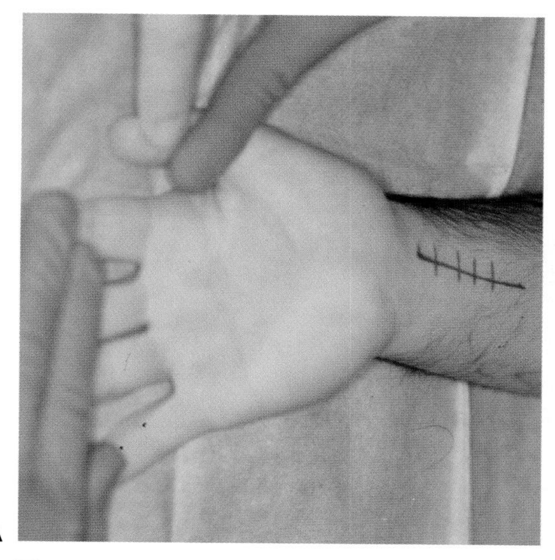

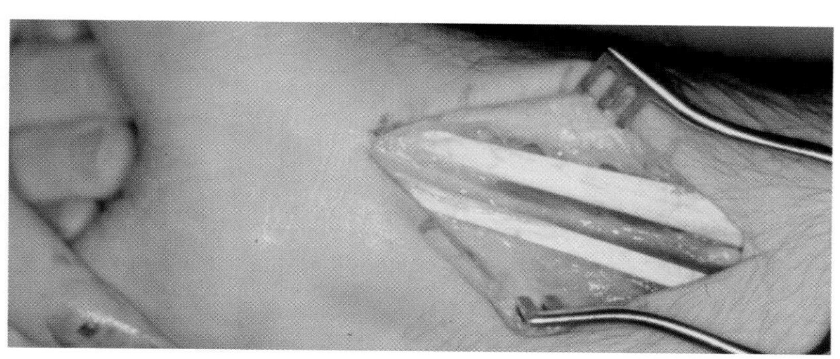

Figure 14.3. A: Incision in the distal volar aspect of the forearm, starting from the wrist flexion crease and extending proximally in a straight line for about 5 cm. **B:** Exposure of the flexor carpi radialis (FCR) and palmaris longus (PL) tendons distally.

SURGERY

Under axillary block or general anesthesia, the patient is placed in a supine position with his arm on a hand table. General anesthesia has the benefit of paralysis, which some surgeons embrace when performing tendon transfers. A tourniquet is applied and the extremity is draped as high as possible to facilitate the surgical procedure and the evaluation of tendon tensioning and function. We first mark all of the appropriate incisions and then exsanguinate the extremity and inflate the tourniquet. We utilize three incisions for our standard transfers. The first is placed distally on the volar aspect of the forearm, starting from the wrist flexion crease and extending proximally in a straight line for about 5 cm (Fig. 14.3A). This incision is made just ulnar to the FCR and will be used to harvest the FCR and PL tendons distally (Fig. 14.3B). Care is taken to avoid injury to the palmar sensory branch of the median nerve.

For the second incision, we palpate the insertion of the PT on the radius and make a lazy-S-shaped incision centered over the radial aspect of the forearm. The proximal limb of the incision is on the volar aspect of the radius, where the PT tendon inserts (Fig. 14.4), and the distal limb is on the dorsal aspect of the radius over the musculotendinous junction of the ECRB (Fig. 14.5A). This incision will be utilized for the harvesting and transfer of the PT

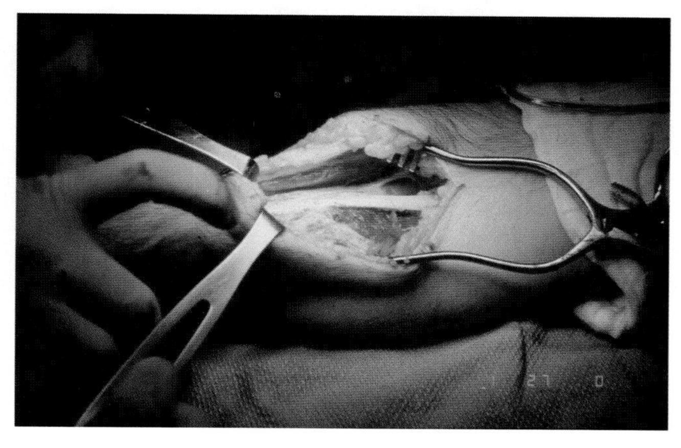

Figure 14.4. Insertion of the pronator teres (PT) tendon into the radius.

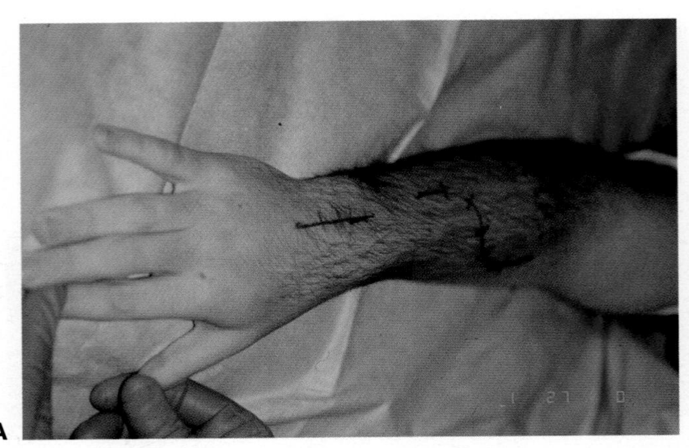
A

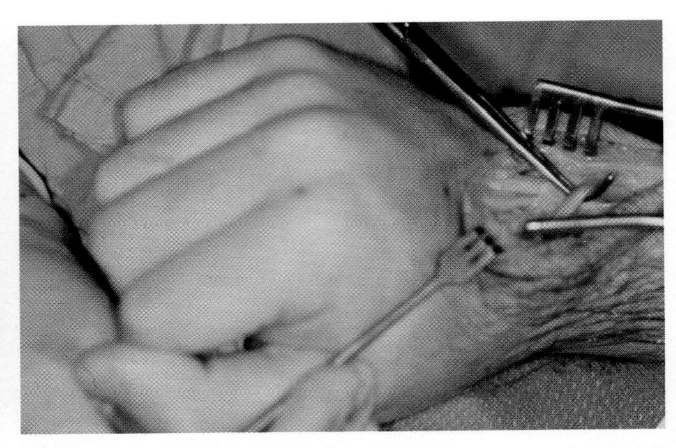
B

Figure 14.5. A: Longitudinal midline incision of the distal dorsal aspect of the wrist and the forearm lazy-S incision. **B:** Exposure of the extensor digitorum communis (EDC) and the extensor pollicis longus (EPL).

to the ECRB (Fig. 14.6, A and B). The third incision is longitudinal and midline over the dorsum of the wrist and distal forearm (Fig. 14.5, A and B). This incision is used to transfer the FCR to the EDC and the PL to the EPL.

Restoration of Wrist Extension

Wrist extension is restored with transfer of the PT to the ECRB. The skin is incised in a lazy-S pattern, as described above, and the subcutaneous fat is dissected down to fascia. Care is taken to protect the lateral antebrachial cutaneous nerve as well as the dorsal sensory branch of the radial nerve. The PT is identified through the FCR/BR interval and followed to its insertion. The PT tendon has a substantial insertion on the radius via Sharpey's fibers, thus limiting the amount of tendinous tissue available. It is thus essential to elevate as much of the insertion as possible subperiosteally, including radius periosteum in the flap that is raised. This step is very important to obtain as much tendon length as possible. An additional 2 to 4 cm of length usually can be obtained.

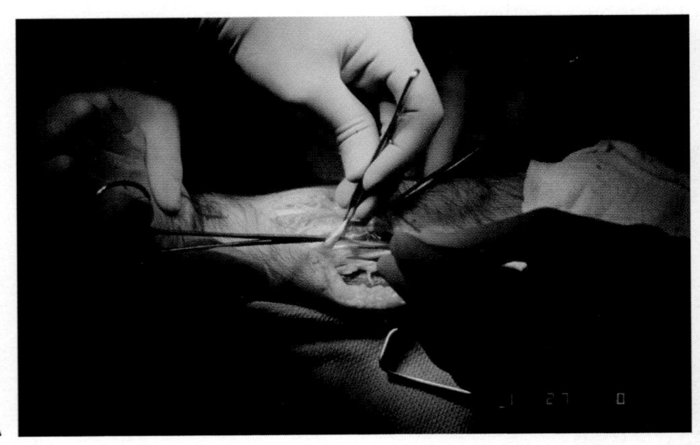
A

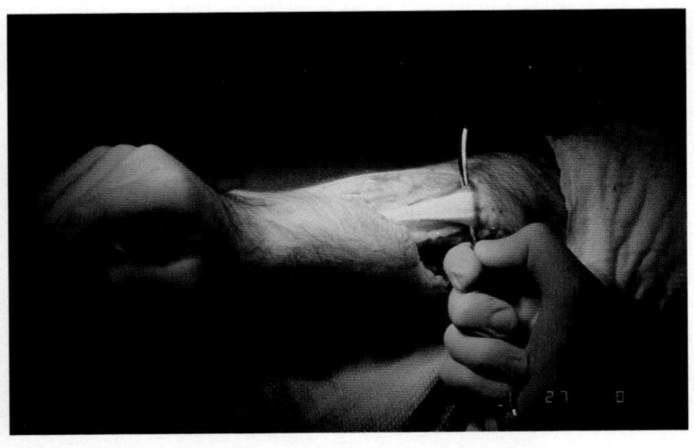
B

Figure 14.6. A: Exposure of the extensor carpi radialis brevis (ECRB) tendon and the pronator teres (PT) tendon through the lazy-S incision and use of a pointed tendon passer to apply the woven Pulvertaft technique. **B:** Identification of the extensor carpi radialis brevis (ECRB), which should extend the wrist without radial deviation, which is noted with the action of the extensor carpi radialis longus (ECRL).

Next, the PT muscle epimysium is divided proximally until the orientation of the muscle allows dorsal rerouting in a straight line. The muscle belly is also bluntly dissected from the adjacent muscles to its origin to obtain a straighter line of traction and to gain more length. The PT tendon is then passed subcutaneously and radiodorsally over the BR and the ECRL to the ECRB tendon. Usually, the length is just adequate for the transfer. If not, the use of additional tissue from the PL or iliotibial band may be required, but we have never encountered that problem.

Once the ECRB is identified from the dorsal aspect of our incision, manual traction of the tendon is applied to assess the gliding ability of the tendon (Fig. 14.6B). If tendon adhesions or scarring is present, these should be released before the PT transfer. Then, with the use of a pointed tendon passer, the PT tendon is weaved through the ECRB tendon several times in accordance with the Pulvertaft technique (Fig. 14.6A). The transfer is then secured with the use of multiple strong-braided nonabsorbable 2-0 sutures with the wrist in at least 40 degrees of extension (Fig. 14.7, A and B). We believe that overcorrection of wrist extension is essential to prevent stress elongation of the transfer. The first stitch should be placed with great caution, as it is the one that determines the final extended wrist position. In our opinion, transfer of the PT to the ECRB is the most technically demanding of the radial nerve transfers and should be performed first.

Restoration of Finger Extension

This is achieved with transfer of the FCR to the EDC. Through the volar, distal longitudinal incision, the FCR tendon is harvested with the wrist in maximum flexion to gain as

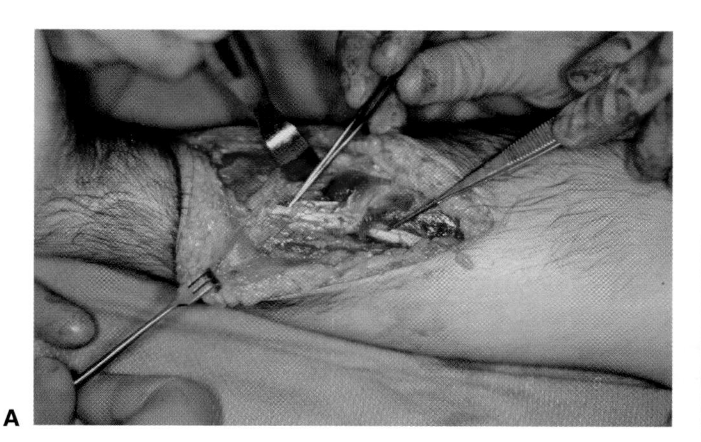
A

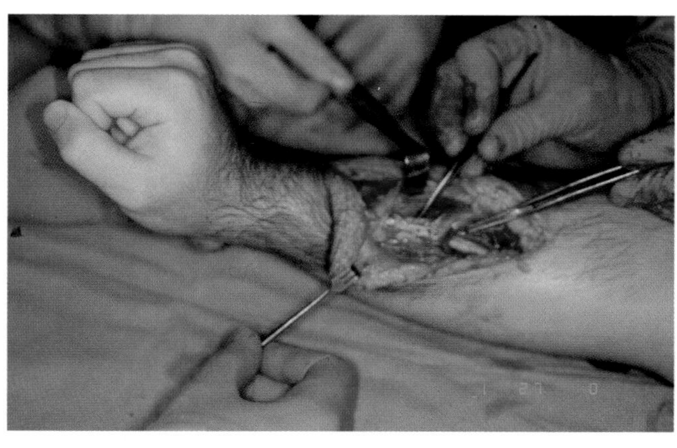
B

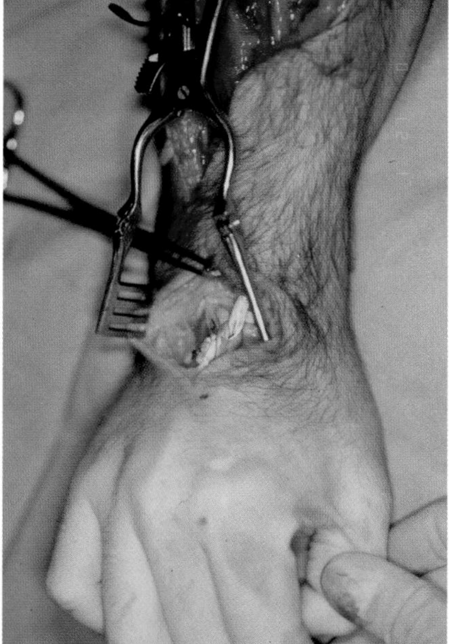
C

Figure 14.7. A: Transfer of the pronator teres (PT) tendon after being secured with a strong-braided nonabsorbable 2-0 stitch. **B:** The wrist in about 40 degrees of extension. **C:** Transfer of the flexor carpi radialis (FCR) to the extensor digitorum communis (EDC).

much length as possible. The FCR muscle is adequately freed from the adjacent muscles and the fascia. The tendon is then delivered subcutaneously over the proximal dorsal aspect of the lazy-S incision to the musculotendinous junction of the ECRB. The third (midline wrist) incision is then made on the distal dorsal aspect of the forearm just ulnar to the Lister's tubercle. The fourth compartment is identified and opened, following the tendons proximally to the EDC musculotendinous junction. The tendons are manually retracted to test for gliding. The FCR tendon, with the help of a tendon passer, is then passed subcutaneously dorsally over the ECRB and ECRL to reach the EDC tendons. Again, a Pulvertaft weave is employed to secure all four extensor tendons. The transfer is then secured with braided 2-0 suture. Finally, the retinaculum of the fourth compartment is repaired.

The tenorrhaphy should be performed well proximal to the extensor retinaculum so that it does not impinge on the fourth compartment in full composite finger and wrist flexion. Although tensioning of a tendon transfer is something that requires surgical experience, the tension of the transfer is adjusted so that full finger extension is restored. It is also important to maintain equal tension to all of the finger extensors. If this is not accomplished with the Pulvertaft weave, the tension of an individual extensor tendon can be fine-tuned with placation just distal to the weave. Smooth and synchronous motion of all of the fingers can be checked with wrist flexion and extension using the tenodesis effect.

Restoration of Thumb Extension

Thumb extension is restored with the PL-to-EPL transfer. We use the same distal volar incision through which we harvested the FCR to harvest the PL, with the wrist in flexion to gain length. The PL is transected distally at its insertion to the palmar fascia. Through the distal wrist dorsal incision, the third compartment is identified and opened to free the EPL, following the tendon proximally to its musculotendinous junction. The EPL is then manually retracted to confirm good gliding of the tendon. The PL is then passed dorsally through a subcutaneous tunnel and is interwoven with the EPL by the method of Pulvertaft, being secured with 3-0 braided sutures. Again, the tension is adjusted to obtain full extension of the thumb by tenodesis with wrist flexion. The retinaculum of the third dorsal compartment is not repaired, thus allowing the EPL tendon to subluxate radially, adding mild thumb abduction to its function.

In cases of PL absence (15–25% of the population), EPL function is restored by including this tendon in the FCR-to-EDC transfer; alternatively, the FDS of the ring finger can be transferred to the EPL.

At the end of the procedure, the tourniquet is released and meticulous hemostasis is obtained. If necessary, drains are utilized (Fig. 14.8, A and B). As a general rule, we prefer

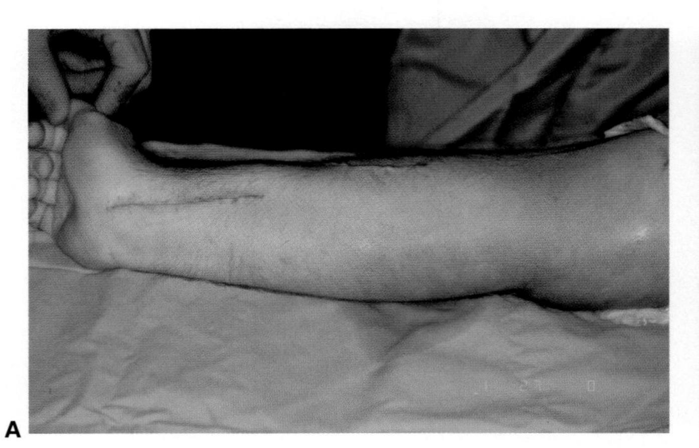
A

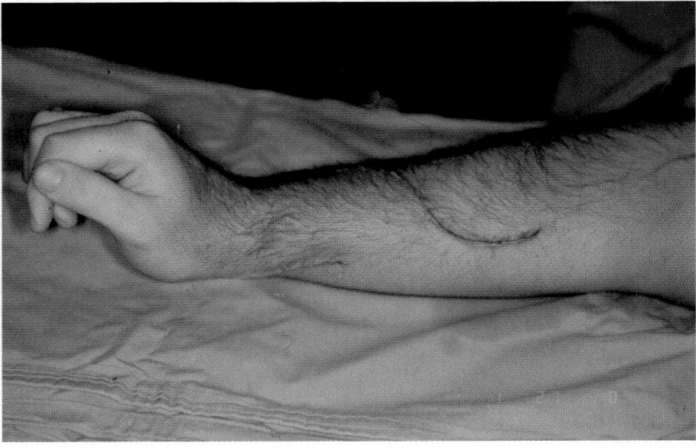
B

Figure 14.8. A, B: Closure of the three incisions.

first to harvest all of the flexor-donor muscles and prepare all of the recipient extensor tendons before performing the transfers. After all donor and recipient musculotendinous units are prepared, we first address wrist extension followed by the fingers and the thumb extension. All three incisions can be extended distally or proximally if necessary. It should be stressed that overtensioning of the transfers is preferred to undertensioning because of inevitable stress relaxation of the transfers over time.

POSTOPERATIVE MANAGEMENT/REHABILITATION

Postoperative long-arm immobilization is applied to reduce tension on the tendon transfers. The splint is applied with the elbow in 90 degrees of flexion, the forearm in neutral rotation, the wrist in 40 degrees of extension, and the fingers in a resting position of about 20 degrees of flexion at the MP and interphalangeal joints. After 2 to 3 weeks, the splint is removed and a short-arm dynamic splint is applied, keeping the wrist in 20 degrees of extension. Individual slings support the fingers with a dorsal outrigger elastic support. Rehabilitation begins with twice-daily passive-motion exercises of the wrist with gentle flexion until the point of resistance is met. The MP and proximal interphalangeal joints are actively flexed and passively extended in the splint. After the 4th week, gentle active extension of the fingers is allowed. As the tenorrhaphies are performed with the strong Pulvertaft weave technique, early active extension is well tolerated. Six weeks postoperatively, the tendon repairs are strong enough to tolerate active flexion of the wrist and the fingers, and the patient is encouraged to make a "loose" fist and the splint is discontinued. We expect the patient to have full range of motion (other than wrist flexion) at 3 months postoperatively with significant strength. From the initiation of the postoperative physiotherapy, the hand therapist teaches the patient how to control the "change of action" (flexors acting as extensors) of the transferred muscles using synergistic motion. Wrist extension is coupled with finger flexion and wrist flexion with finger extension. Usually, the patient returns to full activity 6 months postoperatively.

Before returning to work or sports, muscle strengthening exercises are very important. The time for full recovery and the extensive rehabilitation required should be explained to the patient before surgery. The patient should also consult with the hand therapist before surgery and should be instructed in muscle-strengthening exercises of his flexors, knowing that muscle atrophy will occur postoperatively.

RESULTS

In the authors' experience, tendon transfers with the technique described above for irrecoverable radial nerve palsy have an excellent functional outcome. The ultimate range of motion approximates normal (except for wrist flexion), whereas strength, although adequate, is less than that of the contralateral forearm and hand. Nevertheless, most patients return to their previous daily and work activities with good satisfaction. This does not apply to patients involved in high-demand athletic activities, who have to modify their activities accordingly.

The results are less encouraging in neglected long-standing cases of radial nerve palsies, where the excessive time interval and the inadequate joint mobilization result in muscle shortening and fibrosis of the flexors. This also applies in cases with significant joint contractures.

In cases of acute radial nerve palsies in which the nerve is immediately identified as lacerated, primary nerve repair or nerve grafting should be considered. This has been very rewarding, since the radial nerve is the most suitable for neurorrhaphy of all the major nerves because the fascicles are largely motor and the most common site of injury is not far from the motor endplates. In this scenario, tendon transfer to maintain the wrist splinted in extension should be considered.

COMPLICATIONS

The complication most commonly reported is the formation of tendon adhesions at the site of the tenorrhaphy. If this occurs, the surgeon should not hesitate to perform tenolysis. Usually this is done within 3 to 4 months. If tenolysis is delayed, the functional outcome of the transfer will be at risk because of the limited flexion, delayed joint motion, and significant muscle atrophy. Formation of adhesions at the juncture site will not affect the final outcome if surgical release is performed early and is followed by immediate active and passive range of motion. This complication has been rare in our experience, and a tenolysis was hardly ever necessary, possibly because of the implementation of an early range-of-motion rehabilitation program.

In cases of transfers of the PT to the ECRL or both the ECRL and the ECRB, the complication of radial deviation of the wrist must be considered. Bow-stringing of the EPL after transfer of the PL has been noted but does not need further management.

Inadequate tensioning of tendon transfers can also lead to suboptimal outcomes. This technical error will always result in weakness and limited excursion. If the transfer of the PT to the ECRB is undertensioned, grip strength will be diminished due to wrist position. Secondary plication of undertensioned tendons can be rewarding. In cases of overtensioning, the flexion of the wrist and fingers will be decreased, affecting the functional result and the ability to make a complete fist. Both overtensioning and undertensioning should be avoided intraoperatively, if possible.

Rare cases of tendon ruptures have also been reported as a result of poor surgical technique, the use of inappropriate sutures, or poor tendon quality. A braided 2-0 or 3-0 suture should be used to secure the tendon transfers and avoid this complication. If a tendon juncture ruptures, it should immediately be addressed surgically.

Important neurovascular structures are also in danger during the procedure, and the surgeon should be familiar with anatomy and techniques to avoid iatrogenic neurovascular complications.

Proper patient selection, aggressive preoperative physiotherapy, well-planned and well-executed tendon transfers, and an appropriate rehabilitation program can yield excellent extension of the wrist, fingers, and thumb in radial nerve palsy

RECOMMENDED READING

1. Alnot J-Y, Osman N, Masmejean E, et al. Radial nerve palsy in humeral shaft fractures: a series of 62 cases. *J Bone Joint Surg* 83B(Suppl III):284, 2001.
2. Capener N. The vulnerability of the posterior interosseous nerve of the forearm: a case report and an anatomical study. *J Bone Joint Surg* 48B:770–773, 1966.
3. Chuinard R, Boyes J, Stark H, et al. Tendon transfers for radial nerve palsy: use of superficialis tendons for digital extension. *J Hand Surg* 3A:560–570, 1978.
4. Green DP. Radial Nerve Palsy. In: Green DP, Hotchkiss R, Pederson W, eds. *Green's Operative Hand Surgery.* 4th ed. Philadelphia: Churchill Livingston, 1999:1481–1496.
5. Holstein A, Lewis G. Fracture of the humerus with radial nerve paralysis. *J Bone Joint Surg* 45A:1382–1388, 1963.
6. Kline D, Hudson A. *Nerve Injuries: Operative Results for Major Nerve Injuries, Entrapments, and Tumors.* Philadelphia: Saunders, 2001.
7. Kruft S, von Heimburg D, Reill P. Treatment of irreversible lesions of the radial nerve by tendon transfer: indication and long-term results of the Merle d'Aubigne procedure. *Plast Reconstr Surg* 100:610–616, 1997.
8. Lowe J III, Tung T, Mackinnon SE. New surgical option for radial nerve paralysis. *Plast Reconstr Surg* 110:836–843, 2002.
9. Samardzic M, Grujicic D, Milinovic Z. Radial nerve lesions associated with fractures of the humeral shaft. *Injury* 21:220–222, 1990.
10. Tubiana R. Problems and solutions in palliative tendon transfer surgery for radial nerve palsy. *Tech Hand Upper Extremity Surg* 6:104–113, 2002.

15

Opponensplasty for Low Median-Nerve Deficit

John F. Dalton IV and John Gray Seiler III

> "A great asset to man is the opposable thumb. The hand so useful to all and the livelihood of the manual worker owes much of its efficiency to this pincer action of the thumb."
> —Sterling Bunnell, 1938

INDICATIONS/CONTRAINDICATIONS

Median-nerve deficit resulting in loss of thumb opposition has a debilitating effect on hand function. The inability to rotate the thumb away from the palm and use it as a stable post causes significant impairment of both the pinch and the grasp capabilities. In the broadest sense, tendon transfer to restore thumb opposition is indicated for treatment of patients who have established loss of the native motor capability to oppose the thumb, stable soft tissues, and adequate joint mobility of the thumb ray.

Prior to widespread immunization, polio was the most common cause for the loss of opposition. Today, median-nerve dysfunction more commonly results from nerve entrapment neuropathies, muscular dystrophies (such as Charcot-Marie-Tooth), median-nerve transection, and traumatic conditions that are associated with significant loss of soft tissue about the thumb.

Normal Anatomy

After coursing beneath the lacertus fibrosus, the median nerve innervates the pronator teres (superficial then deep head), gives rise to the anterior interosseous nerve (AIN), and passes deep to the flexor digitorum superficialis (FDS). The AIN continues distally innervating the flexor digitorum profundus (FDP) of the index and tong fingers, the flexor pol-

John F. Dalton IV, M.D.: Department of Orthopaedic Surgery, Emory University, Atlanta, GA
John Gray Seiler III, M.D.: Department of Orthopaedic Surgery, Emory University, Atlanta, GA, and Georgia Hand and Microsurgery, Atlanta, GA

licis longus, the pronator quadratus, and terminates in sensory branches to the wrist capsule.

After the origin of the AIN, the median nerve has no other motor branches in the forearm and travels ulnar to the AIN along the muscle belly of the FDP. Approximately 5 cm proximal to the proximal wrist crease, the palmar cutaneous branch of the median nerve emerges from the volar, radial aspect of the nerve, piercing the antebrachial fascia within 1 cm of the wrist crease to provide sensation to the palmar skin of the hand. The median nerve passes beneath the transverse carpal ligament (TCL), through the carpal tunnel, and divides into several branches.

The recurrent branch of the median nerve usually originates from the body of the median nerve at the level of the distal portion of the TCL, travels distally and radially, and innervates the abductor pollicis brevis (APB), flexor pollicis brevis (FPB), and opponens pollicis (OP). Distal to the origin of the recurrent branch, the remaining motor axons innervate the lumbricals to the index and long fingers. The terminal sensory fascicles innervate the thumb, index, and long fingers as well as to the radial aspect of the ring finger.

Anatomic Variation

Multiple anomalous innervation patterns of the hand and forearm have been described. The median nerve itself has many described variations. Group I variations in the course of the recurrent branch of the median nerve at the carpal canal are well documented and consist of extraligamentous branching distal to the TCL as the most common pattern (46%), followed by subligamentous branching of the recurrent motor branch with (23%), or without (31%) piercing the TCL. Accessory branching of the median nerve in the distal carpal canal is classified as a Group II variation occurring in 7.2% of cases. Group III variations consist of high division of the median nerve in the proximal-to-middle third of the forearm. This anomaly is often seen in association with a persistent median artery or accessory lumbrical muscle belly within the carpal canal. Finally, accessory branching of the median nerve proximal to the carpal tunnel is seen in 1.6% of cases and makes up Group IV variations.

The clinical relevance to the often-performed carpal tunnel release is that when the surgeon detects the origin of the thenar eminence muscles in a location that is significantly more ulnar than is typically seen, the index of suspicion for a transligamentous branch should be heightened.

Communication with the ulnar nerve is another common variation. Communications between the AIN and ulnar nerve occur, accounting for the variable innervation pattern of the FPB. Martin and Gruber both described an interconnection between the median nerve or the AIN and ulnar nerve in the forearm adjacent to the ulnar artery. This communication has an occurrence rate of 15% and supplies motor axons from the median nerve into the ulnar nerve, which innervate the intrinsic muscles of the hand. Riche and Cannieu described a communication between the motor branch of the ulnar nerve in the hand and the recurrent branch of the median nerve.

Due to the various anomalous communications between the median and ulnar nerves, complete injuries to the median nerve may produce a varied clinical picture. Depending upon the patients' actual functional deficit, they may have functional opposition after median-nerve injury. According to Jensen, only 14% of patients with median-nerve palsy require opponensplasty due to dual innervation of the FPB and/or APB.

Classification of Nerve Injury

Median-nerve dysfunction that is localized below the origin of the anterior interosseous nerve is termed "low" median-nerve palsy. Patients with low median-nerve palsy have a deficiency of the intrinsic muscles of the thumb and loss of sensation to the thumb, index and long finger. Median-nerve dysfunction that occurs proximal to the origin of the anterior interosseous nerve is termed "high" median-nerve palsy. In addition to the findings of a low median-nerve palsy, patients with a high median-nerve palsy have loss of FDP function to the index finger and loss of FPL function.

The Motion of Thumb Opposition

The complex motion of thumb opposition is a combination of three movements: thumb metacarpal abduction, pronation of the first metacarpal, and flexion at the metacarpophalangeal (MP) and interphalangeal (IP) joints. The APB, FPB, and OP provide the muscular force to maneuver the thumb into position for opposition. Once maneuvered into this position, the thumb can serve as a dexterous pinch post. The act of pinch is dependent on appropriate balancing of muscular forces and stable MP joints and IP joints. This unique portfolio of muscle and osteoligamentous interactions is sometimes referred to as a "circumduction," and the out-of-plane position that the thumb adopts before activating the flexor components of opposition is considered "anteposotion."

In order to oppose to the other digits, the thumb must abduct and pronate at the carpometacarpal (CMC) joint and then flex at the MP and IP joints. The APB and FPB, as mentioned earlier, are the primary motors coordinating these motions. Antagonizing these motors are the extensor mechanism and adductor pollicis. They function in opposition to stabilize the MCP and IP joints to provide a solid post for pinch. Loss of any of these components will lead to increased contribution of the remaining elements with corresponding deformity and loss of function. In the case of median-nerve palsy, the unopposed pull of the adductor of the thumb contributes to first web space contracture, thereby further diminishing the ability of the thumb to circumduct.

Preoperative Considerations

The accepted general principles of tendon transfer apply to opponensplasty. Successful outcome is based upon adherence to the following basic principles. The joints of the thumb must have adequate passive range of motion, and the skin and soft tissues should be supple and stable. The transfer should not pass through areas of fibrosis that will impede its excursion and promote adhesions. The donor muscle should be under voluntary control with an independent action, and its native function must be expendable.

The transferred motor must have adequate strength to perform its new function. It should also have adequate excursion to reach its new target and allow proper tensioning. If the available donor is unable to reach its target, a tendon graft to extend the transfer may be necessary.

The transferred tendon should have a straight line of pull to perform its new function. Pulleys should be constructed to change the vector of pull, if necessary. Avoiding sharp angles at the pulleys is vital to maximizing donor effectiveness.

Finally, using donor muscles that are "in the same phase" as the target muscle function aids in the rehabilitation and patient re-education while remaining a basic principle of tendon-transfer surgery. However, this concept has less impact on the consideration for opponensplasty donors than it does in other transfer sets. Still, it should be realized that a majority of pinch and cylindrical grasp is performed in a position of relative wrist extension with initial digital extension in the first phase of grasp. Additionally, the act of making a fist requires an element of thumb opposition in addition to digital flexion–these coupled motions should be taken into consideration when choosing among available donors for transfer.

The goal of reconstructive surgery is to restore tip pinch and increase grip strength by transfer of a muscle-tendon unit to replace lost thenar muscle function. Both skeletal stability and extension of the thumb IP joint are necessary to provide effective pinch and must be achieved prior to undertaking any restorative procedure. In addition, flexion of the index and long finger must be present prior to consideration of opponensplasty.

In the case of irreparable damage to the median nerve or traumatic loss of thenar musculature, early opponensplasty is indicated. After repair of median-nerve lacerations, either by primary repair or with cable grafts, opponensplasty may be considered if acceptable function and strength do not return within three months of the expected reinnervation of the target tissues, judged by the level of the nerve injury and by the temporal and biological principles of nerve recovery. Electromyography and nerve conduction velocity are useful tools to follow nerve recovery after repair.

Patients with median-nerve palsies from neuropathies or muscular dystrophies who lose their opposition may also be candidates for opponensplasty; however, several factors complicate their treatment. Selection of a motor unit for transfer depends upon identifying uninvolved donors with adequate strength to perform the needed function. Also, sacrificing the donor from its original function may lead to donor-site sequelae. Finally, progressive neuropathies may lead to diminishing results, as the donor motor unit may become affected by the primary disease process.

PREOPERATIVE PLANNING

There are several considerations in the preoperative evaluation of a potential opponensplasty candidate (Table 15.1). Although a patient may execute many hand functions, even ones requiring dexterity, with only a modicum of motion in the joints of the thumb ray, adequate passive range of motion of the fingers, thumb, wrist, and forearm must be assessed and judged adequate prior to opponensplasty. Advanced median-nerve palsy can lead to an adduction/supination deformity of the thumb. Therefore, thumb CMC joint range of motion and capacity of the first web space must be acceptable.

Prevention of contractures in these patients can be accomplished with appropriate splinting and aggressive therapy. Once contractures develop, however, they must be corrected prior to considering tendon transfer. In the case of dorsal skin contracture of the first web space that is refractory to splinting, surgical release is indicated and can be accomplished with the use of conventional flaps (Z-plasty) or a dorsal rotational flap and skin graft. Loss of pronation with intact abduction is possible and may be due to contracture of the capsule of the trapeziometacarpal joint, which can be treated by simple capsulotomy or additional soft tissue release. Finally, in severe or recalcitrant contractures, metacarpal rotational osteotomy with trapeziectomy may be considered.

A thorough examination of the entire hand and wrist should also be performed. All soft tissue wounds should be stable. Ideally, the tendon transfer should pass through uninjured supple tissues. The IP joint of the thumb must be stable and capable of extension, at least to neutral. Repair or tenodesis of the extensor pollicis longus or fusion of the IP joint should be performed to provide a stable post for pinch grip, if necessary.

Strength and functional excursion of the flexors and extensors of the wrist and fingers must be examined in order to determine the musculotendinous units available for transfer. Important considerations in motor unit selection include donor strength, excursion, and expendability (Table 15.2).

It is well accepted that donor motor units will lose approximately one grade of strength after transfer. Therefore, it is ideal if the donor tendon comfortably reaches the thumb MP joint without lengthening, grafting, or over-tensioning. It is challenging to set appropriate tension through a lengthened system or graft, and over-tensioning may adversely affect the power by altering the length-tension relationship (Blix curve).

Finally, proper patient selection and education is paramount to success. The surgeon should have a detailed discussion with the patient on what is reasonable to expect in terms of potential functional recovery. This discussion should also stress the need for participation in a structured postoperative rehabilitation plan in order to meet these expectations. A patient who is unable or unwilling to actively participate in postoperative therapy should be discouraged from undergoing opponensplasty.

Table 15.1. *General principles for Opponensplasty*

- supple thumb with normal passive range of motion
- stable soft tissues
- available, expendable, strong potential donor muscle and tendon
- educated patient with realistic expectations

Table 15.2. *Common Donor Muscle Choices for Opponensplasty*

Donor muscle	Eponym	Advantages	Disadvantages
Flexor digitorum superficialis (ring)	Royle-Thompson	Excellent tendon length. Sufficient muscular strength and excursion	Can be associated with swan-neck deformity of the PIJ
Palmaris longus	Camitz opponensplasty	Often done at the same time as carpal tunnel release and therefore requires no other incision to harvest the donor tendon	Often requires extension using a tendon graft or the palmar fascia
Extensor Indicis Proprius		Excellent in combined median/ulnar palsies	Metacarpophalangeal joint contracture
Abductor digiti minimi	Huber transfer	Recreates the contour of the thenar eminence	Tentative blood supply may lead to fibrosis

SURGERY

Using the Flexor Digitorum Superficialis (FDS) for Reconstruction of Thumb Opposition

This, the author's preferred method, is done with the patient positioned supine on the operating room table. The shoulder is abducted to 90 degrees, the elbow is extended, the forearm supinated, and the hand and wrist are positioned in a neutral posture on a hand table extension. A non-sterile tourniquet is placed around the brachium, and the arm is sterilely prepared and draped. After exsanguinating the extremity with an Esmarch bandage, the tourniquet is inflated to 100 mmHg above the patient's systolic blood pressure.

Mark the planned incisions on the hand. The preferred incisions are demonstrated in Figure 15.1. Next, harvest the flexor digitorum superficialis to the ring finger. Make a Bruner-type incision centered over the palmar aspect of the ring finger PIP joint. This type of incision is preferred over a transverse incision in the proximal finger flexion crease, as it allows better exposure to the superficialis and its bifurcation. Identify and protect both the radial and ulnar digital neurovascular bundles. A stay suture (5-0 black nylon) should be used to retract the skin flap out of the operative field.

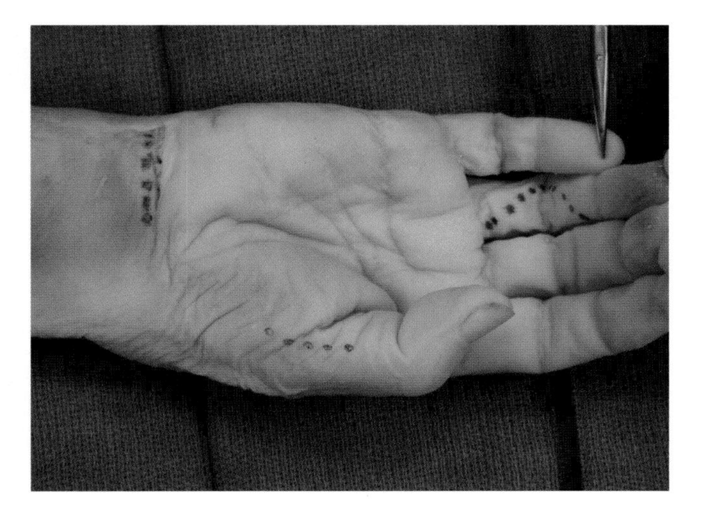

Figure 15.1. Recommended incisions for FDS opponensplasty: (1) Bruner incision centered over the PIP joint flexion crease, (2) tranverse incision at the proximal wrist flexion crease, which may be extended proximally over the FCU from the ulnar corner, (3) longitudinal incision centered over the radial border of the thumb MCP joint.

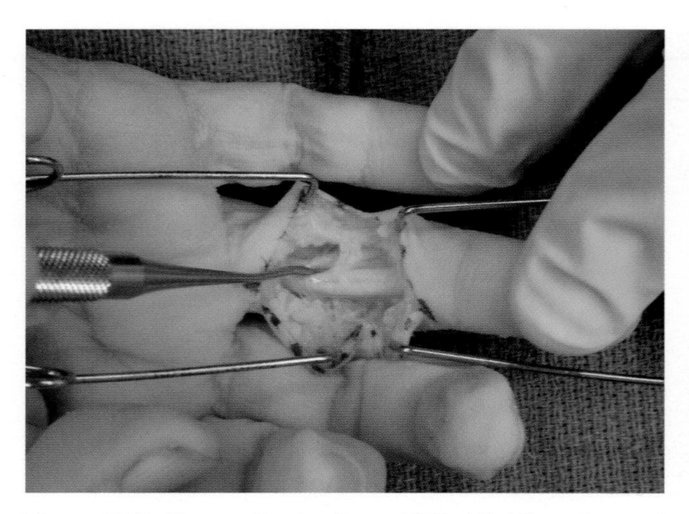

Figure 15.2. Expose the ring finger FDS at its bifurcation and insertion into the base of the middle phalynx.

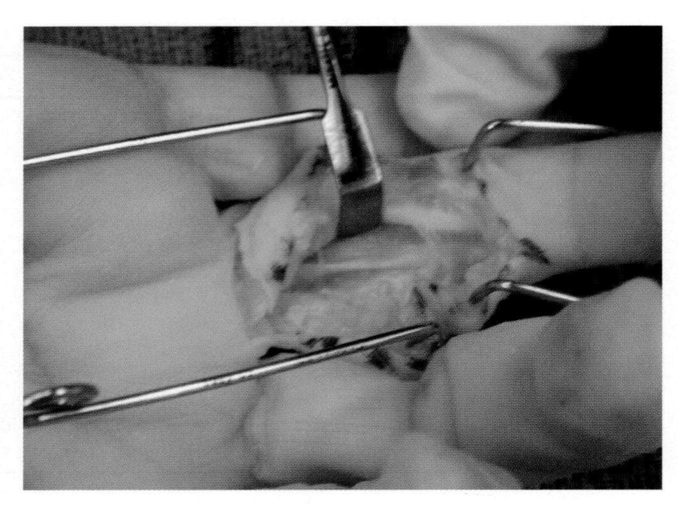

Figure 15.3. The FDP tendon is retracted radially to reveal the ulnar slip of the FDS tendon.

Carry the dissection down to the flexor tendon sheath and open the sheath just distal to the A2 pulley (Fig. 15.2). The flexor digitorum superficialis tendon is easily identified lying lateral to the emerging FDP tendon on both the radial and ulnar aspects of the theca (Fig. 15.3). Divide the two slips of the FDS tendon, leaving approximately 1 cm tails distally that overlie the proximal interphalangeal joint. Cutting the tendon in this area avoids injury to the volar plate and preserves enough of the FDS insertion to heal into the palmar tissues, which helps prevent a hyperextension deformity (swan neck) of the proximal interphalangeal joint (Fig. 15.4).

Next, make a transverse incision along the ulnar aspect of the proximal wrist crease between the palmaris longus and the pisiform. Extend this incision proximally by making a longitudinal limb at 90 degrees from the ulnar corner along the axis of the flexor carpi ulnaris tendon (FCU). In the transverse aspect of the wound, identify the FDS tendon as the most ulnar and the more superficial tendon of the FDS tendon group. The ring finger incision may now be irrigated and closed with a single layer of 4-0 nylon sutures. Using a moistened cotton tape, encircle the FDS tendon and apply proximal traction to deliver the FDS tendon into the proximal incision (Fig. 15.5).

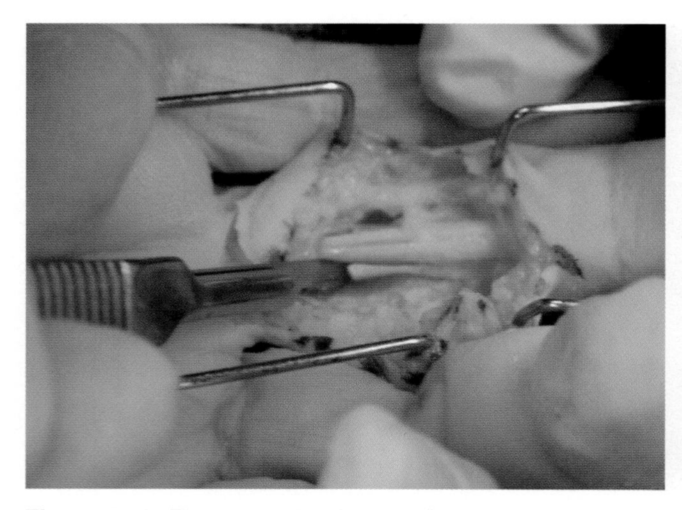

Figure 15.4. The ulnar slip of the FDS tendon is ligated approximately 1 cm from its insertion on the base of the middle phalynx, preventing injury to the volar plate and allowing the distal tails enough length to heal into the palmar soft tissues, preventing hyperextension deformity of the FDS. Repeat this procedure for the radial slip (not shown).

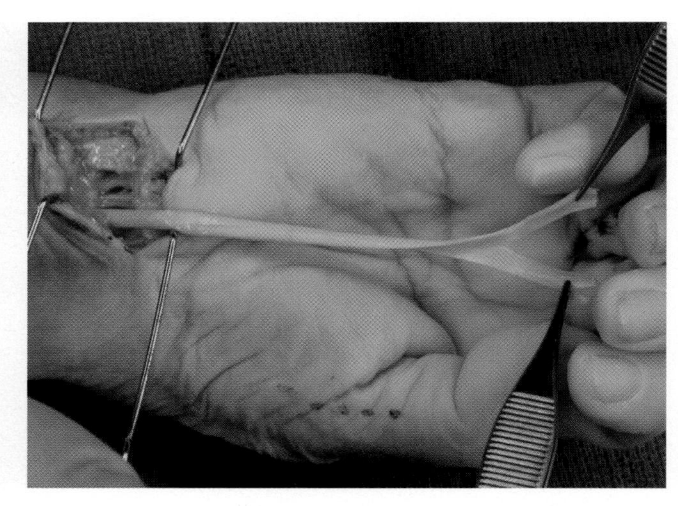

Figure 15.5. The FDS tendon is pulled out of the transverse wrist incision proximal to the transverse carpal ligament.

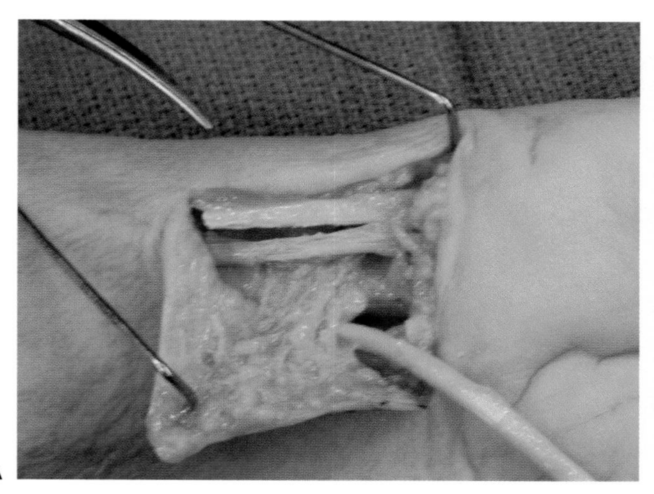
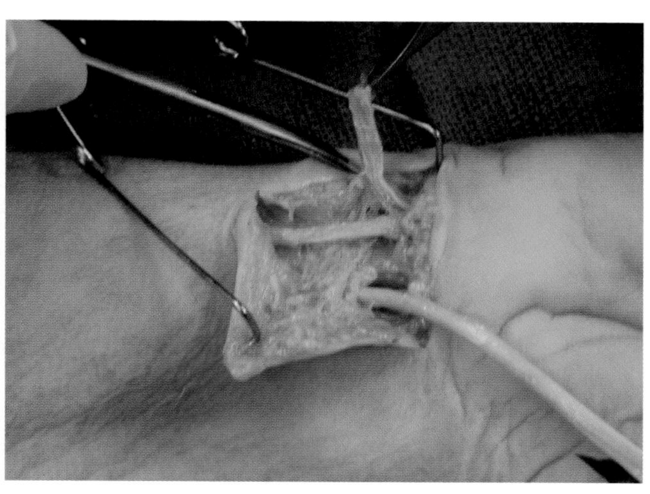

Figure 15.6. A: Expose the distal portion of the FCU tendon and split the tendon longitudinally, leaving the insertion onto the pisiform intact. **B:** Ligate the ulnar limb of the split tendon proximally, leaving a 4-cm, distally-based segment of the FCU for pulley construction.

To improve the vector of the transferred motor unit, we prefer to construct a pulley near the pisiform bone. Multiple options for pulley construction have been described, but have in common their location to optimize the vector of approach of the transfer and the need for stability. The pulley that we utilize in our practice to meet these criteria is constructed by splitting the FCU tendon and creating a distally based tendon loop. Distally based loops are fixed by the insertion of the FCU on the pisiform and are stable. First, dissect the FCU tendon free of surrounding soft tissues. Identify the ulnar artery and ulnar nerve and then encircle them with a silicon vascular tape to mark their position. Using a No. 11 blade scalpel, split the distal 4 cm of the FCU tendon, leaving the insertion intact. Create a distally based loop by dividing the ulnar half of the tendon and flipping the loop distally (Fig. 15.6). Suture the free tendon end to the intact insertion using a 4-0 mattress suture (Fig. 15.7).

Make a 4-cm incision on the dorsal-radial border of the thumb that is centered over the metacarpophalangeal joint. Bluntly dissect out the insertion of the APB and the extensor hood (Fig. 15.8). Take care to protect the branches of the superficial radial nerve and any large dorsal veins.

Inspect the site of APB muscular insertion and the motion of the thumb. Using a large hemostat, create a generous subcutaneous tunnel between the proximal end of the thumb

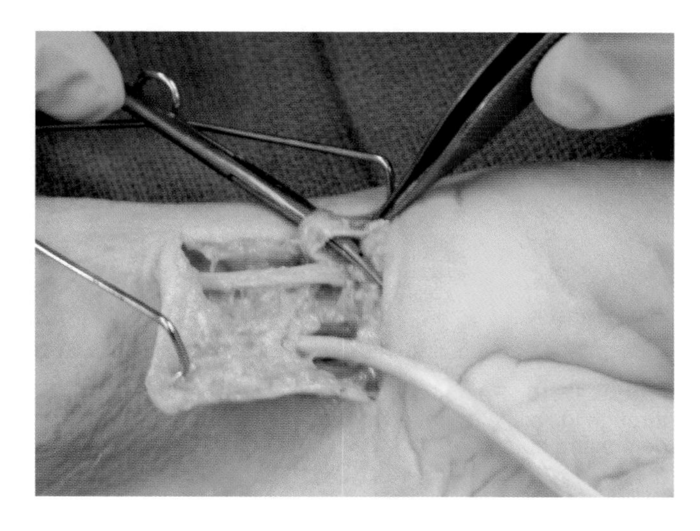

Figure 15.7. Suture the ulnar limb of the FCU back to itself at the pisiform to create the pulley.

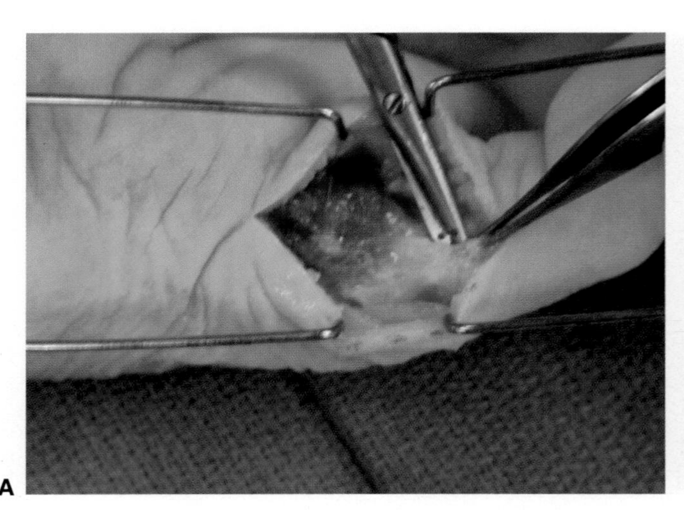
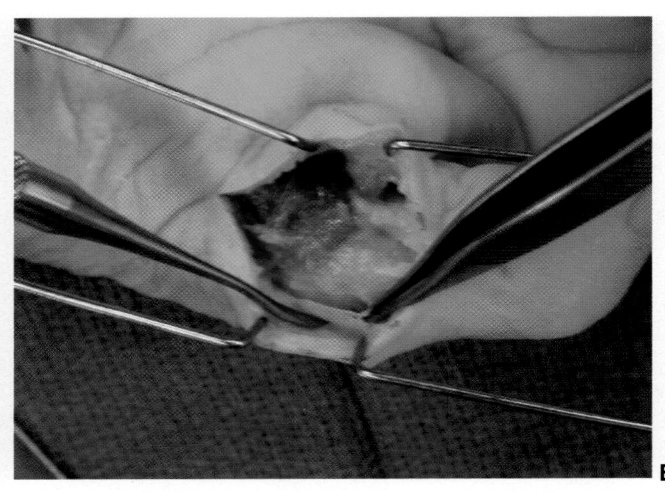

Figure 15.8. A: Expose the APB expansion and (**B**) the extensor hood through the longitudinal thumb incision.

incision and the distal forearm incision (Fig. 15.9). The channel must be sufficient to allow free FDS tendon excursion.

Pass the FDS tendon deep to the FCU and through the distally based FCU pulley, and examine the proposed reconstruction to ensure free tendon excursion and stability of the pulley (Fig. 15.10). This arrangement should prevent the tendon transfer from both radial and proximal migration and ensures an appropriate force vector from the pisiform to the thumb.

Place a tendon passer through the subcutaneous tunnel and withdraw the donor tendon into the thumb wound (Fig. 15.11). Again, check the transfer to ensure free excursion through the pulley and the subcutaneous channel.

To inset the transfer passively, place the thumb in full opposition. Tension the FDS tendon by first placing it in a position of maximum tendon excursion and then relaxing it. Choose a position of approximately 75% of maximum tendon excursion as the point to insert the transfer. With an assistant holding the thumb in opposition and the wrist at neutral, suture one slip of the superficialis to the abductor expansion (Fig. 15.12) at the proximal

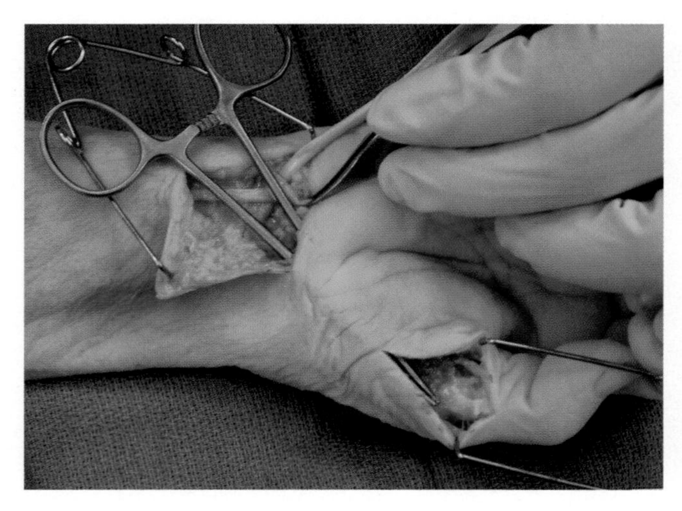

Figure 15.9. Create a generous subcutaneous tunnel for the FDS tendon between the forearm incision and the thumb incision using a hemostat.

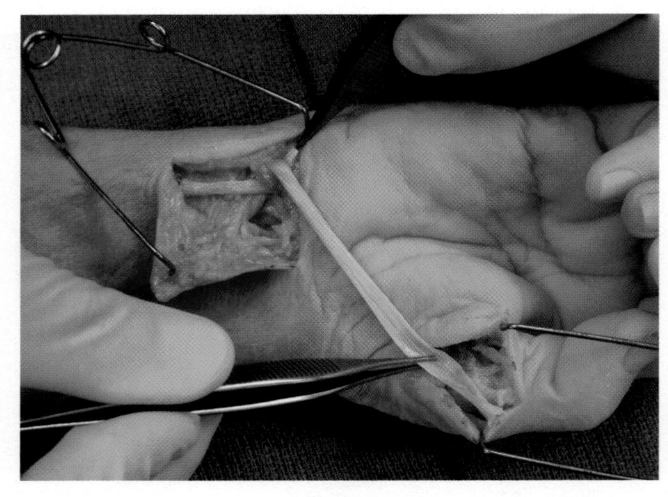

Figure 15.10. Pass the FDS tendon deep to the FCU and through the pisiform-based pulley. The path for the transfer is demonstrated.

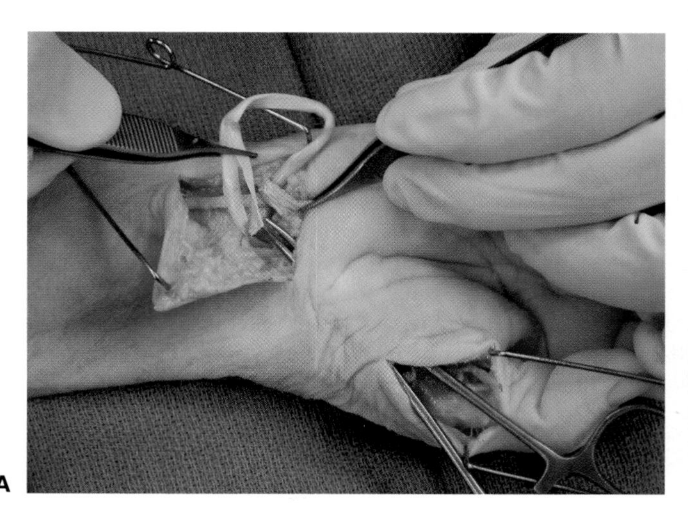

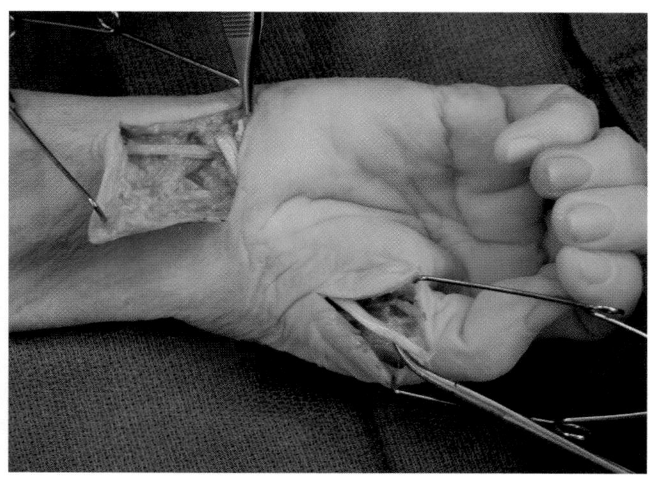

Figure 15.11. A: Insert a hemostat or tendon passer from distal to proximal in the tunnel previously created between the thumb and forearm incisions. **B:** Pull the FDS tendon through the subcutaneous tunnel and out of the thumb incision.

metacarpal and the other dorsal-ulnarly to the extensor hood. We prefer to use a modified Pulvertaft-type weave secured with a 4-0 braided non-absorbable suture to stabilize the tendon repair sites. The ABP insertion location promotes positioning of the thumb away from the palm, and the extensor insertion facilitates pronation of the thumb by directing the thumb pad toward the palm. Proper tensioning of the transfer will allow for some opposition during wrist extension and clearing of the thumb from the palm with wrist flexion.

Deflate the tourniquet and obtain hemostasis with bipolar electrocautery. Administer an anesthetic block of the superficial radial and median nerves for postoperative pain control, irrigate the wounds, and close the incisions, everting the skin edges using interrupted 5-0 nylon sutures. After the wound is closed and prior to application of the dressing, check the transfer position to ensure that the position is appropriate. Apply non-adherent wound coverage, soft dressing, and place the thumb in a well-padded thumb spica splint with the IP joint free. When molded, the splint should keep the thumb in mid-range opposition that we have described as anteposition (the "Coke can" position).

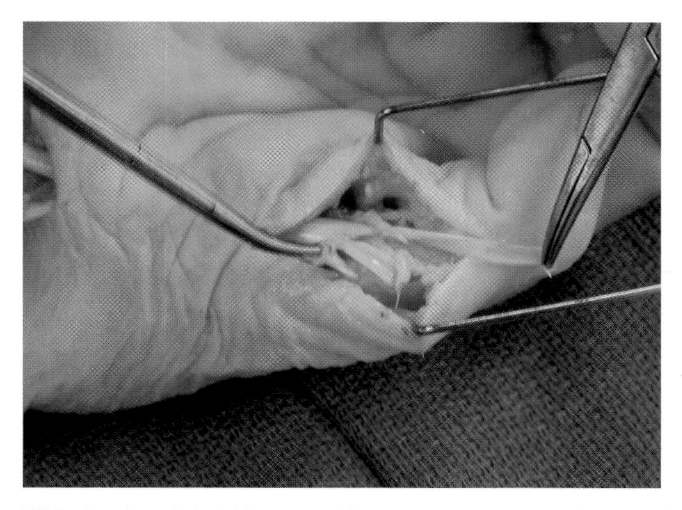

Figure 15.12. With the thumb held in opposition, suture one slip of the FDS into the APB expansion and the other slip into the extensor hood.

POSTOPERATIVE MANAGEMENT

The patient remains in his or her postoperative splint for 10 to 14 days and then in a thumb spica cast for an additional three weeks. After discontinuing the cast, begin passive abduction and opposition with active extension under the supervision of an appropriately trained therapist. When not in therapy, protect the thumb with a removable thumb abduction splint that is molded into opposition. At six weeks, begin active opposition, under supervision, with retraining of the transferred motor unit.

Abduction splinting is continued until the patient has adequate strength in the transferred motor through a near full range of motion. This may take several months. Failure to maintain abduction throughout the rehabilitation process may result in recurrent first web space adduction contracture caused by adduction imbalance.

RESULTS

Restoration of thumb opposition using a transferred tendon is a relatively common tendon-transfer procedure. Our preferred procedure has been to use the flexor digitorum superficialis from the ring finger as the motor for the transfer. This particular transfer, modified slightly from Royle-Thompson's procedure, uses a strong motor to provide thumb abduction and opposition. We've used this transfer in over 20 cases and have been pleased with the results. Because of the method of tendon harvest and after-care, donor site complications have been infrequent. The transferred tendon is consistently long enough for the transfer, and has two stout limbs that can be woven into the APB to ensure a satisfactory distal juncture. Usually, the tendon transfer is easily activated by the patient.

COMPLICATIONS

Proper patient selection is paramount. One of the most common "complications" following tendon-transfer surgery is the patient's disappointment with the outcome of the procedure. Tendon transfers are elective procedures, and ample time usually exists to discuss the goals of the procedure, the anticipated outcome, and the potential complications. Patients must have both a clear understanding of the goals of the procedure and have a willingness to participate in their rehabilitation. Combined nerve palsies and progressive neuropathies should be expected to have less-favorable results.

Failure to adequately address preoperative adduction and supination contractures is a common cause of a poor outcome. A transferred muscle cannot provide enough strength to overcome and correct ulnar-sided thumb deformity that is caused by contracted skin and soft tissues. The key to avoiding this pitfall is prevention. Splinting and passive range-of-motion exercises should be initiated early in patients with median-nerve dysfunction. Once established, these contractures should first be treated with progressive (serial, static) splinting and intensive occupational therapy. Not uncommonly, they will require operative release. Full passive range of motion of the thumb throughout the arc of opposition should be obtained prior to undertaking opponensplasty.

Donor site morbidity is seen in the form of both proximal interphalangeal joint fixed flexion contractures and swan-neck deformity. Flexion contracture of the PIP may develop secondary to scarring and adhesion of the FDS stumps, or secondary to volar plate injury with resultant scarring. Swan-neck deformity of the donor finger may be seen after FDS harvest in patients with a hyperelastic diathesis, but is rare. A hyperextension deformity develops secondary to unbalanced extensor pull at the central slip. Postoperative treatment that employs early ring finger range of motion usually prevents secondary proximal interphalangeal joint deformity.

Postoperative diminution or cessation of function may occur secondary to adhesions and scarring, attenuation, or rupture of the transferred musculotendinous unit. Exploration of the transfer with lysis of adhesions is indicated approximately four months following tendon transfer if it is deemed to have failed. Attenuation may be secondary to pulley rupture, pulley migration, or improper tensioning, and these situations should be identified and addressed at the time of exploration. An abrupt cessation of transfer function is indicative of repair site rupture. Exploration and reconstruction is warranted; however, results cannot be expected to be as good as with a primary procedure.

RECOMMENDED READING

1. Anderson GA, Lee V, Sundararaj GD. Opponensplasty by extensor indicis and flexor digitorum superficialis tendon transfer. *J Hand Surg* 17B:611–614, 1982.
2. Brandsma JW, Ottenhoff-De Jonge MW. Flexor digitorum superficialis tendon transfer for intrinsic replacement. Long-term results and the effect on donor fingers. *J Hand Surg* 17B:625–628, 1992.
3. Bunnell S. Opposition of the thumb. *J Bone Joint Surg* 20:269–284, 1938.
4. Davis TRC, Barton NJ. Median-nerve palsy. In: Green DP, Hotchkiss RN, Pederson WC, eds. *Green's Operative Hand Surgery.* 4th ed. New York: Churchill Livingstone, 1999;1497–1525.
5. Jacobs B, Thompson TC. Opposition of the thumb and its restoration. *J Bone Joint Surg* 42A:1015–1026, 1960.
6. Jenson EG. Restoration of oppostition of the thumb. *Hand* 10:161–167, 1978.
7. Michelinakis E, Vourexakis H. Tendon transfer for intrinsic-muscle paralysis of the thumb in Charcot-Marie Tooth neuropathy. *Hand* 13:276–278, 1981.
8. Omer GE Jr. Timing of tendon transfers in peripheral nerve injury. *Hand Clin* 4:317–322, 1988.
9. Omer GE Jr. Combined nerve palsies. In: Green DP, Hotchkiss RN, Pederson WC, eds. *Green's Operative Hand Surgery.* 4th ed. New York: Churchill Livingstone, 1998:1526–1555.
10. Omer GE Jr. Tendon transfers for combined traumatic nerve palsies of the forearm and hand. *J Hand Surg* 17B:603–610, 1992.
11. Omer GE Jr. Tendon transfers for combined nerve injuries. In: Gelberman RH, ed. *Operative Nerve Repair and Reconstruction.* Philadelphia: JB Lippincott, 1991:747–762.
12. Royle ND. An operation for paralysis of the intrinsic muscles of the thumb. *JAMA* 111:612–613, 1938.
13. Schmidt HM, Lanz U. Anatomy of the median nerve in the carpal tunnel. In: Gelberman RH, ed. *Operative Nerve Repair and Reconstruction.* Philadelphia: JB Lippincott, 1191:889–898.
14. Thompson, TC. A modified operation for opponens paralysis. *J Bone Joint Surg* 26:632–640, 1942.

16

Ulnar Nerve Paralysis

Hill Hastings II

INDICATIONS/CONTRAINDICATIONS

Paralysis of the ulnar nerve at a low level (below the level of innervation of the flexor digitorum profundus) impairs nearly every component contributing power and precision to hand function. The greatest disability results from paralysis of the four dorsal interossei, three volar interossei, abductor digiti quinti, and deep head of the flexor pollicis brevis. The net effect is to diminish the volume within which the digits can be placed in space, creation of deformity to the ring and small digits, disturbance of precision and fine motor coordination, and severe impairment of power pinch and grasp (Fig. 16.1). Functional capacity of the hand is reduced by one-half.

Ideally, tendon transfer should correct clawing deformity, asynchronous pattern of finger flexion, and weakness of grasp. The choice of transfer will depend on the patient's (a) age, (b) relative suppleness of the hand, (c) level of palsy (high or low), and (d) relative needs for strength. Limited tendon transfers, such as the Zancolli "lasso" procedure or Stiles-Bunnell, are capable of correcting clawing deformity and restoring synchronous finger flexion but do not correct the loss of strength. Although clawing of the index and middle fingers is not seen in isolated low ulnar-nerve palsy by virtue of continued function of the radial two lumbricals, patients do complain of loss of radial hand dexterity and strength. For these reasons, I usually recommend tendon transfer to all four digits (index, middle, ring, and small). Persons who require maximum strength for day-to-day activities should have a transfer chosen that will further contribute to strength by adding the power of another muscle/tendon unit to the hand rather than merely redistributing the power to tendon function within the hand, best accomplished by transferring to the hand a muscle/tendon unit that normally powers the forearm or wrist with the use of tendon grafts to prolong such transfer.

Absolute contraindications include the noncompliant patient, with poor motivation or an unreliable nature, who will not appropriately follow through with postoperative immobilization and rehabilitation program. The patient must have an expendable, normal-functioning donor-muscle tendon unit suitable for transfer. The metacarpophalangeal (MCP)

Hill Hastings II, M.D.: Orthopaedic Surgery, Indiana University Medical Center, Indiana Hand Center, Indianapolis, IN, and Orthopaedic Surgery, St. Vincent's Hospital, Indianapolis, IN

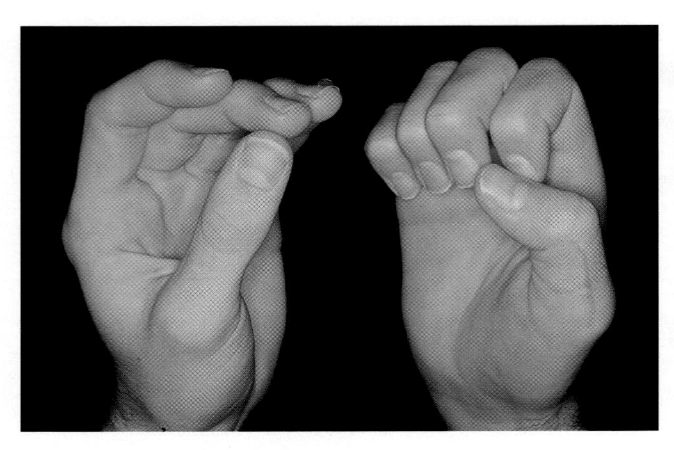

Figure 16.1. Patient with low intrinsic median and ulnar nerve-combined palsy demonstrates loss of precision pinch and balanced finger flexion.

joints and interphalangeal (IP) joints should be supple with full passive range of motion. The extensor digitorum communis (EDC) function to all digits should be intact.

PREOPERATIVE PLANNING

All patients should have supple, full digital range of motion before surgery. The tendon transfer will not overcome flexion contracture of the proximal interphalangeal (PIP) joints or tendon adhesions. When present, contractures must be corrected by splinting, surgical release, or tenolysis before tendon transfer. The MCP joints ideally have full range of motion.

The recipient bed for the tendon transfer must be supple and free of active wound-healing processes. If a poor soft-tissue bed exists, it should be corrected by healthy fascial or composite flap replacement. Silicone tendon rods may be used to create gliding sheaths for the subsequent transfer and tendon grafts.

Potential donor muscle/tendon units must have active volitional control and be of nearly normal strength, as some loss of strength following transfer can result from mild adhesions. Most commonly the extensor carpi radialis brevis (ECRB) is chosen. Other potential donor tendons include the flexor carpi radialis (FCR), brachioradialis (BR), or the extensor carpi radialis longus (ECRL). The BR holds the greatest excursion and work potential, but to achieve the required excursion, the muscle-tendon unit must be freed up back to the proximal forearm. The remaining donor choices are simpler to use, and I consider all to present adequate excursion and force potential. The potential excursion of a muscle relates to its mean fiber length. The BR has a resting fiber length of 16.1 cm, the ECRL 9.3 cm, the ECRB 6.1 cm, and the FCR 5.2 cm. The potential force of a muscle can be expressed as a unit of tension fraction. The ECRB has a tension fraction of 4.2%, FCR 4.1%, ECRL 3.5%, and BR 2.4%.

Finally, the patient's expectations must be clearly understood, realistic, and capable of being met. It is not uncommon for the patient to misunderstand the potential and intent of the tendon-transfer reconstruction and likewise for the surgeon to misunderstand the patient's expectations.

SURGERY

Surgery is usually performed with the patient under a regional anesthetic block, supine, and the arm positioned on a hand table. After preparation and draping, the involved extremity is exsanguinated, and a brachial tourniquet is inflated to 50 mm Hg above systolic pressure.

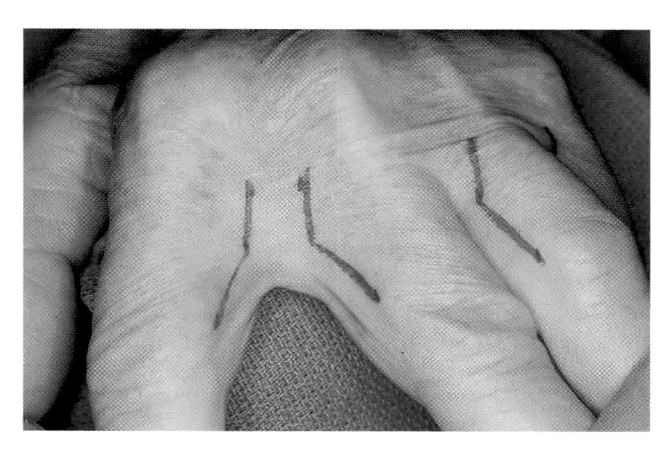

Figure 16.2. Hockey-stick proximal phalangeal incisions for tendon graft distal insertions. Note: All are placed over the radial aspect of the proximal phalanges except that to the index.

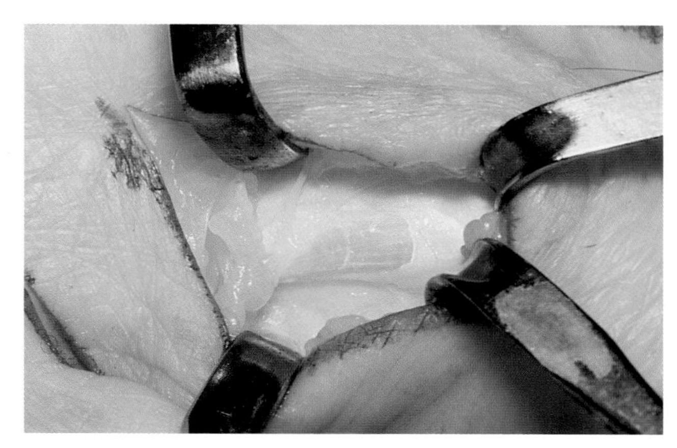

Figure 16.3. Exposure of intrinsic mechanism.

Incision/Dissection

A hockey-stick-shaped incision is made at the radial proximal phalangeal bases of the middle, ring, and small digits with short proximal limbs extending along the dorsal side of the web spaces. A similar incision is made over the ulnar aspect of the index proximal phalanx (Fig. 16.2). Dissection is followed down to the volar edge of the intrinsic expansion (Fig. 16.3), which is retracted dorsally (Fig. 16.4). A longitudinal incision is made in periosteum and a small area subperiosteally exposed for attachment of the tendon grafts (Fig. 16.5). The subsequent tendon grafts are most easily attached to bone by way of a drill hole. To do so, a 2.0-mm drill is used to make a hole in the frontal plane through both cortices (Fig. 16.6). The near cortex then is enlarged with a 2.7-mm drill and curette (Fig. 16.7). The drill holes should be made just dorsal to the distal origin of the second annular pulley (Fig. 16.8), providing for a strong moment arm to contribute to MCP joint flexion.

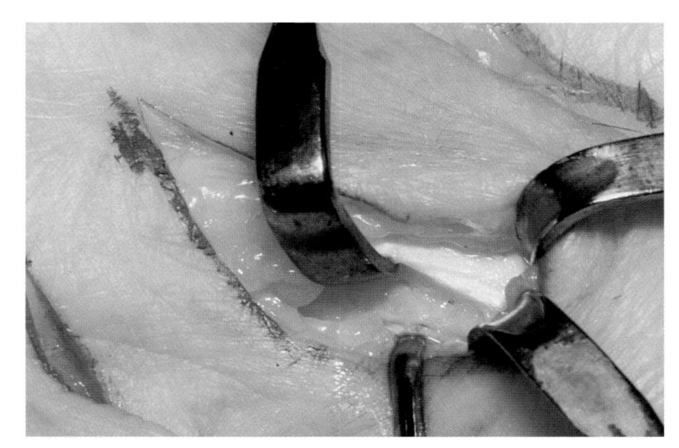

Figure 16.4. Dorsal retraction of intrinsic mechanism at proximal phalangeal level to expose site for drill hole.

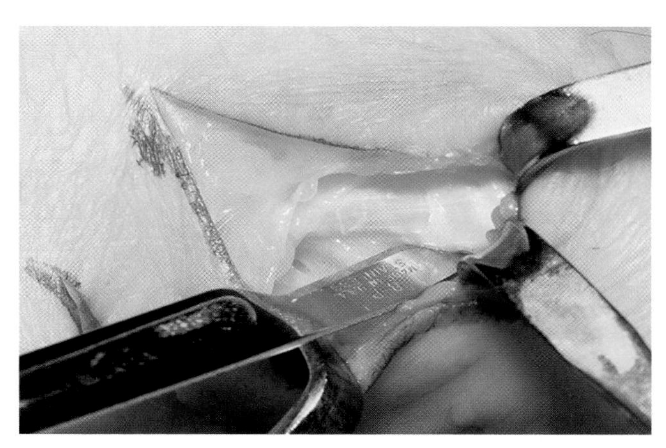

Figure 16.5. Periosteal longitudinal incision dorsal to distal edge of second annular pulley.

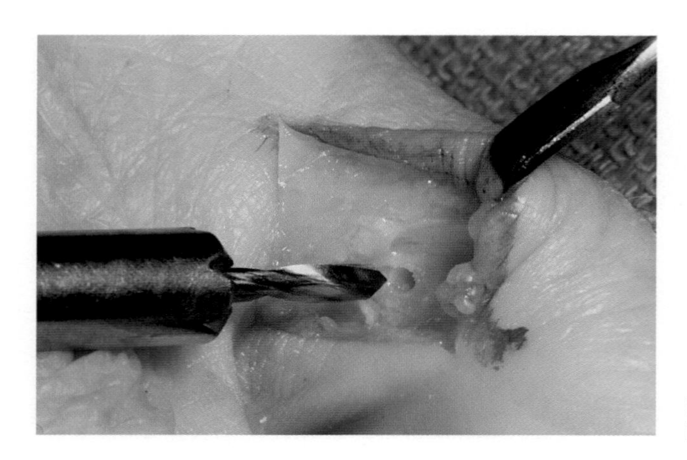

Figure 16.6. Placement of bicortical 2.0-mm frontal plane drill hole.

A transverse incision is made at the midmetacarpal level between the second and third metacarpals, and a second similar incision is centered over the fourth metacarpal (Fig. 16.9). Through these incisions, a window of interosseous fascia is excised from between each metacarpal (Fig. 16.10). The incision over the fourth metacarpal provides access to the interosseous compartments on either side.

The final incision is made in a chevron fashion over the second extensor compartment (Fig. 16.9). The ECRB is exposed at its insertion and divided (Fig. 16.11). The tendon is withdrawn proximal to the second dorsal compartment (Fig. 16.12), and redirected distally to lie superficial to the wrist retinaculum (Fig. 16.13). The chevron incision allows for enough extensile exposure to perform the subsequent ECRB to tendon-graft weave

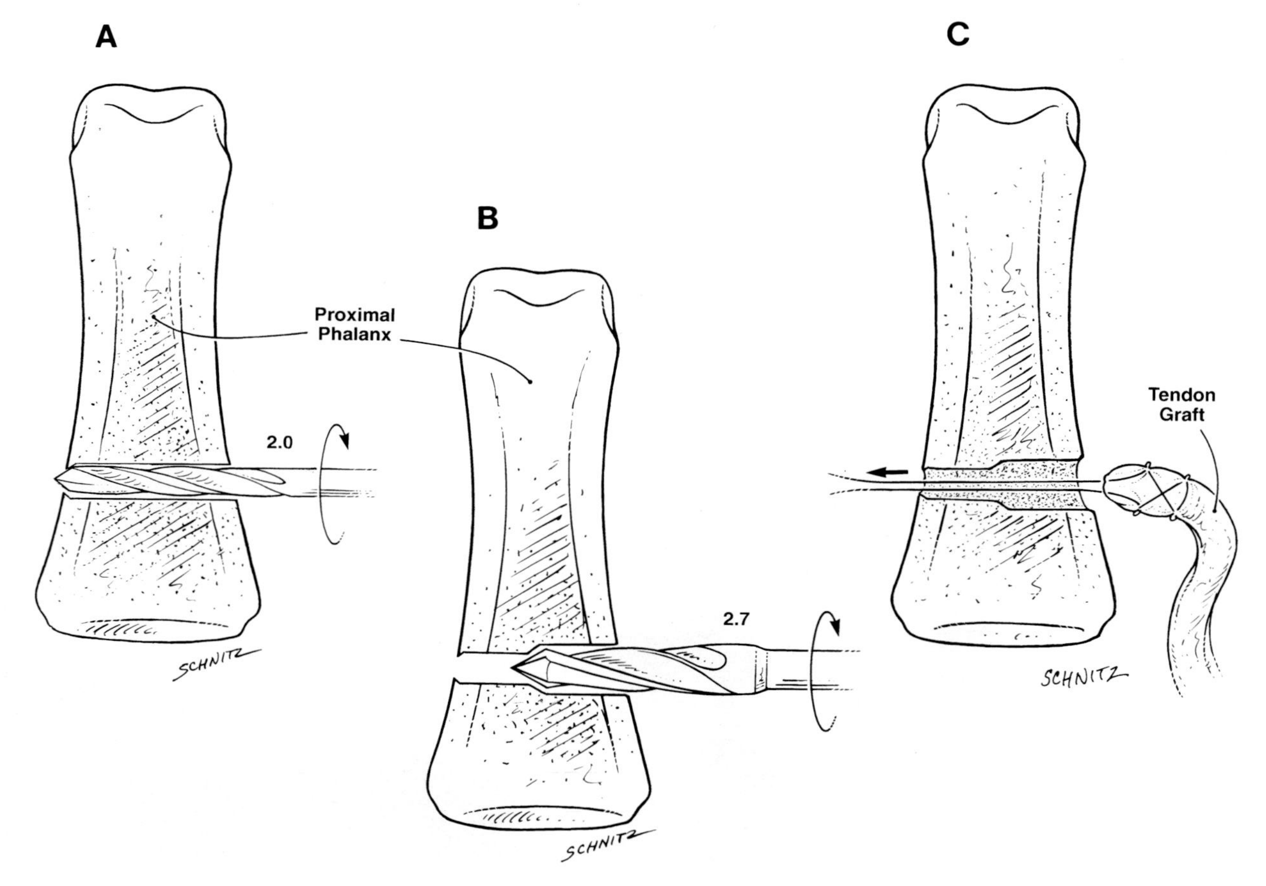

Figure 16.7. A–C: 2.0-mm drill hole is used for both cortices, with the near cortex further enlarged with a 2.7-mm drill.

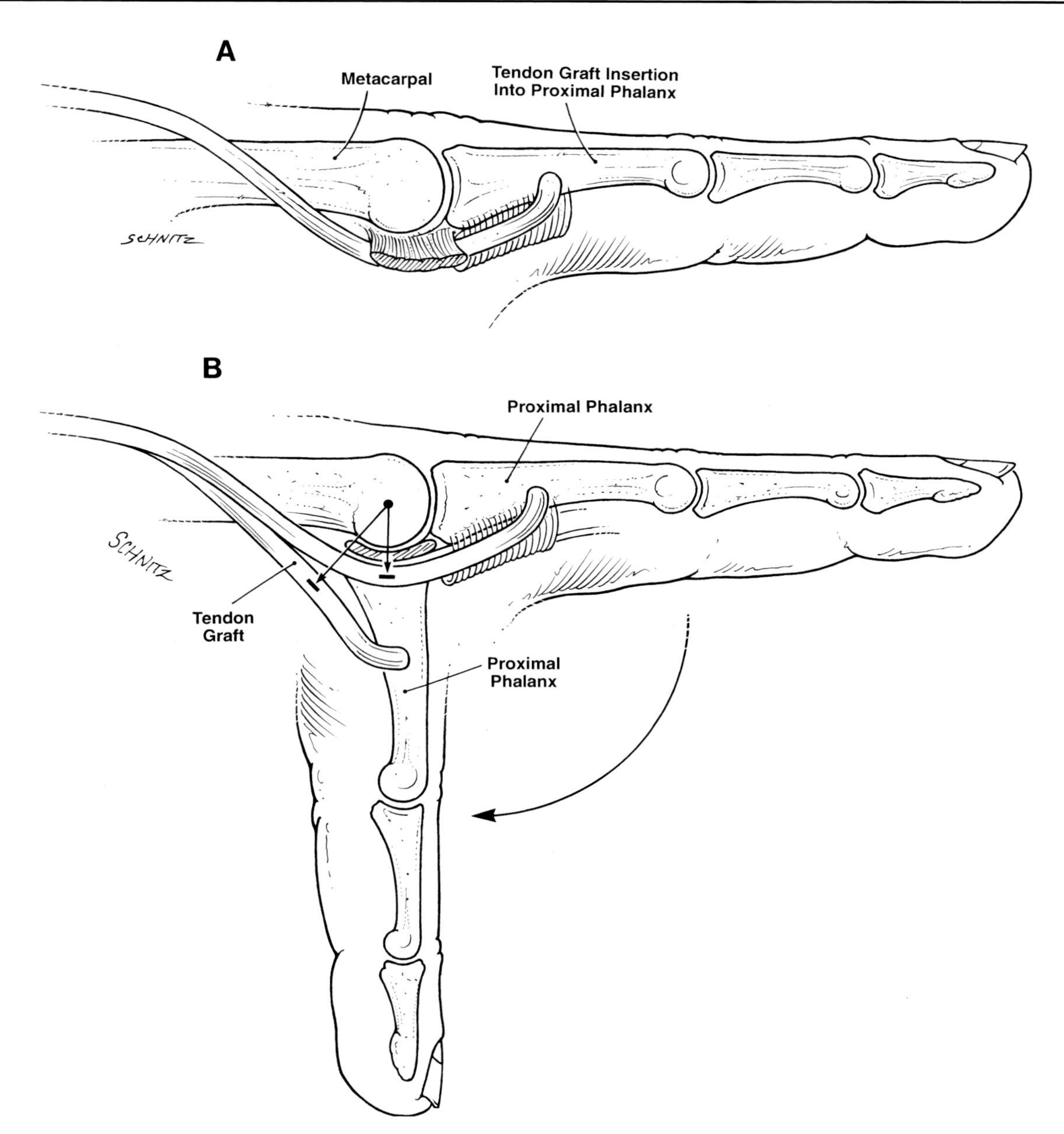

Figure 16.8. Distal attachment of tendon graft allows for strong flexion moment arm.

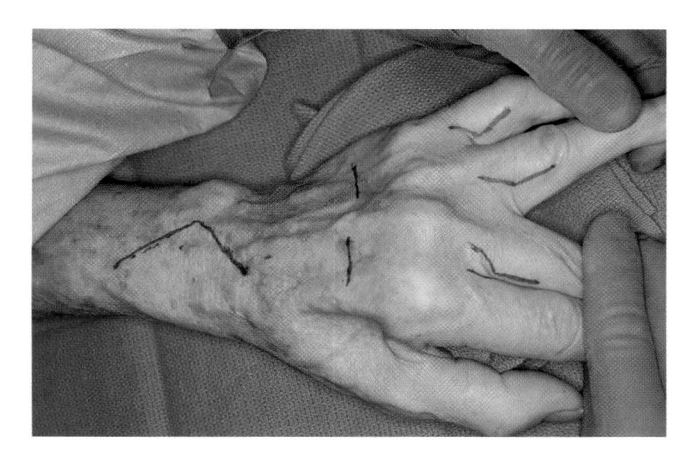

Figure 16.9. Two transverse metacarpal incisions are made, one centered between index and middle metacarpals and a second over the ring metacarpal. The extensor carpi radialis brevis (ECRB) is exposed through a chevron incision centered over the retinacular level and extending out to the base of index metacarpal.

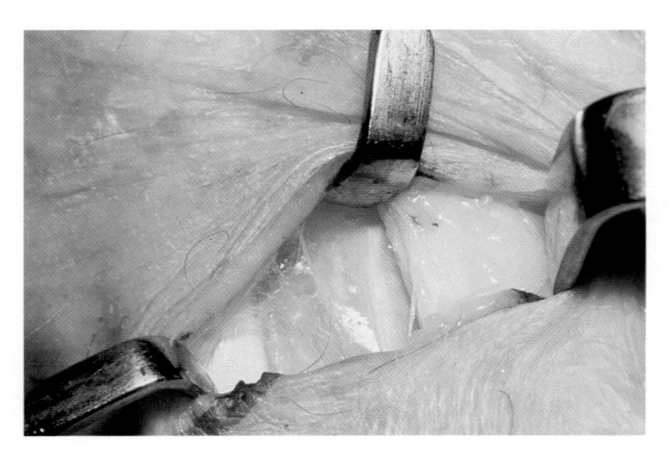

Figure 16.10. Excision of dorsal interosseous fascial window.

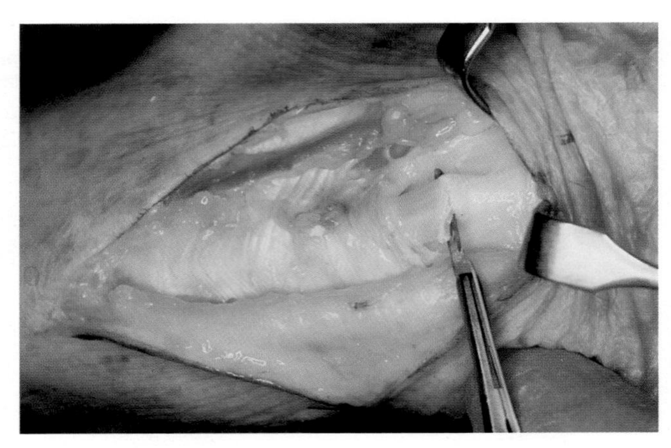

Figure 16.11. Division of extensor carpi radialis brevis (ECRB) distal insertion.

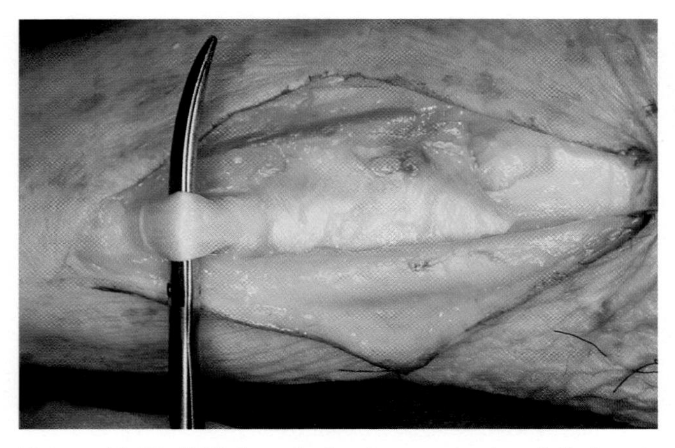

Figure 16.12. Withdrawal of extensor carpi radialis brevis (ECRB) tendon proximal to extensor retinaculum.

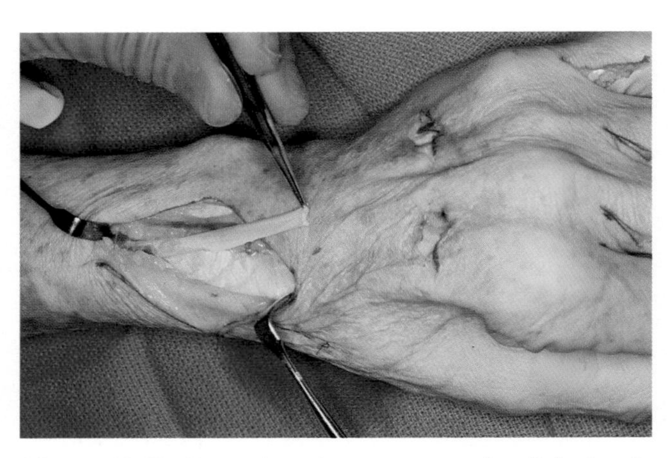

Figure 16.13. Rerouting of extensor carpi radialis brevis (ECRB) superficial to extensor retinaculum.

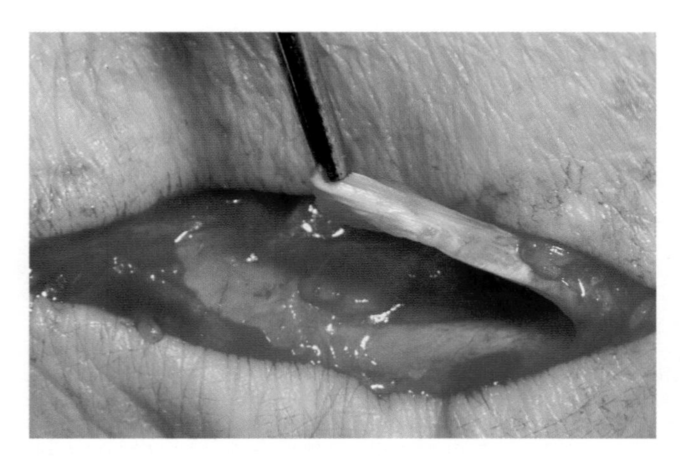

Figure 16.14. Exposure of plantaris tendon adjacent to medial aspect tendon Achilles.

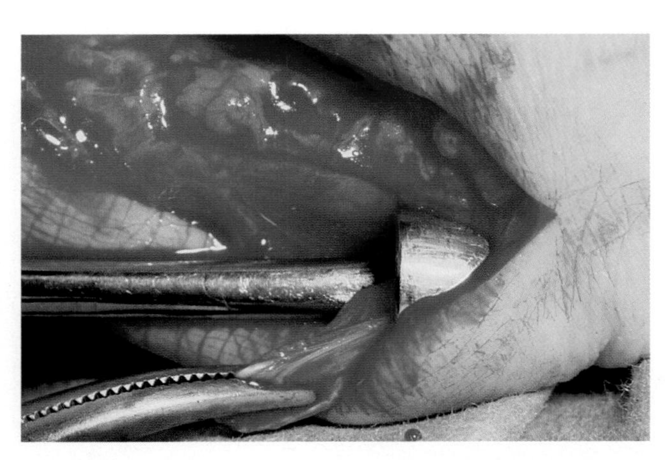

Figure 16.15. Plantaris tendon threaded through Brand tendon stripper.

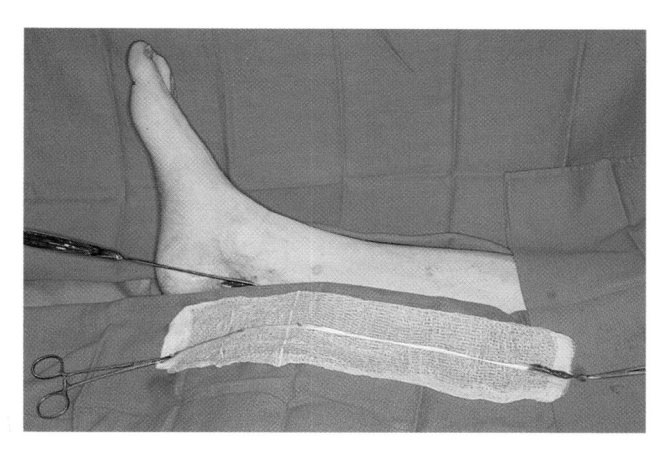

Figure 16.16. Completed harvest of plantaris tendon.

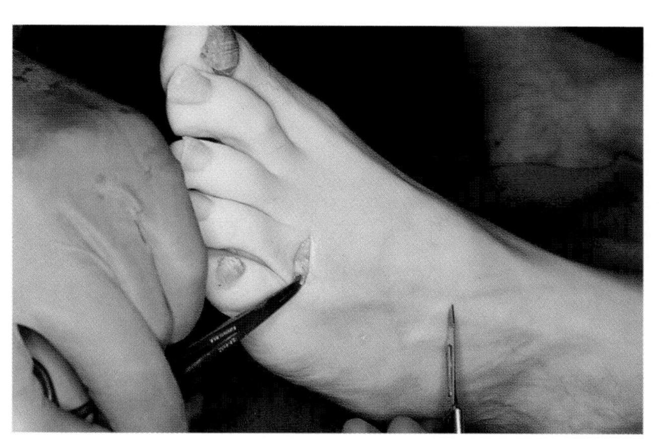

Figure 16.17. Alternative harvesting of long digital toe extensor tendons grafts.

connections easily. The flap created by the chevron incision will subsequently cover and protect the tendon weave connections from skin adhesions.

Tendon grafts are required to prolong the ECRB. Usually, this step is obtained most expediently by harvesting the plantaris tendon from each leg. To do so, a brief general anesthetic is administered. The lower leg is elevated and exsanguinated, and a thigh tourniquet is inflated to 350 mm Hg. A 5-cm incision is made just anterior to the medial border to the Achilles tendon at the ankle level; the plantaris tendon is identified and transected distally (Fig. 16.14). The distal end of the plantaris is passed through the ring of a Brand tendon stripper (Padgett Instruments, Kansas City, MO, U.S.A.) and grasped firmly with a hemostat (Fig. 16.15). It is essential to release the fascia proximally enough to ensure that the tendon stripper passes easily beneath the fascia and up the lower-leg compartment. Traction is applied to the tendon through the grasping hemostat, and the stripper is advanced proximally to the musculotendinous origin, where the stripper will meet resistance. The tendon is then stripped away from the muscle by further firm but controlled advancement of the stripper. The tendon is laid on a saline-moistened sponge, care being taken to avoid digital or instrument manipulation that would induce formation of subsequent adhesions (Fig. 16.16). The incision is closed with 4-0 resorbable polyglactin 910 Dexon resorbable suture (Davis and Geck, Danbury, CT, U.S.A.), the skin with 4-0 nylon, a light compressive dressing applied, and the tourniquet deflated. The same procedure is repeated for harvesting of the plantaris tendon from the second leg.

In the event the plantaris is absent, the second and third and/or fourth long digital toe extensor tendons are used (Fig. 16.17). Palmaris longus tendons usually are not of sufficient length. In most cases, each plantaris tendon is long enough to supply two tendon graft lengths.

Extra muscle is trimmed from the tendon grafts, preserving a thin layer of peritendinous fat (Fig. 16.18). The shortest tendon is divided halfway along its length to provide two segments

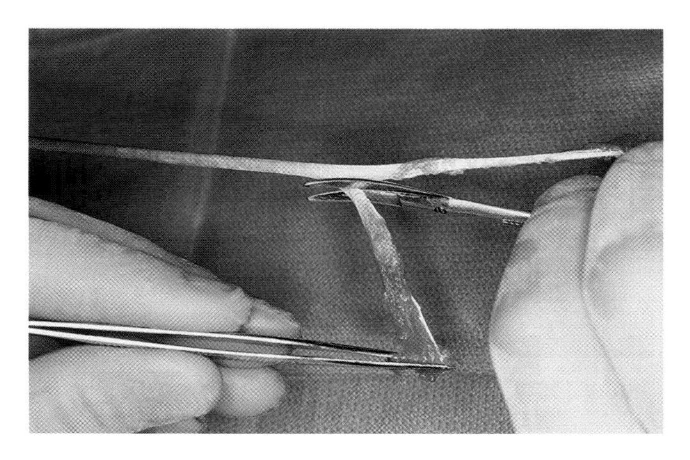

Figure 16.18. Debridement of muscle from tendon graft.

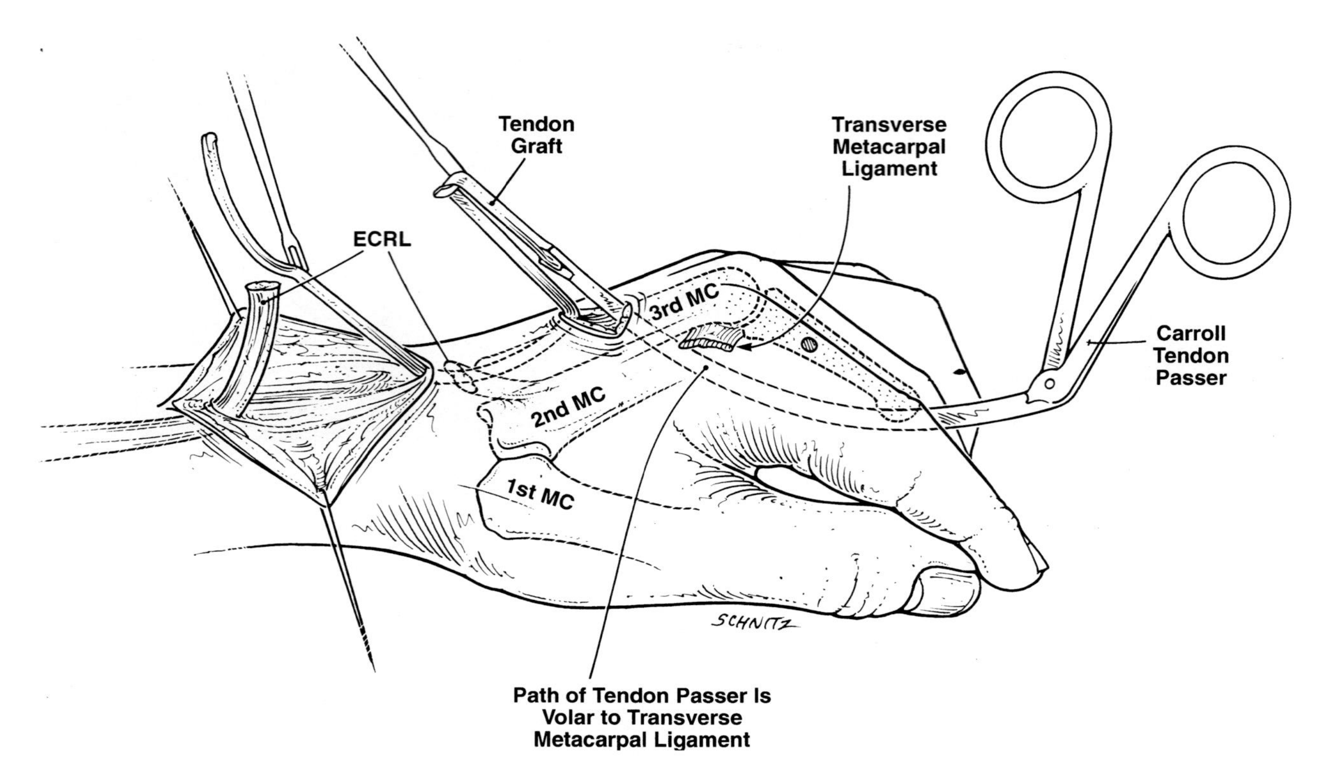

Figure 16.19. Passage of tendon graft through interosseous window and volar to deep intermetacarpal ligament is facilitated by a Brand tendon passer.

for reconstruction of the ring and small digits. Each tendon graft requires separate passage. The longer graft is folded in half, with both limbs passing through the second intermetacarpal space. Whereas the grafts may be passed from distal to proximal, I find it easier to pass the grafts from proximal to distal using a tendon passer to seek the pathway of least resistance from the web space, volar to the intermetacarpal ligament, to the more dorsal intermetacarpal space (Fig. 16.19). Passage volar to the intercarpal ligament is facilitated by holding the MCP joints in flexion. As an intermetacarpal ligament is required to maintain the tendon grafts in a volar position, the index graft passes through the second intermetacarpal space along with that proceeding to the middle finger. As each is to exit through separate distal incisions, each limb of the folded tendon graft is passed separately (Fig. 16.20).

The distal ends of the tendon grafts are secured with 2-0 monofilament nylon Bunnell sutures on straight Keith needles (Figs. 16.21 and 16.22). The Keith needles then are passed

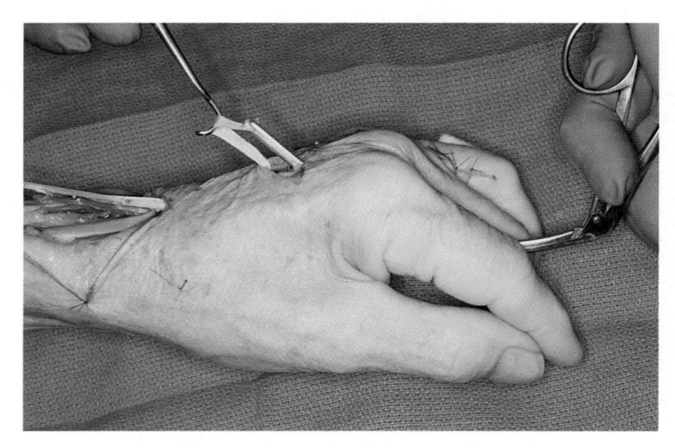

Figure 16.20. Passage of tendon grafts from dorsal hand, through interosseous space, volar to deep intermetacarpal ligament, with exit through proximal phalangeal skin incisions.

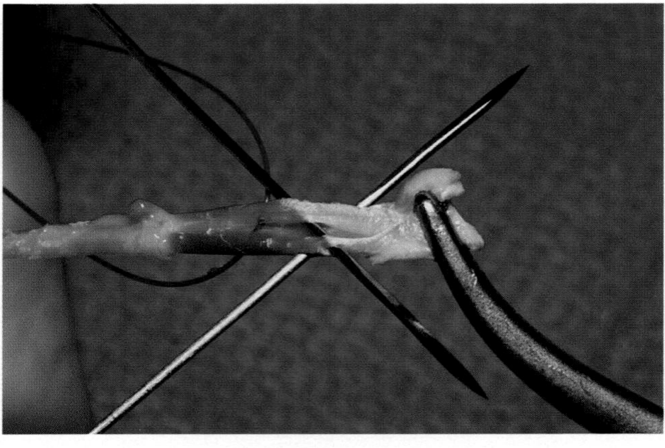

Figure 16.21. Placement of Bunnell crisscross 2.0 monofilament nylon sutures through tendon graft.

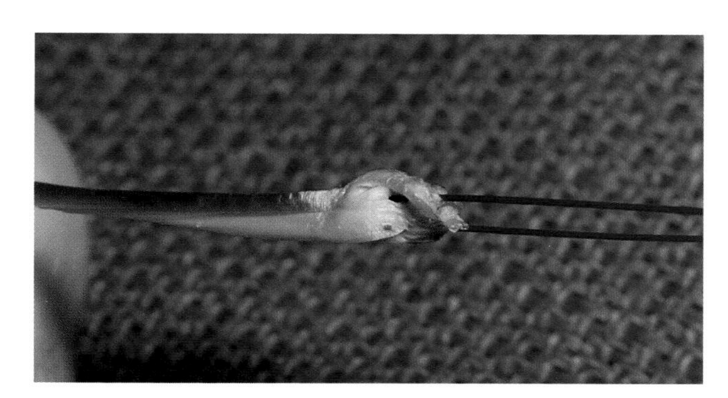

Figure 16.22. Completed suture fixation of tendon graft.

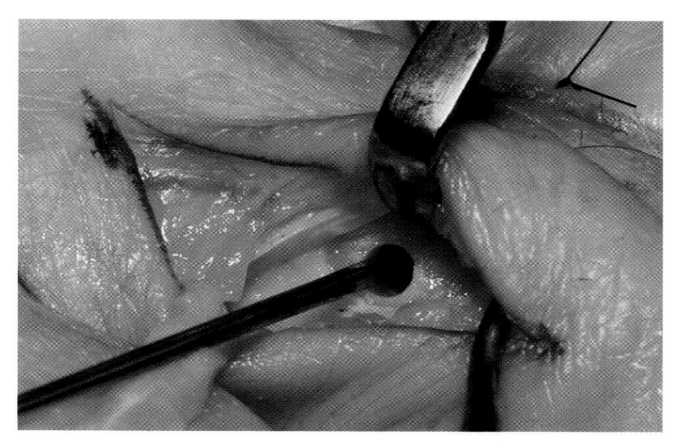

Figure 16.23. Passage of Keith needles and tendon graft into proximal phalangeal bony tunnel.

through the proximal phalangeal drill hole (Fig. 16.23) to exit on the opposite side of the digit (Fig. 16.24). By pulling on the suture, the tendon graft is pulled into the proximal phalangeal medullary cavity, where it butts inside against the smaller drill hole on the far side of the phalanx (Fig. 16.25). The suture then is tied over a padded button (Fig. 16.26). Following fixation of the first tendon graft, a similar sequence is repeated for the remaining digits.

Closure

Distal incisions should be closed at this point before completion of the tendon transfer, as closure is facilitated by extending and spreading the digits apart. Closure of these incisions is difficult after the transfer has been completed (Fig. 16.27). The tendon grafts next are passed through a subcutaneous plane to the dorsal wrist incision. The midmetacarpal incisions are closed at this point.

The relative tension of each transfer is set most easily by suturing all four tendon grafts together before suture to the donor tendon (Fig. 16.28). To do so, the wrist is held in neutral alignment and the converging tendons sutured sequentially to each other with 3-0 braided nylon. The ECRB is routed superficial to the dorsal wrist extensor retinaculum. The tendon grafts then are woven in Pulvertaft fashion into the ECRB tendon (Figs. 16.29–16.31). Alternatively, the ECRB can be split with a scalpel and the tendon grafts inserted into the split tendon like an inner part of a sandwich and sutured.

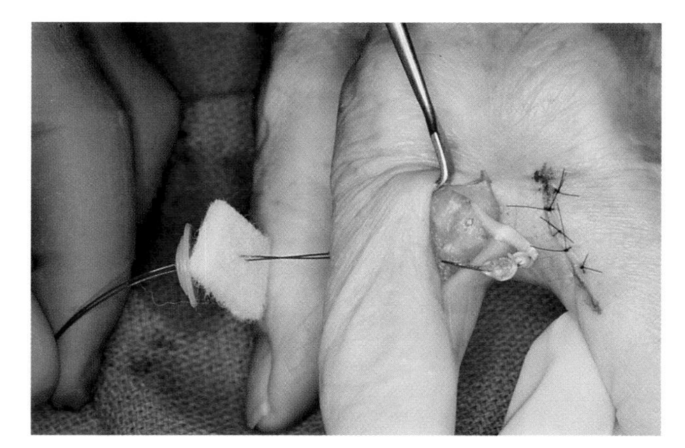

Figure 16.24. Needles pass out opposite side of the proximal phalanx, with suture tied over a slid padded button.

Figure 16.25. **A:** Final appearance of tendon graft firmly seated within proximal phalanx. **B:** Tendon graft secured within bony tunnel in proximal phalanx.

A

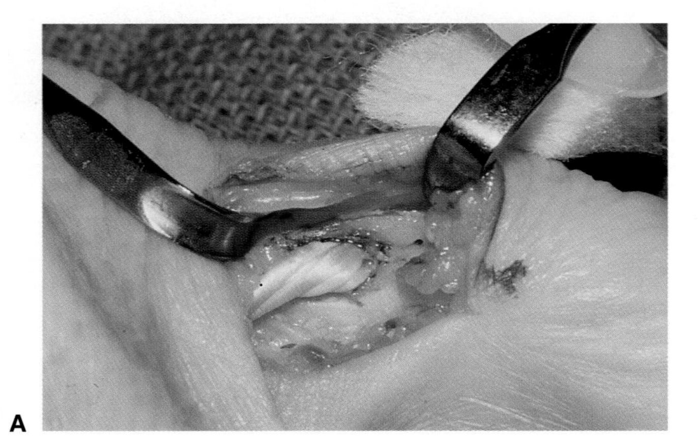

B

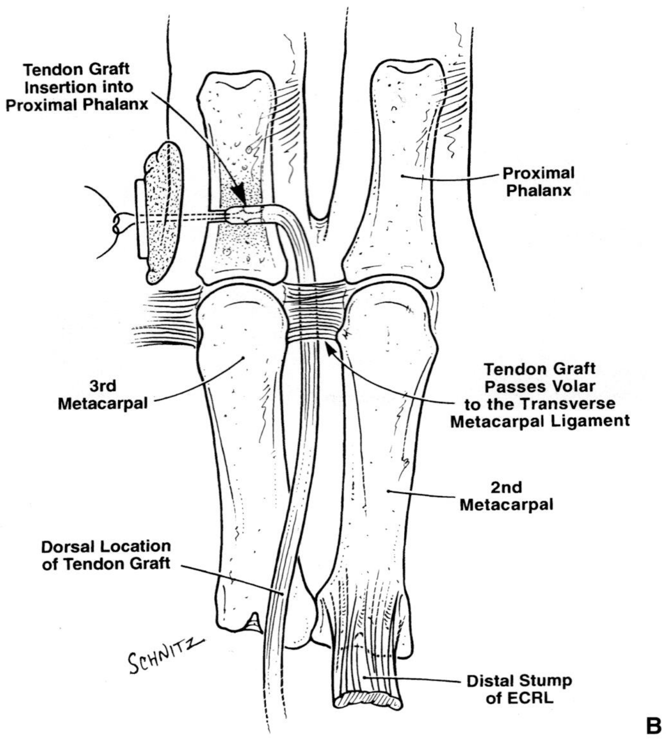

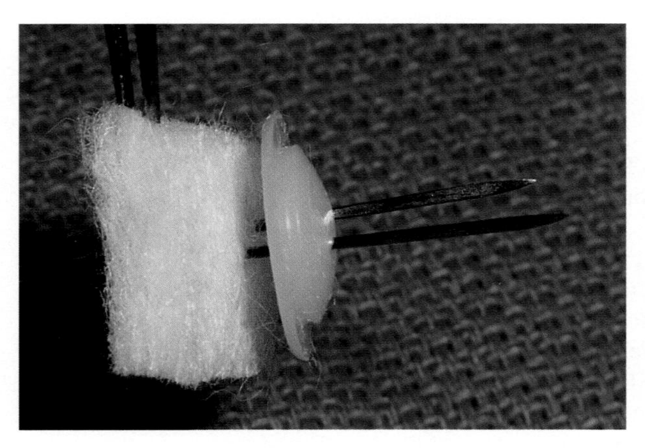

Figure 16.26. Needle and suture placement through felt pad and button.

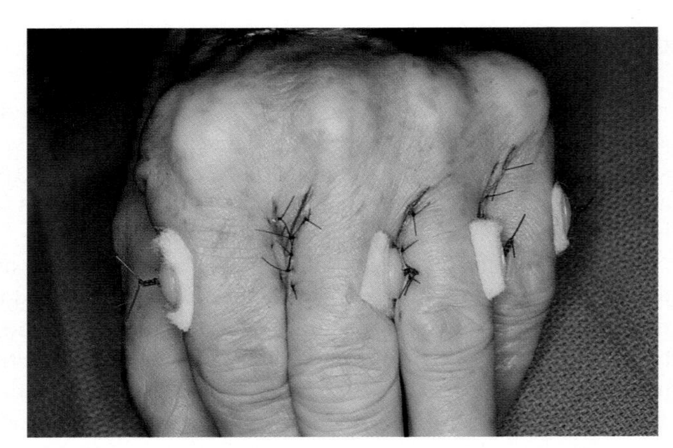

Figure 16.27. Completed wound closure and appearance of button.

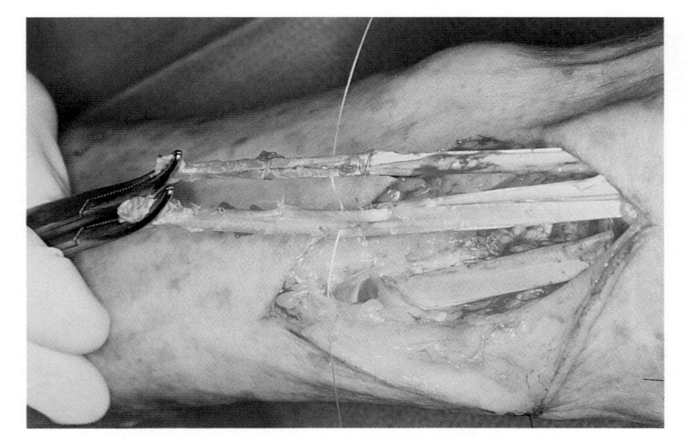

Figure 16.28. Side-to-side suture of tendon grafts of small to ring and index to middle is followed by side-to-side suture of all four together.

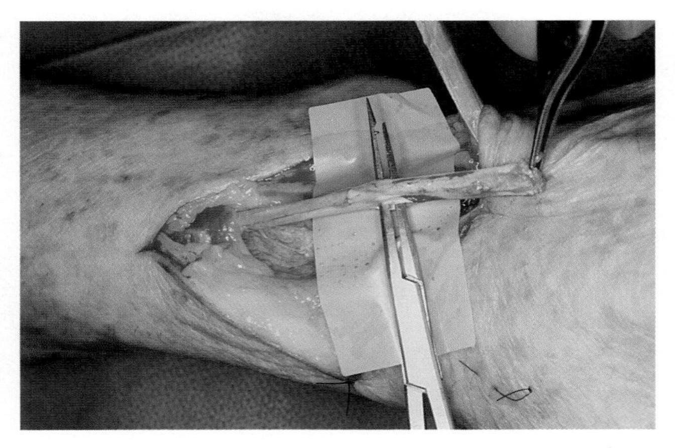

Figure 16.29. Proximal tendon weave is facilitated by Link tendon weaver.

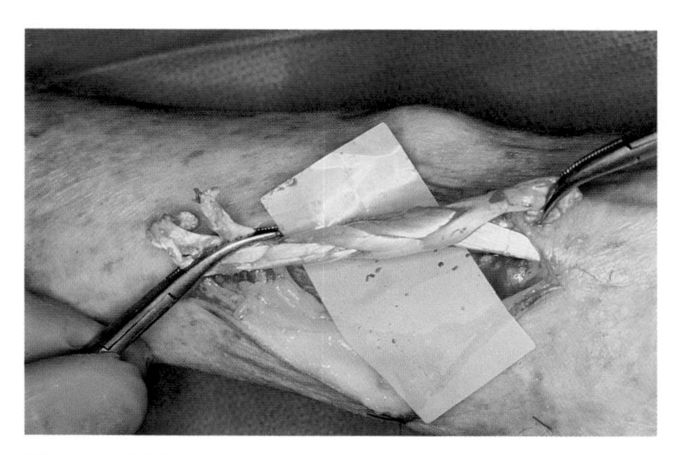

Figure 16.30. The tendon grafts are woven through the extensor carpi radialis brevi (ECRB) in three passes (Pulvertaft weave).

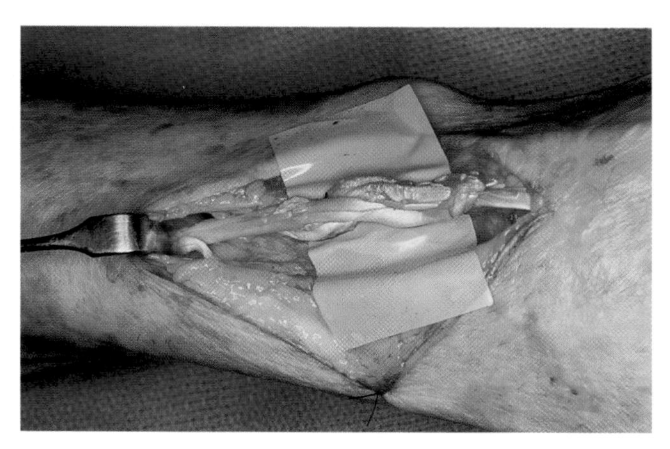

Figure 16.31. Completion of Pulvertaft weave tendon connection.

To set the correct tension properly, the wrist is held in full dorsiflexion, the MCP joints held in complete flexion, and the transfer set at normal resting tension. The first suture (or two) is cut long and divided short only after testing to confirm that the correct tension has been obtained. The wrist is taken through a complete range of motion. In dorsiflexion, passive full extension of the digits should be possible (Fig. 16.32). Wrist palmar flexion should provide a strong tenodesis that flexes fully the MCP joints (Fig. 16.33). When the BR tendon is used, tension is set with the elbow in 90 degrees of flexion. Tension is set at resting fiber length holding the elbow in 90 degrees of flexion and the wrist and digits in extension. With the wrist in dorsiflexion, full passive extension of the digits should be possible. With the elbow at 30 degrees of extension and the wrist in neutral position, the MCP joints should be strongly flexed. In 30 degrees of elbow extension and full wrist dorsiflexion, the MCP joints should be mildly flexed. A light compressive, bulky dressing is applied with a volar plaster splint, which holds the wrist in 45 degrees of flexion, the MCP joints in full flexion, and the IP joints in extension (Fig. 16.34). The proximal tendon weave connection and distal bony insertion are secure enough to be protected by a short-arm splint when the FCR, ECRL, or ECRB tendons are used. Only in the case of the more powerful and proximally arising BR is a long-arm immobilizer applied with the elbow in 90 degrees of flexion.

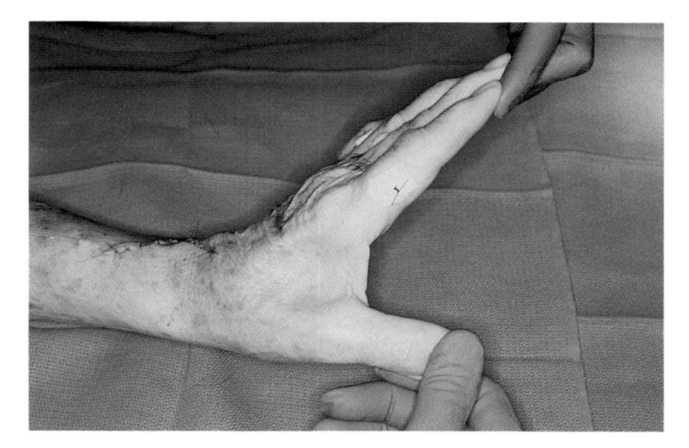

Figure 16.32. Dorsiflexion of wrist relaxes the tendon transfer and allows for full passive digital extension.

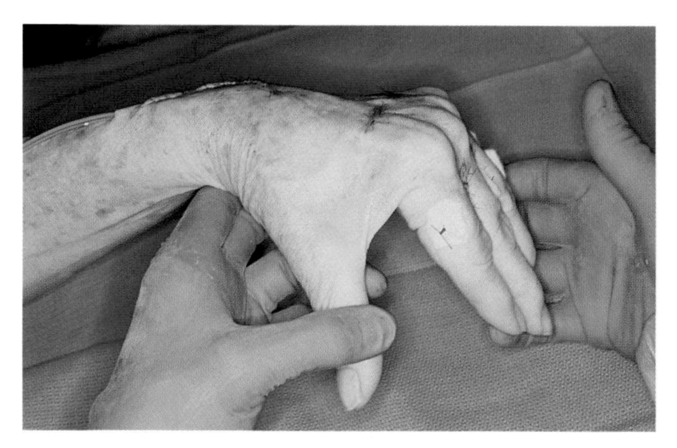

Figure 16.33. Wrist palmar flexion tightens the transfer and imparts a tenodesis function, strongly flexing the metacarpophalangeal joints.

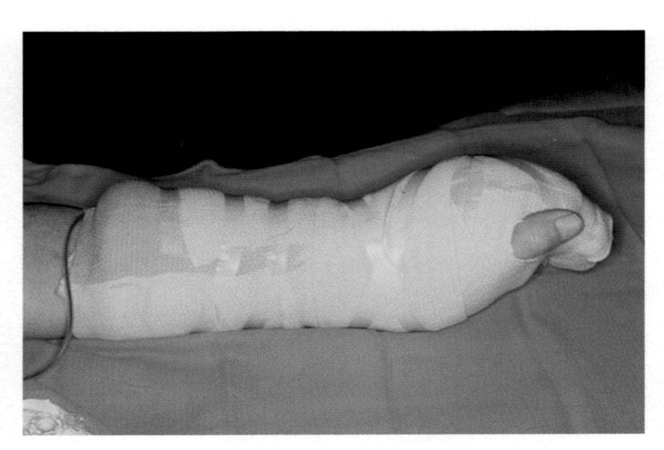

Figure 16.34. Application of short-arm light compressive dressing in volar splint holding the wrist in dorsiflexion, the metacarpophalangeal joints in flexion, and the interphalangeal joints in extension.

POSTOPERATIVE MANAGEMENT

The dressing is changed at 10 to 14 days for suture removal and a thermoplastic molded splint reapplied to hold the wrist in 45 degrees of extension, the MCP joints in full flexion, and the IP joints in extension. At 21 days, active range of motion is initiated to the wrist and digits and performed on an hourly basis. Protective splinting is continued between exercises until 6 weeks postoperatively, when the buttons are removed. Light strengthening is initiated with putty at 8 weeks postoperatively and by a hand helper at 10 weeks. Fully unrestricted use is allowed at 12 weeks postoperatively.

The tendon transfer corrects the clawing deformity of MCP joint hyperextension and IP joint extensor lag (Figs. 16.35 and 16.36). Full digital flexion should be maintained (Fig. 16.37). Strong and independent MCP joint flexion is restored (Fig. 16.38) and grip strength enhanced (Fig. 16.39).

COMPLICATIONS

Tendon Adhesions

Tendon adhesions can occur through the level of the interosseous windows. The risk of adhesions at this level is minimized by meticulous surgical technique that avoids disruption of the dorsal metacarpal arteries and maintains a hemostatically dry wound at the time of

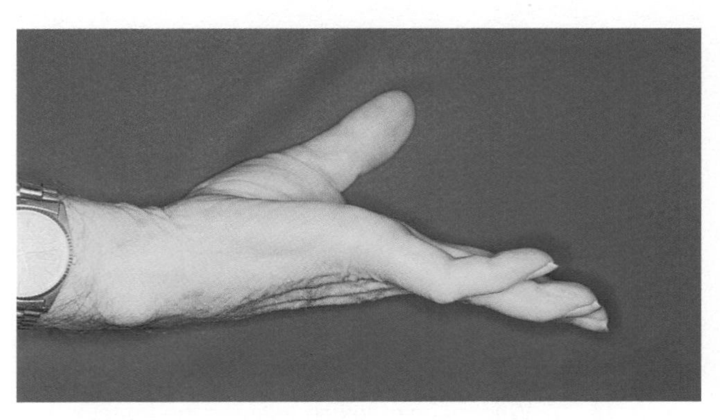

Figure 16.35. Preoperative claw-hand deformity.

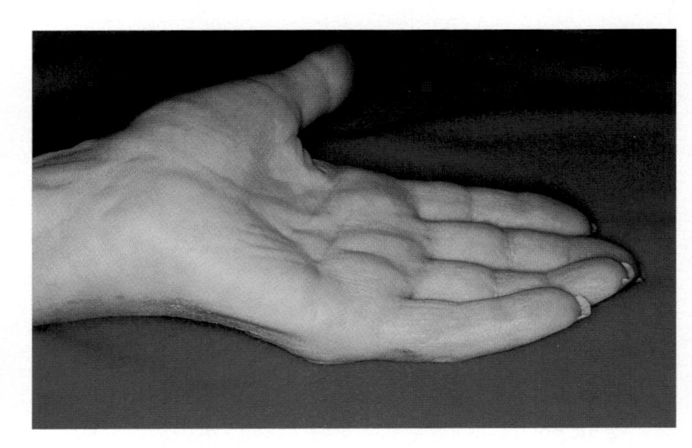

Figure 16.36. Postoperative correction of claw-hand deformity.

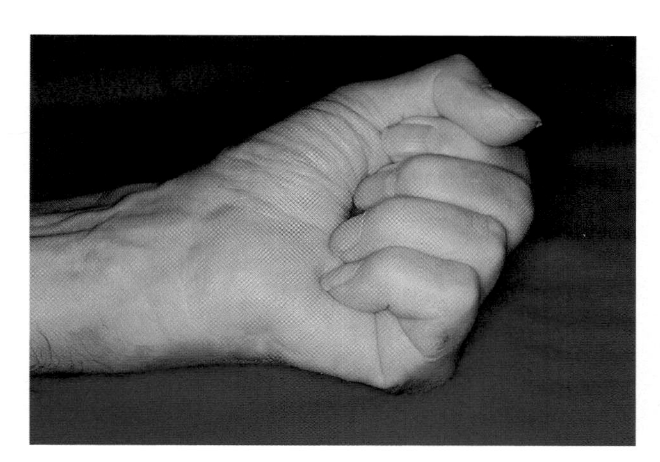

Figure 16.37. Postoperative digital flexion.

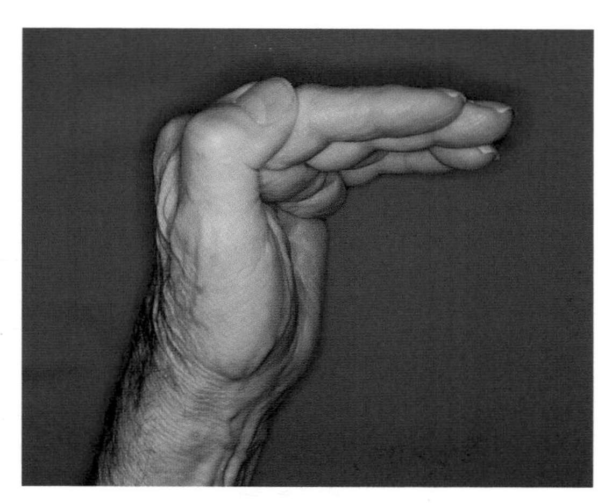

Figure 16.38. Transfer allows for positioning in "safe position" with metacarpophalangeal joint flexion independent of interphalangeal joint flexion.

transfer. Wide fascial excision is required to allow the tendon grafts to pass through muscle planes, which yield and deform to allow tendon gliding. Distal adhesions are present when an MCP joint flexion contracture is present that does not improve by full wrist dorsiflexion. Early adhesions may respond to dynamic extension splinting. Late and rigid adhesions require tenolysis.

Adhesions can occur at the wrist level, where the tendon grafts are woven and sutured into the motor tendon. The risk of adhesions at this level is minimized by atraumatic technique and creation of a smooth tendon juncture. It is essential that the donor wrist tendon be directed superficial to the wrist extensor retinaculum, with the chevron skin incision placed such that the repair site lies under the very base of the flap. Tendon adhesions at this level are diagnosed by restricted wrist palmar flexion and MCP joint extension. It may be impossible to differentiate tightness caused by proximal adhesions or by the combined presence of both proximal and distal restrictions (Figs. 16.40 and 16.41). Early wrist adhesions are corrected most safely by taping the digits in full flexion, followed by passive stretching of the wrist into palmar flexion. Late adhesions require formal tenolysis.

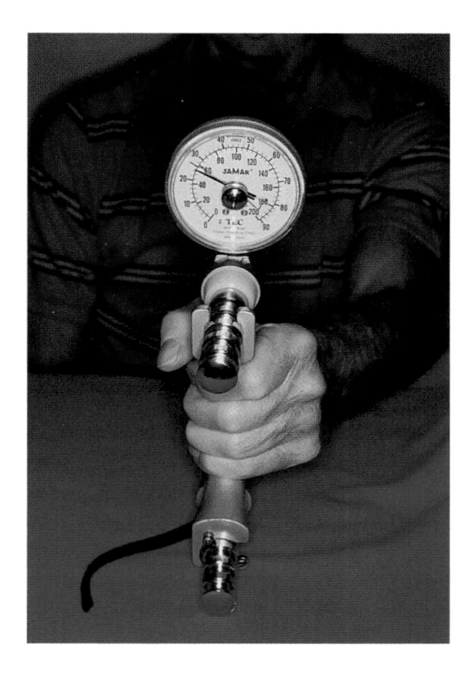

Figure 16.39. Transfer to all four digits provides improved power grasp.

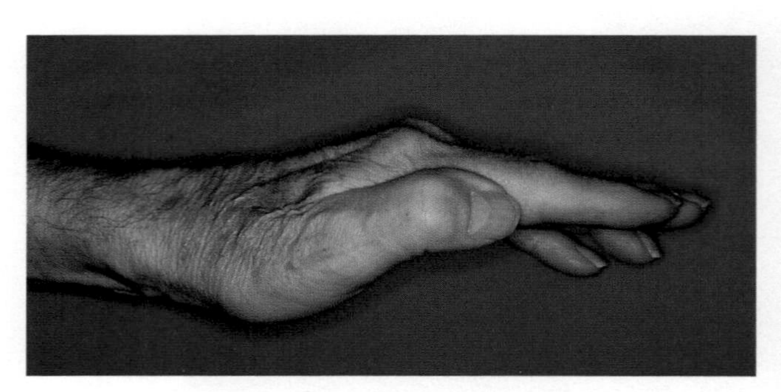

Figure 16.40. Metacarpophalangeal (MCP) joint passive flexion contracture secondary to tendon graft adhesions.

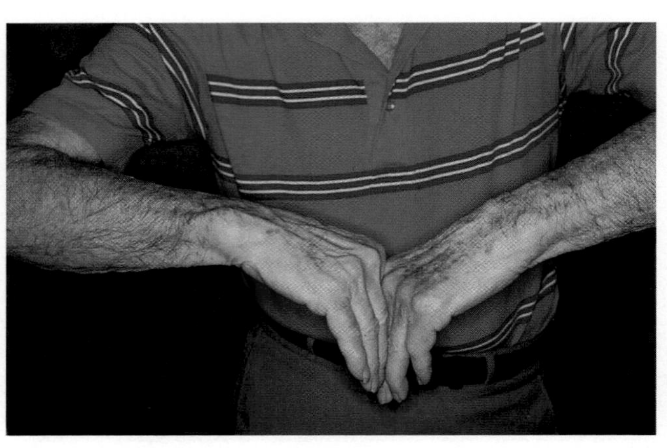

Figure 16.41. Limited wrist palmar flexion secondary to dorsal tendon graft/transfer adhesions at distal forearm/wrist.

Tendon-Transfer Tension Deficiencies

As with all tendon transfers, there is potential for setting the transfer either too tightly or too loosely. Most tendon transfers will adjust by either lengthening or shortening muscle sarcomere length. It is usually better to err by setting the tension too high than too loose. Transfers that have been set too tight may respond to stretching exercises and functional use, but transfers that have been set too loose rarely correct sufficiently. Transfers that are too tight and do not respond to stretching activities will require Z-lengthening of the wrist tendon proximal to the tendon graft junctures.

Inadequate Correction or Overcorrection of a Single Digit

All four tendon grafts connect to a single muscle tendon motor unit proximally. All have slightly different excursion requirements and pass in differing direction to coverage proximally. The more proximal the convergence point, the more forgiving the setting of correct tension will be. Undercorrection or overcorrection of a single digit can occur either from adhesions of the tendon graft to that digit or from incorrect tension set to that digit. Incorrect tension usually results when side-by-side transfer of two digits is accomplished, with the respective tension grafts held in a direction different from the one they will later assume when connected to the motor tendon unit. Incorrect tension also can result when suturing has been accomplished with the wrist held in either radial deviation or ulnar deviation. It is essential in the conjoined suturing of adjacent distal tendon grafts that the wrist be aligned in neutral position, with all grafts converging to the proximal aspect of the second dorsal compartment. Verification intraoperatively that the correct tension has been set is obtained by wrist palmar flexion and assurance that all MCP joints by tenodesis flex fully and with equal force. Also, all digits should be extended passively with the wrist in dorsiflexion to ensure that equal extension is possible with equal passive resistance.

When tension has been incorrectly set, only surgery will correct the problem. The involved tendon graft is taken down at its point of suture to the motor tendon. It is either tightened or relaxed and sutured with appropriate tension to the adjacent extensor graft.

Extensor Tightness

When the tension of tendon transfer has been excessive, tightness may preclude a full-wrist palmar flexion. Passive stretching exercises, as in the case of wrist extensor adhesions, may eradicate the problem.

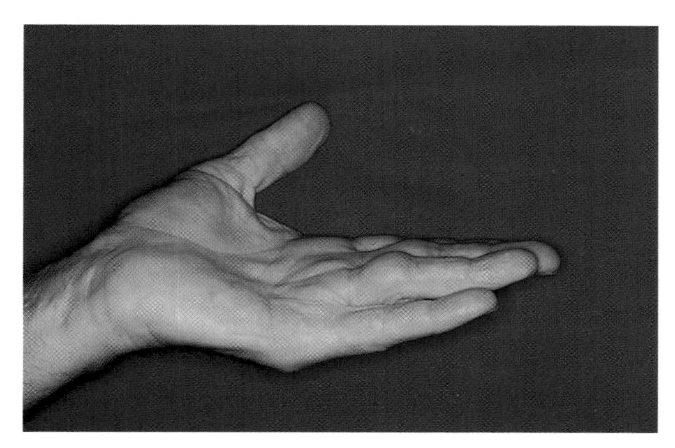

Figure 16.42. Swan-neck deformity of ring finger secondary to excessive tension of tendon graft to ring finger.

Unresponsive to Stretching Exercise

Z-lengthening of the donor tendon proximal to the graft juncture is required.

Swan-Neck Deformity

Excessive tension of one or more digital grafts will result in a MCP joint flexion contracture (Fig. 16.42). In this position, the EDC power is maximized and, over time, may lead to mild hyperextension deformity at the PIP joint. This problem is best corrected by adjusting the tension of the overly tight tendon graft. A second alternative correction is to perform a volar PIP tenodesis.

RECOMMENDED READING

1. Brand PW. Biomechanics of tendon transfer. *Ortho Clin North Am* 5:205–230, 1974.
2. Brand PW. Tendon transfers for median and ulnar nerve paralysis. *Orthop Clin North Am* 1:447–454, 1970.
3. Brand PW, Beach RB, Thompson DE, et al. Relative tension and potential excursion of muscles in the forearm and hand. *J Hand Surg* 6:209–219, 1981.
4. Bruser P. Motor replacement operations in chronic ulnar nerve paralysis. *Orthopade* 26(8):690–695, 1997.
5. Bunnell S. Surgery of the intrinsic muscles of the hand other than those producing opposition of the thumb. *J Bone Joint Surg* 24A:1–31, 1942.
6. Gault DT, Quaba AA. The role of cross-finger flaps in the primary management of untidy flexor tendon injuries. *J Hand Surg* 1313:62–65, 1988.
7. Hastings H, Davidson S. Tendon transfers for ulnar nerve palsy—evaluation of results and practical treatment consideration. *Hand Clin* 4:167–178, 1988.
8. Hastings H, McCollam SM. The flexor digitorum superficialis lasso tendon transfers—a functional evaluation. *J Hand Surg* 19A:275–280, 1994.
9. Micks JE, Reswick JB, Hager DL. The mechanism of the intrinsic-minus finger: a biomechanical study. *J Hand Surg* 3:333–341, 1978.
10. Riordan DC. Intrinsic paralysis of the hand. *Bull Hosp Jt Dis* 44:435–441, 1984.
11. Riordan DC. Surgery of the paralytic hand. *Instr Course Lect* 16:79–90, 1959.
12. Riordan DC. Tendon transfers for nerve paralysis of the hand and wrist. *Curr Pract Orthop Surg* 2:17–40, 1964.
13. Riordan DC. Tendon transplantations in median nerve and ulnar nerve paralysis. *J Bone Joint Surg* 35A:312–320, 1953.
14. Smith RJ, Hastings H. Principles of tendon transfers to the hand. *Instr Course Lect* 29:129–152, 1980.
15. Zancolli E. Correccion de la "garra" digital por paralisis intrinseca; la operacion del "lazo." *Acto Ortopedica Latinoamericana* 1:65–72, 1974.

17

Repeat Decompression of the Median Nerve at the Wrist with Hypothenar Fat Pad Coverage

Kevin Plancher

INTRODUCTION

Idiopathic carpal tunnel syndrome has become one of the most commonly diagnosed and surgically treated peripheral neuropathies in the upper extremity. The incidence of failure or complication after open carpal tunnel decompression varies, but it has been reported to be as high as 10% to 25%. The most commonly cited causes for recalcitrant carpal tunnel syndrome or failure of open decompression include incomplete release of the transverse carpal ligament or volar antebrachial fascia, recurrent tenosynovitis, reformation of the flexor retinaculum (late recurrence), postoperative adhesions, and intraneural fascicular scarring.

Persistent numbness and proximal pain as well as palmar hypersensitivity have been reported infrequently but can be disabling sequelae of open carpal tunnel decompression. Some authors have stated that the most common pathologic finding at re-exploration of the median nerve was tenosynovitis or a fibrous proliferation surrounding and compressing the median nerve; we believe otherwise. Although that may occur, we believe that recurrence often is the result of a median nerve that becomes fixed at the volar and radial side of the carpal canal or to the thin skin at the level of the volar wrist crease. It is this adherence of the nerve to the surrounding tissues that results in traction neuritis and dysesthesias that accompany wrist motion.

Nonoperative treatment for recalcitrant carpal tunnel syndrome (splinting, injection, therapy modalities, and nonsteroidal anti-inflammatory drugs) may provide relief of symptoms but usually fails to give all patients a long-term benefit because of the inability to

Kevin Plancher, M.D., M.S., F.A.C.S., F.A.A.O.S.: Orthopaedics, Beth Israel Medical Center, New York, NY, and Orthopaedics, Albert Einstein College of Medicine, Bronx, NY.

reverse the cause of the nerve compromise. Although there is controversy in the literature, the results of repeat decompression and neurolysis are often disappointing. Unfortunately, some patients undergo multiple explorations and repeat neurolyses only to have the symptoms return as the nerve adheres again to the skin and adjacent structures, resulting in a traction or adhesive neuritis.

Of course, it is critical to fully evaluate and rule out any concurrent pathologies that may contribute to the symptom complex consistent with compression or traction neuropathy. These would include pronator syndrome, cervical radiculopathy, vascular pathology, or even tumor. Thorough physical examination and electrical interrogation may assist in making these differentiations.

In an attempt to address this complex problem, several surgical procedures have been described, all of which attempt to minimize or prevent intraneural fascicular scarring and adherence of the median nerve to the surrounding tissues. All of these procedures provide coverage of the liberated median nerve and attempt to provide an improved tissue environment that hopefully will discourage additional scarring and adherence of the nerve to the surrounding structures. Many of these procedures are technically demanding, use muscles of insufficient size or excursion, are fraught with complications, and may require the sacrifice of normal functioning tissue.

The hypothenar fat pad flap mobilizes local adipose tissue as a pedicled flap from the hypothenar eminence. The flap is interposed between the freed median nerve and the radial wall of the carpal canal, after the radial leaf of the transverse carpal ligament has been isolated and excised. The fat pad prevents readherence and returns favorable mechanics and biology for the median nerve. This procedure has been used for more than 15 years and was modified in 1987 from its original description by Cramer.

INDICATIONS

The hypothenar fat pad flap has been successfully used by experienced surgeons who understand the anatomy and indications. Each of our patients must have two or more of the following criteria to be a candidate for this surgery.

1. Persistent or recurrent median nerve symptoms at the wrist or fingers after adequate open surgical decompression.
2. Significant palmar hypersensitivity or proximal pain migration without permanent damage to the palmar cutaneous branch of the median nerve.
3. A progressive neurologic deficit, including thenar muscle atrophy or expanded two-point sensory discrimination as determined by the Weber two-point discrimination test using a dull pointed eye caliper applied in the longitudinal axis of the digit without blanching the skin.
4. Failure of conservative treatment, including splinting, injection, and the passage of time.
5. No concomitant major wrist surgery, either soft tissue or bony in nature.

ALTERNATIVES TO THE HYPOTHENAR FAT PAD FLAP

Open carpal tunnel release is one of the most frequently performed procedures in hand surgery. It often is the procedure of choice for those who have not responded to conservative management for compression of the median nerve at the wrist. Satisfactory relief of paresthesias, dysesthesias, and hypesthesias, as well as patient satisfaction because of lasting alleviation of symptoms, often result. In fact, alleviation of symptoms from idiopathic carpal tunnel syndrome has been achieved in more than 80% of patients.

It is disappointing for both patient and surgeon that approximately 20% of patients do not have their symptoms relieved by carpal tunnel release. These patients with recurring or persistent symptoms require additional diagnostic and therapeutic consideration. At surgery, the finding of perineural and intraneural scarring with adherence of the median

Table 17.1. *Surgical Procedures Used for Median Nerve Coverage in Recalcitrant Carpal Tunnel Syndrome*

Flap procedure	Author
1 Abductor digiti minimi muscle flap	(Milward, 1977)
2 Lumbrical flap	(Wilgis, 1984)
3 Pronator quadratus muscle flap	(Dellon, 1984)
4 Free flap of gliding tissue	(Wintsch, 1986)
5 Ulnar pedicle synovial flap	(Wulle, 1987)
6 Palmaris brevis turnover flap	(Rose, 1991)
7 Hypothenar fat pad flap	(Cramer 1985, Strickland 1996)

nerve to the radial leaf of the transverse carpal ligament is predictable. Nonoperative treatment and re-exploration with neurolysis frequently fail to provide long-term benefits because the median nerve again becomes trapped in scar that adheres to the transverse carpal ligament. The hypothenar fat pad flap is an alternative operative procedure designed to decrease the morbidity associated with a failed decompression of the median nerve.

Several surgical procedures (Table 17.1) have been described and used to relieve the symptoms of recalcitrant carpal tunnel syndrome. These techniques try to provide a healthy, vascularized pedicle of tissue with size sufficient to allow complete coverage of the median nerve and to prevent readherence to the transverse carpal ligament.

The palmaris brevis flap, as described by Rose, although stated to be absent in only 2% of patients, has proved to be absent or of insufficient size in a much higher percentage of hands. Dellon has detailed the use of the pronator quadratus muscle flap to bring a vascularized muscle distal for coverage of the median nerve. This flap, based on its proximal pedicle, is difficult to mobilize and transfer on a vascular pedicle of length sufficient to provide coverage of the entire median nerve in the proximal palm.

Wulle described the use of an ulnar pedicle synovial flap in conjunction with neurolysis of the median nerve. This flap, like the recommendations of Wintsch, creates a gliding bed for the released median nerve but may not provide adequate padding; to date, its long-term status is unknown. The free flap of gliding tissue of Wintsch requires a large and technically demanding dissection from a tissue that is not available locally.

Hagen has recommended a widening Z-plasty to reconstruct the flexor retinaculum to avoid palmar subluxation of the median nerve. Hagen and coauthors admit that this finding is present only 60% of the time and, therefore, may not be practical in all patients with recalcitrant carpal tunnel. Wilgis promoted the lumbrical flap as a reliable technique for coverage of the median nerve in the carpal tunnel. The lumbrical flap relies on a small muscle that must be mobilized on its pedicle and, in our experience, cannot always provide sufficient proximal coverage of the nerve. Finally, Milward et al. and, later, Reisman and Ruby as well as Buck-Gramcko, all have used the abductor digiti minimi muscle flap for improved coverage of the neurolyzed median nerve. This flap does provide a thick, well-vascularized muscle for coverage but requires an extensive dissection and sacrifices an important hypothenar muscle. The technique requires a long arc of rotation, and the patient postoperatively may have a partial limitation of small finger abduction.

In contrast to the aforementioned procedures, the hypothenar fat pad flap is locally available and expendable. Its mobilization is technically simple and safe and yields few, if any, postoperative complications. This flap provides a healthy tissue environment to prevent readherence of the median nerve to the transverse carpal ligament. The hypothenar eminence is a rich reservoir of well-vascularized adipose tissue that can easily be raised as a flap on its ulnar pedicle and, because of its sufficient size, can be advanced to cover the median nerve completely.

Although the hypothenar fat pad flap is not difficult technically, there are several points that should be emphasized.

PREOPERATIVE PLANNING

There is no special preoperative planning, other than verification that the patient's symptom complex is consistent with median nerve embarrassment at the level of the carpal canal and that the tissues overlying the hypothenar eminence are robust. An Allen's test to verify a patent ulnar artery is suggested. There is probably little indication for formalized study of the vascular tree. Although it has not been typically needed, the surgeon should counsel the patient about the potential need for skin graft.

PERTINENT ANATOMY OF THE HYPOTHENAR FAT PAD FLAP

The hypothenar muscles are consistently covered with a generous layer of adipose tissue of sufficient width and thickness to provide coverage of the carpal tunnel contents. The hypothenar fat pad is supplied by arterial branches arising directly from the ulnar side of the ulnar artery in Guyon's canal and, more distally, from branches of the ulnar artery to the small finger and fourth web space (Fig. 17.1). There are additional arterial branches to the fat pad arising from the arterial branches to the hypothenar muscles and palmaris brevis muscle. The skin overlaying the hypothenar fat pad is supplied by an additional plexus of arteries running through the superficial adipose tissue.

Another critical anatomic relationship that must be appreciated in dissection of the fat pad is the proximity of the ulnar digital nerve of the small finger, which runs deep to the distal third of the fat pad after branching from the ulnar nerve in Guyon's canal.

SURGERY

The procedure is carried out under regional or general anesthesia. Standard positioning and sterile draping are employed. Respect for previous scars is exercised. Through a linear incision with proximal and distal oblique extensions, as necessary, a fat flap is raised by sharp subcutaneous dissection from the distal wrist crease to midpalm (Figs. 17.2, A and B,

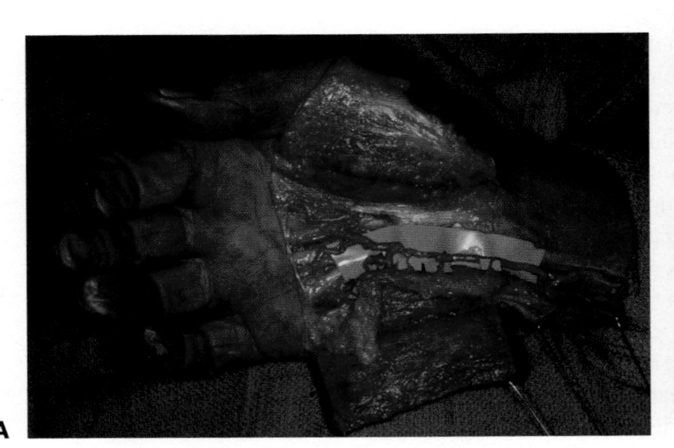

A

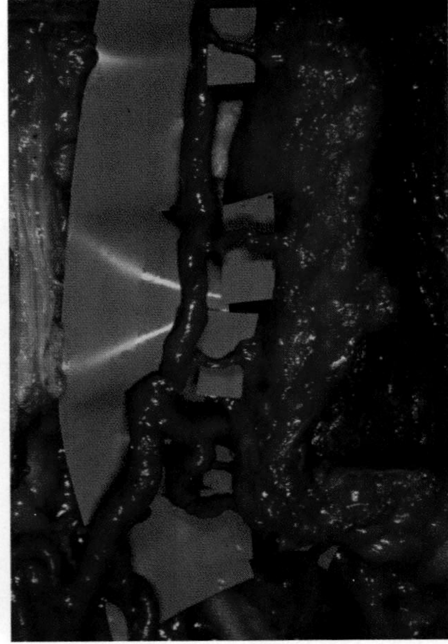

B

Figure 17.1. Latex arterial injection confirming multiple transverse branches arising from the ulna artery in Guyon's canal to provide a rich plexus to the hypothenar fat pad flap (HTFPF).

A

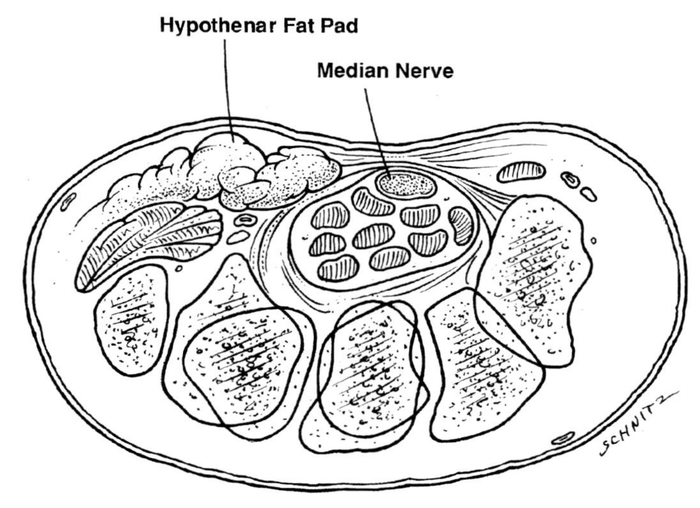

B

Figure 17.2. A: Linear incision between the thenar and hypothenar creases on the radial side of the ring finger with a gentle curved incision through the antebrachial fascia. **B:** Relationship of the hypothenar fat pad and median is seen in this axial illustration. (Courtesy of Gary Schnitz, Indiana Hand Center.)

and 17.3, A and B). Care is taken not to injure the digital nerves to the ring and small fingers while the undermining continues ulnarward to a level in line with the fifth ray. Deep mobilization of the flap is accomplished by first elevating the fat from the ulnar leaf of the transverse carpal ligament, then excising a segment of the ulnar leaf until the ulnar nerve and vessel are visualized in the canal of Guyon (Fig. 17.4, A and B). The flap mobility is tested to determine whether it can be advanced easily over the median nerve to the radial wall of the carpal canal (Fig. 17.5).

If it has not been mobilized sufficiently, additional dissection is carried out, with care taken to preserve the ulnar pedicle of the flap and to not damage the ulnar nerve or artery. This often requires sharp division of fibrous attachments of the adipose tissue to the skin. When adequately prepared, the fat pad flap is draped over the median nerve and secured to the radial wall of the carpal canal.

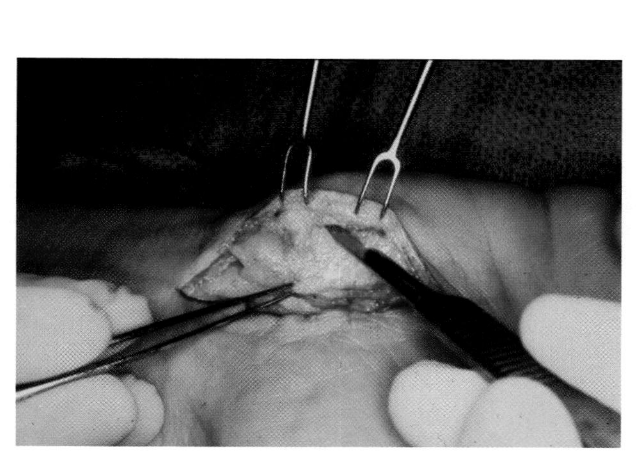

A

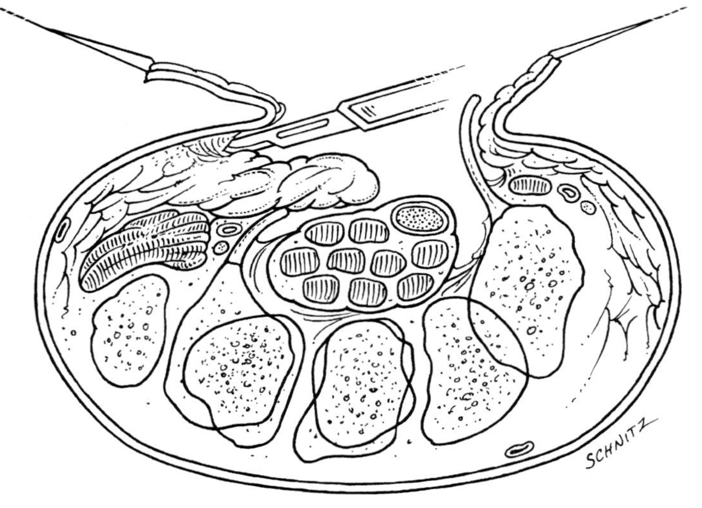

B

Figure 17.3. A: The hypothenar fat is raised in a subcutaneous dissection in an ulnar direction. The median nerve is pictured at the bottom of the incision. Guyon's canal contents are just deep to the developed fat pad. **B:** Subcutaneous dissection of the fat pad with an axial illustration of the anatomy described above. (Courtesy of Gary Schnitz, Indiana Hand Center.)

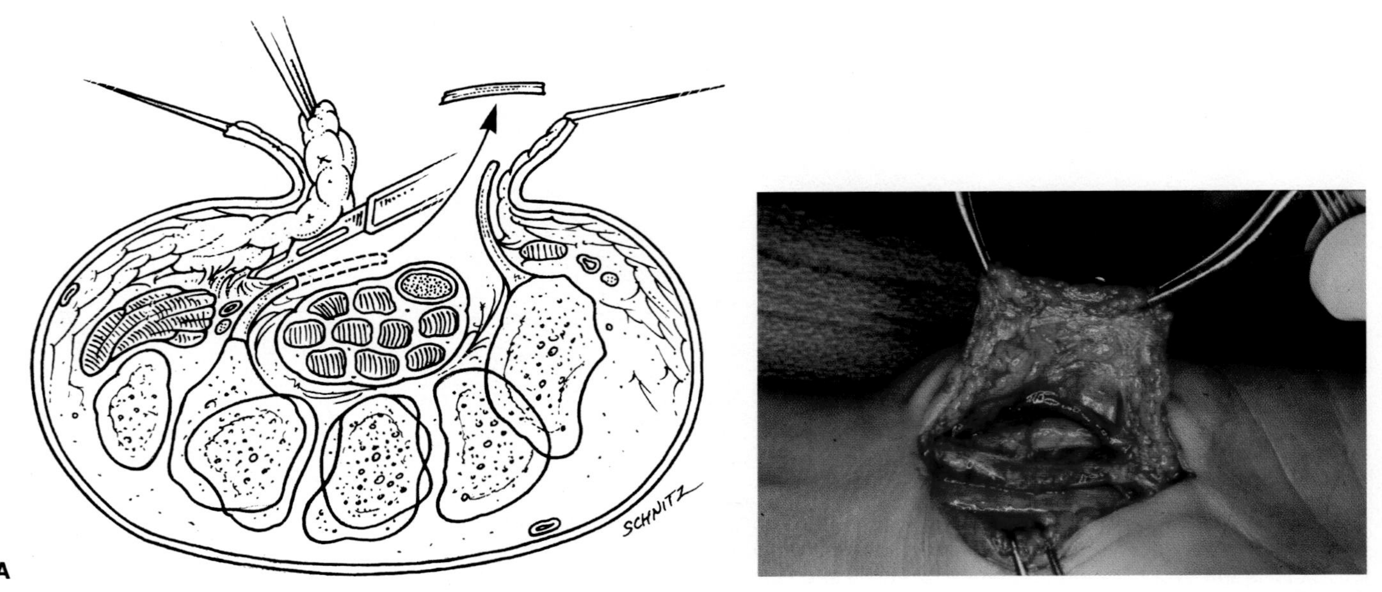

Figure 17.4. **A:** Deep mobilization of the fat pad flap is accomplished by excising a segment of the ulnar leaf of the transverse carpal ligament in an axial illustration of the anatomy described. (Courtesy of Gary Schnitz, Indiana Hand Center.) **B:** Elevating the fat pad flap by blunt and sharp dissection until the ulnar nerve and vessel are visualized in the canal of Guyon.

The contents of the canal are retracted ulnarward while three nonabsorbable horizontal mattress sutures are passed through the edge of the fat pad (Fig 17.6A). These sutures are then passed through the radial wall of the carpal tunnel adjacent to the flexor pollicis longus tendon and, finally, back through the fat pad. Sutures are tagged temporarily with a hemostat to facilitate the placement of all stitches before tying them in sequence (Fig. 17.6B).

When the sutures are tied, the radial and ulnar borders of the hand are compressed gently to ease the delivery of the flap down onto the radial side of the tunnel (Fig. 17.7, A and B). After the hypothenar fat pad is secured, routine skin closure is completed (Fig. 17.8, A and B) and the wrist and hand are immobilized.

Postoperatively, the hand is immobilized with gentle radial ulnar compression for 2 weeks with the wrist in neutral or slight dorsiflexion and the thumb abducted to relieve tension on the repair. Digital motion is encouraged during the course (4 weeks) or immobi-

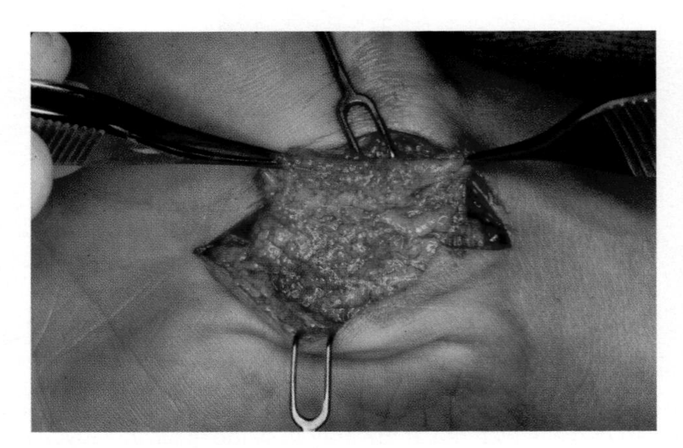

Figure 17.5. The flap is tested to determine whether it can be advanced easily over the median nerve to the radial wall of the carpal canal. Avoid stretching the flap because this will put undue stress on its vascularization and jeopardize graft survival.

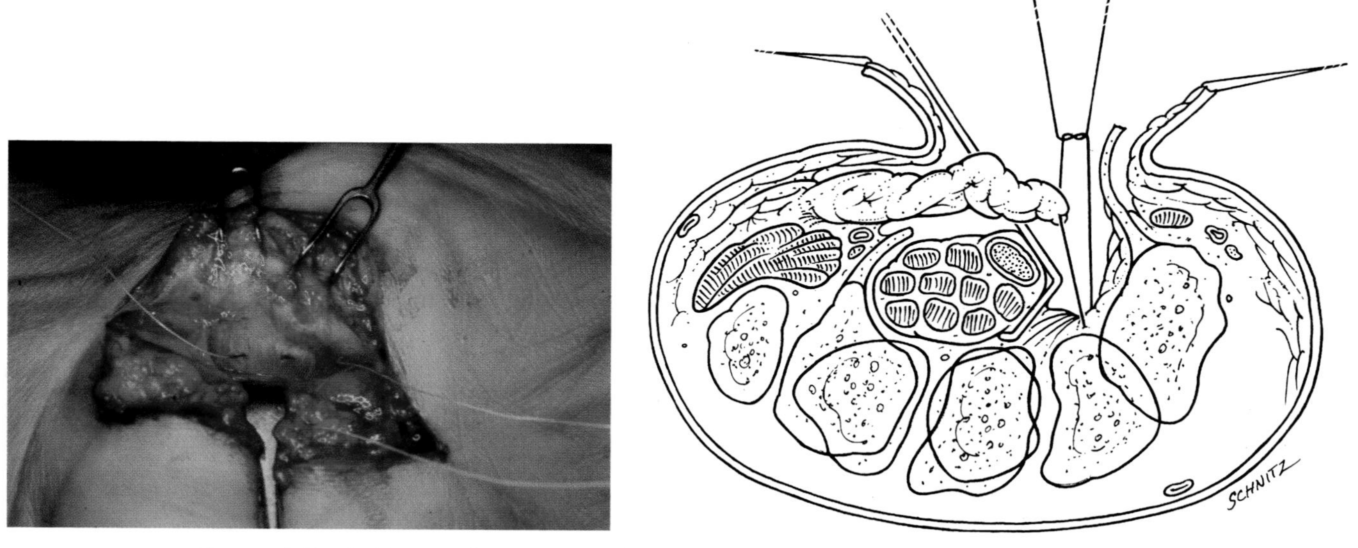

Figure 17.6. A: Retract the contents of the carpal canal ulnarward and place three horizontal mattress nonabsorbable sutures passed through the edge of the fat pad. These sutures are passed through the radial wall of the carpal tunnel adjacent to the flexor pollicis longus tendon and then back through the fat pad. Sutures are tagged temporarily with a hemostat to facilitate the placement of all stitches before tying them in sequence. **B:** An axial illustration identifies the location and placement of the sutures into the carpal tunnel canal. (Courtesy of Gary Schnitz, Indiana Hand Center.)

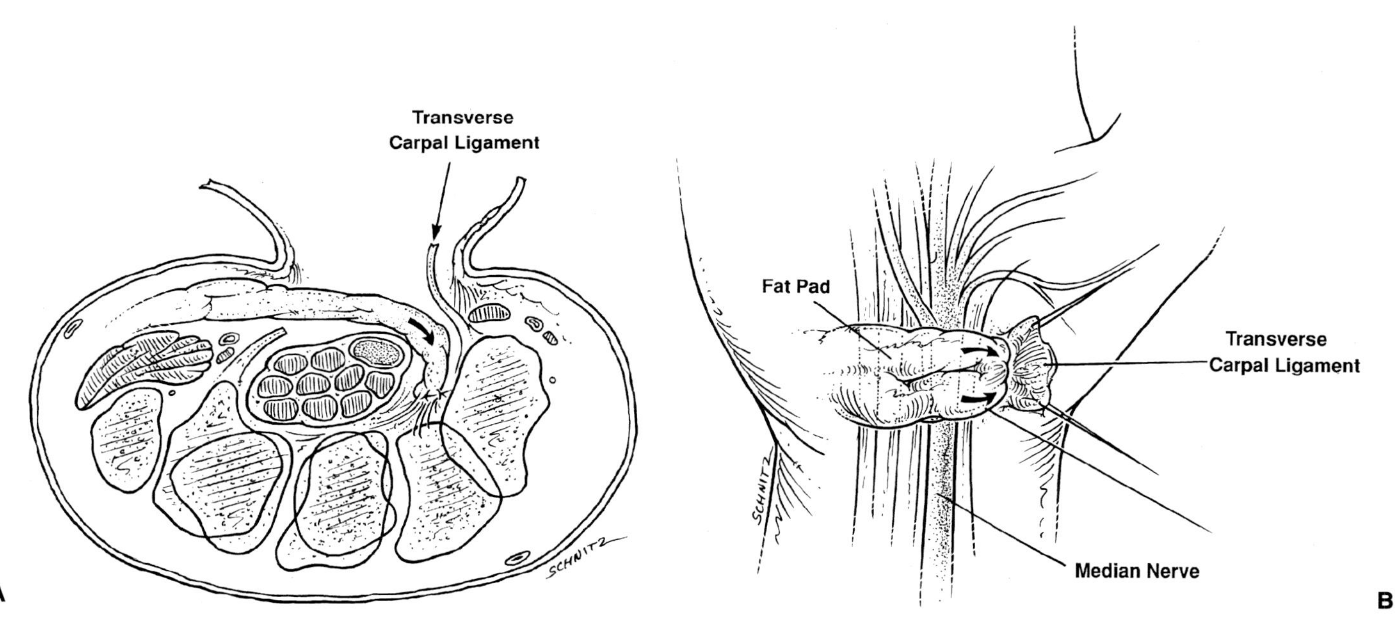

Figure 17.7. A: The fat pad is placed palmar to the median nerve and dorsal to the radial leaf of the transverse carpal ligament. When the sutures are tied, the radial and ulnar borders of the hand are compressed gently to ease the delivery of the flap down onto the radial side of the tunnel. (Courtesy of Gary Schnitz, Indiana Hand Center.) **B:** A sagittal illustration showing the fat pad flap covering the median nerve and acting as a cushion. (Courtesy of Gary Schnitz, Indiana Hand Center.)

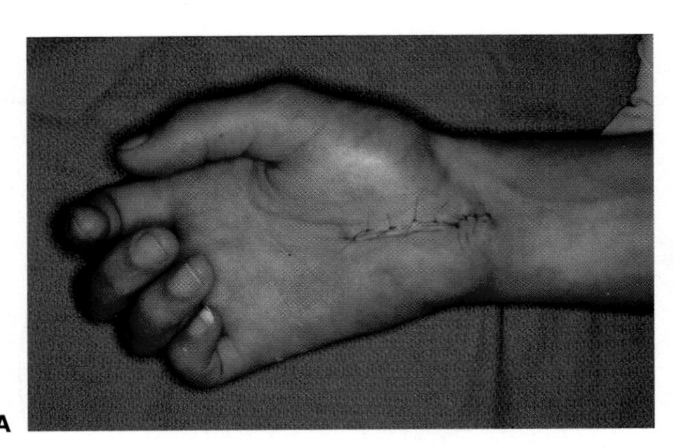

A

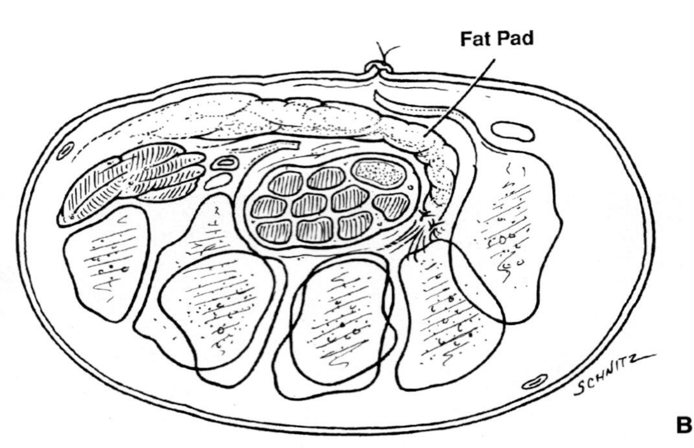

B

Figure 17.8. A: Routine skin closure is done and preparation to immobilize the wrist and hand for postoperative care is completed. **B:** Axial illustration showing the fat pad flap placed between the remnants of the radial aspect of the carpal ligament and a cushion for appropriate sliding and protection between the median nerve and the skin. (Courtesy of Gary Schnitz, Indiana Hand Center.)

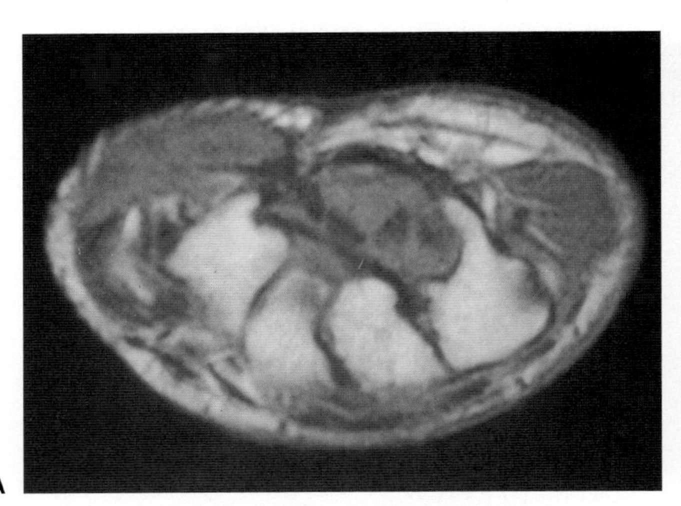

A

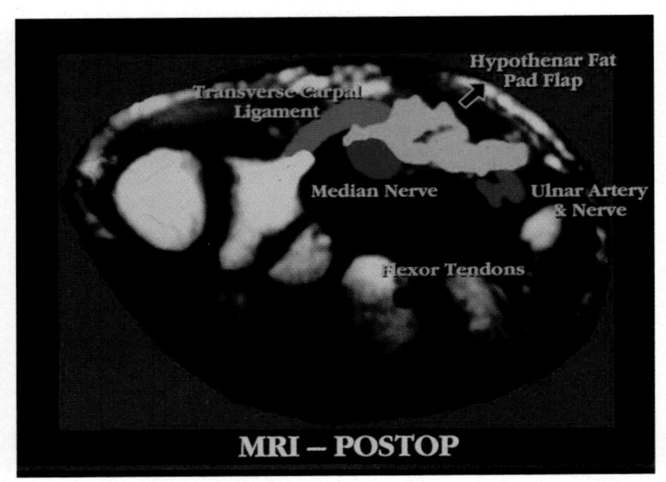

B

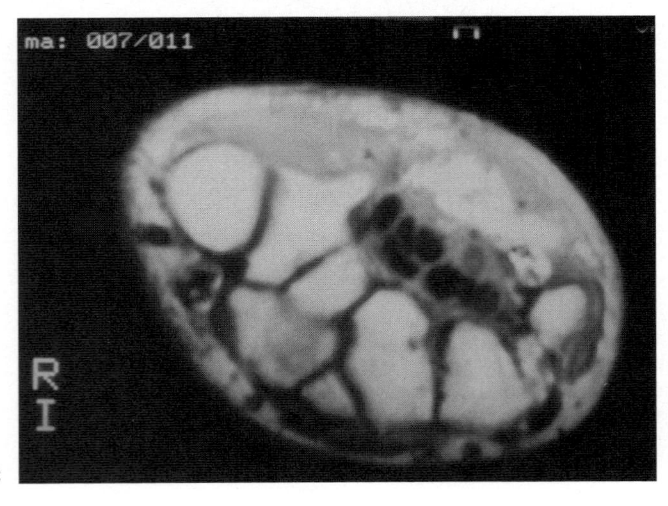

C

Figure 17.9. A: T1-weighted MRI studies performed preoperatively, showing the superficial position of the median nerve, the transverse carpal ligament, and the rich reservoir of hypothenar fat. **B:** The same patient postoperatively, showing the median nerve well within the carpal canal and protected by the hypothenar fat pad flap. **C:** MRI study 2 years postoperatively, showing the persistence and viability of the hypothenar fat pad flap.

lization of the wrist. A protected range of motion with intermittent wrist splinting is continued for an additional 2 weeks, at which time full, unrestricted motion is permitted. Heavy lifting is not allowed until 6 weeks, and supplemental rehabilitation for strengthening, promotion of scar suppleness, and desensitization are instituted as necessary.

T1-weighted magnetic resonance imaging (MRI) studies were performed on our patients, with the use of this flap, early in our experience. The MRI scan shown confirms the position of the fat pad above the median nerve and below the radial leaf of the transverse carpal ligament at 3 days and more than 2 years (Fig. 17.9, A–C). These findings help verify that the fat pad remains vascularized after it is transferred.

SUMMARY OF PERTINENT TECHNICAL POINTS

1. Dissection of the fat pad flap dorsal requires knowledge that the ulnar digital nerve of the small finger runs deep to the distal one-third of the fat pad after branching from the ulnar nerve in Guyon's canal.
2. Palmar undermining should be kept in the subcutaneous plane to avoid thinning of the fat pad flap, which could lead to skin necrosis.
3. A portion, if not the entirety, of the ulnar leaf of the previously divided transverse carpal ligament must be resected to allow for mobilization of the fat pad.
4. Deep mobilization requires visualization of the ulnar nerve and artery in Guyon's canal. Care must be taken to avoid direct injury, but the artery must accommodate the radial mobilization of the fat pad it supplies.
5. The flap should be raised until its radial margin easily reaches the floor of the radial wall of the carpal canal.
6. The hand needs to be immobilized with a gentle amount of radial ulnar compression for 2 weeks postoperatively. A slight amount of palmar corrugation is suggested to minimize tension on the transposed pedicled flap, but it must be minimized to avoid excessive scarring or postoperative stiffness.

COMPLICATIONS

The safety of a technique is always a major concern for a surgeon when selecting a procedure to add to his or her armamentarium. Although dissection of a nerve in a previously operated bed can be technically challenging, hypothenar fat pad coverage can feasibly be performed by those who are familiar with nerve anatomy and surgery. Since this procedure does not require microsurgical techniques, it is an appealing alternative for complex cases.

Because extensive dissection must be carried out in the vicinity of a compromised, multiply operated nerve, inadvertent nerve injury is a potential complication. Even if iatrogenic injury of the nerve is avoided, the possibility of nerve embarrassment from traction and ischemia is still possible.

Skin complications such as focal necrosis or dehiscence may result from the dissection that must be performed to mobilize the fat flap. Another complication is a superficial cellulitis that usually resolves with wound treatment and oral antibiotics.

SUMMARY

Open decompression of the median nerve generally is effective in relieving the symptoms of compressive neuropathy of the median nerve. For cases in which conventional surgical treatment has failed, and the reason appears to be adhesive neuritis, the hypothenar fat pad flap has been shown to be a reliable local source of well-vascularized adipose tissue that can be used for coverage of the median nerve. The hypothenar fat pad flap is a procedure that allows well-vascularized adipose tissue to be mobilized over a released median nerve, effectively preventing readherence in a majority of cases.

This flap improves the tissue environment for the median nerve, promoting normal excursion during wrist motions. Lanz and others feel that this procedure restores a sliding pathway and cushion for the median nerve. Our results to date have been better than previously described for other techniques. Recent reviews recounted that since 1996, when Strickland et al. described their results, others have used the technique and reported great patient satisfaction and excellent clinical results. The hypothenar fat pad flap should be considered in the hand surgeon's armamentarium for recalcitrant median nerve symptoms due to adhesive neuritis.

RECOMMENDED READING

1. Bloem JJ, Pradjarahardja KMC, Vuursteen PJ. The post-carpal tunnel syndrome: causes and prevention. *Neth J Surg* 38:52–55, 1996.
2. Connolly WB. Pitfalls and carpal tunnel decompression. *Aust N Z J Surg* 48:421–425, 1978.
3. Cramer LM. Local Fat Coverage for the Median Nerve. In: Lankford LL, ed. *Correspondence Newsletter for Hand Surgery.* Chicago, Ill.: ASSH, 1985:35.
4. Cseuz KA, Thomas JE, Lambert EH, et al. Long-term results of operation for carpal tunnel syndrome. *Mayo Clin Proc* 41:232–241, 1966.
5. Dellon AL, Mackinnon SE. The pronator quadratus muscle flap. *J Hand Surg* 9A:423–427, 1984.
6. De Smet L, Vandeputte G. Pedicled fat flap coverage of the median nerve after failed carpal tunnel decompression. *J Hand Surg* 27B:350–353, 2002.
7. De Smet L. Recurrent carpal tunnel syndrome: clinical testing indicating incomplete section of the flexor retinaculum. *J Hand Surg* 18B:189–193, 1993.
8. Engber WD, Gmeiner JG. Palmar cutaneous branch of the ulnar nerve. *J Hand Surg* 5A:26–29, 1980.
9. Guinta R, Frank U, Lanz U. The hypothenar fat-pad flap for reconstructive repair after scarring of the median nerve at the wrist joint. *Chir Main* 17(2):107–112, 1998.
10. Hagen VK, Senwald G. Das Karpaltunnelsyndromrezidiv: Problematik und behandlug. *Hanchir Mikrochir Plast Chir* 22:309–311, 1990.
11. Hunter JM. Recurrent carpal tunnel syndrome, epineural fibrous fixation and traction neuropathy. *Hand Clinics* 7:491–504, 1991.
12. Kulich MI, Gordillo G, Javidi T, et al. Long-term analysis of patients having surgical treatment for carpal tunnel syndrome. *J Hand Surg* 11A:59–66, 1966.
13. Langloh ND, Linscheid RL. Recurrent and unrelieved carpal-tunnel syndrome. *Clin Orthop* 83:41–47, 1972.
14. Learmonth GR. The principles of decompression in the treatment of certain diseases of peripheral nerves. *Surg Clin North Am* 13:905–913, 1933.
15. LeDouble AF. *Traite des Variations du Systeme Musculaire de l'Homme et Leur Signification au Point de vue de l'Arthopologie Zoologigue.* Paris: Schleicher Freres, 1987:170–171.
16. Leslie BM, Ruby LK. Coverage of a carpal tunnel wound dehiscence with the abductor digiti minimi muscle flap. *J Hand Surg* 13A:36–39, 1988.
17. Louis DS, Greene TL, Noellert RC. Complications of carpal tunnel surgery. *J Neurosurg* 62:352–356, 1985.
18. MacDonald RI, Lichtman DM, Hanlon JJ, et al. Complications of surgical release for carpal tunnel syndrome. *J Hand Surg* 3A:70–76, 1978.
19. Mackinnon SE. Secondary carpal tunnel surgery. *Neurosurg Clin North Am* 2:75–97, 1991.
20. Marie F, Foix C. Atrophie isolee de l'eminence thenar d'orgin nevritique: role du ligament annulaire anterieur du carae dans la pathegenie de la lesion. *Rev Neurol* 26:647–649, 1913.
21. Milward TM, Stott WG, Kleinert HE. The abductor digiti minimi muscle flap. *Hand* 9:82–85, 1977.
22. Mathoulin C, Bahm J, Roukoz S. Pedicled hypothenar fat flap for median nerve coverage in recalcitrant carpal tunnel syndrome. *Hand Surg* 5(1):33–40, 2000.
22. Novelino F, Goncalves J. The fasciocutaneous hypothenar flap: preliminary anatomical and clinical study. *Ann Chir Plast Esthet* 47(1):9–11, 2002.
24. Paget J. *Lectures on Surgical Pathology.* Philadelphia: Lindsay and Blakestone, 1854:42.
25. Phalen GS. Spontaneous compression of the median nerve at the wrist. *JAMA* 145:1128–1132, 1951.
26. Phalen GS. Carpal tunnel syndrome: 17 years' experience in diagnosis and treatment of 654 hands. *J Bone Joint Surg* 48A:211–228, 1966.
27. Phalen GS. Reflections on 21 years' experience with the carpal-tunnel syndrome. *JAMA* 212:1365–1367, 1970.
28. Phalen GS. The carpal-tunnel syndrome: clinical evaluation of 598 hands. *Clin Orthop* 83:29–40, 1972.
29. Reisman NR, Dellon AL. The abductor digiti minimi muscle flap: a salvage technique for palmar wrist pain. *Plast Reconstr Surg* 72:859–863, 1983.
30. Rose EH, Norris MS, Kowalski TA, et al. Palmaris brevis turnover flap as an adjunct to internal neurolysis of the chronically scarred median nerve in recurrent carpal tunnel syndrome. *J Hand Surg* 16A:191–201, 1991.
31. Strickland JW, Idler RS, Lourie GM, et al. The hypothenar fat pad flap for management of recalcitrant carpal tunnel syndrome. *J Hand Surg* 21A:840–848, 1996.
32. Ulmer J, Buck-Gramcko D. Der neurovaskular gestielte abductor digiti minimi-muskellappen zur abdeckung des n. medianus oder seiner aste. *Handchirurgi* 20:338–341, 1988.

33. Urbaniak JR. Complications of Treatment of Carpal Tunnel Syndrome. In: Gelberman R, ed. *Operative Nerve Repair and Reconstruction.* Vol 2. Philadelphia: JB Lippincott, 1991:967–979.
34. Werner JL, Omer GE. Evaluating cutaneous pressure sensation of the hand. *Am J Occup Ther* 24:347–356, 1970.
35. Wilgis EFS. Local muscle flaps in the hand anatomy as related to reconstructive surgery. *Bull Hosp Joint Dis* 44:552–557, 1984.
36. Wintsch K, Healy P. Free flap of gliding tissue. *J Reconstr Microsurg* 2:143–151, 1986.
37. Wulle C. Treatment of reoccurrence of the carpal tunnel syndrome. *Ann Chir Main Membr Surper* 6:203–209, 1987.

PART V

Tendon Surgery

18

Flexor-Tendon Injuries

James W. Strickland

INDICATIONS/CONTRAINDICATIONS

Although the results of primary flexor-tendon repairs in the digits have improved considerably, controversy about the best methods of tendon suture and the most effective post-repair protocols remains. Techniques based on anecdotes, hearsay, and personal experience have been gradually replaced with programs incorporating meaningful laboratory and clinical information relating to flexor-tendon anatomy, nutrition, structure, function, excursion, biomechanics, and the biologic response to injury, repair, and stress application. Table 18.1 summarizes a large volume of published information that I have incorporated into the flexor-tendon repair technique and postoperative rehabilitation program described in this chapter.

Restoration of function to a digit following flexor-tendon interruption may be a long and tedious undertaking. Strong rapport must be developed between surgeon, patient, and therapist. When initiating the care of a patient with such an injury, I always spend considerable time with the patient to explain the nature of the injury, the problems associated with restoring function, and the possibility of needing several operations to achieve success.

The concept that flexor-tendon repair should be considered a surgical emergency also has been dispelled by several studies that demonstrated that equal or better results usually can be achieved by delayed primary flexor-tendon suture. It also has been effectively shown that it is better to repair both the flexor digitorum profundus (FDP) and superficialis (FDS) tendons rather than the profundus alone, once thought to be the wiser option. This chapter concentrates on flexor-tendon severance in zones I and II (distal palm and digit), where recovery of function is the most difficult to achieve.

The primary repair of severed flexor tendons may be contraindicated when there are severe multiple tissue injuries to the involved fingers or palm, when the wounds are badly contaminated by potentially infecting materials, or when there has been significant skin loss over the flexor system. Concomitant fractures or neurovascular injuries are not necessarily contraindications to primary or delayed primary suture. If the fracture can be

James W. Strickland, M.D.: Reconstructive Hand Surgery of Indiana, Carmel, IN, and Indiana University School of Medicine, Indianapolis, IN

Table 18.1. *Flexor Tendon Repair: Tips and Pearls*

Tendons heal by a combination of extrinsic and intrinsic cellular activity.
Stressed tendons heal faster, gain tensile strength faster, and have fewer adhesions and better excursions than unstressed tendons.
There may be minimal decrease in repair strength when subjected to early motion stress. A conservative estimate of a 25% decline between the first and third weeks should be safe.
Gapping at the repair site results in a weakening of the repair and may result in adhesions.
Synthetic braided sutures are probably best for tendon repair.
Each larger suture caliber increases the repair strength.
The strength of a tendon repair is roughly proportional to the number of suture strands that cross the repair site, provided there is equal load sharing between the strands.
The number of suture knots in the repair site should be minimized.
Flexor tendon repairs are stronger when the core sutures are placed dorsally.
Repaired tendons usually rupture through the suture or through the knot.
Locking loops contribute modestly to repair strength but may collapse and lead to gapping at moderate loads.
A strong peripheral epitendinous suture (running lock or horizontal mattress) results in an increase in repair strength and a significant reduction in the tendency for gapping at the repair site.
Extrapolations (admittedly imperfect) from a considerable quantity of research have permitted some reasonable suppositions with regard to the strength of various flexor repairs during the healing process and their safety when subjected to passive, light active, and strong active motion stresses (Fig. 18.1). These suppositions indicate that four- and six-strand flexor tendon repairs with a horizontal mattress or running lock peripheral epitendinous suture enjoy relative safety for both passive and light active digital motion during the entire healing process in the unswollen digit.
Repairing the sheath following tendon suture seems to have a theoretical advantage of providing a barrier for adhesion formation, restoring synovial fluid nutrition, and restoring the sheath mechanics.
The ability to bring the wrist synergistically into extension provides the greatest excursion of repaired flexor tendons.
If an active motion protocol is used, the least tensile demand on a zone II during active digital flexion occurs when the wrist is extended.
Ibuprofen or indomethacin improve functional recovery.

anatomically reduced and stabilized with strong fixation, it is almost always better to proceed with flexor-tendon repair and microscopic nerve and vessel suture, recognizing that the ultimate results of these combined tissue injuries are not as good as those following tendon severance with no associated injuries. The ability to rejoin the tendon at its normal length in the acute or subacute setting is usually preferable to delaying the repair for several

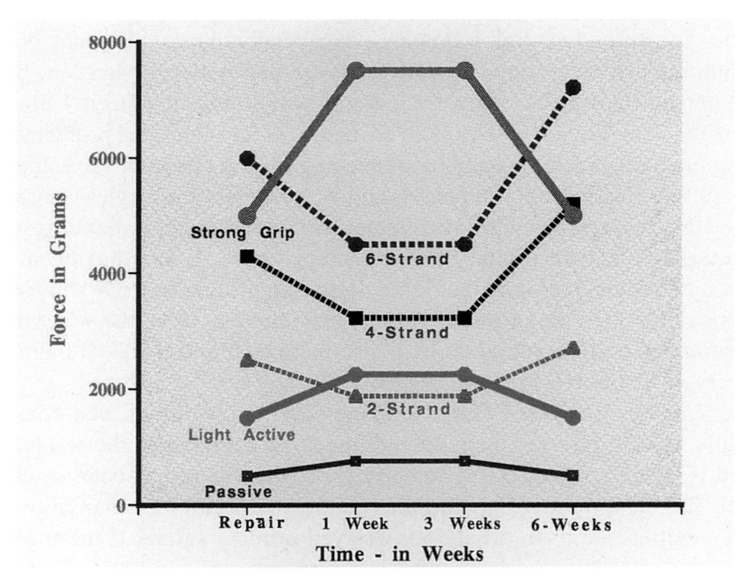

Figure 18.1. Flexor-tendon repair: strength versus force. Two-, four-, and six-strand repairs plotted against passive, light active flexion and strong grip. Adjusted for friction, edema, and stress.

weeks with the inevitable deterioration of the tendon ends and shortening of the extrinsic muscle/tendon system. When infection is a possibility, tendon repair should be delayed for several days until a clean wound can be established.

PREOPERATIVE PLANNING

A thorough examination and radiographic study of the involved hand are extremely important in recognizing all aspects of an injury that has resulted in disruption of the digital finger flexors. The surgeon must examine the injured patient's hand carefully in an effort to determine the total extent of the injury. Alterations in the normal resting flexion posture of the digits will help identify the loss of continuity of one or both flexor tendons, and well-known functional tests will confirm the loss of FDP or FDS function or both. Lacerations on the palmar aspect of the fingers will always injure the profundus before severing the superficialis, and the absence of profundus function alone does not rule out the possibility of a near complete superficialis division.

A careful sensory examination of the distal phalanx allows the examiner to identify injuries to the digital nerves and to plan incisions to facilitate their exposure and repair. A deep laceration with lacerations of both digital nerves almost surely indicates division of the digital arteries as well. Although the digit probably will survive the loss of both vessels, the viability of the skin flaps used for exposure may be in jeopardy, and the inevitable digital ischemia may impair tendon and nerve healing and create severe cold intolerance for the patient. In this era of microvascular competence on the part of almost all hand surgeons, there is no excuse for not repairing one or both digital arteries in these complex injuries.

When planning the surgical exposure, one must appreciate the fact that the severed flexor-tendon ends will retract well away from the laceration site. Particularly when the digit is in flexion at the time of injury, the distal stumps of the severed tendons will come to lie a centimeter or more distal to the level of sheath disruption. Whereas there is no fixed rule for the incisions that should be used to expose the flexor tendons, there is no advantage in trying to carry out these complicated repairs through existing unextended wounds or through small incisions along the length of the digit. Incisions should be selected that will not compromise the viability of skin flaps and that, when healed, will not create contracting or cosmetically unsightly scars. Zigzag or midaxial incisions are often used, and the decision as to which to use will be determined by the position, length, and direction of the original laceration; the need to gain access to other injured structures, and personal experience and preferences.

SURGERY

The author prefers to carry out flexor-tendon repairs on an outpatient basis with the patient under axillary block anesthetic. The blocks are administered by an anesthesiologist, most often with the use of bupivacaine (Marcaine) so that the patient will experience prolonged postoperative anesthesia, permitting a comfortable return home before any postoperative discomfort occurs. The block is carried out in a separate area with additional sedation provided, depending on the patient's desires.

The patient is brought into the regular operating room, where preparation and draping are carried out as described in Chapter 12 on Subcutaneous Palmar Fasciectomy. As the procedure begins, the author would emphasize the time-honored advice of Sterling Bunnell that tendon repair be carried out using meticulous, atraumatic technique in an effort to lessen adhesion formation. Reckless flexor-tendon surgery can result in a greater functional impairment than would have occurred if no repair had been attempted at all. Inadvertent nerve or vessel interruption, the propagation of abundant digital scar, and the development of postoperative joint contractures all may result from ill-advised efforts at tendon repair by the untrained surgeon. The use of two to four X-loupe magnifications is a great technical aid in performing flexor-tendon and sheath repair, and small delicate instrumentation is a prerequisite for this type of surgery. Pinching, crushing, or excessive touching of the tendon sheath or flexor tendons must be avoided, and it is usually not advisable to debride or shorten tendon ends.

It is always necessary to extend the wound of injury in both proximal and distal directions to provide wide visibility of the area of injury. Whenever possible, I prefer midaxial wound extensions in an effort to return well-nourished subcutaneous tissue over the repair site and to minimize the proximity of skin scarring to the underlying tendon repairs. An adequate view of the surgical field must be created to avoid the need to carry out delicate tendon repairs within the constraints of a small surgical wound. Although T extensions of transverse lacerations generally should be avoided, I may use them on occasion to gain access to digital nerves or vessels. In zone I (distal to the superficialis insertion over the middle phalanx), when only the FDP has been severed, there is usually little difficulty finding the proximal tendon end, which is at least temporarily retained in the finger by its vinculum and usually can be located in the distal portion of the proximal phalanx or at the level of the proximal interphalangeal (PIP) joint. Careful dissection will expose the entire distal half of the flexor-tendon sheath, and the entire A4 annular pulley should be preserved. If the distal interphalangeal (DIP) joint was flexed at the time of injury, the tendon probably will have a short distal stump over the base of the distal phalanx and can be exposed by opening the C3-A5 pulley complex. It will also be necessary to open the C2 or C1 cruciate-synovial segments proximal to the A4 pulley to retrieve the proximal stump of the divided profundus tendon.

After the proximal profundus is delivered into the appropriate cruciate-synovial interval, a core suture is placed in the tendon allowing it to be passed distally under the A4 annular pulley without the need for further instrumentation of the tendon. Usually, the proximal tendon is maintained in position by passage of a transversely oriented 25-gauge hypodermic needle, and the repair is completed distal to the A4 pulley by an end-to-end tendon suture if enough distal tendon remains to accept a suture. If the distal stump is short or nonexistent, the profundus stump may be reattached by first elevating an osteoperiosteal flap from the base of the distal phalanx and then drilling an oblique hole beneath the flap, directed to penetrate the dorsal cortex just beneath the proximal fingernail. A double-armed (straight needles) 3-0 suture is placed in the proximal tendon stump and passed through the bone hole. In this instance, it is better to use a synthetic monofilament suture placed in a crisscross (unlocked) fashion so that the suture can be pulled out after bone-tendon healing has occurred. The sutures then are used to pull the tendon beneath the periosteal flap and are tied over a cottonpad-button combination over the nail. In my view, pullout wires are now unnecessary for any type of tendon repair. An alternate method is to use a bone anchor suture, such as the Mytec or Sta-Tec, to anchor the distal stump. When possible, the tendon attachment should be supplemented by sutures through an adjacent sheath or periosteum.

For zone II (from the origin of the flexor-tendon sheath to the insertion of the superficialis tendon over the midportion of the middle phalanx) flexor-tendon repairs, it is again necessary to make proximal and distal extending incisions that provide satisfactory exposure of the repair site. Dissection proceeds with identification and protection of the digital nerves and arteries, and, if they have been severed, the ends are mobilized and brought into proximity for subsequent suturing. At this point, I gently clear off the flexor sheath, which allows an assessment of the level and extent of sheath injury and the position of the tendon ends. Depending on the level of injury, I will open either the C1 (between A2 and A3) or C2 (between A3 and A4) cruciate-synovial windows using connecting incisions along one end and one side. When opening the intact components of the sheath, every attempt must be taken to preserve the annular components (A1, A2, A3, and A4), which are almost impossible to repair. Tendon suture should be performed in the cruciate-synovial sheath "windows," which usually can be restored following tendon suture. By acutely flexing the DIP joint and, to some extent, the PIP joint, it is usually possible to deliver the profundus and superficialis stumps into a cruciate window, and, if at least 1 cm of the distal tendons can be exposed in this manner, core sutures can be placed in the profundus tendon and two superficial slips without great difficulty (Fig. 18.2).

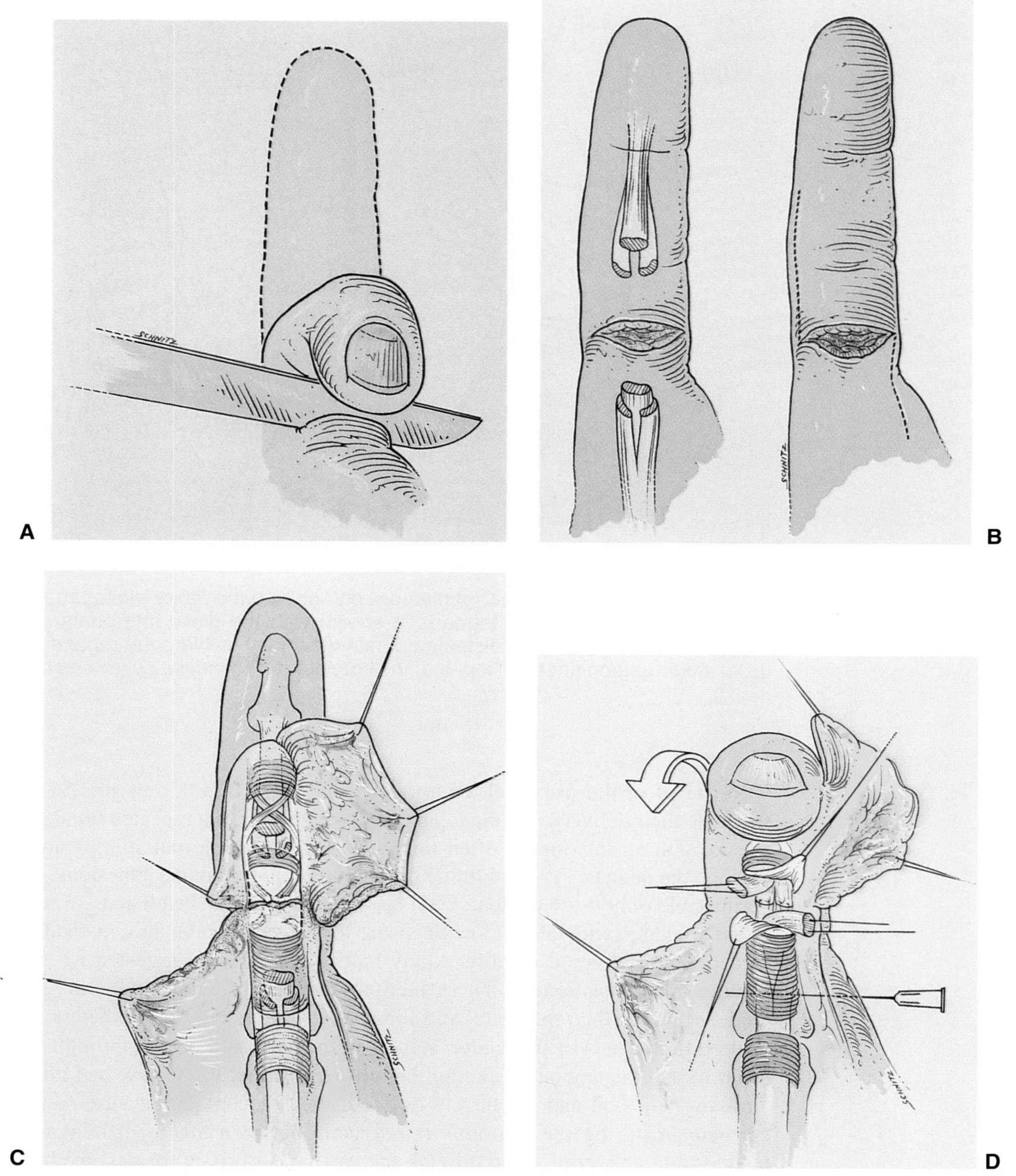

Figure 18.2. The author's technique of flexor-tendon repair in zone II. **A:** A knife laceration through zone II with the digit in full flexion. **B:** The level of flexor-tendon retraction of the same finger following digital extension. Dotted lines indicate the radial and ulnar extending incisions used to allow wide exposure of the flexor-tendon system. **C:** The appearance of the flexor-tendon system of the involved finger after reflection of skin flaps. The laceration occurred through the C1 cruciate area. Note the proximal and distal position of the flexor-tendon stumps. Dotted lines indicate the lateral incisions into cruciate-synovial portions of the sheath used to provide exposure for tendon repair. **D:** Reflection of small triangular flaps at the cruciate-synovial sheath allows the distal flexor-tendon stumps to be delivered into the wound by passive flexion of the distal interphalangeal joint. The profundus and superficialis stumps are retrieved and maintained at the repair site by means of a transversely placed small-gauge hypodermic needle.

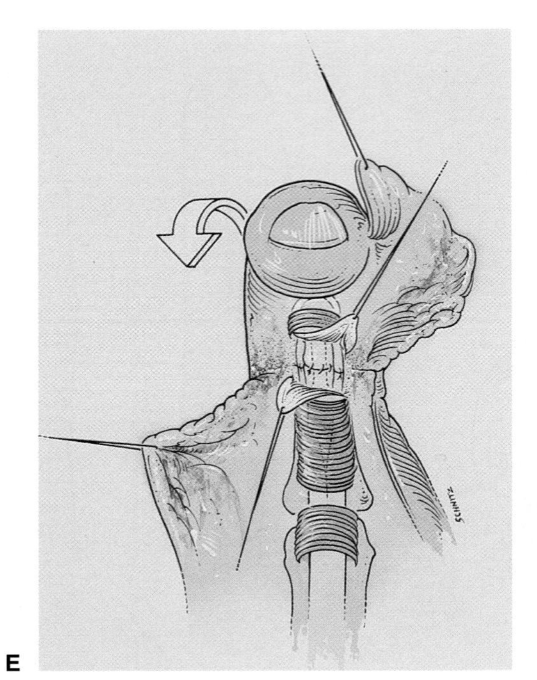

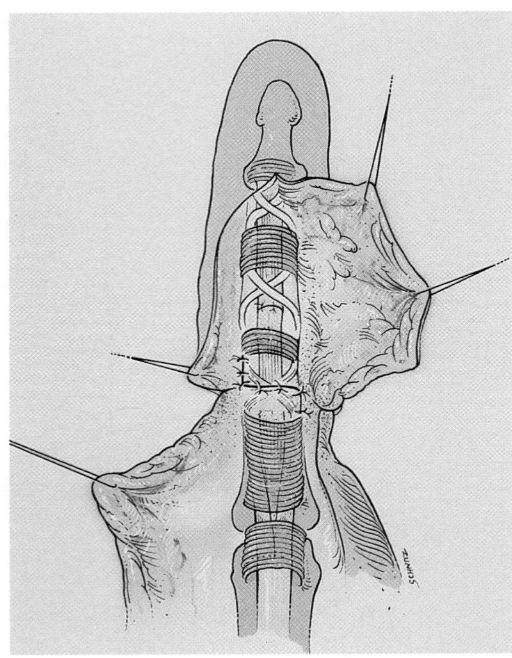

E F

Figure 18.2. *Continued.* **E:** Completed repair of both the flexor digitorum superficialis and flexor digitorum profundus tendons is shown with the distal interphalangeal joint in full flexion. **F:** Extension of the distal interphalangeal joint delivers the repairs under the intact distal flexor-tendon sheath. Repair of the cruciate (C1) synovial pulley has been completed.

Retrieval of the proximal tendon ends may be difficult, and several techniques can facilitate their delivery into the repair site. I emphasize that repeated blind grasps down the sheath with an instrument often fail to retrieve the proximal stumps and, in fact, may damage the delicate synovial lining of the pulleys and provoke adhesions. Such efforts are permissible only if the tendon(s) can be visualized in the sheath and are sufficiently close to the cruciate-synovial window to ensure that an end can be atraumatically pinched with forceps and delivered distally. Many tactics have been suggested to facilitate tendon capture and repositioning. These methods include proximal-to-distal "milking" of the tendons toward the repair site, and the use of various types of catheters or silicone rods sutured to the ends of the tendon stumps in the palm and passed through the sheath in an effort to pull the tendons back into their distal position. I have also had little luck with the "milking" method and rarely rely on the catheter technique because of the difficulty in correctly restoring the anatomic relationship between the superficialis and profundus tendons and delivering them through the narrow A1 orifice for passage from the palm to the digit. Two clever techniques have eased this dilemma:

1. If the tendon end is visible in the sheath, a skin hook may be used, as described by Morris and Martin. The hooked end is slid along the surface of the sheath until it is past the tendons, and the hook is then turned toward the tendons and pressed into the most superficial one. When the hook engages a tendon, the instrument is pulled distally, and both tendons usually follow. They then can be held in position by a 25-gauge hypodermic needle.
2. More frequently, the author employs a method described by Sourmelis and McGrouther. A small catheter is passed from the distal wound into the palm (or vice versa) beneath the annular pulleys. An important feature of this method is that the flexor tendons are left in situ in the sheath, and through a midpalmar incision, the catheter is sutured to both tendons several centimeters proximal to the A1 pulley. Then the catheter is pulled distally and easily delivers the tendon stumps into the distal repair site. A transversely

oriented needle secures the tendons for repair, and the connecting suture can be severed in the palm and the catheter withdrawn. Core sutures then can be placed in the proximal profundus stump, and the superficialis slips and the tendons usually can be brought into juxtaposition with the distal stumps for repair (Fig. 18.3).

When the proximal tendon ends have retracted into the palm, it is extremely important to reestablish the proper anatomic relationship of the profundus and superficialis tendons. To accomplish this step, the profundus will have to be passed back through the hiatus created by the superficialis slip so that it will lie palmar to Camper's chiasma and recreate the relative positioning present at the level of tendon laceration. Failure to restore the correct relationship will create an impediment to unrestricted tendon gliding following repair. Once the proper tendon anatomy has been reestablished, a catheter passed retrograde from the cruciate window is attached to the tendons, and, usually with some difficulty, the tendons are entered into the sheath and delivered distally, where they can be maintained with a transverse-oriented hypodermic needle.

Although several methods of four-strand flexor-tendon repair have been described, most are somewhat complicated or require a doubled suture. The method the author uses consists of a simple two-strand core stitch that enters and exits through the tendon ends and has locking grasps on the side of the tendon. For the repair, the author usually employs 3-0 braided synthetic suture material for the core sutures, but may elect to use 4-0 or 5-0 for children's tendons. An additional horizontal mattress suture is inserted across the tendon ends to complete a four-strand repair. A running horizontal lock stitch is used as a peripheral epitendinous stitch, and the author has found it easier than some of the more complicated methods described in recent articles (Fig. 18.4).

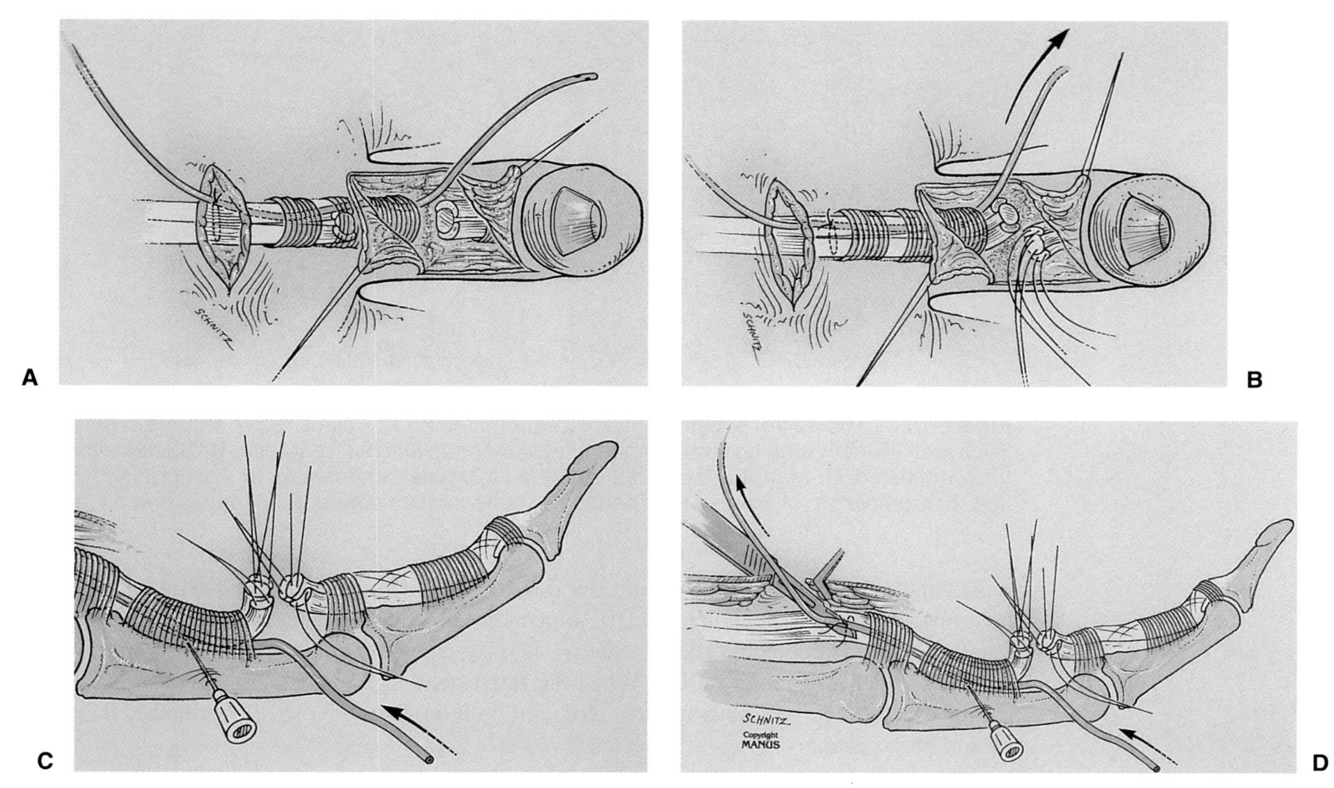

Figure 18.3. Sourmelis and McGrouther's method of retrieving flexor tendons. **A:** Polyethylene catheter passed (distal to proximal) alongside flexor tendons, which are left in situ. Catheter sutured to both tendons 2 cm proximal to A1 pulley through palmar incision. **B:** Catheter advanced distally to deliver tendon ends into repair site. **C:** A 22-gauge hypodermic needle passed transversely through the annular sheath to maintain tendon position. **D:** Catheter-tendon suture cut in palm and withdrawn.

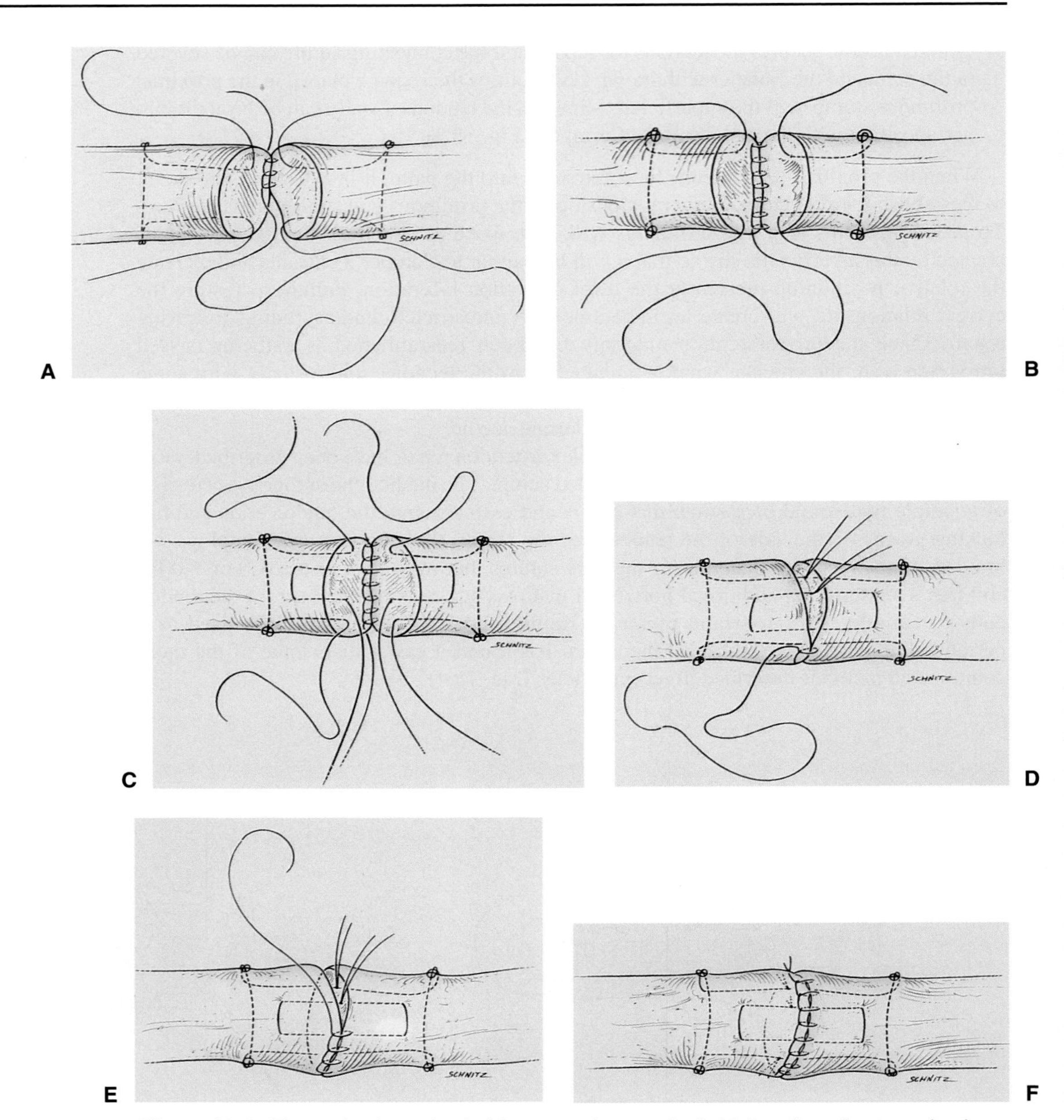

Figure 18.4. The author's method of flexor-tendon repair. **A:** Tajima "core" sutures in place. Back-wall (dorsal) running lock peripheral epitendinous stitch in progress. **B:** Back-wall suture completed. **C:** Mattress "core" suture added in palmar tendon gap. **D:** All "core" sutures tied. **E:** Completion of running lock peripheral epitendinous suture. **F:** Repair is complete.

At conclusion of the tendon repair, the flexor sheath is repaired using 6-0 nylon suture on a small needle. At this point, the DIP joint can be extended, a maneuver that delivers the repair distally. The repaired sheath usually serves as a smooth conduit for the repair site as it moves under an annular pulley. When the flexor tendon sheath cannot be repaired, the author usually elects to leave it open, although no more than 1.5 cm of continuous sheath should be excised.

When it is not possible to place core sutures in both the proximal and distal tendon ends in the proximal cruciate-synovial window, the next cruciate-synovial interval must be opened for distal core suture placement. The final repair is carried out in the most appropriate "window" after the proximal or distal stumps have been delivered into position by passing their core suture ends under the intervening annular pulley (usually A3) and pulling the tendon ends into position (Fig. 18.5).

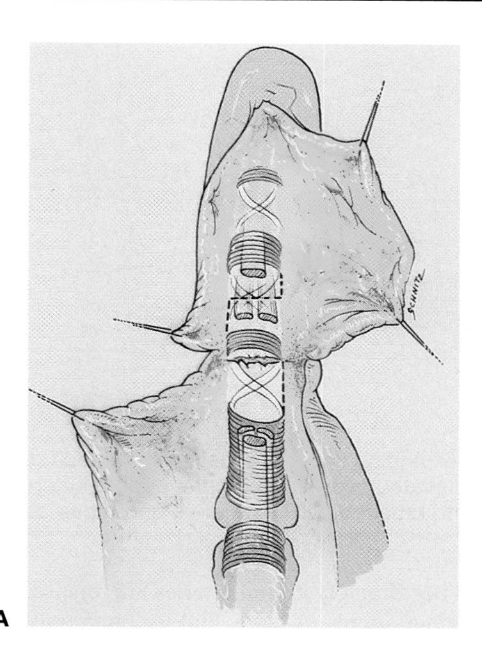

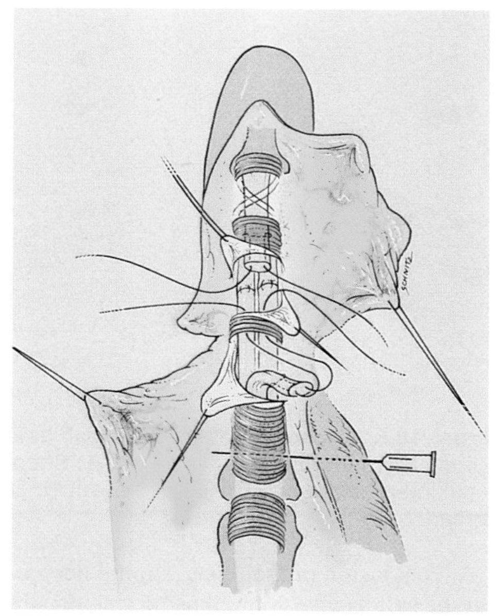

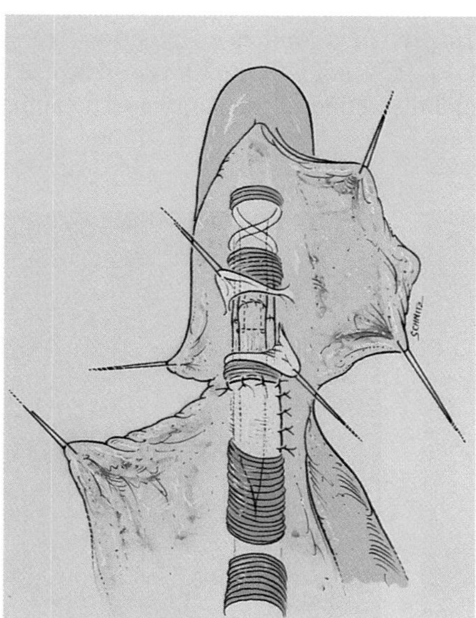

Figure 18.5. More distal severance of the flexor digitorum profundus (EDP) and flexor digitorum superficialis (FDS) tendons resulted in the ability to deliver 1 cm of the distal stumps into the C1 window. Incisions in both the C1 and C2 intervals are necessary to provide adequate exposure for suture placement and repair. **A:** Appearance of the flexor sheath after flexor-tendon interruption at a level just proximal to the proximal interphalangeal joint and the A3 pulley. Passive flexion of the distal interphalangeal joint does not provide adequate length of the distal stump in the C1 window for placement of the core sutures and repair. Dotted lines indicate the appropriate incisions in both the C1 and C2 windows. **B:** After placement of sutures in the distal tendon stumps in the C2 window and in the proximal stumps in the C1 opening, proximal tendon stumps can be delivered distally beneath the A3 pulley. (The FDS tendon stumps have been repaired.) **C:** Appearance of the digit after repair of both the FDP and FDS tendons and the C1 cruciate-synovial sheath. Repair of the C2 sheath should now be possible.

Flexor sheath repair is facilitated if the bulk of the tendon juncture can be minimized and careful sheath incisions have been used. To facilitate the passage of tendon repair beneath the annular pulleys, the author usually elects to close the overlying synovial sheath before extending the interphalangeal joints (Fig. 18.6). A series of clinical photographs illustrate a flexor-tendon repair in zone II (Fig. 18.7).

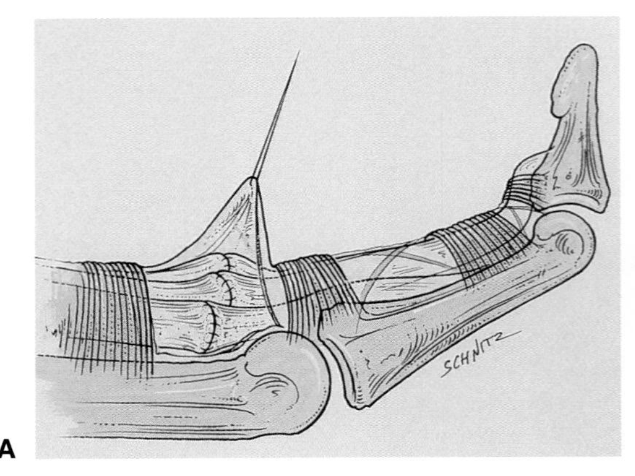

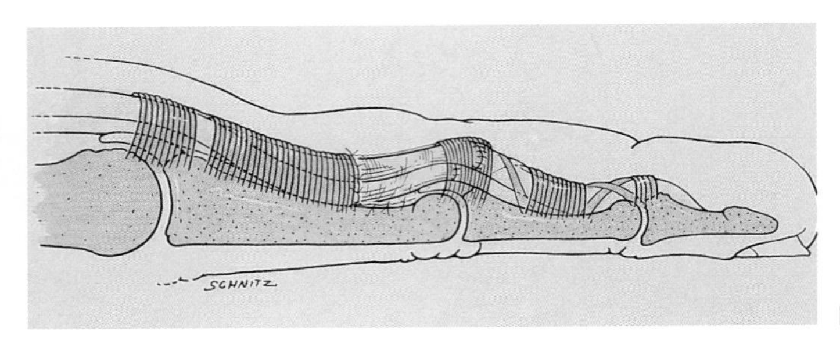

Figure 18.6. Technique of sheath repair before extending finger and delivering tendon repair distally under an annular pulley. **A:** Sheath elevated over tendon repair prior to suture. Distal interphalangeal (DIP) joint flexed. **B:** Sheath repaired, DIP extended, and repair advanced.

At conclusion of the repair, digital nerves and occasionally digital arteries are repaired, and the skin is then sutured using fine nonabsorbable sutures. A large, bulky, compressive dressing immobilizes all the digits, and the thumb is used postoperatively with the wrist in midflexion and the fingers in a "balanced position" of moderate flexion of the metacarpophalangeal (MCP), PIP, and DIP joint levels. The use of antibiotics depends on the personal philosophy and discretion of the surgeon. The author's own preference is to use them in the acute setting.

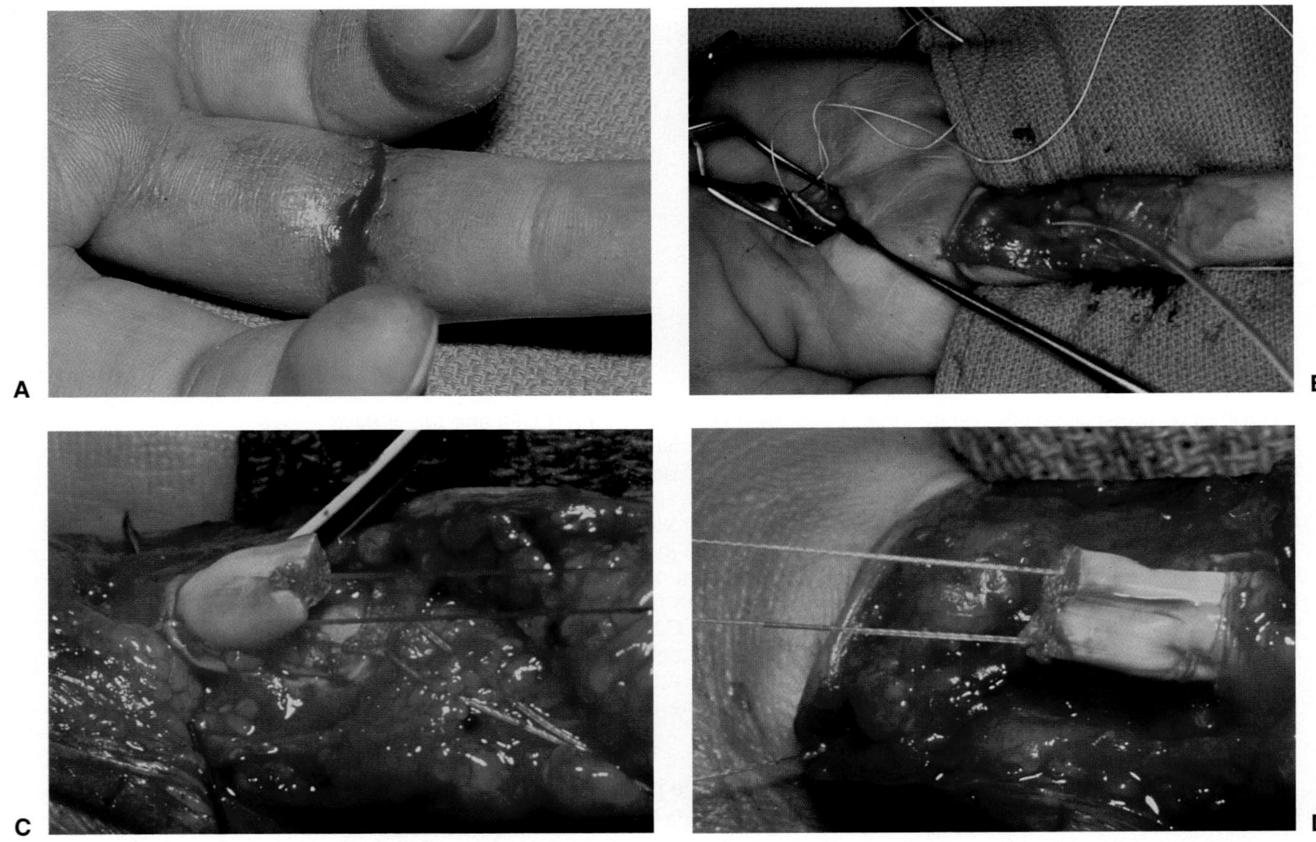

Figure 18.7. A: Appearance of digital laceration. **B:** Tendon retrieval using the method of McGrouther and Sourmelis. **C:** Tajima core suture in proximal stump. **D:** Tajima core suture in distal stump.

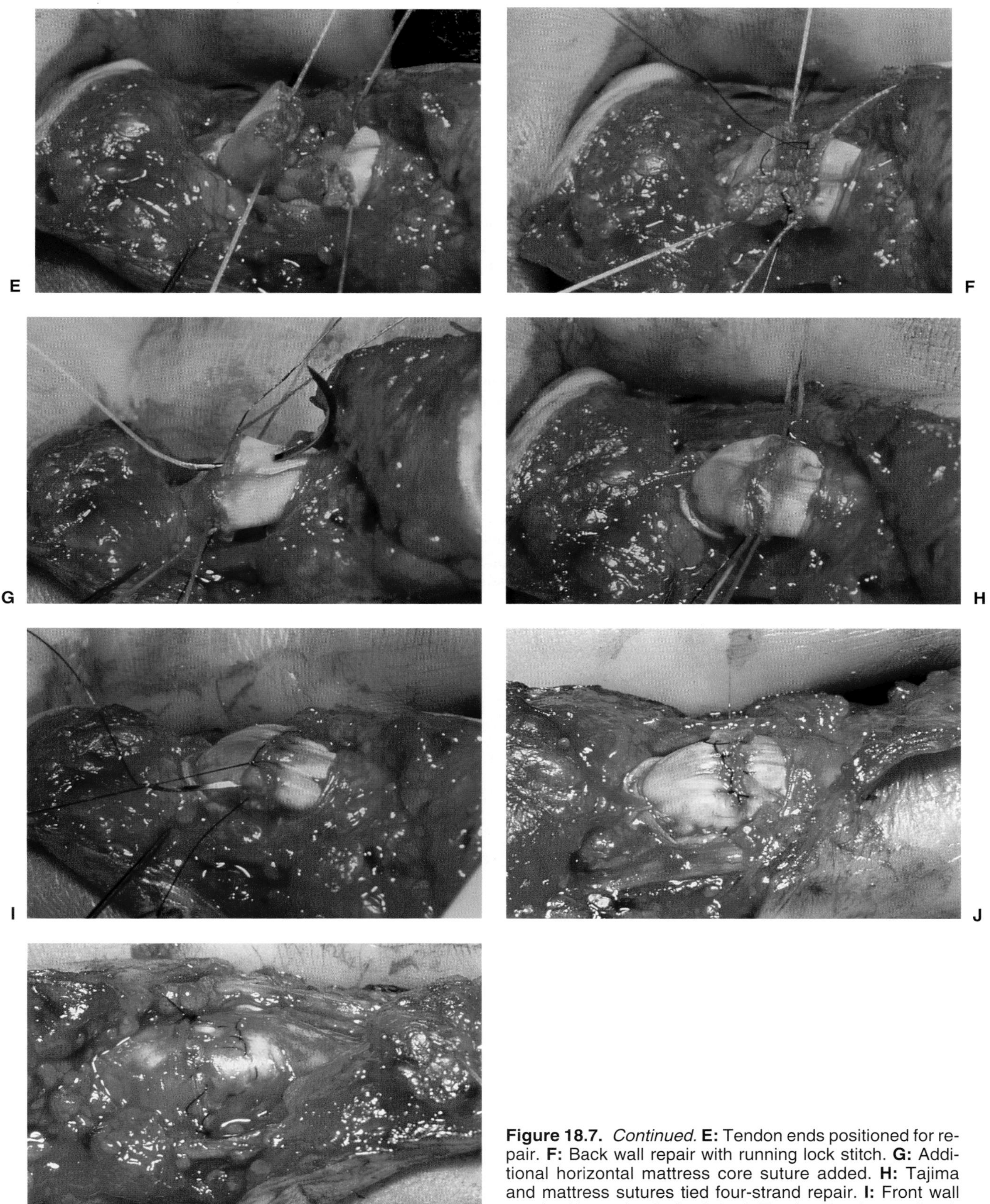

Figure 18.7. *Continued.* **E:** Tendon ends positioned for repair. **F:** Back wall repair with running lock stitch. **G:** Additional horizontal mattress core suture added. **H:** Tajima and mattress sutures tied four-strand repair. **I:** Front wall repair with running lock stitch. **J:** Tendon repair completed. **K:** Sheath repaired.

POSTOPERATIVE MANAGEMENT

Our post-flexor-tendon repair rehabilitation program emphasizes techniques that employ not only a near complete range of composite digital motion, but also the use of "synergistic" wrist extension, in an effort to gain the greatest amount of excursion of the repaired tendon. It was demonstrated that light active finger flexion carried out with the wrist in extension should be relatively safe for tendons repaired with a four- or six-strand core suture augmented by some type of strong running-lock peripheral epitendinous suture. Because our repair protocol uses a four-strand method, the postoperative program permits the active maintenance of digital flexion once the wrist is brought from flexion to extension. The details of this method were worked out by Nancy Cannon, OTR, CHT, and Karen Harmon Gettle, OTR, CHT, at the Indiana Hand Center, and have worked extremely well for patients who are well-motivated and demonstrate a serious desire to maximize their recovery. The therapists spend a great deal of time with the patient explaining the details of the therapy program and ensuring that he or she comprehends all the details of the somewhat rigorous regimen. The program can be summarized as follows.

Several splints or combinations of splints adhere to the principle that at rest the wrist and MCP joints should be in flexion and the IP joints in extension. The motion program begins by passively flexing all three digital joints while the wrist is in flexion, and then actively maintaining that composite flexion after the wrist is brought into extension. The resting splint is a traditional dorsal blocking splint that positions the wrist in 20 degrees of palmar flexion, the MCP joints in 50 degrees of flexion, and the IP joints in neutral. The passive flexion (wrist flexion), active hold (wrist extension) phase then may be achieved by removing the resting splint and assisting the patient through the exercise sequence. For more sophisticated splint fabricators, an articulated splint may be designed that maintains wrist flexion at rest and, by means of either a hinged component or a dorsal, removable section, allows the wrist to be brought into 30 degrees of dorsiflexion during active flexion (Fig. 18.8). By removing restricting Velcro straps, the PIP and DIP joints may achieve a full range of passive and active PIP and DIP flexion and extension while the MCP joints are maintained in 60 degrees of flexion.

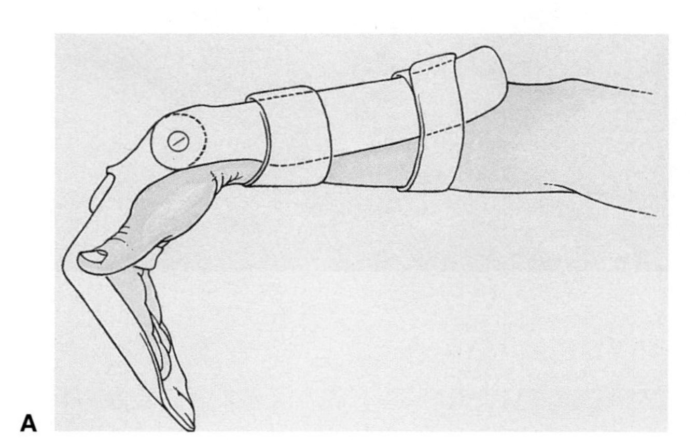

A

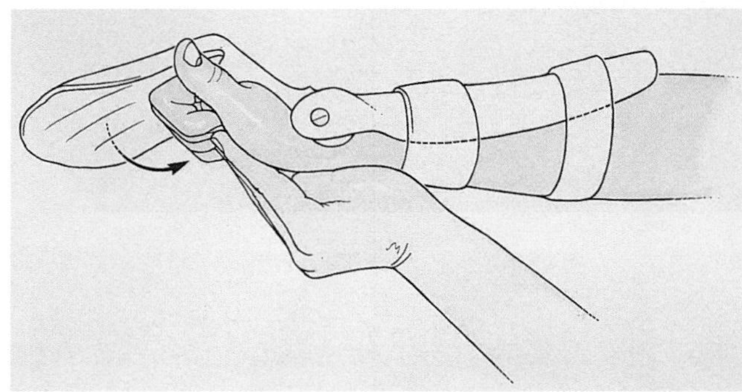

B

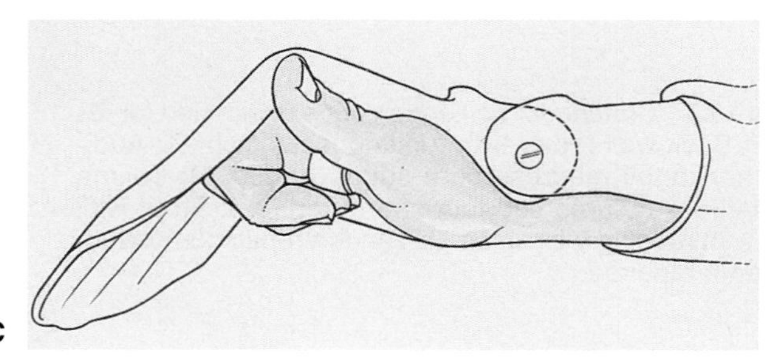

C

Figure 18.8. Postflexor-tendon repair motion protocol. **A:** Following removal of the surgical bandage, a traditional dorsal blocking splint that positions the wrist in 20 degrees of palmar flexion, the metacarpophalangeal (MCP) in 50 degrees of flexion, and the interphalangeal joint in extension are applied. **B:** A tenodesis splint with a wrist hinge is fabricated to allow full wrist flexion and wrist dorsiflexion to 30 degrees, maintaining MCP flexion of at least 60 degrees. **C:** Following composite passive digital flexion, the wrist is extended as passive flexion is maintained. The patient actively maintains digital flexion and holds that position for about 5 seconds. Patients are instructed to use the lightest muscle power necessary to maintain digital flexion.

The formal therapy program consists of efforts to maximize independent and combined gliding of the FDS and FDP tendons during each exercise session. Fifteen repetitions of passive flexion and extension of the PIP joint, the DIP joint, and the entire digit are carried out during each hour, and these exercises are performed within the restraints of the dorsal blocking splint, which immobilizes the wrist and MCP joints in flexion. The patient is instructed to flex the digits passively and completely and then to extend the wrist. He or she then is asked to contract the long flexor muscles gently and to hold the position achieved by passive flexion for at least 5 seconds (Fig.18.9). After 5 seconds, the patient relaxes the muscle contraction and allows the wrist to drop back into flexion, which will automatically allow the digits to straighten within the confines of the splint. Twenty-five repetitions of this exercise sequence are performed each hour throughout the day.

This protocol is followed for 4 weeks, with adjustments made depending on problems the patient may experience, particularly with regard to digital edema and joint stiffness. The development of any flexion contractures at either the PIP or DIP joint is closely monitored, and appropriate splinting and exercise programs are designed to ensure the recovery of full digital extension. At 4 weeks, the tendons should have regained sufficient strength to allow the splints to be removed for gentle active and passive exercises. The dorsal block splint is worn between exercises, and the program continues to emphasize passive digital flexion with the wrist flexed, followed by active maintenance of that flexion with the wrist extended. The patient then drops the wrist into flexion and extends the digits to complete the tenodesis sequence. Active flexion and extension exercises of the digits and wrist are performed with a light muscle contraction, and the patient is instructed not to extend the wrist and digits simultaneously.

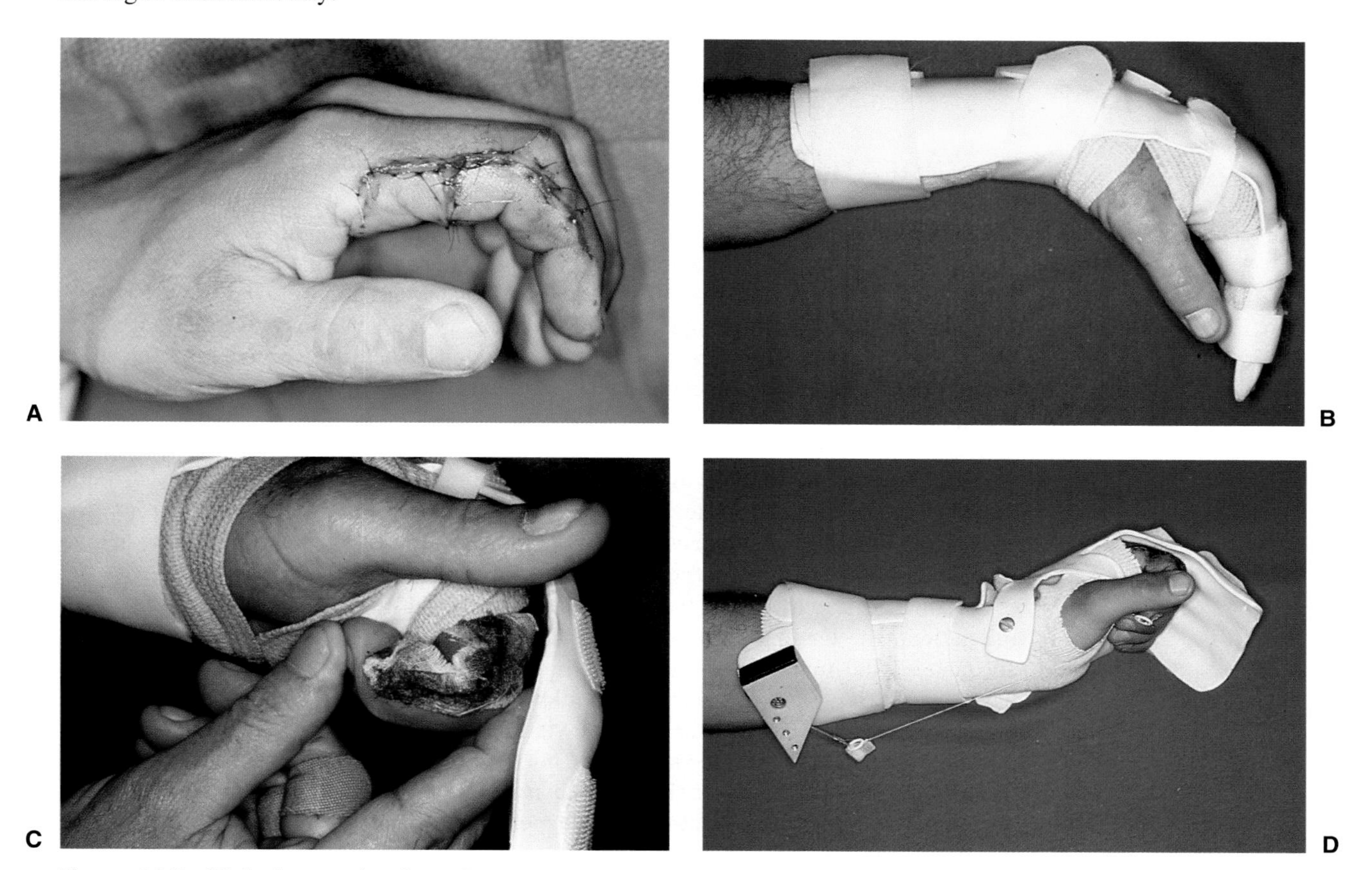

Figure 18.9. Clinical example of postflexor-tendon repair program. **A:** Index finger following four-strand repair of the flexor digitorum superficialis (FDS) and the flexor digitorum profundus (FDP). **B:** Resting splint with wrist and metacarpophalangeal (MCP) joints flexed, interphalangeal (IP) extended. **C:** Digit is passively flexed with wrist in flexion. **D:** Wrist extended while maintaining passive digital flexion. Patient then holds this position with light active flexion.

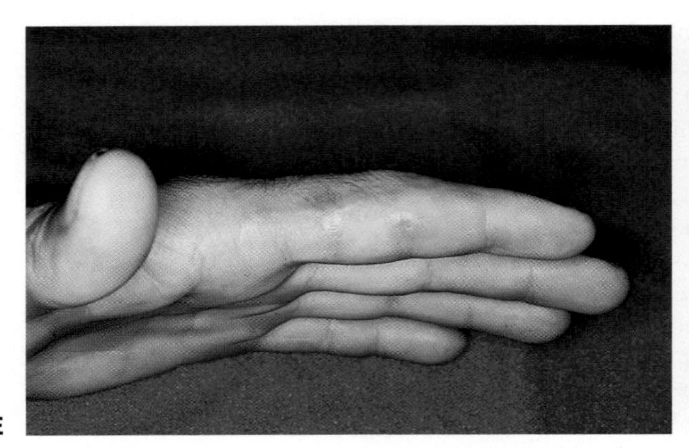
E

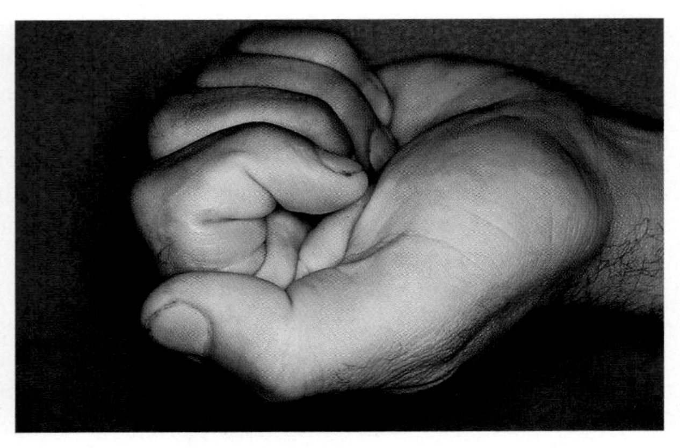
F

Figure 18.9. *Continued.* **E:** Extension at 10 weeks. **F:** Flexion at 10 weeks.

At 5 to 6 weeks, more vigorous exercises are permitted, including isolated tendon excursion exercises, blocking exercises, and passive extension exercises. Strengthening is initiated at 8 weeks in a gradual, progressive manner.

It should be emphasized that this protocol will not work for everyone. I believe it is important for the surgeon to spend some hours in the cadaver lab to develop the technical skills for the four-strand repair and the running lock peripheral epitendinous stitch. Success also requires a well-trained therapist who thoroughly understands the rationale for the rehabilitation program and its pitfalls. Finally, the method cannot succeed without an intelligent, motivated, and cooperative patient.

COMPLICATIONS

Rupture of one or both flexor-tendon repairs is a significant complication. It may occur during therapy, with inadvertent strong gripping or lifting, or while a patient is sleeping. Ruptures after four-strand repairs have been infrequent and almost always are related to overenthusiastic use of the injured hand because a good early range of motion breeds overconfidence in the strength of the healing tendon. When one receives the sickening news that a repaired flexor tendon or tendons have ruptured, the preferred treatment is prompt re-exploration and repair.

The most frequent late complication following early postoperative mobilization programs is the development of flexion contractures at the PIP or DIP joints or both. Prompt recognition of the development of contractures, modification of the motion program to permit greater extension, and the judicious use of dynamic splints can help to prevent or overcome those deformities before they progress too far.

On some occasions, despite the best possible repair and strong cooperation on the part of the patient, the tendons may become adherent and fail to glide sufficiently to return adequate digital function. The decision to carry out a secondary tenolysis procedure is based on serial joint measurement indicating that there has been no appreciable improvement for several months despite a vigorous therapy program and the conscientious efforts of the patient. The procedure should not be considered until all wounds have reached "equilibrium" with soft pliable skin and subcutaneous tissues and minimal reaction around the scars. Joint contractures must have been mobilized and a normal or near-normal passive range of digital motion achieved.

RECOMMENDED READING

1. Aoki M, Manske PR, Pruitt DL, et al. Work of flexion after tendon repair with various suture methods. *J Hand Surg* 20:310–313, 1995.

2. Aoki M, Pruitt DL, Kubota H, et al. Effect of suture knots on tensile strength of repaired canine flexor tendons. *J Hand Surg* 20:72–75, 1995.
3. Bright DS, Urbaniak JS. Direct measurements of flexor-tendon tension during active and passive digit motion and its application to flexor-tendon surgery. *Orthop Trans* 1:4–5, 1977.
4. Cannon NM. Post flexor-tendon repair motion protocol. *The Indiana Hand Center Newsletter* 1:13–17, 1993.
5. Carstadt CA, Madsen K, Wredmark T. The influence of Indamethacin on biomechanical and biochemical properties of the plantaris longus tendon in the rabbit. *Arch Orthop Trauma Surg* 106:157–160, 1987.
6. Chow JA, Thomes LJ, Dovelle SW, et al. A combined regimen of controlled motion following flexor-tendon repair in "no man's land." *Plast Reconstr Surg* 79:447–453, 1987.
7. Chow JA, Themes LJ, Dovelle S, et al. Controlled motion rehabilitation after flexor-tendon repair and grafting: a multi-centre study. *J Bone Joint Surg* 70:591–595, 1988.
8. Cohert JH, Uchiyama S, Amadio PC, et al. Flexor tendon-pulley interaction after tendon repair: a biomechanical study. *J Hand Surg* 2013:573–577, 1995.
9. Cooney WP, In GT, An KN. Improved tendon excursion following flexor-tendon repair. *J Hand Surg* 2:102–106, 1989.
10. Defino HLA, Barbieri CH, Goncalves RP, et al. Studies on tendon healing: a comparison of suturing techniques. *J Hand Surg* 11B:444–450, 1986.
11. Duran RH, Hauser RG. In: *American Academy of Orthopaedic Surgeons: Symposium on Flexor Tendon Surgery in the Hand.* St. Louis: C.V. Mosby, 1975:105–114.
12. Duran RH, Hauser RG, Stover MG. Management of flexor lacerations in zone 2 using controlled passive motion postoperatively. In: Hunter JM, Schneider L, Macking EJ, et al., eds. *Rehabilitation of the Hand.* St Louis: CV Mosby, 1978.
13. Eiken O, Holmberg J, Ekerot L, et al. Reconstruction of the digital tendon sheath: a new concept of tendon grafting. *Scand J Plast Reconstr Surg* 14:89–97, 1980.
14. Garlock JM. The repair process in wounds of tendons and in tendon grafts. *Ann Surg* 85:92, 1927.
15. Gelberman RH, Amiel D, Gonsalves M, et al. The influence of protected passive mobilization on the healing of flexor tendons: a biochemical and microangiographic study. *The Hand* 13:120–128, 1981.
16. Gelberman RH, Butte MJ, Spiegelman JH, et al. The excursion and deformation of repaired flexor tendons treated with protected early motion. *J Hand Surg* 11A:106–110, 1986.
17. Gelberman RH, Jayasanker M, Gonsalves M, et al. The effects of mobilization on the vascularization of healing flexor tendons in dogs. *Clin Orthop* 153:283–289, 1980.
18. Gelberman RH, Vande Berg JS, Lundborg GN, et al. Flexor tendon healing and restoration of the gliding surface. *J Bone Joint Surg* 65A:70–80, 1983.
19. Gelberman RH, Woo SLY, Lothringer K, et al. Effects of early intermittent passive mobilization on healing canine flexor tendons. *J Hand Surg* 7A:170–175, 1982.
20. Harmer TW. Cases of tendon and nerve repair. *Boston Medical and Surgical Journal* 194:739–747, 1926.
21. Harmer TW. Injuries to the hand. *Am J Surg* 42:638–658, 1938.
22. Harmer TW. Tendon suture. *Boston Medical and Surgical Journal* 177:808–810, 1917.
23. Kleinert HE, Kutz JE, Ashbell TS, et al. Primary repair of flexor tendons in "no man's land." *J Bone Joint Surg* 49A:577, 1967.
24. Kubota H, Pruitt DL, Manske PR. In: *Meeting Abstracts of the American Society for Surgery of the Hand, 50th Annual Meeting*, San Francisco, 1995:65.
25. Kulick MI, Smith HS, Hadler K. Oral ibuprofen: evaluation of its effect on peritendinous adhesions and the breaking strength of a tenorrhaphy. *J Hand Surg* 11A:110–120, 1986.
26. Lee H. Double loop locking suture: a technique of tendon repair for early active mobilization. Part I. Evolution of technique and experimental study. *Am J Hand Surg* 15:945–952, 1990.
27. Lin GT, An KN, Amadio PC, et al. Biomechanical studies of running suture for flexor-tendon repair in dogs. *J Hand Surg* 13A:553–558, 1988.
28. Lister GD. Incision and closure of the flexor-tendon sheath during tendon repair. *Hand* 14:123–135, 1983.
29. Lister GD. Pitfalls and complications of flexor-tendon surgery. *Hand Clin* 1:133–146, 1985.
30. Lister GD, Kleinert HE, Kutz JE, et al. Primary flexor-tendon repair followed by immediate controlled mobilization. *J Hand Surg* 2:441–451, 1977.
31. Manske PR. Review article: flexor-tendon healing. *J Hand Surg* 13B:237–245, 1988.
32. Mashida ZB, Arms AA. Strength of the suture in the epitenon and within the tendon fibres: development of stronger peripheral suture technique. *J Hand Surg (Br)* 17:172–175, 1992.
33. McGrouther DA, Ahmed MR. Flexor-tendon excursions in "no man's land." *The Hand* 13:129–141, 1981.
34. Morris RJ, Martin DL. The use of skin hooks and hypodermic needles in tendon surgery. *J Hand Surg* 1813:33–34, 1993.
35. Peterson WW, Manske PR, Dunlap J, et al. Effect of various methods of restoring flexor-sheath integrity on the formation of adhesions after tendon injury. *J Hand Surg* 15A:48–56, 1990.
36. Pruitt DL, Manske PR, Fink B. Cyclic stress analysis of flexor-tendon repairs. *J Hand Surg* 16A:701–707, 1991.
37. Robertson GA, Al-Quattan MM. A biomechanical analysis of a new interlock suture technique for flexor-tendon repair. *J Hand Surg* 17B:92–93, 1992.
38. Saldana MJ, Ho PK, Lichtman DM, et al. Flexor-tendon repair and rehabilitation in zone II open-sheath technique versus closed-sheath technique. *J Hand Surg* 12A(6):1110–1113, 1987.
39. Savage R. In vitro studies of a new method of flexor-tendon repair. *J Hand Surg* 10B:135–141, 1985.
40. Savage R. The influence of wrist position on the minimum force required for active movement of the interphalangeal joints. *J Hand Surg* 13B:262–268, 1988.
41. Schuind F, Garcia-Elias M, Cooney WP, et al. Flexor-tendon forces: in vivo measurements. *J Hand Surg* 17A:291–298, 1992.
42. Seradge H. Elongation of the repair configuration following flexor-tendon repair. *J Hand Surg* 11A:106–110, 1986.
43. Silfverskiöld KL, May EI. Flexor-tendon repair in zone II with a new suture technique and an early mobilization program combining passive and active flexion. *J Hand Surg* 19A:53–60, 1994.

44. Soejima O, Diao E, Lotz JC, et al. Comparative mechanical analysis of dorsal versus palmar placement of core suture for flexor-tendon repairs. *J Hand Surg* 20A:801–807, 1995.
45. Sourmelis SG, McGrouther DA. Retrieval of the retracted flexor tendon. *J Hand Surg* 12B:109–111, 1987.
46. Strickland JW. Biologic rationale, clinical application, and results or early motion following flexor-tendon repair. *J Hand Ther* 71–83, 1989.
47. Strickland JW. Flexor-tendon repair—symposium on flexor tendon surgery. *Hand Clin* 1:55–68, 1985.
48. Strickland JW. Flexor-tendon surgery—Part 2: flexor-tendon repair. *Orthop Rev* 11:701–721, 1986.
49. Strickland JW. Flexor-tendon repair: Indiana method. *Indiana Hand Center Newsletter* 1:1–12, 1993.
50. Strickland JW. Flexor-tendon injuries: I. Foundations of treatment. *JAAOS* 3:44–54, 1995.
51. Strickland JW. Flexor-tendon injuries: II. Operative technique. *JAAOS* 3:55–62, 1995.
52. Strickland JW. Management of acute flexor-tendon injuries—Symposium on rehabilitation after reconstructive hand surgery. *Orthop Clin North Am* 14:827–849, 1983.
53. Strickland JW. Results of flexor-tendon surgery in zone II. *Hand Clin* 1:167–179, 1983.
54. Strickland JW. In: Taras JS, Schneider LH, eds. *Atlas of the Hand Clinics.* Phildelphia: WB Saunders, 1996:77–103.
55. Strickland JW, Glogovac SV. Digital function following flexor-tendon repair in zone II: a comparison of immobilization and controlled passive-motion techniques. *J Hand Surg* 5:537–543, 1980.
56. Taras JS, Raphael JS, Marczyk S, et al. The double grasping and cross-stitch in flexor-tendon repair. In: Meeting Abstracts of the American Society for Surgery of the Hand, 50th annual meeting. San Francisco, CA, 1995:42.
57. Trail IA, Powell ES, Noble J. The mechanical strength of various suture techniques. *J Hand Surg* 17B:89–91, 1992.
58. Urbaniak JR. Replantation in children. *Pediatric Plastic Surgery* 2:1168, 1984.
59. Urbaniak JR, Cahill JD, Mortenson RA. In: *American Academy of Orthopaedic Surgeons Symposium on Tendon Surgery in the Hand.* St Louis: CV Mosby, 1975:70–80.
60. Wade PJF, Muir IFK, Hutchenon LL. Primary flexor-tendon repair. The mechanical limitations of the modified Kessler technique. *J Hand Surg* 11B:71–76, 1986.
61. Wade PJF, Wetherall RG, Amis AA. Flexor-tendon repair: significant gain in strength from the Halsted peripheral suture technique. *J Hand Surg* 14B:232–235, 1989.
62. Wagner WF, Carroll C, Strickland JW, et al. A biomechanical comparison of techniques of flexor-tendon repair. *J Hand Surg* 19A:1–5, 1994.

19

Treatment of the "Jersey Finger": Repair and Reconstruction of Flexor Digitorum Profundus Avulsion Injuries

Brian M. Katt and Joseph P. Leddy

INDICATIONS/CONTRAINDICATIONS

Avulsion of the flexor digitorum profundus (FDP) tendon from its insertion on the distal phalanx is a relatively common flexor tendon injury. The so-called "jersey finger" is one of the few closed injuries in the hand for which the timing of presentation may have a profound effect on the reconstructive plan and eventual outcome. The level of retraction of the untethered FDP within the flexor tendon sheath, the maintenance or loss of the vincular blood supply and nutrition through synovial bathing, and the capacity of the sheath itself are variables that are influenced by the interval between the injury and the reconstruction.

Although there is no firm chronology that dictates the treatment options, it is more likely that anatomic reconstruction can be performed if the interval between injury and surgery is abbreviated. If this interval is prolonged, the viability of the tendon, the likelihood of advancement without excessive digital flexion, and the ability of the sheath to accommodate the tendon all diminish.

In most patients in whom the tendon remains in the sheath or is easily retrieved and advanced, primary repair back to the anatomic location on the metadiaphysis of the distal phalanx is indicated. In circumstances in which the advancement and repair is prohibited by any of the multiple factors discussed, other reconstructive alternatives must be entertained.

Brian M. Katt, M.D.: Department of Orthopaedic Surgery, University of Medicine and Dentistry of New Jersey, Robert Wood Johnson Medical School, New Brunswick, NJ

Joseph P. Leddy, M.D.: Department of Orthopaedic Surgery, University of Medicine and Dentistry of New Jersey, Robert Wood Johnson Medical School, New Brunswick, NJ

In some patients, the ability to independently and actively flex the distal interphalangeal (DIP) joint is mandatory for vocational or avocational pursuits (the violinist is the common example). Primary repair is obviously the most desirable option in these patients. Reconstructive alternatives, such as staged tendon grafting and pulley reconstruction, must be part of the hand surgeon's armamentarium when treating these populations.

Not all patients will require FDP reattachment and are comfortable with the loss of DIP flexion ability. Potential or relative contraindications to anatomic repair or complex staged reconstruction include medical illness, advanced age, and inability to accept the risks of operation or the rigors of rehabilitation. If there are patient factors or anatomic factors that preclude primary repair, the portfolio of options that may be available include volar soft-tissue imbrication (capsule, volar plate, skin) or DIP arthrodesis.

The jersey finger is a common problem that all hand surgeons will encounter. Primary repair will be chosen for a majority of patients who recognize the injury early and present promptly. In some forms, tethering of the tendon within the flexor sheath can substantially prolong the interval during which primary repair can be affected. If the tendon has retracted from the sheath and can no longer be advanced without adversely affecting digital or hand function, then other reconstructive alternatives must be entertained. This chapter covers the recognition and treatment of the acute injuries and details the treatment alternatives for remote FDP avulsion injuries.

MECHANISM OF INJURY

Flexor digitorum avulsion from the distal phalanx is caused by forcible extension against a flexed DIP joint. Avulsion of the FDP tendon insertion commonly involves athletes; football and rugby are two of the more common sports in which this entity is seen in the act of tackling the opponent.

Von Zander was the first to describe avulsion of a flexor tendon from its insertion, namely in the flexor pollicis longus. McMaster performed clinical and experimental studies on the causes and locations of subcutaneous ruptures of tendon and muscle. His work showed that the tendon is the strongest unit in the musculoskeletal chain and that rupture occurs at the insertion or musculotendinous junction rather than midsubstance. However, a recent study showed "normal" tendon rupturing in midsubstance in two cases.

Roughly 75% of FDP avulsions occur in the ring finger. In a laboratory study using cadaveric tendons, Manske and Lesker found the breaking strength of the FDP insertion of the ring finger significantly less than that of the middle finger.

Dynamic factors may also play a role in why this finger is more likely to be injured; when the metacarpophalangeal (MCP) joints of the middle and little fingers are flexed down to 90 degrees, the ring finger is unable to fully extend at the MCP joint. The ring finger extensor tendon is pulled distally via its attachment to the extensor tendons of the long and little fingers through the junctura tendinae. The distal position of the ring extensor tendon prevents full extension. This mechanism causes the extended finger to encounter resistance earlier in its arc of motion. Rupture can occur when the flexed finger is forced into extension.

The athlete may be grabbing the opposing player's jersey and flexing the digit, thus the term "jersey finger." The little finger loses its grip and continues to flex, simultaneously flexing the ring through the juncturae. As the opposing player moves away, the attached ring finger is forced into extension, causing avulsion of the tendon insertion. Additionally, the ring fingertip becomes the most prominent and absorbs the most force during grip. This is due to the shorter length of the fourth metacarpal and the increased mobility of the fourth MCP joint.

CLASSIFICATION

The classification of this injury, contributed by Leddy and Packer, is based on a review of 36 athletes with an avulsion of the FDP. Unlike so many attempted classification systems, this logical descriptive matrix defines pathoanatomy succinctly and assists the sur-

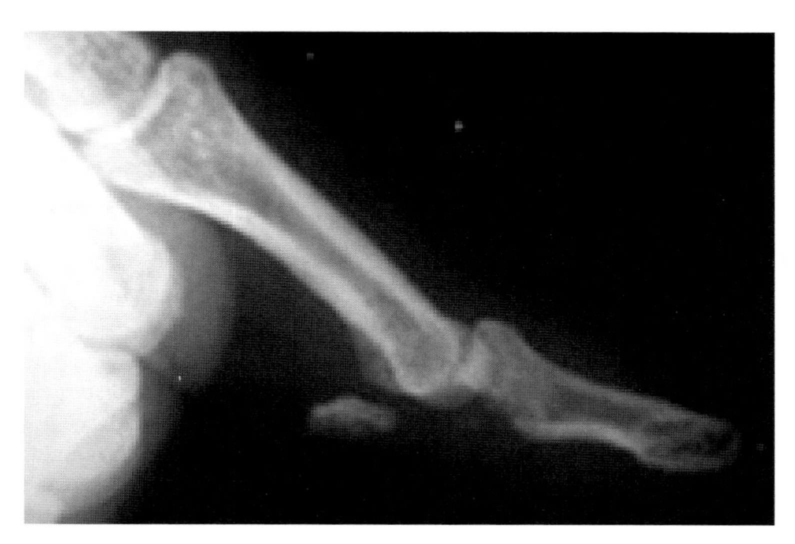

Figure 19.1. Type III injury. The tendon is attached to the bony fragment, which is held up by the A4 pulley.

geon in choosing a treatment course. The classification was initially divided into three types. More recently, the classification has been expanded to include a variation of the type III injury and a type IV.

- Type I: the tendon retracts into the palm and is held by the lumbrical origin. The blood supply is disrupted because both vinculae are ruptured. There is no diffusion of nutrients from the synovial fluid.
- Type II: the tendon retracts to the level of the proximal interphalangeal (PIP) joint and may still be attached to the long vinculum. There remains diffusion of nutrients through synovial fluid.
- Type III: the tendon is avulsed with a piece of bone and is held at the level of the A4 pulley (Fig. 19.1). Both vinculae are intact, as is diffusion from synovial fluid.
- Type IIIB: fracture of the distal phalanx combined with an avulsion of the tendon from the fractured bone.
- Type IV: comminuted intra-articular fracture of distal phalanx (Fig. 19.2).

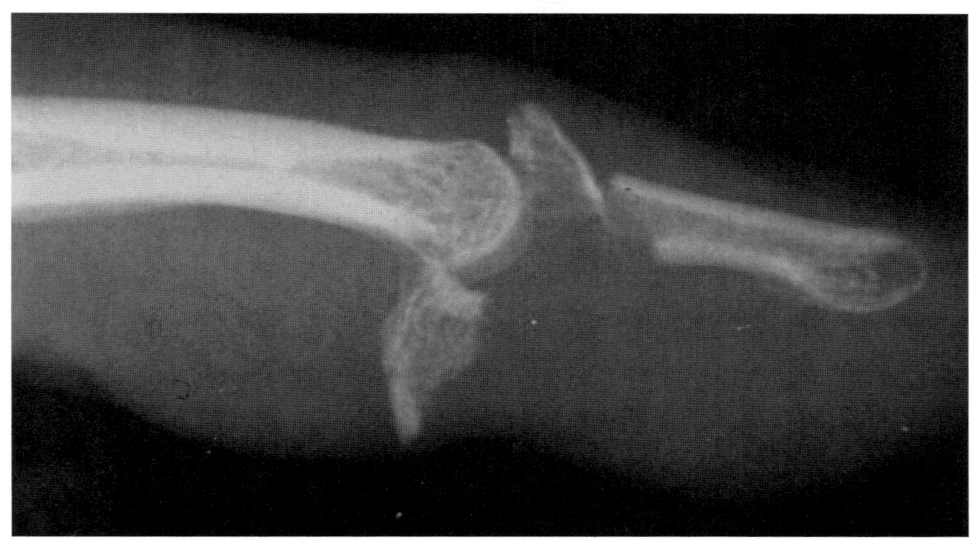

Figure 19.2. X-ray of a type IV injury. The extensor insertion is on the dorsal fragment, and the FDP insertion is on the palmar fragment held up at the A4 pulley.

PREOPERATIVE PLANNING

Four prognostic factors will dictate the appropriate treatment:

(1) level of tendon retraction;
(2) remaining blood supply to the tendon and synovial fluid diffusion;
(3) length of time between injury and treatment; and
(4) the presence and size of the bony fragment.

Blood supply to the tendon comes from both the short and long vinculae. The short vinculum is at the distal portion of the flexor tendon and is usually ruptured in type I and II injuries. The long vinculum is at the level of the middle phalanx and may be the sole structure preventing retraction into the palm in type II injuries. The tendon also receives nutrition through diffusion from the synovial fluid in the flexor tendon sheath.

The diagnosis of tendon avulsion is often delayed. Although Carroll thought there was "universal unawareness" of this injury, in his series, in 26 of 35 patients, the diagnosis was made more than 1 month after injury. For these reasons, it is important to educate those individuals, such as football coaches and rock-climbing instructors, about the injury and to emphasize the timing elements and the relationship between recognition, treatment, and ultimate outcome.

It is imperative to specifically test for flexion of the DIP joint, and young athletes need to be educated and made to feel comfortable about bringing forth a "minor hand injury" when they recognize the inability to flex the DIP joint of a triphalangeal digit. Pain, swelling, and ecchymosis are not always present. Tenderness on the volar side of the digit or in the palm will give a clue to where the tendon has retracted.

The pathognomonic feature is inability to actively flex the DIP joint of the affected finger. A patient with a type I injury most often will present with pain in the palm and is able to fully flex the PIP joint (Fig. 19.3). Patients with type II injuries will have pain and swelling at the DIP and PIP joints. Additionally, loss of PIP motion due to swelling and the presence of the tendon will be identified (Fig. 19.4).

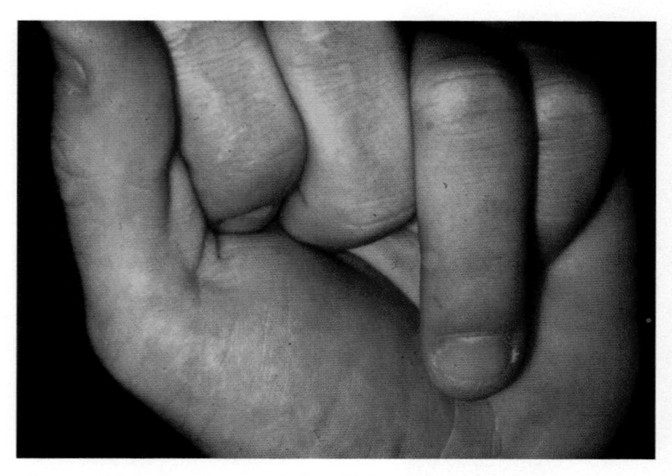

Figure 19.3. Avulsion of the FDP of the ring finger with the tendon retracted into the palm.

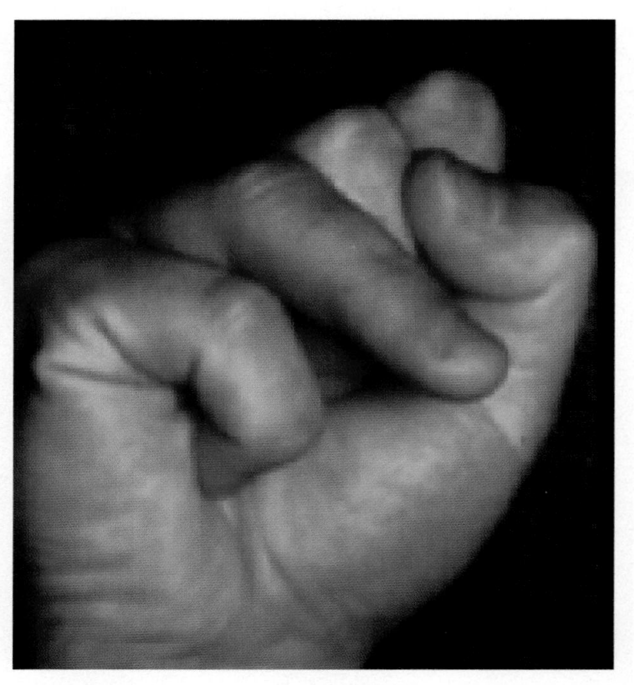

Figure 19.4. Avulsion of the FDP of the ring finger with retraction to the level of the PIP joint. Note the inability to fully flex at the PIP joint.

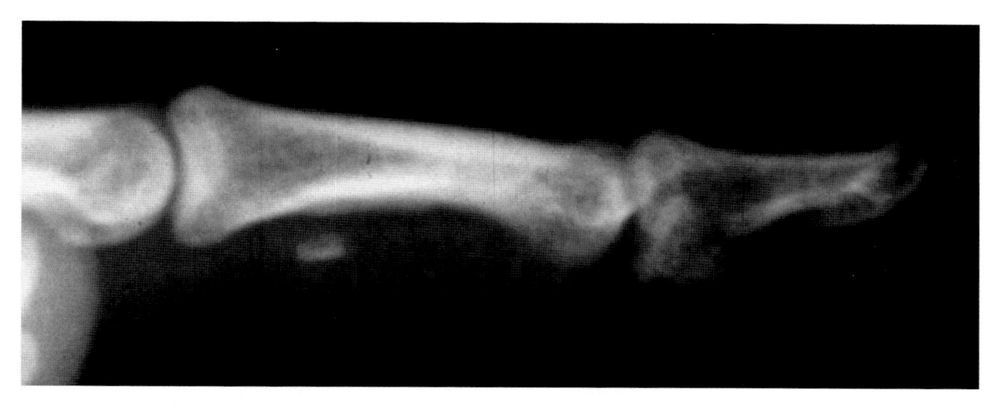

Figure 19.5. X ray of a type II injury. Note the small fleck of bone just distal to the PIP joint. The tendon was found at this level.

X-rays are often normal for type I and II injuries. However, it may be possible to see a fleck of bone at the distal end of the tendon with a type II injury (Fig. 19.5). In type III injuries, the x-ray shows a large fragment of bone held up at the A4 pulley. In type IIIB injuries, that fragment is still seen but a smaller fragment may be visualized more proximally at the PIP joint, indicating the true level of retraction. In type IV injuries, the displaced comminuted intra-articular fracture is easily visible.

Magnetic resonance imaging and ultrasound have both been reported to help locate the distal end of the tendon. These modalities are not commonly used by the senior author. Trumble reported on six cases in which the tendon retracted farther than the fracture pattern suggested. He stated that fracture patterns are not reliable in predicting the location of the retracted tendon end preoperatively. We agree with this assessment.

ACUTE TREATMENT

Type I and II FDP Avulsions

Surgery for a type I avulsion depends on the timing of the diagnosis. First, it must be recognized that these temporal guidelines are not firm and that the capability to advance a viable tendon to its anatomic insertion may be inexplicably prolonged well beyond the 7- to 10-day period in some patients. This phenomenon seems to be particularly prevalent in younger patient populations.

If the lesion is noticed within 7 to 10 days, primary repair is recommended. If repair is not carried out in this timeframe, the tendon may become necrotic and shortened. It gets swollen and edematous and cannot be pulled back through the pulley system. If repair is attempted after 10 days, the tendon may be too short, resulting in the inability to obtain full extension. Reattaching this foreshortened tendon may result in flexion deformities or the quadrigia effect on adjacent digits.

In a type II injury, some diffusion and perfusion are preserved. Reinsertion can be attempted up to 6 weeks or more after injury. These injuries should be surgically repaired as soon as possible. If the injury is more than a few weeks old and the tendon is at the level of the PIP joint, excising granulation tissue and obtaining full passive motion during reinsertion will improve functional outcome. The motor unit does not shorten dramatically with a type II injury. A type II injury may convert to a type I injury with continued participation in athletics or use of the injured finger.

The Surgical Technique for Type I and II Injuries

Either general, regional, or Bier block anesthesia is acceptable for the operation. Make a midaxial or volar zigzag (Bruner) incision on the affected finger, exposing the flexor

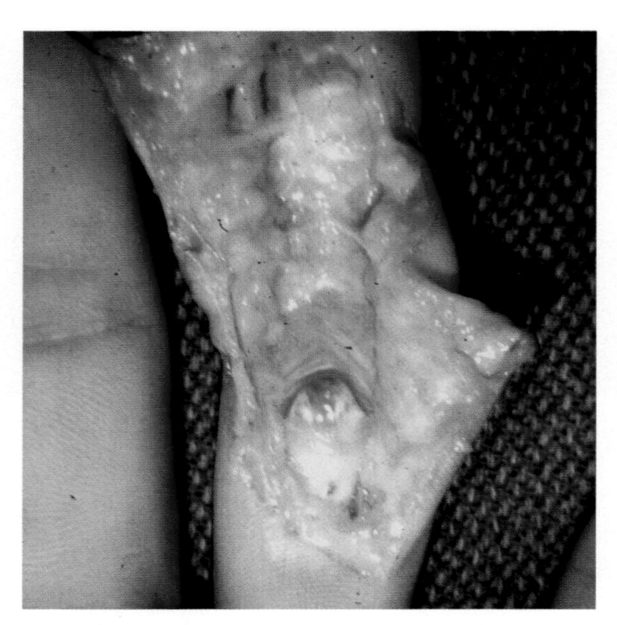

Figure 19.6. Type II injury. The distal stump is held at the A3 pulley. The incision is just distal to the A2 pulley.

sheath from the level just proximal to the PIP joint to the insertion of the FDP tendon on the distal phalanx. The advantage of the midaxial incision is that there is no skin scar directly over the flexor tendons and, therefore, less risk of adhesions. The advantage of the Bruner incision is equivalent visibility and familiarity to most surgeons treating hand problems.

Once the flexor tendon mechanism is exposed, make a transverse incision in the sheath just distal to the A2 pulley to look for the tendon end (Fig. 19.6). If it is not at this level, turn your attention to the palm. Make a small incision just proximal to the A1 pulley, and the tendon should be right in that vicinity and often coincident with the level of greatest palmar tenderness to palpation, a location that can be identified and marked before anesthetizing the patient (Fig. 19.7).

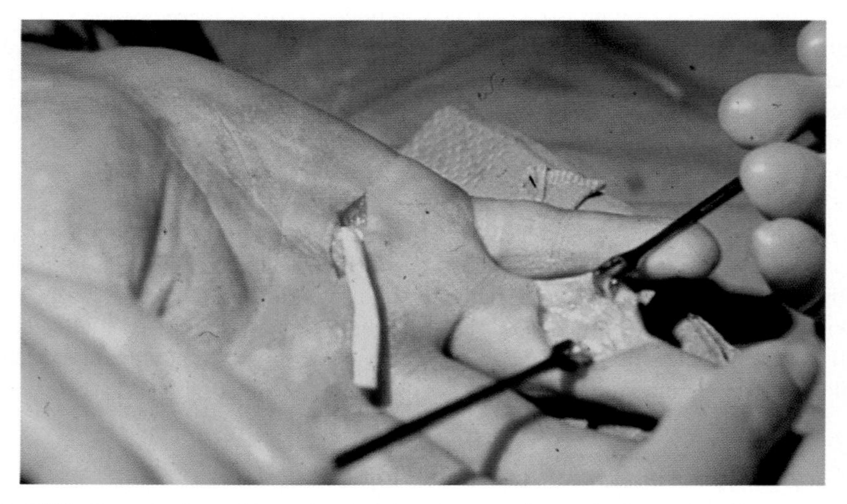

Figure 19.7. Type I injury. The retracted tendon was found in the palm. Exposure of the flexor sheath is now being performed.

Preserve all annular pulleys and sacrifice a cruciform pulley only when absolutely necessary. Pulleys A2 and A4 are extremely important and should not be injured (Fig. 19.8). These pulleys prevent bowstringing of the tendons. Incise the sheath proximal to the A1 pulley. Identify the retracted flexor tendon and pull the tendon end into the wound.

Pass a small pliable catheter, such as an infant-feeding gastrostomy tube, from the PIP joint to exit proximal to the A1 pulley. Pass the catheter through the superficialis decussation. Take care not to damage the pulley system as the catheter is inserted. Attach the distal end of the retracted tendon to the proximal end of the gastrostomy tube with nonabsorbable sutures. Take care to minimize handling of the distal end of the tendon. Minimal handling will decrease the risk of adhesion formation. Pull the catheter distally to slide the tendon under the pulleys and through the superficialis decussation to exit distal to the A2 pulley (Fig. 19.9). Then pass the tendon end beneath the sheath and under the A4 pulley to the level of the distal phalanx using the same tube.

Reinsert the tendon into the base of the distal phalanx through a raised osteoperiosteal flap using the standard pullout suture-and-button technique. We use a synthetic monofilament such as 4-0 Prolene. Elevate an osteoperiosteal flap on the distal phalanx just distal to the volar plate. Take special care to not injure the volar plate of the DIP while inserting the tendon. Pass the ends of the suture through the distal phalanx to exit through the nail plate using a Kirschner wire and Keith needles. With the tendon in the osteoperiosteal flap, tie the sutures over a button on top of the nail plate (Fig. 19.10). Some authors prefer using suture anchors to attach the tendon to bone. Do not directly suture the tendon to the periosteum or soft tissues of the distal phalanx. In our opinion, this is an inadequate way of anchoring the tendon.

The end result should have each finger with the natural arcade restored (Fig. 19.11). Apply a dorsal splint with the wrist in slight flexion, MCP joints in 70 degrees of flexion, and the PIP and DIP joints in relative extension.

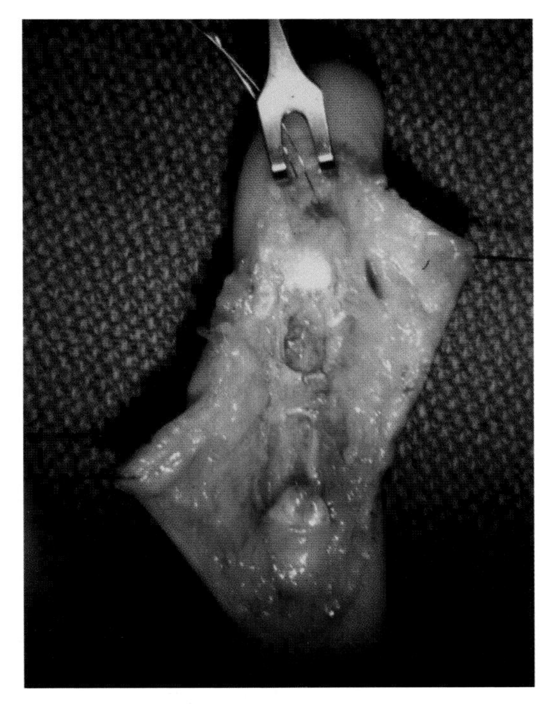

Figure 19.8. Type II injury. The tendon is found at the level of the PIP joint under the A3 pulley. The cruciform pulleys have been removed. An osteoperiosteal flap has been made just distal to the volar plate in the distal phalanx.

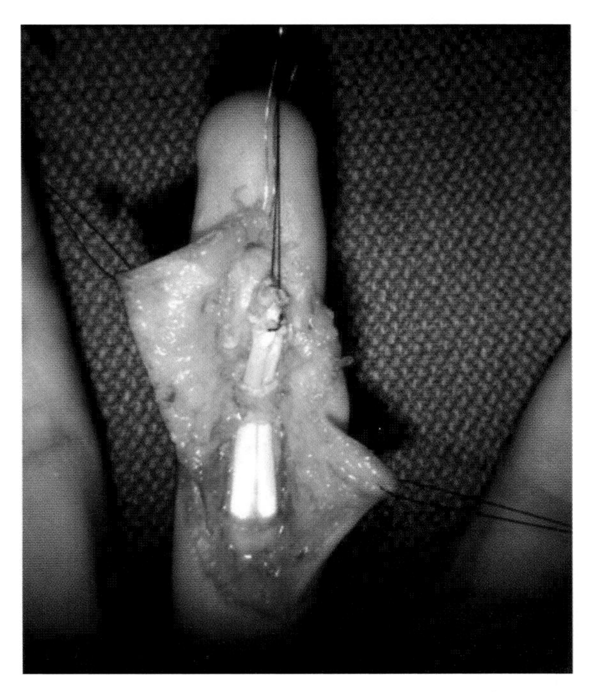

Figure 19.9. FDP threaded under the A3 and A4 pulleys.

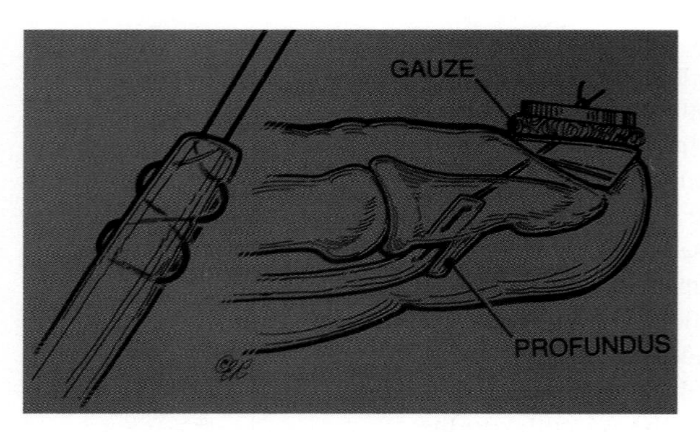

Figure 19.10. Distal juncture technique. The suture is done with 3-0 or 4-0 Prolene. It is removed distally by pulling on one of the ends of the Prolene suture at the time of button removal. (Reprinted with permission from Schneider LH: Flexor Tendons: Late Reconstruction. In: Green DP, Hotchkiss RN, Pederson WC, eds. *Green's Operative Hand Surgery.* 4th ed. Philadelphia: Churchill Livingstone, 1999:1907.)

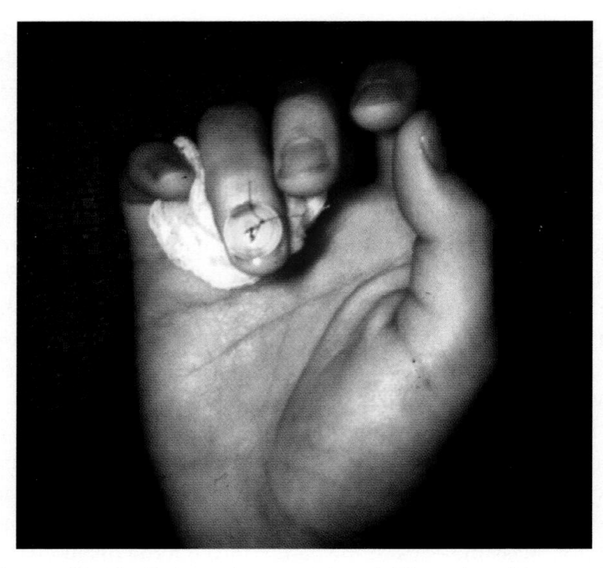

Figure 19.11. Reinsertion completed. There is evidence of a symmetric cascade, with each finger slightly less flexed than its ulnar neighbor. A Prolene suture is tied over a button.

Type III FDP Avulsions

With a type III injury, the bony fragment is held by the A4 pulley. Tendon nutrition and length are preserved, and both vincular systems are still attached. Recognizing both the orientation and position of the fracture fragment is helpful in determining if the tendon is still attached. If the bony fragment is caught at the level of the A4 pulley, the tendon is probably still attached. If the axis of the fragment is transverse, or not at the level of the A4 pulley, then it is likely that the tendon has detached from this piece of bone.

Repair a type III injury by opening and reducing the fracture site. Use either Kirschner wires or mini fragment screws to secure the fragment to bone. If the tendon has separated from the fracture fragment, first fix the fracture by open reduction and internal fixation. Then reattach the tendon to bone in the same way mentioned for type I and II injuries.

Postoperative Management

Aftercare for each type of injury is similar. Passive flexion exercises may be instituted early. Remove the splint at 4 weeks and start protected active motion. Remove the Prolene suture at 3 to 4 weeks. Rehabilitation is then similar to that for other flexor tendon injuries. At the time of suture removal, cut one end of the suture and pull the other through the tendon and bone. An advantage of Prolene is that it slides easily through these tissues. In type III, IIIB, and IV injuries, the hardware can be removed if necessary when the bone is sufficiently healed. No strenuous sports activities or heavy work is permitted for at least 10 to 12 weeks.

TREATMENT OF REMOTE OR CHRONIC FDP AVULSION INJURIES

Optimal treatment is controversial when the patient presents beyond the window for acute treatment of the tendon avulsion. Options include an informed decision to forgo surgical intervention, arthrodesis of the DIP joint, tenodesis of the DIP joint, and tendon grafting in one or two stages. In asymptomatic patients with stable DIP joints and those in whom loss of active DIP flexion will have little or no affect on their pursuits, no surgical intervention is generally recommended. Patients are able to obtain a satisfactory range of composite (PIP, MCP) motion with only superficialis function. Full superficialis function should give a 210 degree total arc of motion. Patients will lack active DIP flexion and some power grip and pinch strength. The pain in the palm from the retracted tendon usually disappears within 6 months, but if not, the tendon can be excised as a short outpatient procedure without undue recovery time and no additional morbidity to the adjacent rays.

The indications for arthrodesis of the DIP joint include instability and recurrent dorsal dislocations of the joint. The advantage of an arthrodesis is that the procedure will produce a stable joint that will not interfere with superficialis tendon function. Tenodesis of the DIP joint, like arthrodesis, is indicated for instability. Tenodesis is a technically difficult procedure with unpredictable outcome. The tendon or volar soft-tissue structures can stretch out over time. In many cases there is no FDP tendon remaining on the distal phalanx, making the operation much more difficult. Therefore, volar plate advancement or a free tendon graft needs to be inserted into both the distal and middle phalanges. We prefer arthrodesis to tenodesis when faced with the proper indications for a stabilizing procedure of the DIP joint.

In a patient who requires increased grip and pinch strength and active flexion of the DIP joint, tendon grafting in one or two stages can be recommended. This might apply to a skilled laborer, a musician, or an athlete. Tendon grafting in the face of an active and functioning superficialis tendon can be a dangerous procedure. If scarring and adhesions limit the function of the superficialis tendon, the patient may lose motion and function and actually be worse off than he/she was before the procedure. McClinton and Curtis recommended passing the graft around the superficialis to prevent this complication. Stark, Goldner, and Coonrad and others have listed their indications for this procedure in a thoughtful manner. We agree with their suggestions and prefer a tendon graft done in two stages, with a silicone rod, when faced with this situation.

There is an extensive discussion of staged flexor tendon grafting offered in companion chapters in this volume.

REHABILITATION

Rehabilitation is the same as for other flexor tendon injuries. When the strength of the repair is adequate, the patient can embark confidently on one of the many documented programs for zone I tendon repairs. Supervision by a skilled therapist and intermittent visits to the surgeon will document milestones and accelerate selected aspects of the program as needed. After motion recovery, and at a logical postoperative time to ensure tendon healing, a strengthening program can commence and return to play or work decisions can be individualized.

RESULTS

In patients who are seen early and treated with reinsertion of the tendon, a satisfactory result can be expected. There may be a 10- to 15-degree loss of extension at the DIP joint, but grip strength is near normal. A fusion or tenodesis will result in a stable joint, but grip strength will not improve. If tendon grafting is successful, the patient will benefit from a stable joint, active range of motion, and improved grip strength.

In patients seen remotely from the time of the injury, the opportunity to restore full digital function, especially DIP motion, diminishes. Optimal results are usually obtained with type II and III avulsions when the tendon was never deprived of its vincular blood supply and intrasynovial nutrition. Of course, complex fractures involving the DIP joint (type IV injuries) have the additional challenges of potential arthrosis or instability.

COMPLICATIONS

Patients treated without operation have few long-term complications. An unstable joint is the most common and can be treated with an arthrodesis if painful or dysfunctional.

Complications of acute repair include loss of fixation, loss of motion, instability of the DIP joint, weak pinch and grip strength, and infection. Loss of motion, if significant, may require tenolysis and/or tendon grafting. Loss of fixation, if seen early, may be treated with reoperation. Infection is treated immediately with wound debridement and appropriate antibiotics. The treatments for instability of the joint and weak pinch and grip strength are already described earlier.

RECOMMENDED READING

1. Bynum DK, Gilbert JA. Avulsion of the flexor digitorum profundus: anatomic and biomechanical considerations. *J Hand Surg* 13A:222–227, 1988.
2. Carroll RE, Match RM. Avulsion of the profundus tendon insertion. *J Trauma* 10:1109–1110, 1970.
3. Davis C, Armstrong J. Spontaneous flexor tendon rupture in the palm: the role of a variation of tendon anatomy. *J Hand Surg* 28A:149–152, 2003.
4. Goldner JL, Coonrad RW. Tendon grafting of the flexor profundus in the presence of a completely or partially intact flexor sublimis. *J Bone Joint Surg* 51A:527–532, 1969.
5. Langa V, Posner MA. Unusual rupture of a flexor profundus tendon. *J Hand Surg* 11A:227–229, 1986.
6. Leddy JP. Avulsions of the flexor digitorum profundus. *Hand Clinics* 1:77–83, 1985.
7. Leddy JP, Packer JW. Avulsion of the profundus insertion in athletes. *J Hand Surg* 2A:66–68, 1977.
8. McMaster PE. Tendon and muscle ruptures: clinical and experimental studies on the causes and location of subcutaneous ruptures. *J Bone Joint Surg* 15:705, 1933.
9. Manske PR, Lesker PA. Avulsion of the ring finger digitorum profundus tendon: an experimental study. *Hand* 10:52–55, 1978
10. Robins PR, Dobyns JH. Avulsion of the Insertion of the Flexor Digitorum Profundus Tendon Associated with Fracture of the Distal Phalanx. In: *American Academy of Orthopaedic Surgeons: Symposium on Tendon Surgery in the Hand.* St. Louis: CV Mosby, 1975:151–156.
11. Schneider LH. Flexor Tendons: Late Reconstruction. In: Green DP, Hotchkiss RN, Pederson WC, eds. *Green's Operative Hand Surgery*. 4th ed. Philadelphia: Churchill Livingstone, 1999:1898–1949.
12. Smith JH. Avulsion of the profundus tendon with simultaneous intraarticular fracture of the distal phalanx: case report. *J Hand Surg* 6:600–601, 1981.
13. Stamos BD, Leddy JP. Closed flexor tendon disruption in athletes. *Hand Clinics* 16:359–365, 2000.
14. Stark HH, Zemel NP, Boyes JH, et al. Flexor tendon graft through intact superficialis tendon. *J Hand Surg* 2:456–461, 1977.
15. Trumble TE, Vedder NB, Benirschke SK. Misleading fractures after profundus tendon avulsions: a report of six cases. *J Hand Surg* 17A:902–906, 1992.
16. Von Zander. *Trommerlahmung Inaug* [dissertation]. Berlin, 1891.

20

Correction of Post-Traumatic Extensor Tendon Ulnar Subluxation of the Metacarpophalangeal Joint with a Dynamic Lumbrical Tendon Transfer

Keith A. Segalman and E. F. Shaw Wilgis

INDICATIONS/CONTRAINDICATIONS

Post-traumatic failure of the sagittal bands at the level of the metacarpophalangeal (MCP) joint results in extensor tendon instability. When the extensor tendon is no longer centered over the MCP joint, there is a resultant loss of extension of the finger. Legoust first described traumatic extensor tendon instability in 1866. Paget, Krukenberg, and Marsh provided later descriptions of the condition. The technique described here has not been previously described.

PHYSICAL EXAMINATION

The sagittal band (SB) is the main stabilizer of the extensor digitorum tendon at the level of the metacarpal phalangeal joint. The SB forms a cylindrical tube surrounding the metacarpal head and the metacarpal phalangeal (MCP) joint (Fig. 20.1). The sagittal fibers are superficial to the MCP joint capsule, and there is no communication between the sagit-

Keith A. Segalman, M.D.: Department of Orthopaedic Surgery, Johns Hopkins Hospital, Baltimore, MD
E. F. Shaw Wilgis, M.D.: Greater Chesapeake Specialists, Lutherville, MD

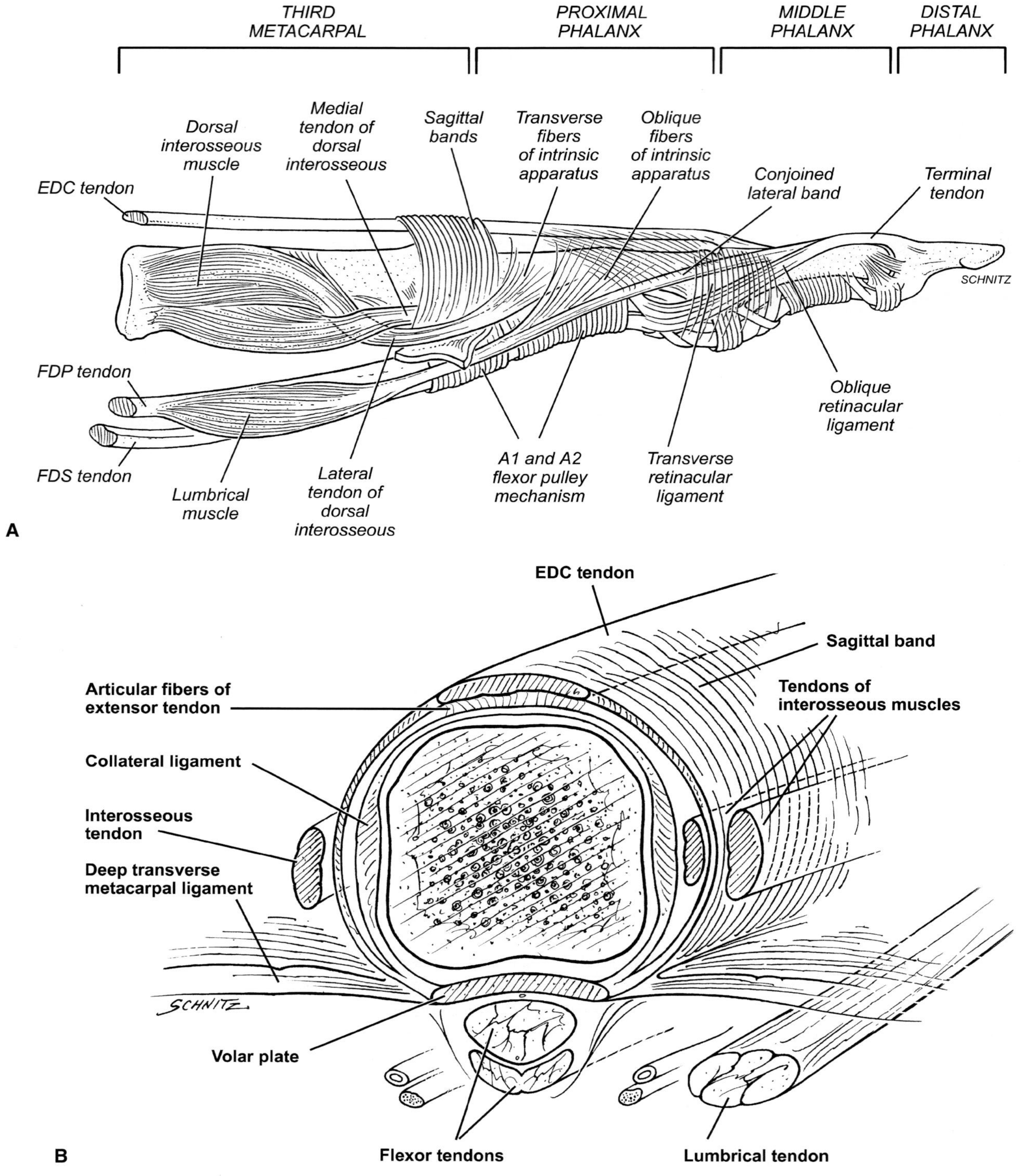

Figure 20.1. Normal anatomy of the MCP joint (**A**) and the sagittal fibers (**B**).

tal fibers and the collateral ligaments. The radial SB is thinner and longer than the ulnar fibers. The SB is thicker in the central digits and thinner in the peripheral digits. The greatest tension in the SB is noted with MCP flexion and radioulnar deviation, with a vast majority of the injuries occurring on the radial side. Biomechanical studies have shown that greater than 50% of the proximal radial fibers must be torn to create extensor tendon instability (Fig. 20.2).

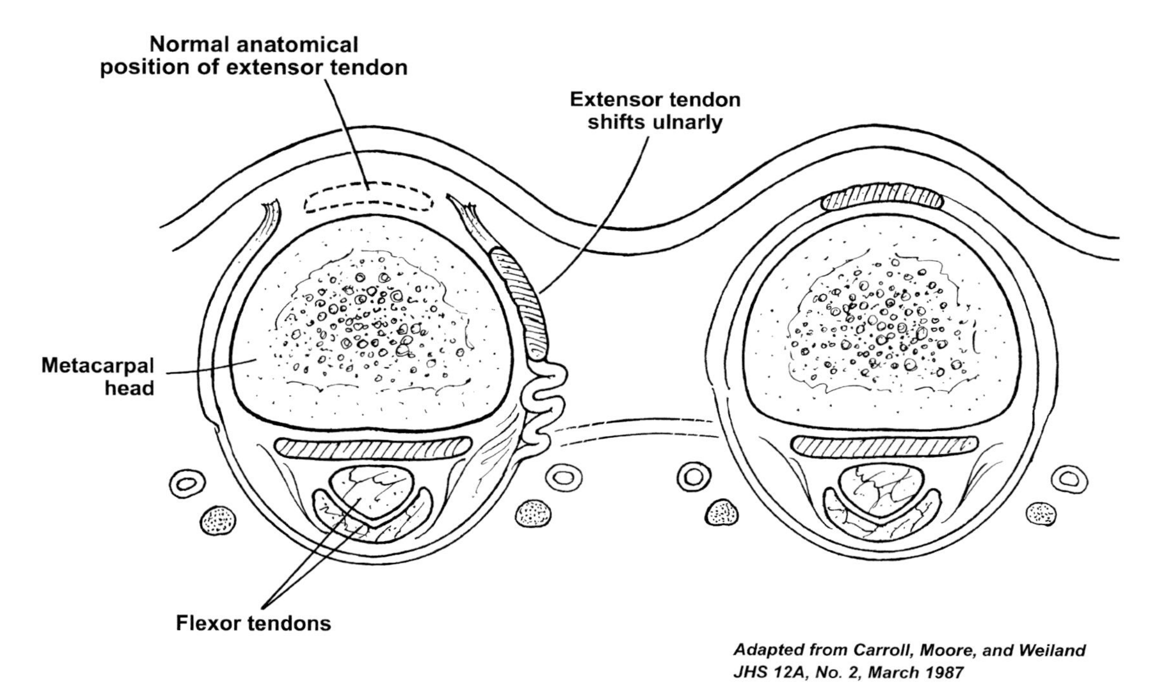

Figure 20.2. Diagram of SB injury.

The usual mechanism of injury is a blow to the hand with the MCPs flexed, such as a boxing injury. SB injuries occur when the finger is forced into flexion with the wrist flexed and ulnarly deviated. Rarely, a SB injury may be associated with collateral ligament injuries. The patient will usually present with swelling and tenderness over the SB and limited or deviated extension of the MCP joint. The most telltale finding is a painful snapping sensation with concomitant ulnar subluxation of the extensor during active MCP flexion (Fig. 20.3). Rayan and Murray described a provocative test for SB injury: resisted finger extension and attempted deviation toward the injured SB elicits apprehension and pain.

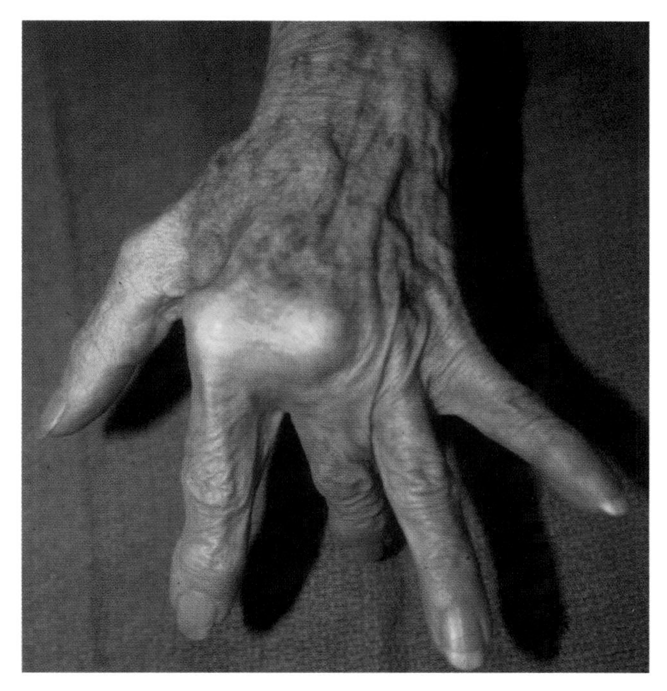

Figure 20.3. Clinical photograph showing the subluxation of the extensor tendon.

Two classification systems have been described, but in our opinion neither fully characterizes the clinical situation. Ishizuki differentiates ruptures of the SB secondary to superficial tears and deep tears. Rayan and Murray have described a more treatment-oriented classification system of three varieties emphasizing whether the SB is torn or there is subluxation of the tendon. What is most important is the assessment of the passive motion in the joint and the stability of the contralateral ligaments.

For acute injuries, immobilization with a cast or Orthoplast splint with the MCP joints in extension and the wrist in neutral is often satisfactory. Rayan and Murray have reported that conservative treatment is most successful when begun within 3 weeks of the injury, whereas Inoue recommended repair or reconstruction when the patient is seen more than 2 weeks after the injury. Occasionally, conservative treatment is unsuccessful, but most patients with SB injuries will present with a chronic condition.

Extensor tendon instability is most common in the middle finger, followed by the small, index, and ring fingers. Various authors have suggested that the middle finger is most often involved because of the cross-sectional thickness of the SB, the distal attachment of the extensor hood, or the increased proximal-distal length of the SB. These authors noted a less well-developed juncture tendinum in the radial two digits and excessive ulnar deviation of the metacarpal head in the middle finger versus the ulnar two digits. In our experience, the middle finger is most often involved.

PREOPERATIVE PLANNING

It is imperative to ensure that there is full passive motion in the digit. Radiographs should be obtained to confirm that there is no underlying fracture or arthritis. There is no role for arthrography or arthroscopy in the treatment of this condition

The lumbrical muscle is chosen for its radial location, ease of harvest, and most importantly its synergistic action to stabilize and radicalize the extensor tendon. The lumbrical muscle inserts in the transverse or oblique fibers of the extensor, with half of the fingers having an additional attachment to tendon or bone (Fig. 20.4). The lumbrical has no role in MCP flexion, whereas the interossei are the main flexors of the proximal phalanx. Electromyographic studies have determined that the lumbrical fires with digital flexion to prevent clawing. Since extensor instability is most pronounced with MCP flexion, transferring the lumbrical will serve as a direct antagonist to the deforming force of the extensor. Thus, the lumbrical acts as a dynamic tendon transfer to correct ulnar subluxation of the extensor.

SURGERY

Local anesthesia with sedation is the preferred choice, but regional anesthesia is an acceptable alternative. The patient is positioned supine on the operating room table. An upper arm tourniquet is applied, and the arm is draped in a standard fashion. After exsanguination of the arm, a dorsal 4-cm incision is centered over the MCP joint (Fig. 20.5). The pathology is confirmed, and the extensor is reduced over the MCP joint.

Reduction of the extensor typically does not require release of the ulnar sagittal fibers. The lumbrical is harvested just proximal to its insertion into the oblique fibers and gently mobilized proximally (Fig. 20.6). Care is taken to avoid detaching the tendon from the muscle belly and separating the lumbrical from the interossei. Because the lumbrical and interossei join into one conjoined tendon, the lumbrical could easily be separated from the muscle belly if the surgeon is not careful.

An isometric point is chosen for passage of the transfer by holding the extensor reduced with a pair of forceps and gently ranging the finger or asking the patient to gently flex the finger. The tendon of the lumbrical is now passed through a small longitudinal slit in the extensor at the isometric point (Fig. 20.7). The tension is set by ranging the finger and ensuring that the extensor does not subluxate ulnarly. If the ulnar sagittal fibers were released and excess tension was applied to the transfer, then radial subluxation would result. A non-

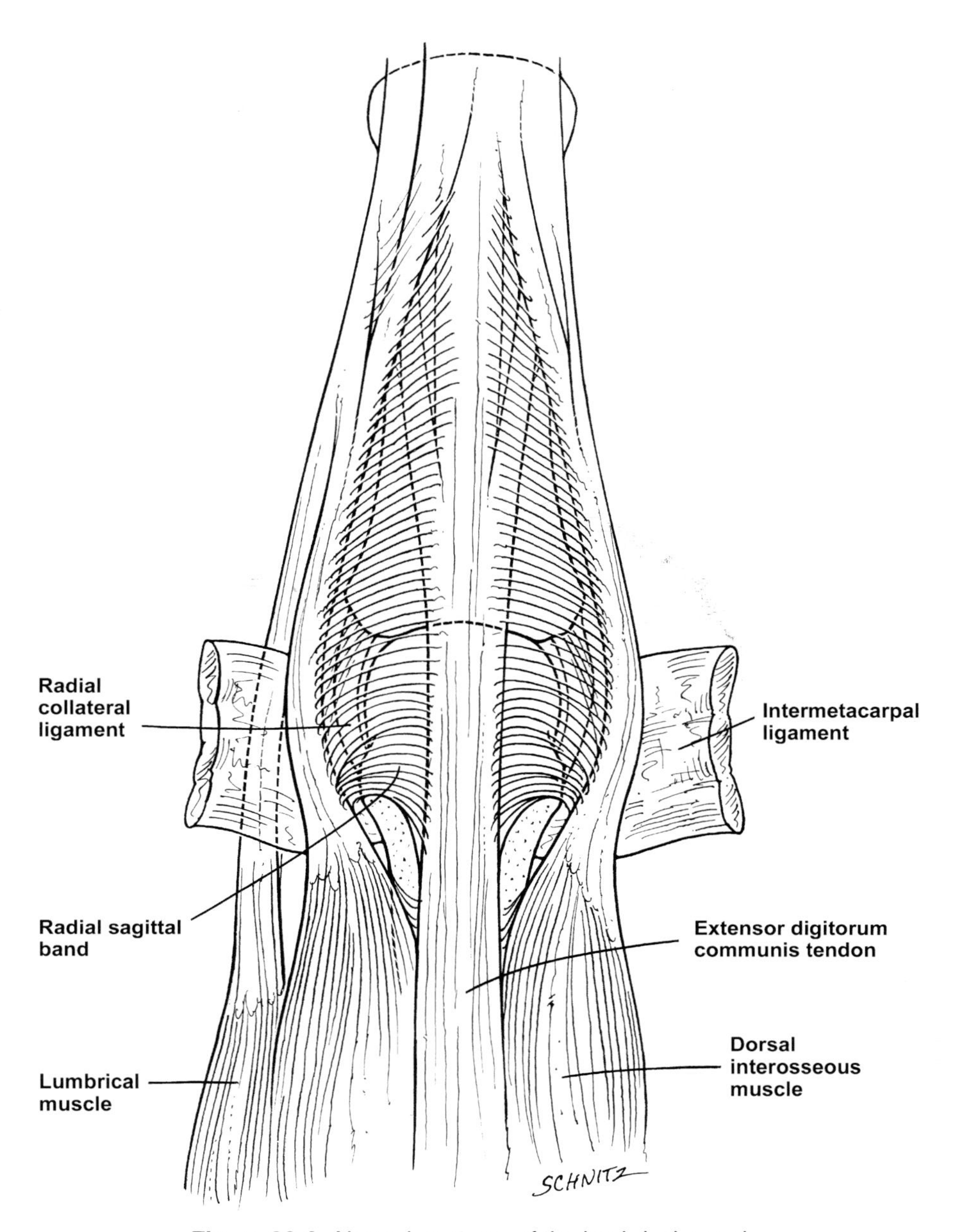

Figure 20.4. Normal anatomy of the lumbrical muscle.

absorbable 4–0 suture is used to secure the transfer. The wound is closed with nonabsorbable sutures, and the patient is immobilized in a short splint with the MCP joints in extension and the proximal interphalangeal joints free.

POSTOPERATIVE MANAGEMENT

The sutures are removed 8 to 10 days after the surgery, and immobilization is continued for a total of 4 weeks after surgery. We prefer a short arm cast with the wrist in neutral and the MCP joints in extension. It is important to leave the proximal interphalangeal joints free. Dynamic extensor splinting is not usually used, but it is a reasonable alternative. The patient is expected to regain nearly full motion and strength.

Active motion is begun 4 weeks after surgery, and strengthening is begun 6 weeks after surgery. The patient will continue with therapy for approximately 6 to 8 weeks (Fig. 20.8).

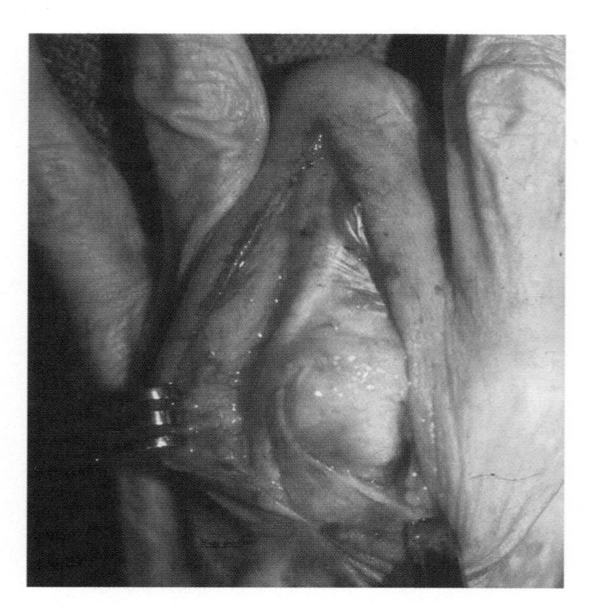

Figure 20.5. Dorsal incision over the MP joint demonstrating ulnar subluxation of the extensor and attenuation of the radial sagittal fibers.

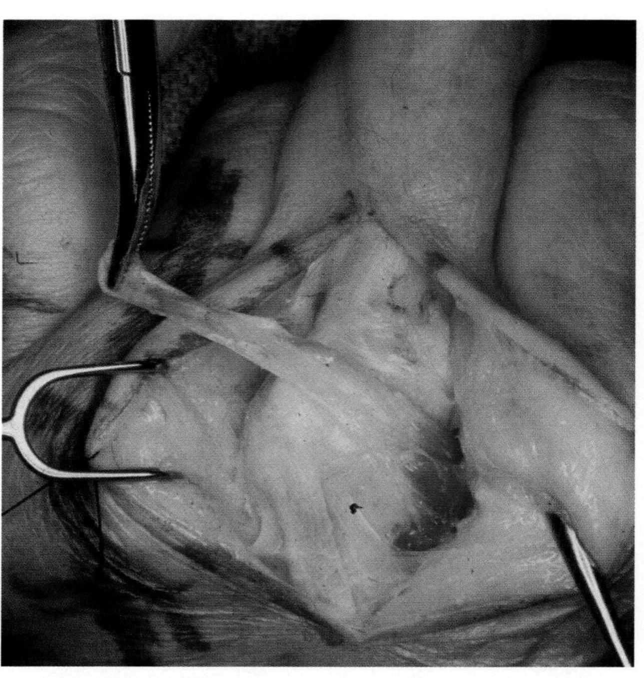

Figure 20.6. Harvesting the lumbrical from just proximal to its tendinous insertion.

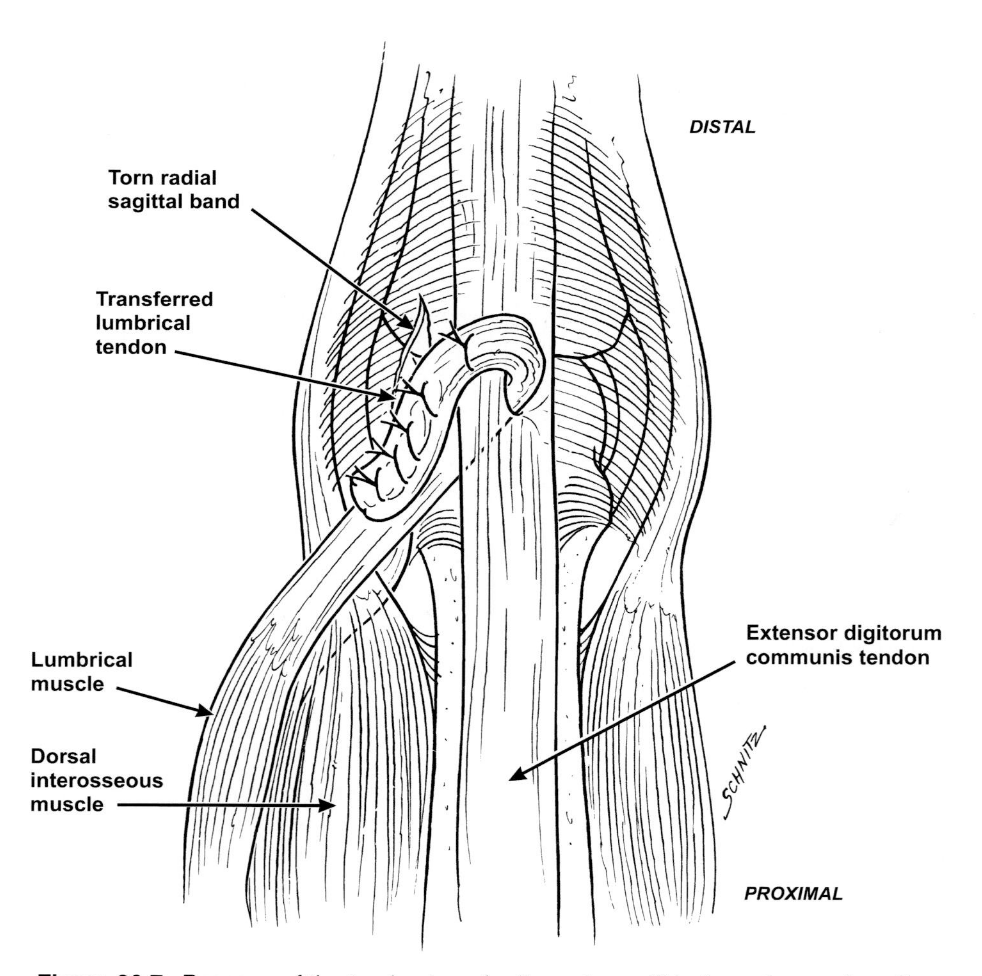

Figure 20.7. Passage of the tendon transfer through a split in the extensor dorsally.

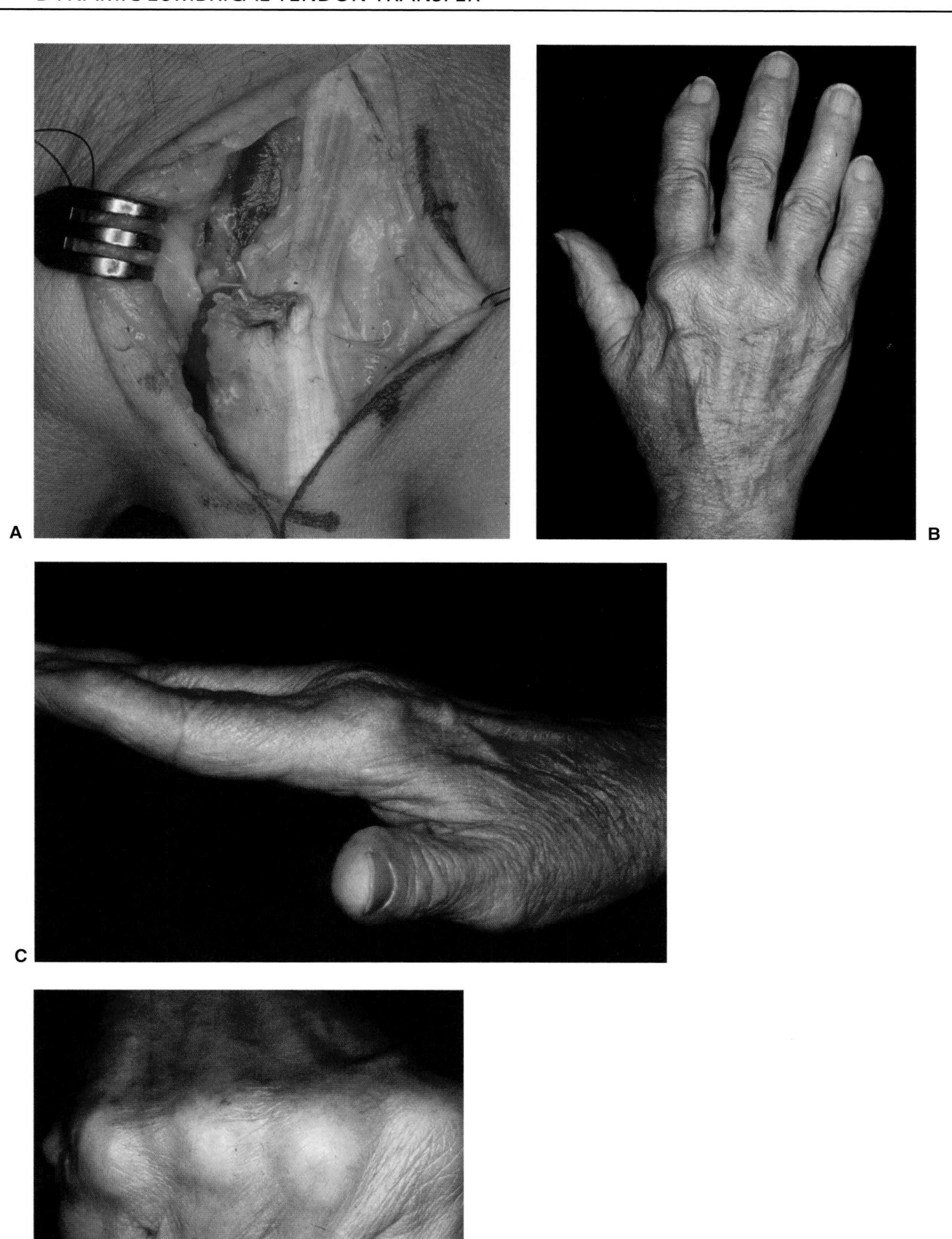

Figure 20.8. Intraoperative photograph (**A**) and postoperative photographs after lumbrical transfer for extensor tendon instability. Postoperative dorsal view (**B**), active extension (**C**), and active flexion and centralization of the tendon (**D**) are shown.

Minimal loss of motion is expected from this technique. The patient should be able to return to normal activities within 3 months. In our experience, there has never been a recurrence.

RESULTS

Stiffness is rarely a problem after the procedure, as the joint capsule is not violated. In our experience, patients have averaged 90 degrees of MCP motion. We have not seen any recurrence of the deformity, and all patients have been satisfied with the procedure. No interphalangeal stiffness has been identified.

COMPLICATIONS

The complication rate is very low. Superficial infection has only occurred in one patient, and this was successfully treated with oral antibiotics without the need for further surgery. No deep infection has been identified, and we feel that there is no indication to routinely use preoperative antibiotics. As noted above, the surgeon should expect minimal stiffness after the surgery. Radial deviation has not been seen and would not occur with normal bony architecture. There has not been any need for secondary surgery, and all patients were satisfied with the procedure. In theory, a failure could result in recurrent subluxation after removal of the cast. If recurrence occurred, we would prefer the technique described by Carroll et al.

CONCLUSIONS

A lumbrical muscle transfer provides excellent correction for SB ruptures of the extensor located over the MCP joint. The lumbrical is a dynamic transfer easily harvested, which minimizes stiffness. Complications are few, and recurrence has not been observed in our series of patients.

RECOMMENDED READING

1. Carroll C, Moore JR, Weiland AJ. Posttraumatic ulnar subluxation of the extensor tendons: a reconstructive technique. *J Hand Surg* 12A:227–231, 1987.
2. Inoue G, Tamura Y. Dislocation of the extensor tendons over the metacarpophalangeal joints. *J Hand Surg* 21A:464–469, 1996.
3. Murray D, Rayan GM. Late reconstruction of sagittal band laceration. *Orthop Rev* 23:445–447, 1994.
4. Rayan GM, Murray D. Classification and treatment of closed sagittal band injuries. *J Hand Surg* 19A:590–594, 1994.
5. Ritts GD, Wood MB, Engber WD. Nonoperative treatment of traumatic dislocations of the extensor digitorum tendons in patients without rheumatoid disorders. *J Hand Surg* 10A:714–716, 1985.
6. Saldana MJ, McGuire RA. Chronic painful subluxation of the metacarpal phalangeal joint extensor tendons. *J Hand Surg* 11A:420–423, 1986.
7. Smith RJ. Intrinsic Muscles of the Fingers: Function, Dysfunction, and Surgical Reconstruction. In: *AAOS Instructional Course Lectures.* Vol 24. St. Louis: Mosby, 1975:200–220.
8. Watson HK, Weinzweig J, Guidera PM. Sagittal band reconstruction. *J Hand Surg* 22A:452–456, 1997.

21

Staged Flexor Tendon and Pulley Reconstruction

John S. Taras, Stephen M. Hankins, and
Daniel J. Mastella

STAGE I SURGICAL TECHNIQUES

Staged flexor tendon reconstruction is a salvage operation that can restore function to a digit that has lost function in its flexor tendon system. The technique requires attention to detail by the surgeon and cooperation of the patient in therapy to maximize outcome.

In the badly scarred flexor tendon system, reconstruction is done in stages. The first stage is excision of the scarred tendon, release of joint contractures, placement of a Dacron reinforced silicone passive tendon implant, and reconstruction of the flexor pulley system.

The second stage is replacement of the tendon implant with a tendon graft. The tendon implant allows passive range of motion of the joints and, by sliding with digital motion, encourages the formation of a smooth flexor tendon sheath to accept the tendon graft.

The importance of an adequate pulley system in achieving full and efficient flexion of the digits has been well documented. The flexor tendon pulley system converts the linear excursion and force of the digital flexors to rotation and torque about the finger joints. Failure of the pulley system results in loss of digital motion and flexion contracture. Reconstruction of the pulley system is crucial to optimize the results of flexor tendon reconstruction.

John S. Taras, M.D.: Department of Orthopaedic Surgery, Drexel University/Thomas Jefferson University, and Division of Hand Surgery, Drexel University/Thomas Jefferson University, Philadelphia, PA

Stephen M. Hankins, M.D.: Department of Orthopaedic Surgery, Drexel University, Philadelphia, PA

Daniel J. Mastella, M.D.: Department of Orthopedics, Thomas Jefferson University Hospital and The Philadelphia Hand Center, Philadelphia, PA

Indications and Contraindications

Ultimately, the indication for reconstruction of the flexor pulley system is significant loss of active motion in the digits (Fig. 21.1). Staged flexor tendon reconstruction is indicated in a compliant patient who lacks flexor tendon function due to loss of tendon continuity, scarring within the fibro-osseous theca, and loss of a competent tendon sheath.

In evaluation of the patient with a dysfunctional tendon system, oftentimes it is difficult to assess the degree of damage until surgical exploration is carried out. The surgeon and patient should be prepared for different courses of action depending on the surgical findings. This typically is a choice between tenolysis, primary tendon grafting from palm to fingertip, or a two-stage tendon graft. If bowstringing is evident, motion can be restored during examination with manual pressure to hold the bowed tendon against the phalanx. The effect of pulley reconstruction can be tested with the use of plastic or metal pulley rings (Fig. 21.2), which mimic the effect of pulley reconstruction but with a significantly longer moment arm.

Contraindications to staged flexor tendon reconstruction are ongoing infection, lack of soft-tissue coverage, paralysis of the flexor musculature, and loss of passive digital motion. Appropriate treatment of overlying skin deficits, including flap coverage, should preclude tendon reconstruction. Reconstruction should be undertaken only after maximum passive range of motion has been achieved through therapy and the tissues have reached equilibrium. Relative contraindications include digits with borderline vascularity, bilateral digital nerve injuries, or severe joint degeneration. These digits may be better treated with amputation.

Preoperative Planning

Planning for flexor tendon reconstruction should include plain X rays to ensure that any fractures have healed and assessment of the joint surfaces. Flexor tendon reconstruction re-

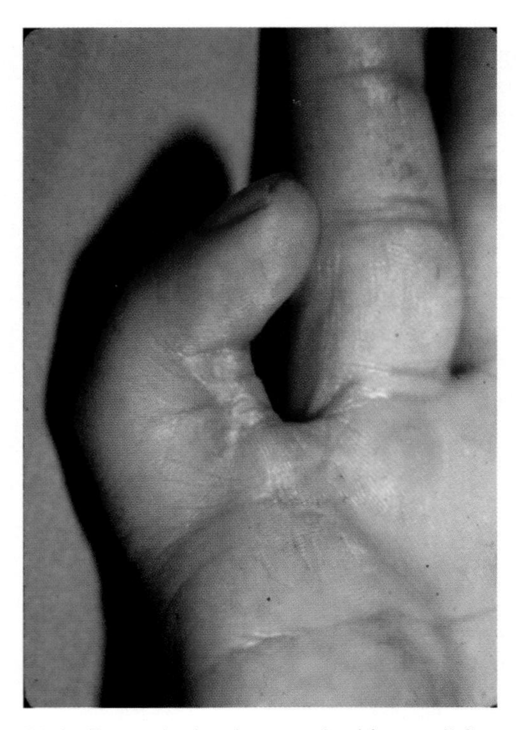

Figure 21.1. Bowstringing is seen in this small finger after primary tendon repair with division of the A2 pulley. The result is loss of active flexion and eventual loss of passive motion.

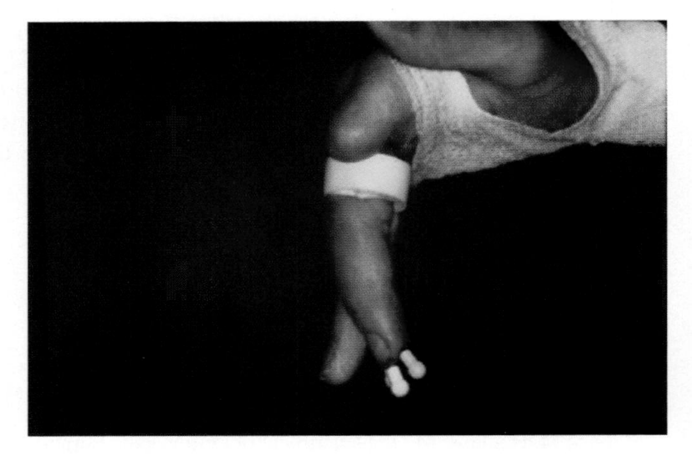

Figure 21.2. A thermoplast pulley ring protects this pulley reconstruction in a severely injured digit.

quires early controlled digit mobilization for success and should not be undertaken during the treatment of fractures.

Preoperative planning requires the location of adequate graft material. The optimal pulley graft would be strong, wide, and have a synovial lining next to the tendon graft and be placed in the optimal position at surgery. Considerable graft material may be needed for pulley reconstruction, and the common sources are the flexor tendons excised at stage I of staged flexor tendon reconstruction or other tendon autograft. Some techniques describe use of the extensor retinaculum (Littler) and the fascia lata as graft material or use of the volar plate as a tendon guide (Karev).

The number of pulleys to reconstruct is a subject of discussion. Barton, Doyle, and Hunter have all confirmed that the A2 and A4 pulleys are the most critical to reconstruct. Further work seems to indicate that A2 and A4 are not more important if the rest of the sheath is intact. Reconstruction of four or five pulleys seems to be optimal, but three or four are typically all that are practical to reconstruct without impairing digit motion. At a minimum, pulleys should be reconstructed at the base of the proximal phalanx, just distal to the metacarpophalangeal (MP) joint, and at the base of the middle phalanx, just distal to the proximal interphalangeal joint.

Surgery

The patient is supine on the operating table, and the index extremity and any limb from which tendon graft will be harvested have deflated pneumatic tourniquets applied and are sterile prepped. A Bruner-type zigzag incision is preferred for tenolysis and excision of tendon, but note that others prefer a midaxial approach. Great care is used to protect the neurovascular bundle and preserve critical native pulleys as much as possible. Joint contractures are then released, and the tendon implant is placed. The tendon implant should never be touched by gloved hands to limit foreign material from adhering to the implant, which will lead to a greater inflammatory response. The implant is handled only with clean smooth forceps to limit injury to the implant. The implant size should approximate the size of the planned graft, with 3- to 4-mm implants used for plantaris and palmaris grafts and 5- to 6-mm implants used for flexor digitorum superficialis and toe flexor grafts.

The implant is sutured to the distal stump of the FDP (Fig. 21.3) and threaded through the intact portions of the sheath to lie in the distal forearm, or palm, depending on the planned length of the graph. Pulleys are then reconstructed over the tendon implant where necessary.

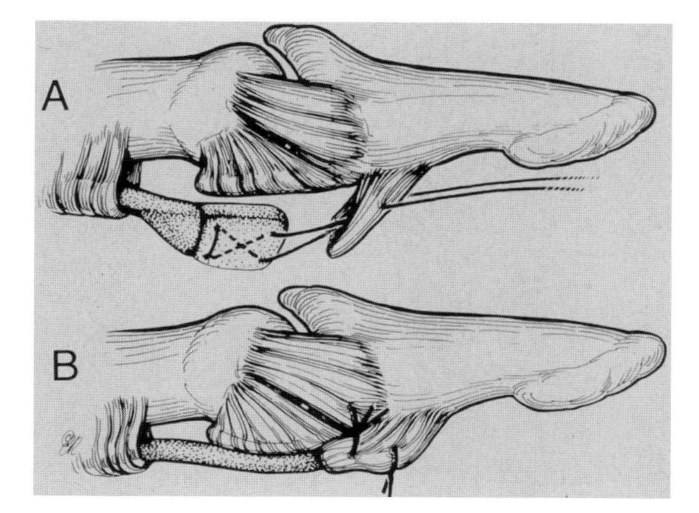

Figure 21.3. The distal tendon implant juncture. Great care must be used to avoid any contamination of the implant with foreign material. Foreign bodies such as talc from surgical gloves can cause a sterile synovitis and compromise staged flexor tendon reconstruction.

A circumferential pulley is created using the method of Bunnell (Fig. 21.4). Either excised flexor tendons or tendon grafts are used as material for reconstruction. At the proximal phalanx level, the tendon is placed deep to the neurovascular bundles and beneath the extensor mechanism to prevent compression of the intrinsic system (Fig. 21.5). At the middle phalanx level, the graft has traditionally been placed over the extensor mechanism; however, we have placed the graft between the tendon and middle phalanx without difficulties.

Several methods can facilitate the placement of tendon material. A curved, small cardiovascular ligature carrier can be used, with sutures placed through the tendon graft attached through the eyelet in the ligature carrier and drawn around the phalanx with the instrument. The graft follows the suture into position and is repaired snugly over the tendon implant. Alternatively, a Penrose drain can be passed around the phalanx using a right-angled hemostat. The graft material is slipped into the drain and carried atraumatically around the phalanx on removal of the drain. This is particularly effective when the material used is extensor retinaculum. Finally, Sanders has described the use of a 0.028-inch Kirschner wire bent into a hairpin loop to facilitate the passage of pulley material.

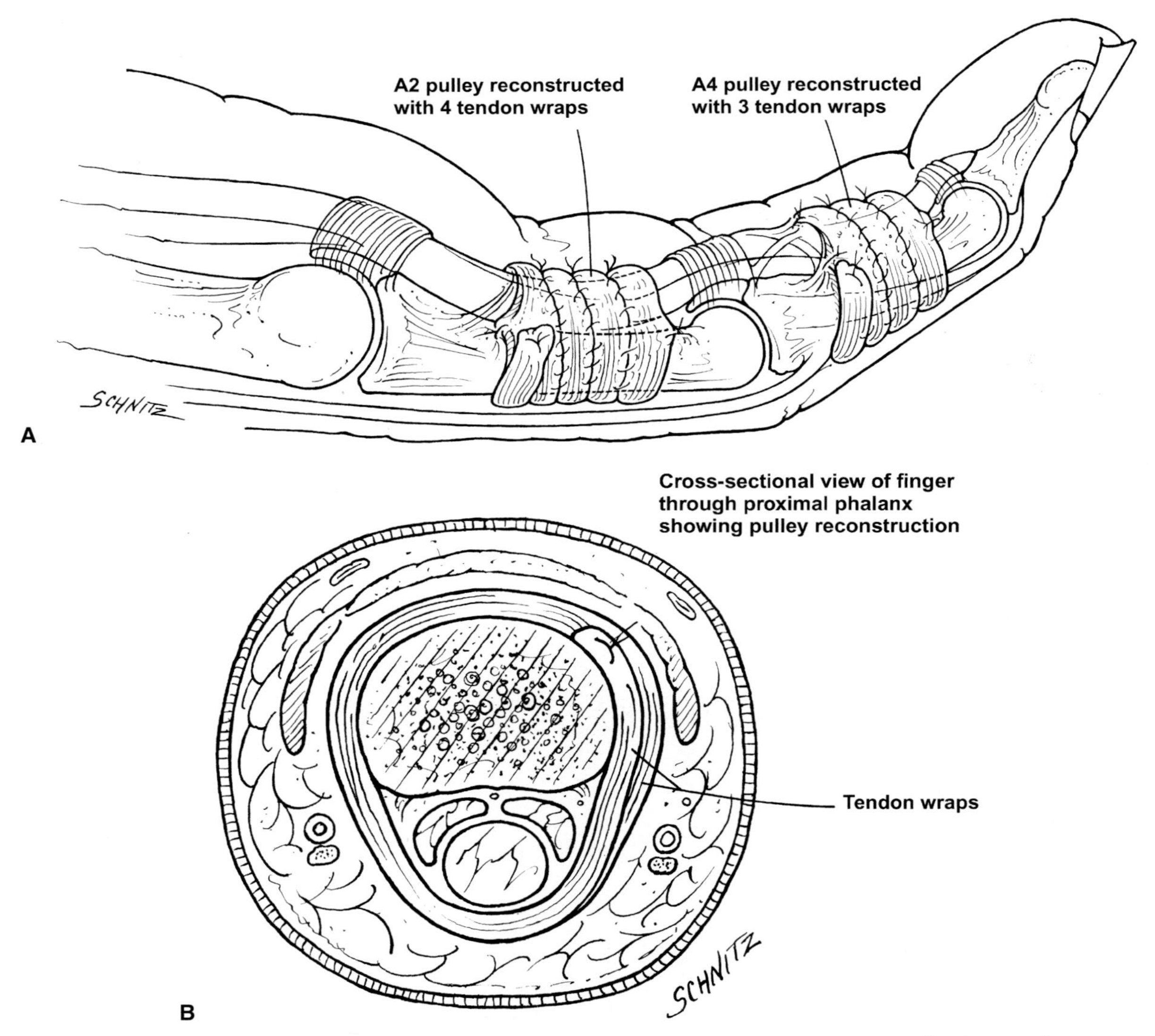

Figure 21.4. Bunnell-type tendon wrap pulley reconstruction. We prefer three to five wraps for the A2 pulley with three to five stitches between and securing the wraps to the pulley remnant.

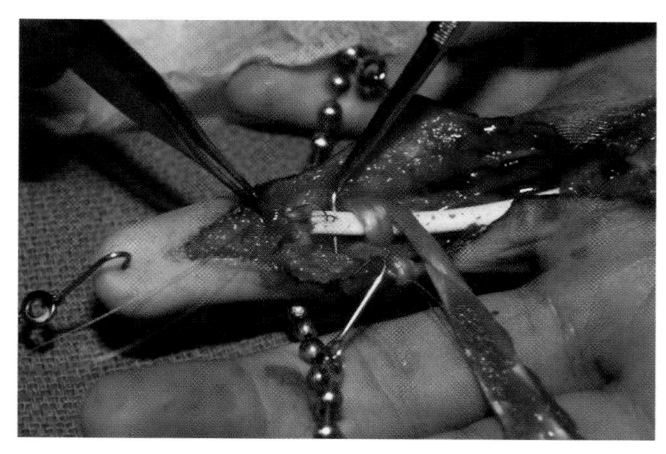
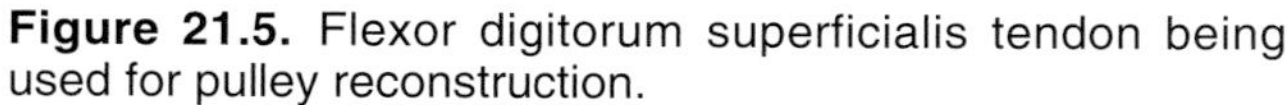

Figure 21.5. Flexor digitorum superficialis tendon being used for pulley reconstruction.

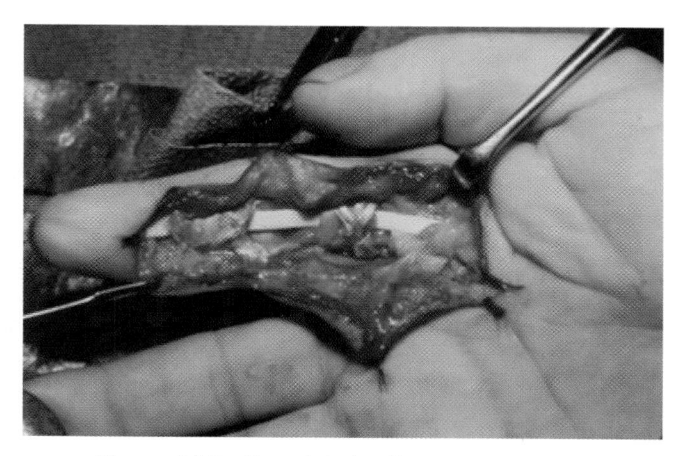

Figure 21.6. Completed pulley reconstruction.

To best simulate the biomechanics of the A2 and A4 pulleys, we recommend at minimum two wraps of the graft around the phalanx. This should provide adequate strength for early digital motion. If possible, up to four wraps can be used for A2 reconstruction. This is especially true with a palmaris longus graft, which is usually 3 to 4 mm wide.

To reconstruct the A2 pulley (which is 18–20 mm in length), four wraps best simulate the normal anatomy. The tendon wraps should be pulled snugly to keep the tendon implant closely applied to the bone. This will increase the active range of motion achieved at the joints by the future tendon graft. After the grafts have encircled the phalanx, they are repaired with 4-0 nonabsorbable sutures connecting each wrap with the remaining rim of the native pulley attached to the phalanx (Fig. 21.6).

The suture and junction site should always be placed away from the palmar portion of the digit so that it provides a smooth palmar sliding surface. The surgeon must be aware that significant tendon material is required to reconstruct pulleys. Approximately 6 to 8 cm of graft is required to circle the phalanx one time. The efficiency of the pulleys can then be tested by traction on the tendon implant (Fig. 21.7).

Rehabilitation

The patient is sent to hand therapy at the first postoperative visit to mobilize the joints with passive range-of-motion exercises. With mobilization, pulleys should be protected with pulley rings to prevent loosening of the reconstruction.

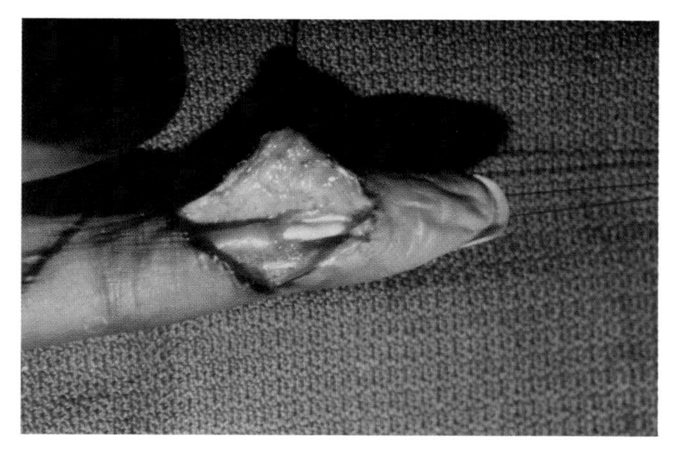

Figure 21.7. The distal tendon implant juncture at stage II with new tendon sheath proximal.

Sutures are removed at 2 weeks, and scar massage is added to the therapy regimen. The passive range-of-motion protocol is continued for 3 months, by which time the wounds have again achieved equilibrium. At this time, the patient is able to proceed with stage II.

STAGE II SURGICAL TECHNIQUES

Timing

In stage II, the Silastic implant is replaced with a tendon graft. This procedure is performed after a fluid nutrition system and normal gliding biomechanics are reestablished. By 3 months after stage I surgery, the pseudosheath has matured, the hand should be supple, and the joints are well mobilized.

Surgical Exposure

Expose the distal juncture by opening the distal finger incision to the midportion of the middle phalanx. Care is taken not to violate the pseudosheath over the middle phalanx (Fig. 21.8). Leave the distal juncture intact and expose the proximal portion of the implant through the previous distal forearm or palmar incision. If soft, portions of the proximal sheath may be retained at the surgeon's discretion. If synovitis has been present, the thickened sheath must be removed from the proximal juncture site to the wrist flexion crease. To determine the excursion necessary to produce maximum finger flexion, lay the hand and finger flat on the table and firmly pull the implant proximally. The surgeon should note: (1) the excursion of the implant to produce the range of motion from maximum extension to maximum flexion, (2) the distance the finger pulp rests from the distal palmar crease, and (3) joints with restricted motion. Carefully pack the wounds and release the tourniquet while the tendon graft is harvested.

Tendon Graft Harvest

The tendons available for use as free grafts include those of the plantaris, long toe extensors, palmaris longus, flexor digitorum superficialis, and proprius extensors.

We have generally preferred using the plantaris tendon because it is reliably long enough for grafting from fingertip to forearm. Make a longitudinal incision anterior to the medial aspect of the Achilles tendon at its calcaneal insertion. Identify the plantaris anterior to the tendoachilles (Fig. 21.9) and divide it near its insertion. Bluntly mobilize the plantaris under direct vision and then use a Brand tendon stripper to free the tendon from its musculo-

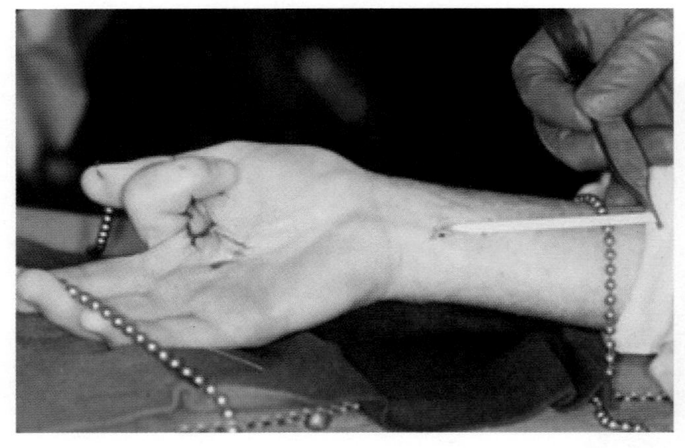

Figure 21.8. Maximum excursion attained by tendon implant after pulley reconstruction. This motion is an assessment of the reconstruction and a gauge of what motion is possible after stage II.

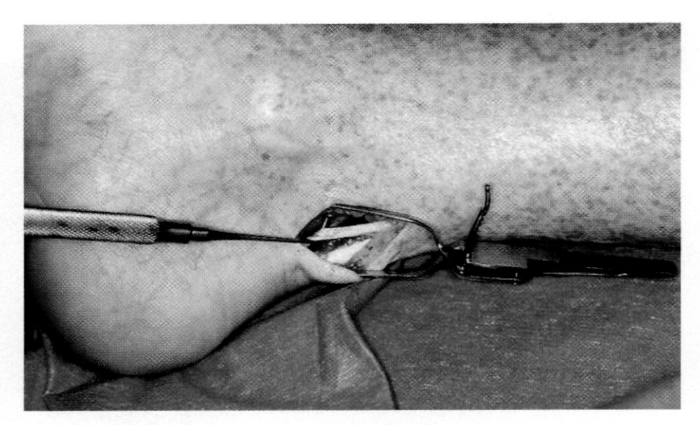

Figure 21.9. Locating the plantaris tendon. Future directions in tendon surgery may show the FDC to the toes as the preferred graft.

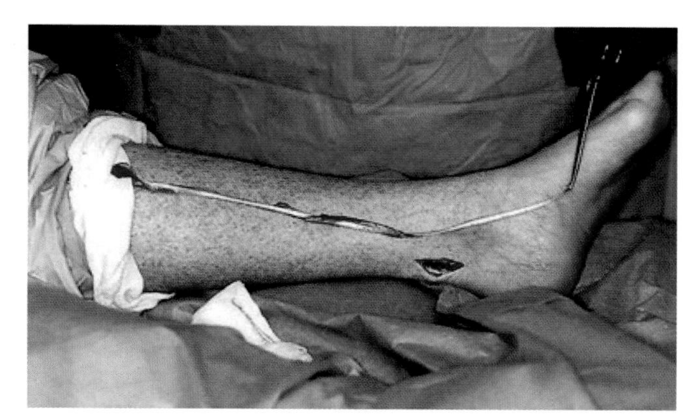

Figure 21.10. Plantaris after harvest. The plantaris tendon is reliably long enough to graft from the distal interphalangeal joint to the distal forearm.

tendinous junction. The tendon stripper must be applied parallel to the longitudinal axis of the tendon to prevent premature tendon severing (Fig. 21.10).

If the plantaris tendon is absent, a long toe extensor can be harvested. It is usually necessary to make three to four transverse incisions to prevent injury to the graft. Make one incision at the metatarsophalangeal joint of the toe, the next just distal to the retinaculum of the ankle, and a third just proximal to the retinaculum. The tendon is stripped and passed through each incision until the musculotendinous juncture is reached. The fifth toe extensor should not be used because the little toe usually has only one extensor.

Shorter tendon grafts (e.g., toe flexors, palmaris longus, extensor indicis, extensor digiti minimi, and segments of superficialis) are removed by standard technique and may be used for: (1) thumb, little finger, and superficialis finger, or (2) index, long, and ring fingers with an attachment to a tendon juncture in the uninjured palm.

Occasionally, several grafts are needed at once. In this situation, the flexor digitorum longus (FDL) to the toes can be used with multiple slips (Fig. 21.11). Recent studies on the use of toe flexors as grafts suggest that these tendon grafts heal with less adhesion formation, and we believe that as experience is gained using this graft it may become the donor tendon of choice for flexor tendon grafting in the future.

Distal Juncture

Suture the tendon graft to the proximal end of the implant (Fig. 21.12) and pull it distally into the new tendon sheath (Figs. 21.13 and 21.14). Next, detach the implant from the graft

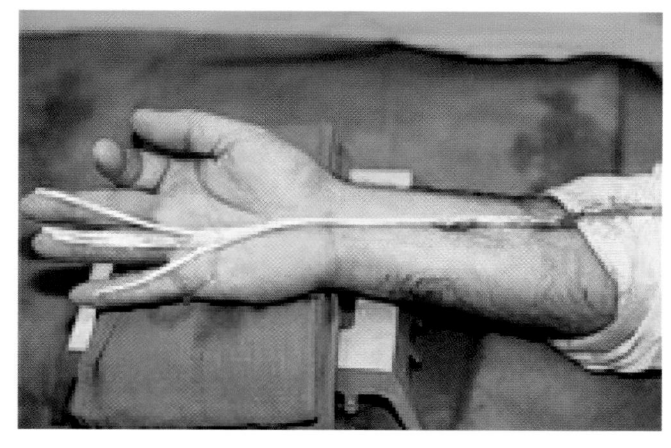

Figure 21.11. Use of a three-tailed FDL to the foot graft for multiple tendon reconstruction. (Photograph courtesy of Dr. David Zelouf.)

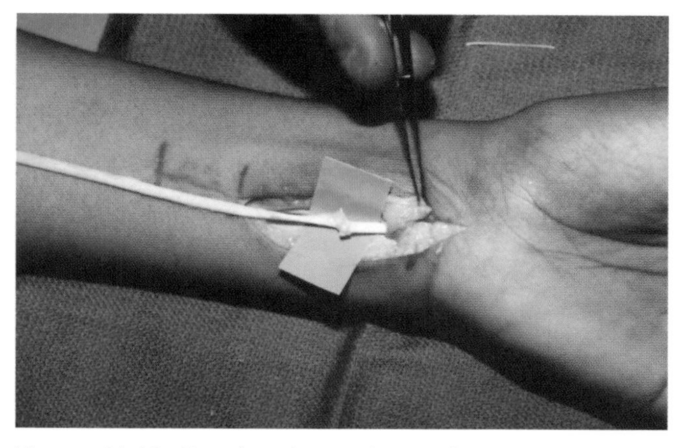

Figure 21.12. Suturing the tendon graft to the tendon implant at stage II.

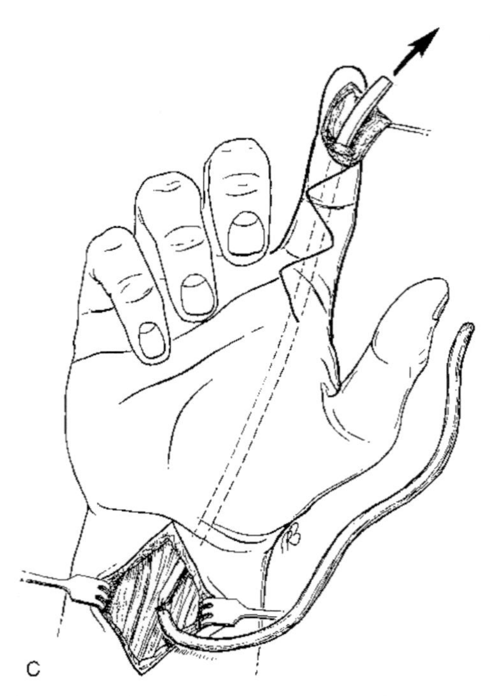

Figure 21.13. Advancing the tendon graft into the reconstructed tendon sheath.

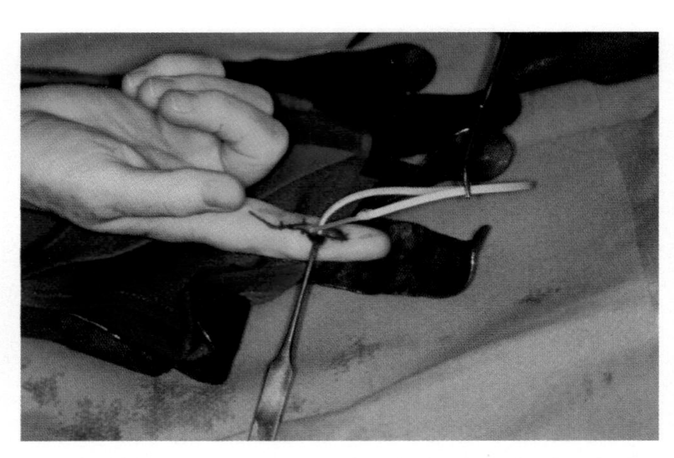

Figure 21.14. The tendon graft is in position in the reconstructed sheath.

and the distal phalanx and discard it. A 3-0 Prolene suture is crisscrossed twice in a Bunnell type of weave through the distal end of the graft and pulled snug.

Two methods can be used to secure the distal tendon graft. One technique involves creating an oblique hole in the volar cortex of the distal phalanx. This is made with a bone awl under the profundus stump remnant and enlarged with a curette. Next, drill two Keith needles in a parallel fashion through the distal phalanx and exit dorsally in the middle of the nail. Pull the suture through the distal phalanx by threading each tail through the Keith needles. It is important to visualize the graft being pulled snugly into the bone on the volar side of the finger as the Keith needles are advanced through the tip of the finger. Tie the suture over the dorsum of the fingernail over a button or stent and reinforce with two 4-0 nonabsorbable polyester sutures that anchor the graft to the profundus stump. The suture is left in place for 6 weeks.

The second technique used to secure the distal tendon graft involves weaving the graft through the profundus stump and placing the tails of the Bunnell suture around the sides of the distal phalanx and through the nail plate (Fig. 21.15). Use a tendon-braiding instrument to weave the tendon graft through the profundus stump once or twice, depending on stump

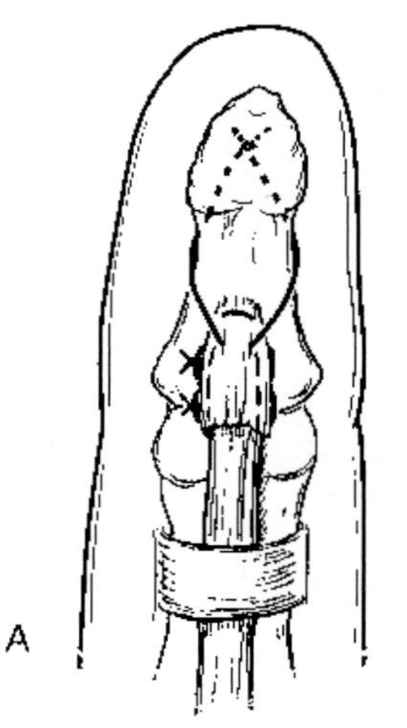

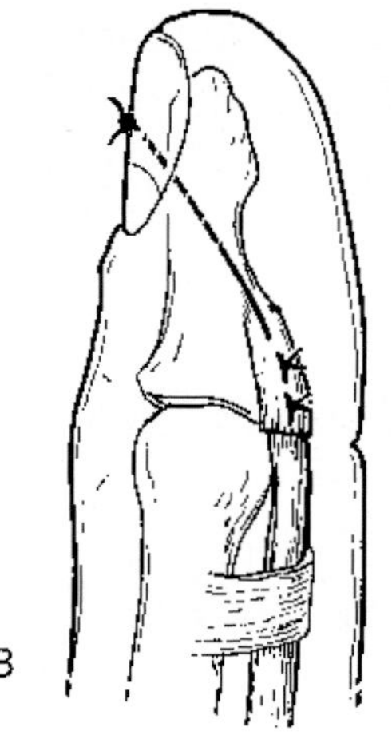

Figure 21.15. Distal insertion of the tendon graft at stage II. We prefer passing the suture around the distal phalanx and tying it over the nail plate without the use of a plastic button.

length. Pass the 3-0 Prolene pullout suture tails in the graft around the midshaft of the distal phalanx. Use a stout needle driver to pass the Keith needles and tie the Prolene suture directly over the nail plate. Tension the graft to remove slack from the bunched-up distal juncture and place reinforcing sutures to secure the graft to the tendon stump. We have seen a handful of complications from the use of plastic buttons tied over the nail plate with skin necrosis at the nail fold, which has led to permanent nail deformities.

Proximal Juncture

We find that the proximal juncture level most favorable for tendon gliding is the distal forearm. Ideally, the profundus of the injured digit is used as the motor tendon for the graft. However, a shorter graft may be used by placing the juncture at the level of the lumbrical origin if the palm is uninjured. If the profundus is inadequate as a motor, the superficialis can be used instead. Keep in mind that the excursion potential of the superficialis is less than that of an intact profundus. Superficialis muscle power may be used to an advantage when grafting to a superficialis finger.

After the motor is selected, anchor the graft to the motor tendon. Use a standard endweave technique (Fig. 21.16) when the graft is woven to only one motor tendon. This

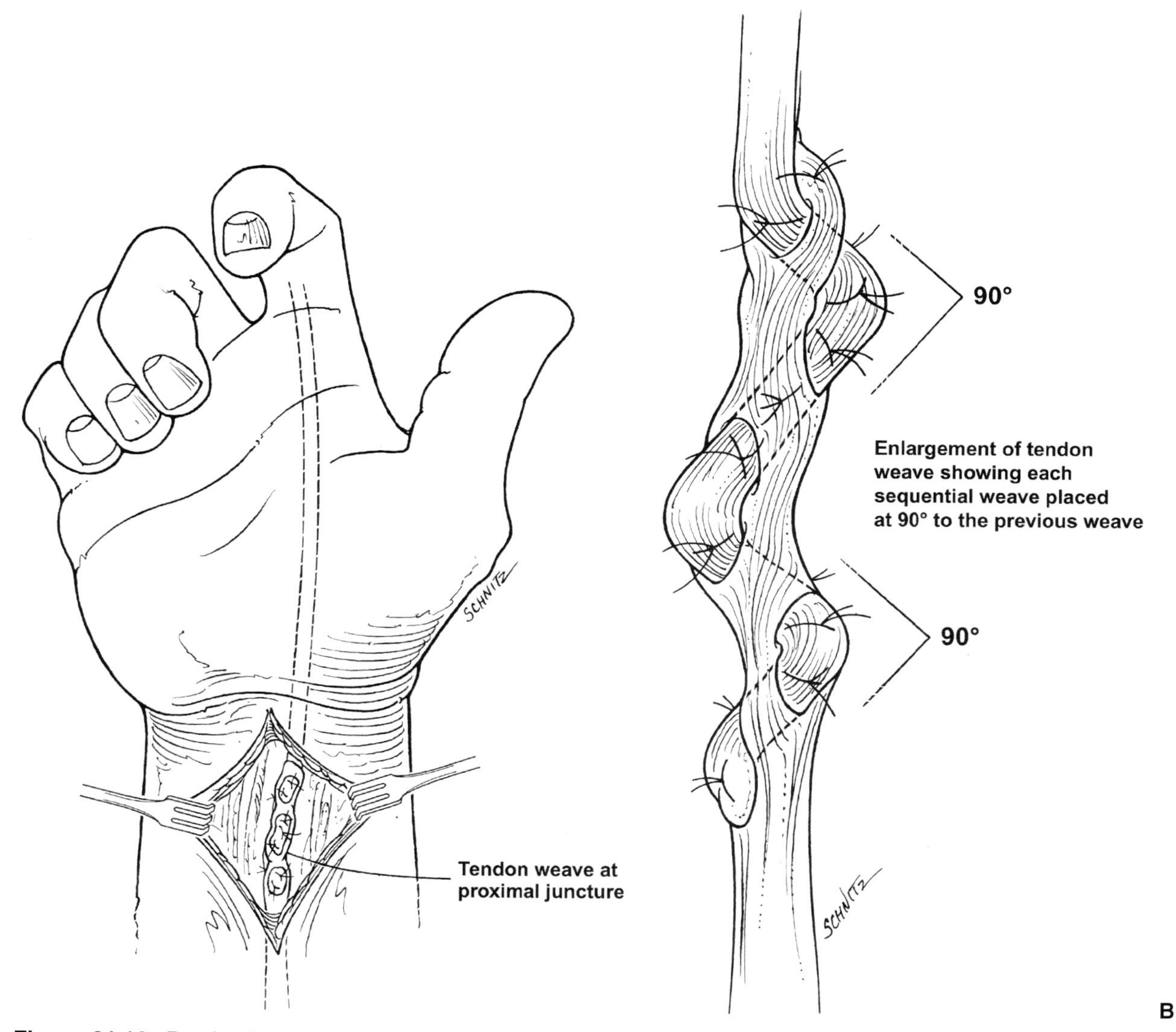

Figure 21.16. Proximal tendon juncture weave in zone 5. Note that each entry into the tendon is 90 degrees to the previous one. We recommend three to five tendon weaves and securing sutures.

is the case when using the flexor pollicis longus, profundus to the index, or a superficialis tendon. A multiple endweave juncture is created when the profundus tendons of the long, ring, and small fingers are chosen as the common motor. Although it is easier to set the correct tension with the endweave technique compared with an end-to-end tenoraplay, the endweave technique creates a bulky juncture; therefore, it should preferably be performed outside the flexor sheath at the level of the distal forearm. Be sure that the pseudosheath does not impede excursion of the tendon graft juncture, and if necessary excise more of the proximal sheath to permit full extension.

Start the endweave by incising the profundus motor tendon near its end. Thread the graft through the slit with a tendon braider, then tension and fix with a buried 3-0 nonabsorbable polyester suture. The position of the finger with the wrist in neutral should be one of slightly more flexion than the adjacent digits. After repeated manipulations, the finger should remain in slightly more flexion than normal. The selected tendon motor must provide at least as much excursion as previously required by the silicone implant to produce maximal flexion. When the tension is correct, thread the graft at least two more times transversely through the motor tendon in alternating 90-degree planes. Complete the juncture by suturing the tendons into place with buried 3-0 nonabsorbable polyester sutures (Fig. 21.17). The multiple endweave is performed in a similar manner, noting that the tendon graft passes through all three ulnar profundus tendons.

After a bulky nonconstrictive dressing is applied, a short-arm posterior splint is fashioned to hold the wrist in 30 degrees of flexion, MP joints in 70 degrees of flexion, and interphalangeal joints in full extension.

Rehabilitation

With our current suture techniques of tendon graft fixation, supervised gentle active flexion in therapy is initiated at the first postoperative visit at 1 to 3 days after surgery. The therapists instruct the patient on passive flexion-active extension and place-and-hold techniques (Fig. 21.18), which the patient performs at home. Active flexion against re-

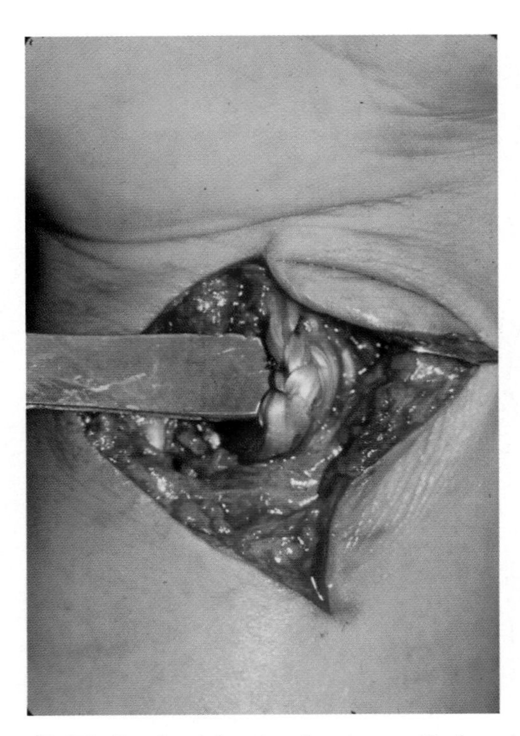

Figure 21.17. Proximal tendon juncture with four tendon weaves and securing sutures. We take great care to ensure that this juncture does not impinge on normal anatomy or on the new tendon sheath when it is in the fully extended position.

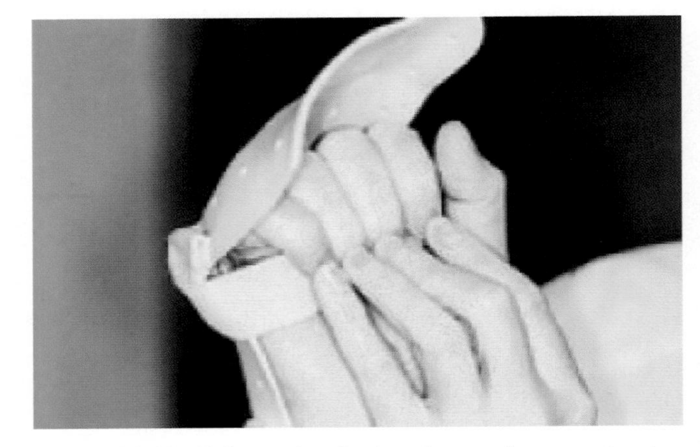

Figure 21.18. Full passive flexion does not ensure tendon gliding. Place-and-hold techniques must be used to move the tendon graft.

sistance is started at 6 weeks after surgery and continues with strength training for 12 to 24 weeks.

RESULTS

Staged flexor tendon reconstruction with a Silastic passive tendon implant has proven to be a consistently reliable technique for salvaging scarred tendon systems. The production of a pseudosheath that provides a fluid nutrition system for the subsequent tendon graft, in concert with early, protected gliding of the graft, has resulted in a significant reduction of postoperative adhesions. Contracture release with pulley reconstruction of appropriate size, quantity, and location, combined with a supervised therapy program, results in maximum postoperative digital motion.

We have found that patient outcome in general is correlated with overall preoperative status, although the range of outcomes can be quite varied for patients presenting with similar clinical circumstances. Poor prognostic indicators include extensive pulley damage, capsular contractures, multiple digit involvement, and prolonged time from injury to stage I. Patients who sustain significant damage to the flexor tendon system should be made aware of the potential for poor outcome. Restoration of finger flexion requires the combined efforts of patient and surgeon to maximize function.

COMPLICATIONS

Adhesions are prone to occur in areas where there is poor graft gliding, an inadequate fluid nutrition system, pulleys are too tight, or there has been dense scarring. Most commonly, adhesions form at the proximal juncture. A tenolysis procedure should be considered if the adhesions at the proximal juncture significantly restrict motion. Tenolysis is performed 4 to 6 months after stage II using local anesthesia and intravenous sedation. The region of the proximal juncture should be explored primarily, with attention directed toward the juncture at the new tendon sheath, then to the distal juncture, and last to the tendon graft within the new sheath. Only adhesions that restrict motion should be treated.

After surgery, immediate active motion of the released tendon graft is necessary to preserve the increased range of motion. Many of these patients return to therapy with an indwelling catheter placed next to the median or ulnar nerve. Bupivacaine is injected through the catheter every 4 to 6 hours postoperatively to minimize pain and maximize active movement. The catheter can be left in place for up to 5 days. These patients require a carefully coordinated management program directed by the surgeon and therapist.

Rupture of the graft can occur at either juncture and may be attributable to faulty operative technique. With the recent emphasis on increasing the strength of tendon junctures, we have not encountered rupture in compliant patients. Early rupture at the proximal juncture may result from faulty weaving and suturing of the tendon graft when one is performing an endweave technique. We advocate three to five interweaves with three to five sutures to create a very strong juncture. Late tendon rupture is unusual but may occur if extreme force is applied. We have seen cases of tendon rupture occur more than 20 years after successful grafting. When rupture of a tendon graft juncture is suspected, immediate exploration is indicated because it is often possible to reattach the graft, particularly in instances in which the patient had good tendon gliding before rupture. Alternatively, the finger can be salvaged by creation of a superficialis finger.

Infection is a disastrous complication after stage I and one that can be difficult to distinguish from sterile synovitis. Early on, it may be possible to treat infection after stage I with antibiotics and irrigation of the tendon sheath with small-caliber catheters. Established infection necessitates removal of the implant, treatment with appropriate antibiotics, and an infection-free interval of 3 to 6 months. After clearing the infection, reconstruction of the tendon may again be considered.

Two complications after stage II tendon grafting deserve discussion. The first is adhesions to the tendon graft. These may occur along the tendon graft or at the proximal tendon juncture. The second is rupture of the tendon juncture.

One unique complication of staged tendon reconstruction is synovitis of the sheath forming in response to the implant. Careful handling of the implant can reduce the occurrence of this complication; gloved hands should never touch the tendon implant. Many instances of synovitis appear to be caused by talc contamination. This can be avoided by only opening the sterile implant at the time of implantation and by not directly handling the implant. Another possible cause of synovitis is irritation from too tight a system of pulleys, causing buckling of the implant. Synovitis has been reduced from 20% in early series to 8% in more recent series. Clinically, the patient presents with increased heat, crepitus, and obvious swelling with fluid in the tendon sheath. These findings will be associated with a thick and less pliable flexor tendon sheath found at stage II. Synovitis is a serious complication that often leads to less successful results after stage II grafting. Cultures have shown no identifiable bacteria in these cases. This sterile synovitis is treated with immobilization and nonsteroidal anti-inflammatory medication.

RECOMMENDED READING

1. Amadio PC, Wood MB, Cooney WP, et al. Staged flexor tendon reconstruction in the fingers and hand. *J Hand Surg* 13A:559–562, 1988.
2. Foucher G, Lenoble E, Ben Youssef K, et al. A post-operative regime after digital flexor tenolysis: a series of 72 patients *J Hand Surg* 18B:35–40, 1993.
3. Frakking KP, Depuydt KP, Werker PM. Retrospective outcome analysis of staged flexor tendon reconstruction. *J Hand Surg* 25B:168–174, 2000.
4. Hunter JM. Staged flexor tendon reconstruction. *J Hand Surg* 8:789–793, 1983.
5. Imbriglia JE, Hunter JM, Rennie W. Secondary flexor tendon reconstruction. *Hand Clinics* 5:395–413, 1989.
6. Okutsu I, Niyomiya S, Hiraki S, et al. Three-loop technique for A-2 pulley reconstruction. *J Hand Surg* 12A:790–794, 1987.
7. Schneider LM. Staged Flexor Tendon Reconstruction. In: Green DP, Hotchkiss RN, Pederson WC, eds. *Green's Operative Hand Surgery*. 4th ed. Philadelphia: Churchill Livingstone, 1999:1898–1949.

22

Free Tendon Grafting

Robert Lee Wilson

INDICATIONS AND CONTRAINDICATIONS

When the flexor tendons have been divided in zone I or II and not repaired, tendon grafting is the recommended treatment to restore digital flexion (Fig. 22.1). The selection of conventional free tendon graft or staged flexor reconstruction will be determined on evaluation of the involved finger, including the condition of the retinacular (pulley) system and the extent of scarring within the flexor-tendon sheath.

To be considered a surgical candidate, the patient's wound must have healed satisfactorily to allow a suppleness of the soft tissues in the hand. Passive flexion and extension of the involved digit should be complete. At least one digital nerve should have normal function. If both digital nerves have been divided at the time of the original injury, nerve repair and regeneration should precede flexor-tendon grafting. The factor with the greatest prognostic significance after flexor reconstructions is age, with the best results occurring in patients aged between 10 and 30 years. Younger children are unable to cooperate with the necessary postoperative immobilization and the rehabilitation program.

The mechanism of injury to the digit has predictive significance. Conventional flexor grafting is often not advised after crush injuries, soft-tissue loss, or severe phalangeal fractures. The presence of a fixed-joint contracture, particularly at the proximal interphalangeal (PIP) joint, is also a contraindication for flexor grafting in a single stage, as is the presence of an insensate digit, one with poor vascularity, or the need for pulley reconstruction.

PREOPERATIVE PLANNING

The patient needs to be evaluated carefully, considering the factors just mentioned. If the injured digit does not meet the standards for conventional tendon grafting, a period of hand therapy might be helpful, particularly when the digit is stiff or contracted. Otherwise, consideration should be given to staged flexor-tendon reconstruction. Preoperative evaluation should include assessment of potential tendon-graft sources, especially testing for the presence of the palmaris longus.

Robert Lee Wilson, M.D.: Phoenix Integrated Hand Surgery Fellowship, Phoenix, AZ

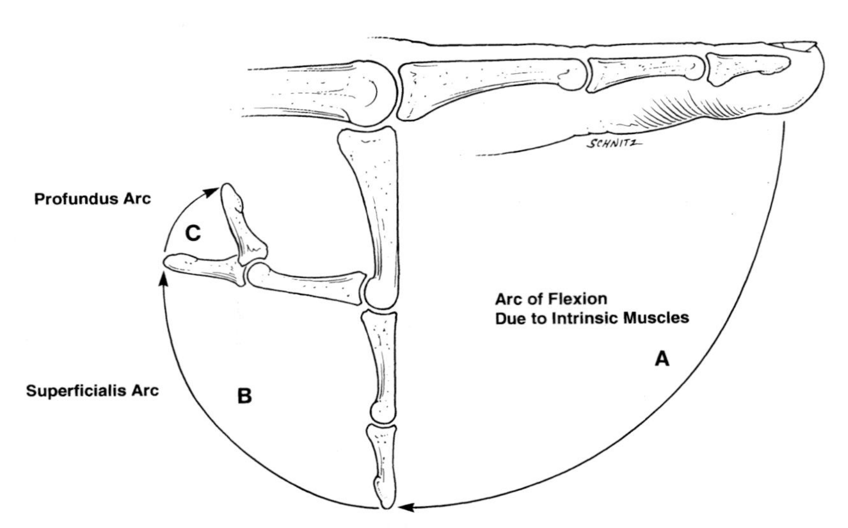

Figure 22.1. Diagram demonstrating the arc of flexion.

SURGERY

The patient is placed supine on the operating table with a tourniquet applied to the extremity. The arm will be shaved in anticipation of obtaining a tendon graft. The use of a plantaris or a toe extensor might be contemplated; if so, the contralateral lower extremity should be similarly prepared. The extremity(s) is prepared and draped in the usual manner, and blood is expressed from the upper extremity with a rubber bandage and application of the pressure tourniquet.

The surgical approach to the injured finger should minimize scar formation. The ideal finger for tendon grafting is one that is supple with minimal scarring and has an undamaged bed. The incision should allow complete exposure of the flexor tendons, the overlying retinacular structures, and the neurovascular bundles. This incision should not produce a scar contracture or limit joint motion. Although the midlateral incision is preferred by many, I recommend a zigzag incision, leaving the neurovascular bundles protected in their normal position (Figs. 22.2 and 22.3). The incision should be located away from the side used for tactile function, which is the radial side of the index, middle, and ring fingers, and the ulnar

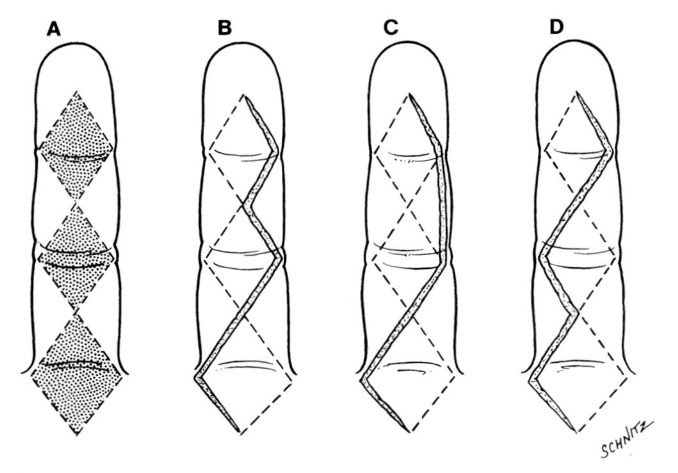

Figure 22.2. Incision should expose the flexor tendons and other important structures but not produce a contracture. Lines of stress sketched along the finger form a diamond pattern. The length of these lines will not change with finger motion. A longitudinal incision should not enter the shaded area. An incision should be designed to avoid these areas and to allow sufficient exposure.

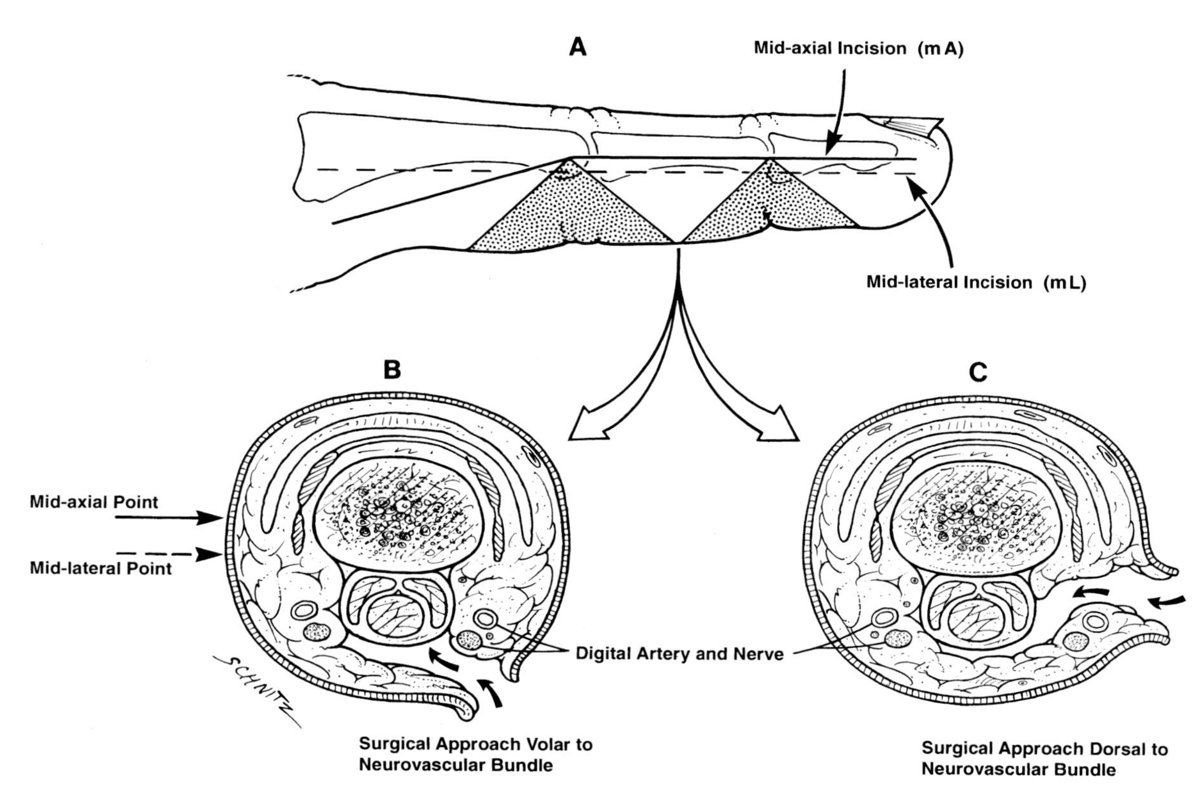

Figure 22.3. A: Lines of midaxial and midlateral incisions. If the lateral approach is selected, the incision should be midaxial, passing through the axes of joint motion (versus a midlateral approach made halfway between the dorsal and palmar surface). The latter incision may produce a flexion contracture and, in a child, will migrate palmward. In the midaxial approach, Cleland's ligament will be divided and the neuromuscular bundle raised with the palmar flap. With the zigzag approach, the neurovascular structures remain with the dorsal tissue. **B, C:** Volar and dorsal approaches to the neurovascular bundle.

side of the little finger. If possible, the incision will not cross the proximal flexion crease of the digit, but it will spare this area, as it is the most frequent site of scar contracture postoperatively. In the palm, the incision should not pass directly over the anticipated site of the proximal tendon juncture (Fig. 22.4). Instead, a skin flap is created so that subcutaneous fat will be situated next to the tendon repair.

Following the incision and exposure, the flexor sheath and associated fibro-osseous pulleys are evaluated for preparation of a satisfactory bed for the tendon graft. Starting at the site of injury, the tendon sheath is opened, but only the traumatized segment is excised. Particular care is taken to spare the critical annular pulleys, and the segments in between are opened in a zigzag fashion. The retracted tendon ends are located and carefully dissected where they are adherent to the damaged sheath. Particular care is taken to preserve the floor of the tendon sheath. One centimeter of the profundus stump is preserved for use in attaching the tendon graft. An oblique hole is placed through the volar cortex of the distal phalanx and enlarged with a series of gouges to receive the distal end of the tendon graft.

During dissection of the proximal part of the tendon from the sheath, meticulous care must be taken to preserve the normal sheath contents and bed. When the superficialis has been divided near the base of the proximal phalanx, the distal portion may have become adherent to the phalanx and the floor of the sheath proximal to the PIP joint. If this segment of tendon does not contribute to a PIP flexion deformity, consideration should be given to leaving it in place, as it may stabilize the PIP joint to prevent a hyperextension deformity and will provide a smooth surface for the tendon graft as well as protect the underlying volar plate.

The incision in the palm is made to expose the retracted flexor tendons and prepare the proximal juncture site (Fig. 22.5). The vertical fascial septum, which separates the flexor

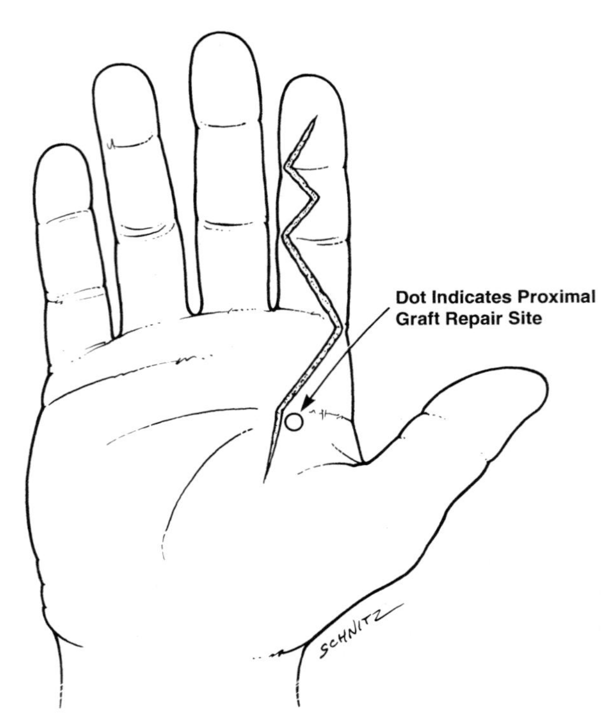

Figure 22.4. The incision is developed on the nontactile side of the index finger. The palmar portion is raised as a flap over the anticipated site of the proximal juncture, marked with a dot.

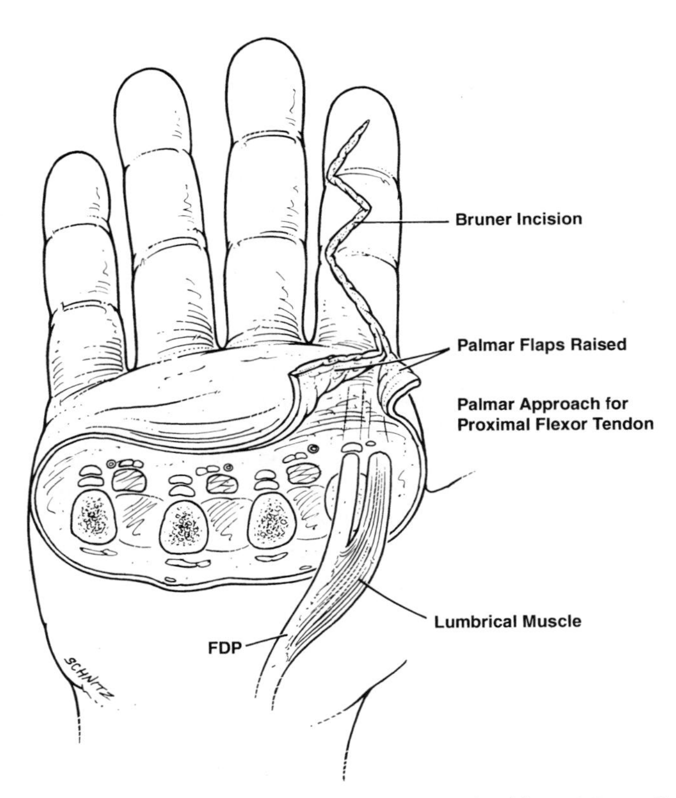

Figure 22.5. In the palm, the flexor tendons are approached by raising a flap of skin and fascia after dividing the vertical septum separating the tendons and the adjacent neurovascular bundle.

tendons from the adjacent neurovascular compartment, is incised and retracted with the overlying skin flap. If this fascia has not been injured, it may be incorporated in the wound closure; however, excision of all rigid palmar fascia is necessary because in this form it will contribute to adhesions around the graft. Exposure of the palm for tendon grafting in multiple digits will require a transverse incision along the distal palmar crease, which swings proximally along its ulnar aspect with complete excision of the exposed palmar fascia. The proximal portions of the flexor tendons are now dissected from their adhesions to the sheath. All reactive tissue about the tendon ends and the adjacent tissues is resected. The relationship between the profundus and lumbrical is defined, and all distal adhesions are lysed to establish a normal relationship between these structures. If the lumbrical is involved with scarring in the palm, it is resected rather than left adherent to the profundus.

The muscle-tendon unit that will motor the flexor graft is usually the profundus tendon. Before this selection is made, however, traction is applied to both the superficialis and profundus tendons with the wrist held in flexion. This maneuver should overcome adhesions that may have occurred within the carpal tunnel or a more proximal myostatic contracture. Thirty-five millimeters of profundus excursion with traction is considered ideal.

The entire flexor sheath system should be reevaluated before obtaining the graft (Fig. 22.6). The unscarred portions of the sheath are retained, with particular attention to the A-2 and A-4 pulleys. Collapse of the sheath occurs after a flexor-tendon injury and increases with time. To allow the graft to be passed through the sheath, distention may be required and can be accomplished with a curved hemostat or by using a series of pediatric urethral dilators. If the remaining portions of the fibro-osseous sheath are insufficient, pulley reconstruction is indicated. The remaining pulleys must measure 5- to 8-mm long. In my opinion, rebuilding any flexor pulleys is an indication for insertion of a tendon implant as a first-stage flexor reconstruction because of the likelihood for formation of adhesions between the graft and the newly constructed pulley.

The donor tendon should be selected after the sheath has been prepared. Important factors are the tendon diameter, length, and ease of suturing. My first choice is the palmaris longus, which is present in 85% of patients; however, sometimes this tendon, even when present, may be too short, atrophic, or have muscle attached distally. Other alternative graft sources are the superficialis in the same digit, toe extensors, and the index finger common extensor tendon. Although the superficialis has a comparable diameter and similar texture, allowing end-to-end approximation, it may be too large to be advanced through the sheath.

After obtaining the graft, the question arises as to whether to remove the paratenon or leave it intact. Recent studies have shown that leaving the paratenon attached allows prompt revascularization. The tendon graft is handled carefully and specifically, and the graft surface is not touched with anything except a smooth surface of an instrument or moistened gauze. The tendon graft then is placed within the sheath (Fig. 22.7). Whether the

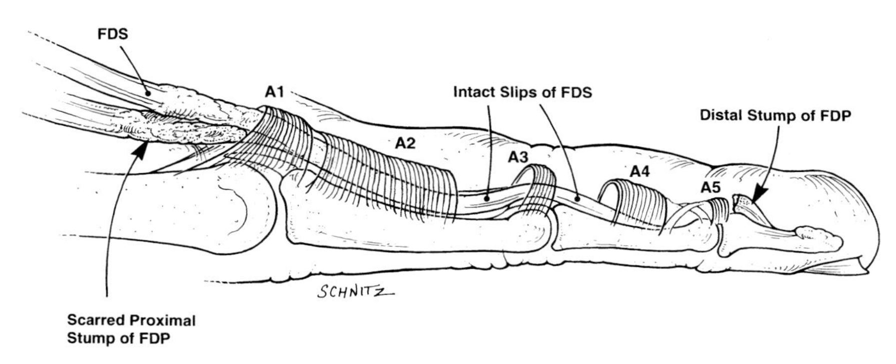

Figure 22.6. Adherence of the divided proximal tendon stump usually occurs over the proximal phalanx. The scarred tendon remnants must be dissected carefully, sparing the pulleys and the floor of the tendon sheath to create a satisfactory bed.

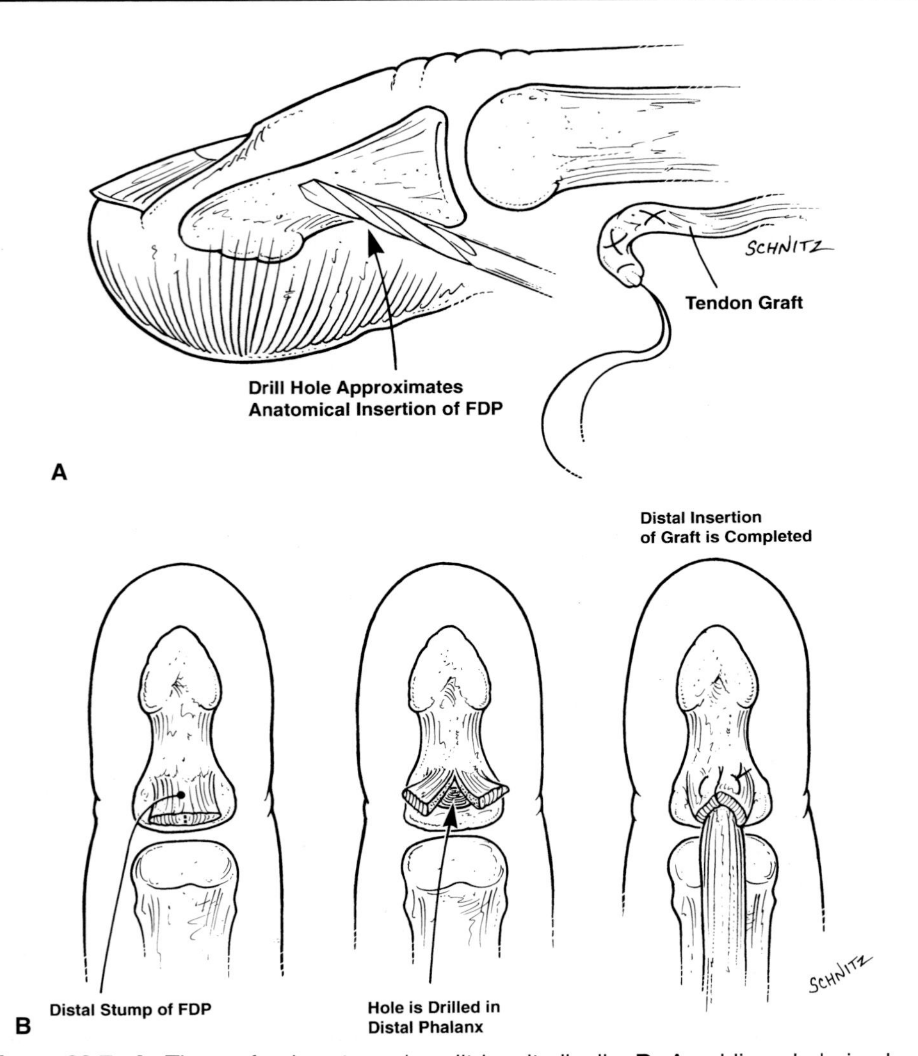

Figure 22.7. A: The profundus stump is split longitudinally. **B:** An oblique hole is placed through the palmar cortex of the distal phalanx. The dorsal cortical bone is thinned. The groove should be designed so that the exit is distal to the germinal nail matrix. The tendon graft then is placed inside the sheath.

proximal or distal juncture is performed first will depend on the diameter of the tendon graft and the preference of the surgeon. When there is a discrepancy between the proximal motor and the graft, such as with a small-diameter tendon (palmaris or plantaris), I prefer performing the proximal repair first with an end-to-side technique (Pulvertaft). If the superficialis or any other large tendon is used as a graft, end-to-end repair using a 4-0 braided polyester or nylon is advised. The lumbrical muscle is not sutured about the repair site (Fig. 22.8).

I prefer to perform the proximal juncture first and determine the appropriate graft length and tension with adjustments distally. If the graft has a small diameter, passage of the end through the pulp close to the bone can facilitate adjustment of the tension. The profundus stump and the distal phalanx drill hole are assessed. The distal end of the graft is clamped at the tip of the digit, and the tension is estimated. The grafted finger should be held in slightly more flexion than the adjacent digits. Overall, the fingers are held in a cascade with progressively more flexion toward the ulnar side of the hand. The wrist is flexed and extended vigorously several times, and the tension is tested again by passively extending all the fingers, including the digit with the graft. After the appropriate length has been calculated, the tendon is marked within the finger in such a way that the excess portion can be removed. The tendon then is secured within the distal phalanx cavity with a pull-through

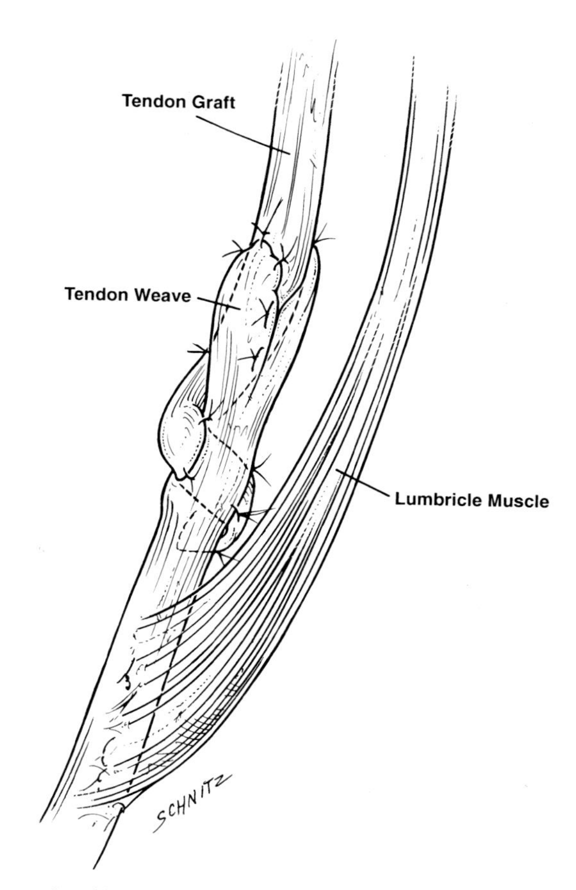

Figure 22.8. The proximal juncture is repaired by first weaving the smaller tendon through the profundus stump and using a distal fishmouth closure.

suture (Fig. 22.9). Additional sutures are placed between the graft and the profundus stump. In children, this latter technique will serve as the sole site of suturing, as passage of the graft through the bone is to be avoided with an open epiphysis.

Hemostasis is achieved after the tourniquet is released. Portions of the sheath that are not scarred should be sutured in place. The palm wound is closed either by returning the fascia to its normal place or by removing it and allowing subcutaneous fat to lie directly over the graft and the proximal juncture. A bulky gauze dressing with anterior and posterior plaster splints for support is applied while maintaining the wrist in 30 to 40 degrees of flexion, and the fingers are flexed 60 to 70 degrees at the metaphalangeal (MP) joints. The IP joints are held in full extension. If a graft has been applied to one of the ulnar three digits, the thumb and index finger are left free for pinch activities. If the long thumb flexor has been reconstructed with a graft, the fingers are not restrained.

POSTOPERATIVE MANAGEMENT

The hand is immobilized for 20 to 25 days after surgery to allow revascularization of the graft and time for healing at the junctures. Following flexion-tendon reconstruction, a single tendon is used to flex both IP joints. It is necessary to have the graft act primarily to flex the PIP joint and to provide power at the distal joint. This difference can be determined at surgery by having different pulley diameters proximally and distally. The postsurgical exercise program should allow early motion at the PIP joint and delayed flexion at the distal joint. The purpose of the rehabilitation program is to establish graft motion while preventing disruption of the junctures.

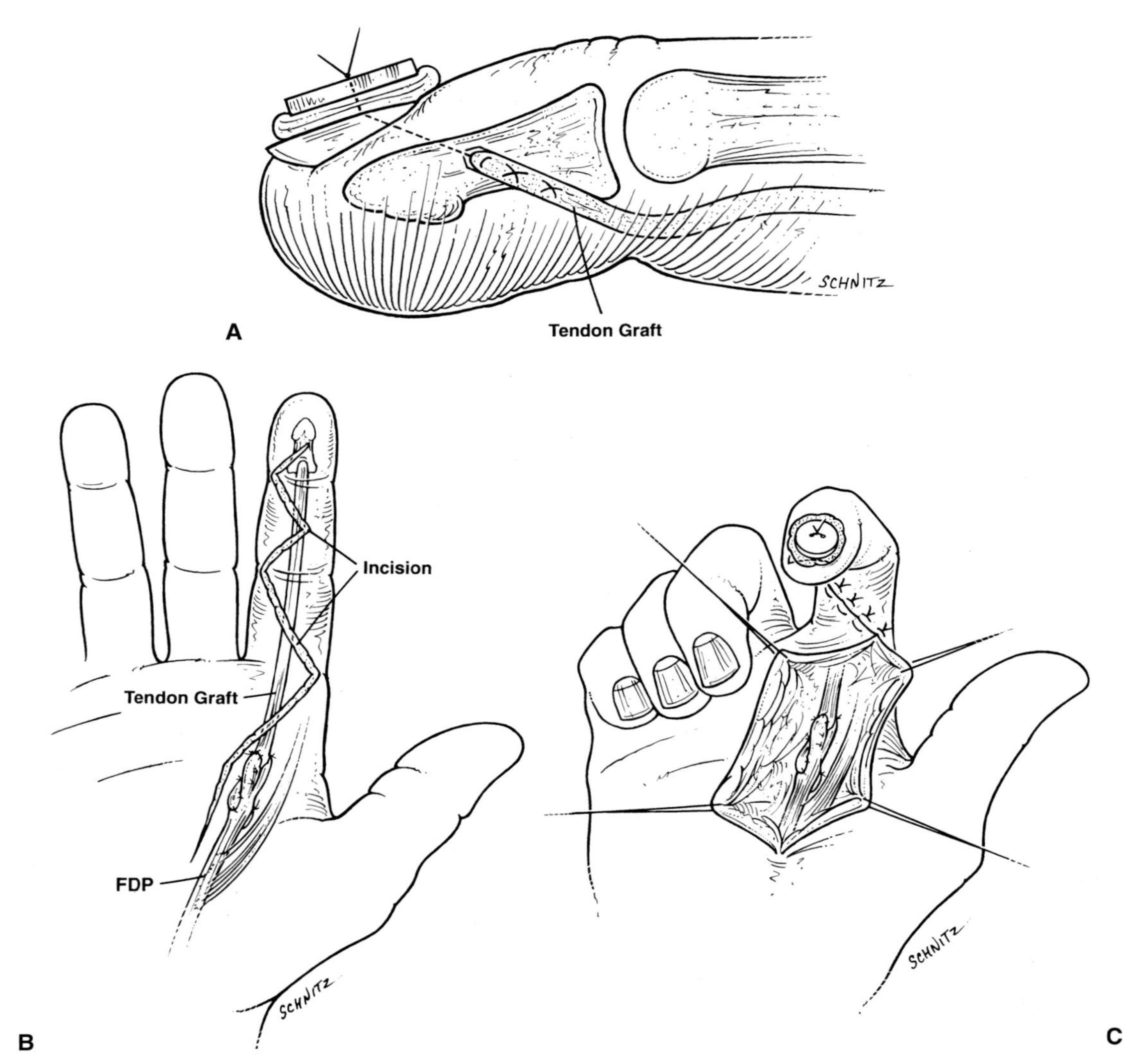

Figure 22.9. A, B, C: After establishing the correct graft length and tension, the distal end of the graft is sutured to the distal phalanx with a pull-through suture.

The results following flexor-tendon grafting depend on numerous factors, including the patient's age, preoperative evidence of scarring, joint involvement, and which digit is involved. The best motion following a flexor-tendon graft is achieved in the little finger and the least motion in the index finger. If conventional tendon grafting is performed in fingers with minimal scar, full passive motion, and no trophic changes, 50–65% should be able to flex to within 1.25 cm of the distal palmar crease. In digits with scarring, joint contractures, or multiple associated problems, fewer than half of the patients will have a similar degree of flexion. Patients should be expected to improve their motion for 4–5 months after surgery, and by 22 weeks will have achieved 90% of their eventual motion. A tenolysis to improve motion should not be considered until 6 months after a conventional flexor-tendon graft.

In the fourth postoperative week (the first week of the exercise program), the digit is remobilized to obtain full passive flexion to the proximal palm. It is important to prevent flexion contractures at the IP joints; while the wrist and MP joints are held in maximal flexion, the IP joints are passively extended. The PIP joint should not be fully extended, to prevent a swan-neck deformity. Active PIP flexion is initiated while stabilizing the MP joint in progressively more extension. Some patients have difficulty with the exercising of a single finger, and simultaneous contraction of adjacent digits may prove beneficial.

The pull-through sutures are removed the following week, and active PIP flexion and extension are increased. The distal IP passive flexion exercises are continued. In the third week of rehabilitation, active flexion is initiated at the distal joint, with the more proximal joints stabilized in extension. Exercise at the PIP joint is more vigorous, with active simultaneous flexion of both IP joints. In the seventh week, the finger is extended both actively and passively, and resistance is initiated. The patient should be protected in a posterior splint for at least 50 days after surgery. In the 18th postoperative week, dynamic extension is begun. The hand should not be used for extremely heavy activities for at least three months after surgery.

COMPLICATIONS

Problems that can occur following flexor-tendon grafting include adhesions that will limit graft motion as well as produce flexion contractures and joint stiffness. Other problems include graft rupture, a swan-neck deformity, bowstringing, and a lumbrical plus deformity.

The surgeon can prevent some of these problems. It is most important to locate the tendon junctures outside the tendon sheath. The repair site must gain sufficient strength to prevent dehiscence. Although all grafts will develop adhesions, the quality of these is best controlled through meticulous surgical technique. In particular, the tendon bed should be preserved, the pulley system sufficiently constructed to prevent bowstringing, and proper length of the graft achieved, as well as satisfactory hemostasis. The patient must strictly adhere to the rehabilitation program and be reexamined on a weekly basis.

Rupture of a flexor graft usually occurs within the first eight weeks and is related to the strength of the repair and the method of immobilization. Disruption occurs more commonly at the proximal juncture, whereas distal ruptures are found 1 cm proximal to the bony attachment. Options for treatment once rupture occurs are prompt resuture, placement of a new graft, or insertion of a tendon implant with flexor reconstruction in two stages.

An imbalance in the extrinsic flexor and intrinsic systems can occur, with the intrinsics flexing the MP joint and all the extensor forces being concentrated at the PIP joint, producing a swan-neck deformity. Detachment of the superficialis stump proximal to the PIP joint at surgery or erroneous release of the volar plate proximally from the phalanx can contribute to this abnormal posture. During the postoperative exercise program, it is important to maintain the PIP joint in slight flexion. It is far preferable to allow a 10-degree PIP flexion contracture than to create a swan-neck deformity. A figure-of-eight splint holding the middle joint slightly flexed may prevent development of a permanent swan neck.

If the tendon-graft length is excessive, the profundus will retract proximally in the palm, producing increased tension on the lumbrical muscle and creating an intrinsic/extrinsic imbalance, termed the lumbrical plus deformity. The patient demonstrates this problem by initiating flexion normally at the MP joint but then extends the IP joints when further flexion is necessary. Such a deformity can be prevented by accurately determining the length of the tendon graft. Should this problem occur, tenotomy of the lumbrical tendon may resolve it.

RECOMMENDED READING

1. Boyes JH, Stark HH. Flexor-tendon grafts in the fingers and thumb: study of factors influencing results in 1,000 cases. *J Bone Joint Surg* 53A:1332–1342, 1971.
2. Gelberman RH, et al. Genetic expression for type I procollagen in the early stages of flexor-tendon healing. *J Hand Surg* 17A:551, 1992.
3. Littler JW. Free tendon grafts in secondary flexor-tendon repair. *Ann J Surg* 74:315, 1947.
4. Parkes A. "Lumbrical plus" finger. *Hand* 2:164–165, 1970.
5. Pulvertaft RG. Tendon grafts for flexor-tendon injuries in the fingers and thumbs: a study of technique and results, *J Bone Joint Surg* 38B:175–194, 1956.
6. Tubiana R. Postoperative care following flexor-tendon grafts. *Hand* 6:152–154, 1974.
7. Weeks PM, Wray RC. Rate and extent of functional recovery after flexor-tendon grafting with and without silicone rod preparation. *J Hand Surg* 1:174–180, 1976.
8. Wilson RL. Flexor-tendon grafting. *Hand* 1:97–107, 1985.

PART VI

Elective and Traumatic Microsurgery and Amputations

23

Capsulectomies of the Metacarpophalangeal and Proximal Interphalangeal Joints

Richard S. Idler

INDICATIONS/CONTRAINDICATIONS

Capsulectomy is a surgical procedure commonly employed to restore motion in the stiff metacarpophalangeal (MCP) and proximal interphalangeal (PIP) joints of the hand. The surgical procedure involves excision of noncompliant or contracted portions of the joint capsule combined with mobilization or release of its specialized components that normally provide joint stability, that is, the collateral ligaments and palmar plate. Because the loss of joint motion is usually multifactorial, capsulectomy frequently is combined with other surgical procedures, such as tenolysis and release of soft-tissue contractures. Results of capsulectomy are most favorable when applied to pathology involving solely the joint capsule.

Management of the patient with a stiff MCP or PIP joint begins with a thorough understanding of the pathology that has produced the loss of joint motion and the tissues directly affected by the process. The original provocative pathology must be in a quiescent rather than an evolving phase before surgery can be considered. The normal inflammatory reaction that occurs in response to injury includes elements such as pain, edema, and fibrosis, which of themselves may compromise joint motion. Adding additional insult to injury from surgery in the presence of an ongoing pathologic process will serve only to compromise the ultimate results of surgery. Efforts at conservative management to restore joint motion should be continued until the pathologic process has reached a quiescent state.

It is critical that all conservative therapeutic efforts to regain joint motion are exhausted before considering surgical intervention. There are no absolutes that define a functional range of motion for the MCP or PIP joints. As a rule, when the arc of joint motion falls within 30 degrees of normal, surgery is unnecessary, and concerted efforts should be made at continuing therapy until a plateau in joint motion is achieved. In cases where inadequate

Richard S. Idler, M.D.: Hand Surgery Associates of Indiana, Indianapolis, IN

or no therapy has been provided, it is incumbent on the surgeon to assess the patient carefully in regard to the potential for improvement with conservative management and aggressive therapy. Therapy should include active assisted range of motion, passive range of motion, joint taping, and dynamic splinting. Measures should be taken to address edema and pain. The patient's own efforts at active motion may be assisted with functional electrical stimulation. For conservative treatment to succeed, the patient must understand the importance of frequent daily exercise sessions independent of those sessions conducted with a therapist.

As Curtis clearly pointed out, surgical capsulectomy rarely produces a return of normal joint motion but, in most cases, can offer functional improvement. Surgical capsulectomy, therefore, should be recommended only when therapy has failed and the gains likely to be realized from surgery will be of functional benefit to the patient.

The presence of arthritis is a contraindication to capsulectomy. The arthritis itself may be the explanation for the loss of joint motion. Even in the absence of acute inflammatory changes occurring within the joint capsule, one can anticipate a poor outcome following joint mobilization surgery if there has been any compromise in the quality of the articular surfaces. This particular pathology is frequently exacerbated after surgical challenge of capsulectomy and postoperative therapy.

PREOPERATIVE PLANNING

Before proceeding with capsulectomy, it is important that all potential causes for the loss of joint motion are taken into consideration and identified. Pathologic changes occurring within the joint capsule include loss of compliance, capsular contracture, or adhesion of its gliding surfaces. Capsulectomy should be part of the surgical release only if it is determined preoperatively to be one of the causative factors for loss of joint motion.

To perform surgery with the least impact on the surrounding soft tissues and the joint capsule, the surgeon must have a thorough understanding of the regional anatomy and the specific structure of the joint capsule to be approached. It is critically important that the surgeon understand that other causes may contribute to the loss of joint motion. The surgeon must be prepared to differentiate these other causes of joint dysfunction and to deal with them should they exist concurrently with capsular pathology.

The joints to be surgically released should be inspected carefully for signs of swelling or erythema, which may indicate an ongoing inflammatory process that has not reached a quiescent state. The periarticular tissue should be palpated for evidence of deeper soft-tissue contractures, such as Dupuytren's cords. Occasionally, the presence of an extra-articular exostosis is identified. Scars should be examined to ensure that they do not compromise a normal surgical approach to the joint capsule. If they are contracted as part of the pathologic process, release of the contracture and excision of the scar with appropriate coverage must be planned. Such combined procedures may not permit initiation of immediate motion, potentially compromising the final result.

Because motion at the MCP and PIP joints can be influenced by intrinsic contractures, an intrinsic tightness test should be performed to rule out this pathology. Loss of joint motion also may occur with pathology affecting the excursion of the adjacent flexor and extensor tendons. In assessing the flexor system, particular attention should be paid to evaluation of the status of the flexor sheath and its pulleys. Bowstringing across either the MCP or PIP joints may be a contributing factor to flexion contractures, and will continue to be so following capsulectomy if not dealt with appropriately. Finally, careful radiographic evaluation should be performed of the joints in question to assess the status of the joint surfaces and to rule out any mechanical blocks to motion, such as joint incongruity, fracture malunions, or periarticular exostoses.

The results after capsulectomy will be influenced greatly by postoperative management. To achieve a successful result, the surgeon must be prepared to provide the patient during the postoperative period of rehabilitation with an aggressive and comprehensive therapy program using necessary modalities to maximize and maintain the joint motion gained at surgery.

SURGERY

Capsulectomy at either the MCP or PIP joint level may be performed with the patient under local anesthesia. Use of local anesthesia allows the patient to move the joint undergoing surgical release actively to assess the adequacy of the release. It is also helpful in identifying other causes of limited joint motion, such as tendon adhesions or mechanical blocks to joint motion, such as obliteration of the palmar recess. The limiting factor to working with the patient under local anesthesia tends to be the duration of tourniquet time, which can be somewhat diminished by using a wrist-block anesthetic and sterile wrist tourniquet. Additional patient comfort can be achieved using short-acting intravenous sedatives administered by an anesthesiologist. If a more extensive surgical procedure is required, a reversible regional anesthetic in the form of a Bier block supplemented with local anesthetic can be used, which allows multiple joints to be approached with a longer tourniquet time.

The patient is positioned in the supine position on the operating table. A well-padded, pneumatic tourniquet is placed about the upper aspect of the arm. The desired anesthetic is administered. The extremity is prepared and draped in a sterile fashion. As needed, a sterile wrist tourniquet may be used. The extremity is exsanguinated by dependent positioning or the use of an elastic wrap, following which the tourniquet is inflated to 250 mm Hg.

Dorsal Metacarpophalangeal Capsulotomy

If approaching a single MCP joint, a linear incision is made directly over the dorsal aspect of the joint. If multiple joints are being approached, linear incisions over the dorsum of the web space between two adjacent joints, or a transverse incision across all joints at the MCP level, may be used (Fig. 23.1A). Dissection is carried down sharply through the skin and subcutaneous tissues, taking care to avoid injury to the larger longitudinal veins and the dorsal sensory nerves. The extensor mechanism is split longitudinally through the central tendon (Fig. 23.1B). The dorsal joint capsule then is mobilized from the central tendon and sagittal bands. If necessary, a local extensor tenolysis is performed. Assessment is made of the location of the radial and ulnar collateral ligaments. The dorsal joint capsule is sharply excised (Fig. 23.1C) to allow visualization of the articular surfaces. Using a small elevator, the collateral ligaments are freed of any adhesions between their synovial surface and the condylar recess of the joint. At this point, an attempt is made to flex the MCP joint passively. It is important to translate the articular surface of the base of the proximal phalanx along the curvature of the corresponding articular surface of the metacarpal head. If full joint motion is not possible or there is a tendency of the joint to open like a hinge, as opposed to gliding on the head of the metacarpal, adhesions of the palmar capsular recess may be present. This space can be released by passing a blunt elevator through the recesses of each collateral ligament to reach the palmar surface of the metacarpal head and the palmar plate (Fig. 23.2). If incomplete joint motion persists, recession of the collateral ligaments is indicated and is done with a scalpel blade placed in the collateral ligament recess and sharply releasing the ligament from the head of the metacarpal (Fig. 23.3A). It is possible to stage the amount of release beginning dorsally and progressing palmarly until full passive joint motion is present (Fig. 23.3B). Whenever possible, a portion of the radial collateral ligament is preserved, particularly in the index finger, to prevent ulnar drift with pinch and power grasp.

At this point, the central extensor tendon is reapproximated with interrupted white braided nonabsorbable 3-0 suture. The pneumatic tourniquet is released, and wound hemostasis is achieved using electrocautery. Wound hemostatic agents, such as thrombin or gelfoam, may be helpful. Once tourniquet paresis has passed, the patient is permitted to flex and extend the involved joint actively. If active motion does not equal the passive motion gained by capsulectomy, assessment must be made as to whether the problem relates to a lack of excursion in the flexor/extensor tendons or there are other potential causes for this absence of motion.

Assuming satisfactory motion has been achieved, final wound hemostasis is obtained. If excessive bleeding persists, the tourniquet may be reinflated for wound closure over a

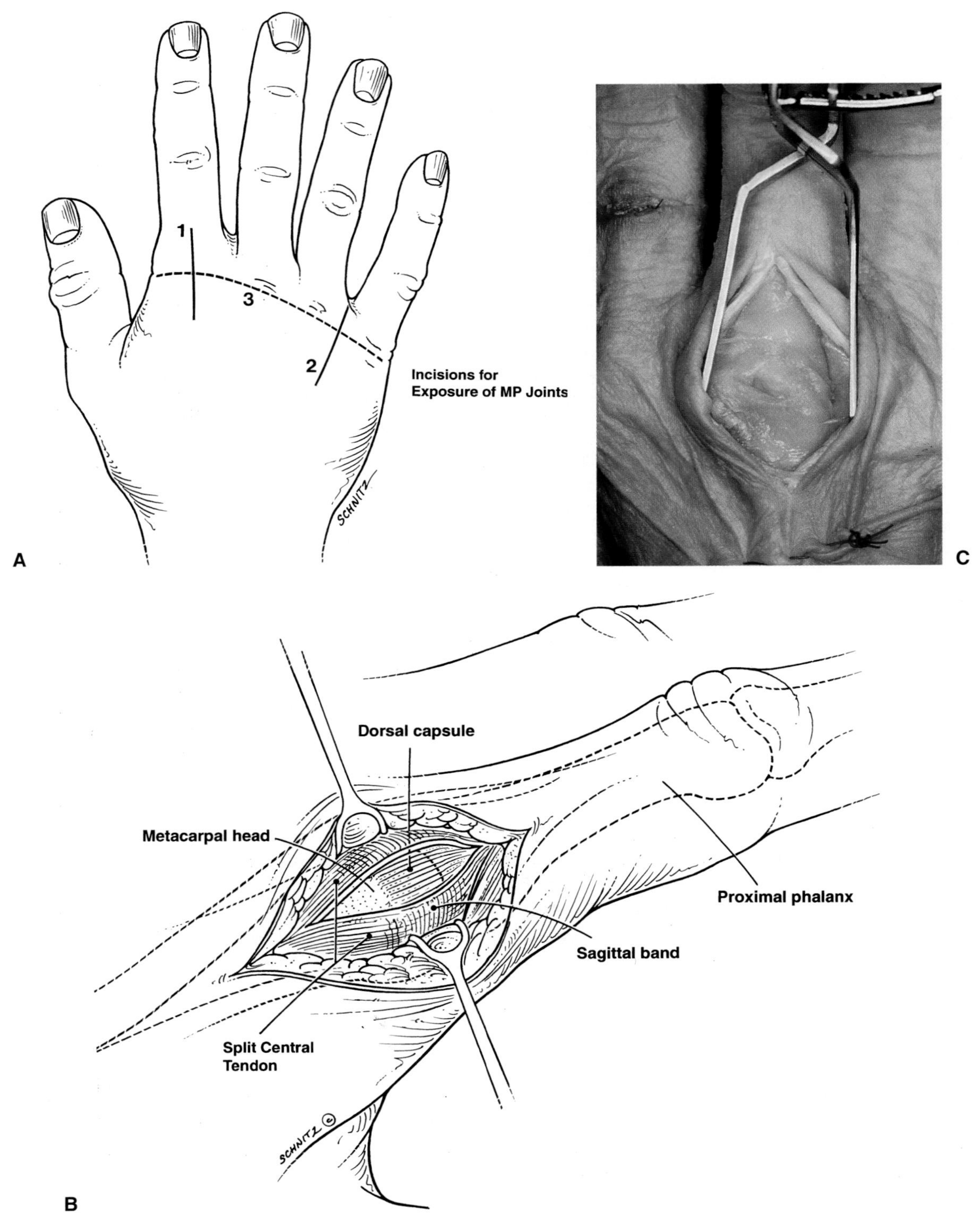

Figure 23.1. A: Potential approaches for a dorsal metacarpophalangeal (MCP) capsulectomy. 1. Midline dorsal approach to single MCP joint. 2. Dorsal web-space incision to the approach to adjacent MCP joints. 3. Transverse incision to approach multiple MCP joints. **B, C:** After exposure of the extensor mechanism, the central tendon is split longitudinally over the MCP joint. The extensor hood and sagittal bands are mobilized from the dorsal capsule if necessary; an extensor tenolysis proximal and distal to the MCP joint can be performed at this time.

drain. Skin closure is accomplished with interrupted sutures of 4-0 or 5-0 monofilament suture. Active and passive motion is checked a final time after completing wound closure if there is any concern regarding the influence the surrounding soft tissues might have on joint motion. Once the wound is closed, a well-padded dressing with a dorsal splint is applied to the hand, holding the MCP joints in approximately 60 to 80 degrees of flexion. Once the dressing is in place, the pneumatic tourniquet is released.

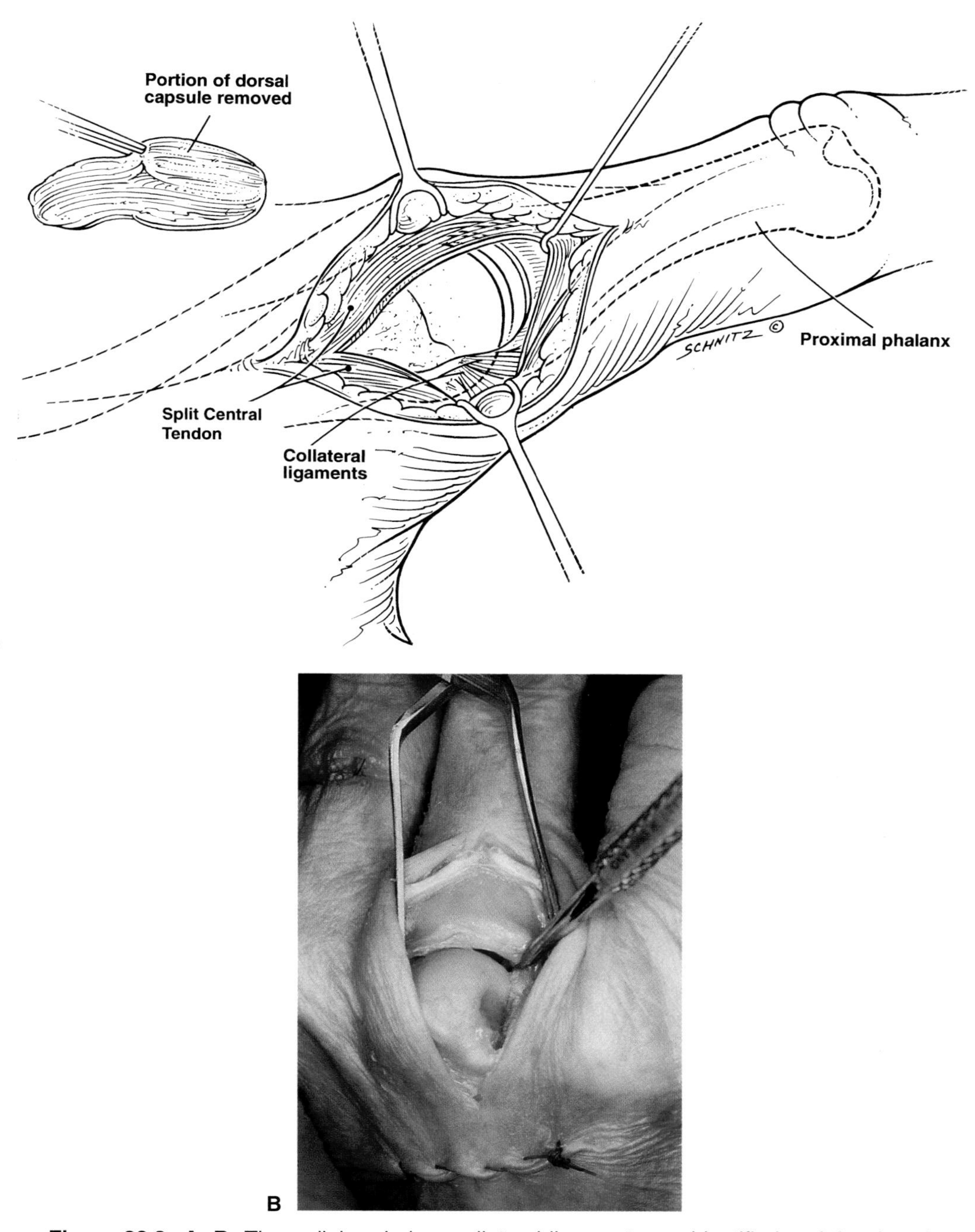

Figure 23.2. A, B: The radial and ulnar collateral ligaments are identified and the dorsal capsule excised. It is now possible to introduce a small periosteal elevator along the collateral recess on each side of the metacarpal head to release any adhesions. The same technique is used to reach the palmar recess.

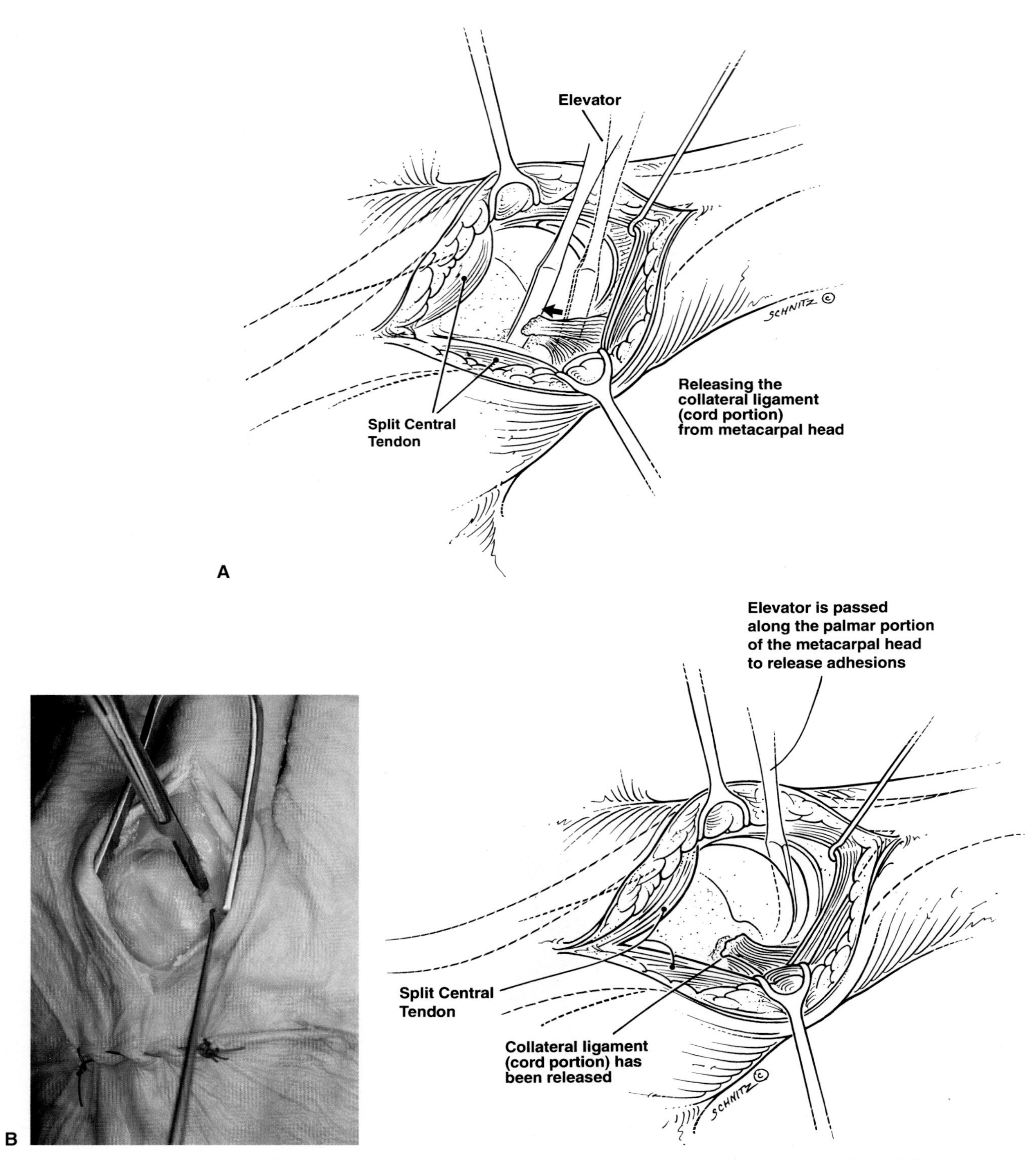

Figure 23.3. A, B: If full passive flexion is still not possible, the collateral ligaments are released from the metacarpal origin.

Proximal Interphalangeal Dorsal Capsulotomy

A linear incision is made over the PIP joint (Fig. 23.4). Dissection is carried down sharply through the skin and subcutaneous tissue, with hemostasis achieved using electrocautery. Care is taken to avoid dorsal sensory nerve branches in the area. The overlying soft tissue is mobilized, exposing the extensor mechanism. The extensor mechanism is visualized laterally until the transverse retinacular fibers at the level of the PIP joint can be identified. The transverse retinacular fibers then are released along the palmar margin of the lateral bands at the level of the PIP joint. Once the transverse retinacular ligament has been released along the radial and ulnar sides of the extensor mechanism, a blunt elevator or scalpel blade is used to lyse and define the plane between the lateral band and the capsule of the PIP joint. Proximal to the joint, a plane is developed between the deep surface of the extensor mechanism and the shaft of the proximal phalanx. If necessary, tenolysis can be applied to the terminal extensor tendon. It is now possible to elevate the lateral bands to visualize the joint capsule. Once the location of the collateral ligaments is determined, an arthrotomy is made just dorsal to the collateral ligaments to permit visualization of the joint space and the dorsal aspect of the condylar head of the proximal phalanx. A small scalpel blade is inserted into the joint space and directed along the dorsal margin of the head of the proximal phalanx, releasing the dorsal capsule from its attachments to the head of the proximal phalanx (Fig. 23.5). This release is repeated from the opposite side of the joint. Care is taken to release and, if necessary, to excise the entire dorsal joint capsule. Using a small blunt-tipped elevator, the recess between the collateral ligaments and head of the proximal phalanx is mobilized. Through this same approach, it should be possible to mobilize any adhesions in the palmar capsular recess. Then the joint is passively flexed. If there is a tendency of the joint to hinge open, there may not be complete clearance of the palmar recess, or there may be obliteration of the retrocondylar space.

If it is still not possible to flex the joint fully, it is necessary to ensure that there are no proximal adhesions of the extensor mechanism that might be limiting its excursion. If not, recession of the collateral ligaments is indicated. A scalpel blade is inserted within the collateral recess, and by subperiosteal dissection the collateral ligament is released from its attachments to the head of the proximal phalanx. Recession of the collateral ligaments can be done in stages, beginning dorsally and progressing palmarly until full digital flexion is achieved (Fig. 23.6). As the joint is passively flexed, the extensor mechanism is observed to

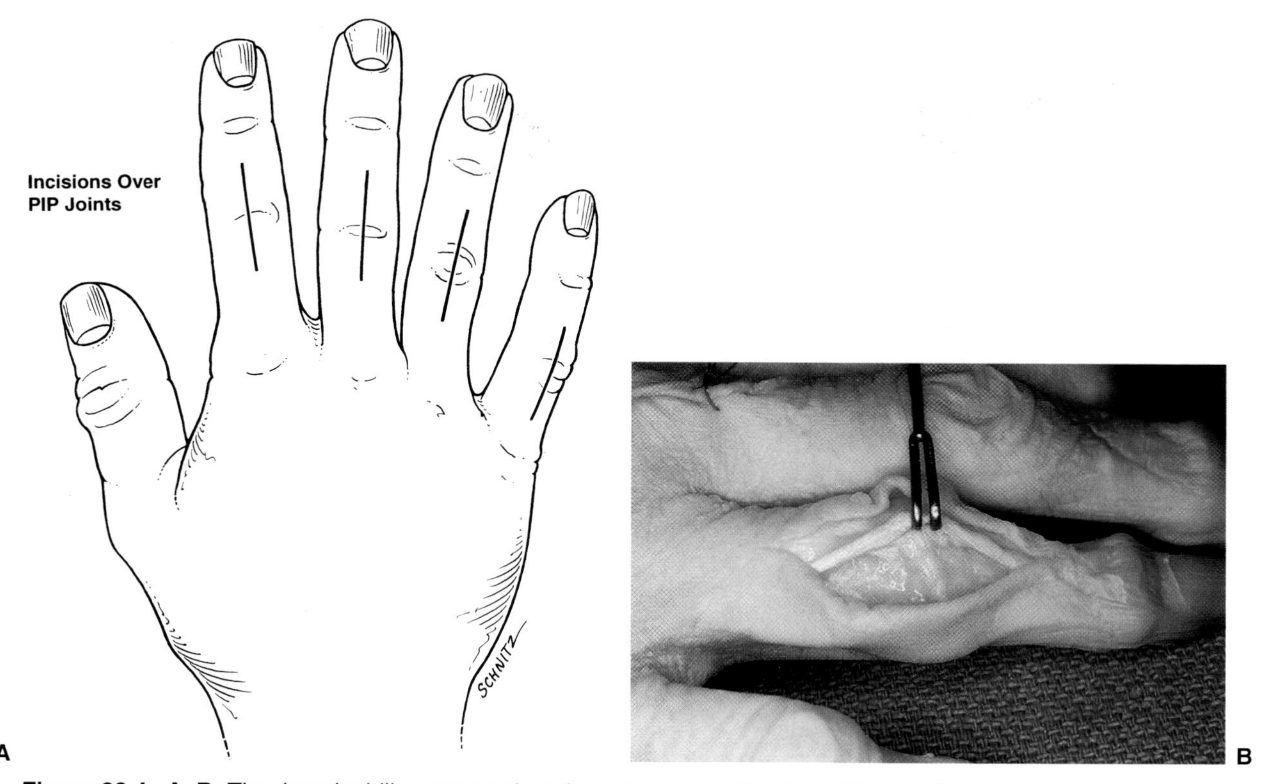

Figure 23.4. A, B: The dorsal midline approach to the extensor mechanism at the proximal interphalangeal (PIP) joint. After identifying the palmar margin of the lateral bands, they are sharply released from the transverse retinacular fibers. The lateral bands and extensor mechanism proximal and distal to the PIP joint are tenolysed as needed.

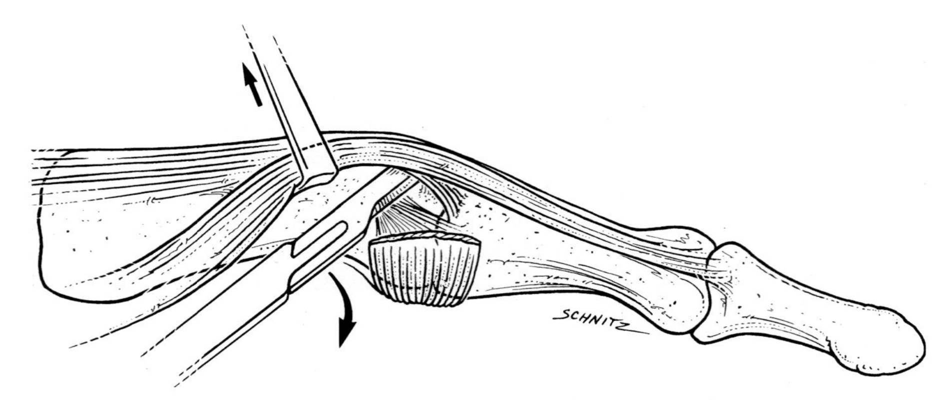

Figure 23.5. With the extensor mechanism elevated with a retractor, the joint is entered just dorsal to the collateral ligament on each side of the joint. Keeping the articular surface in view, the dorsal capsule is excised. A small periosteal elevator may now be introduced into the collateral and palmar recesses to lyse any adhesions.

A

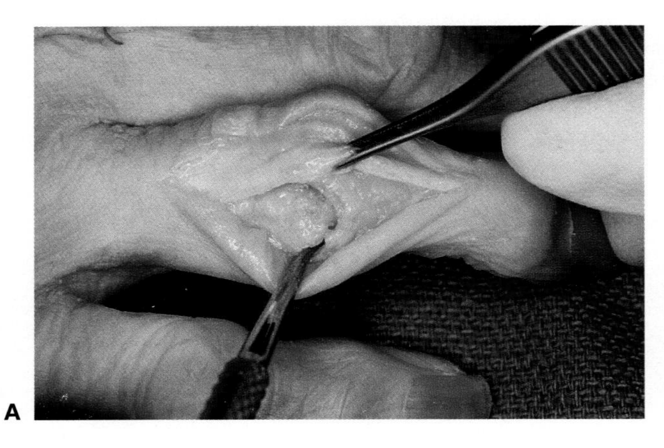

Figure 23.6. A, B: If required, the collateral ligaments are released from their proximal phalangeal origin and the palmar recess cleared again. If full passive flexion is not present, then proximal adhesions of the extensor mechanism or contracture of its contributing muscle groups must be considered.

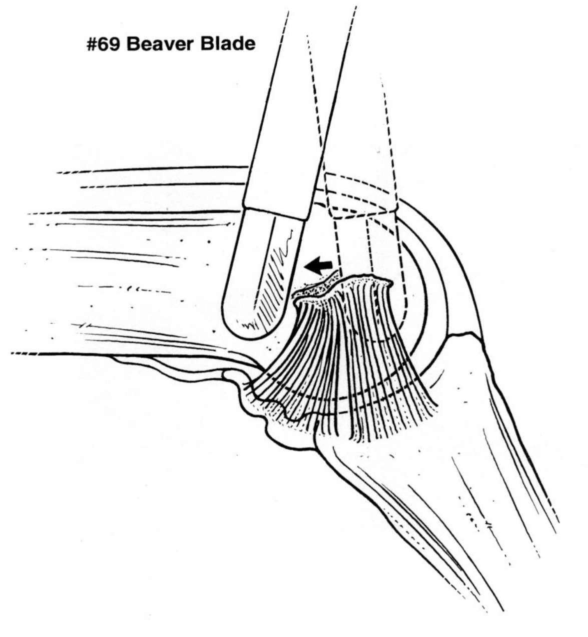

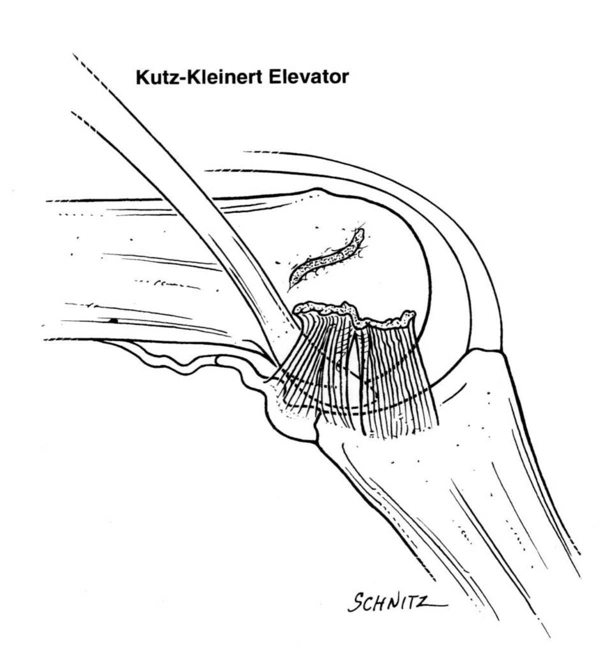

B

ensure that it remains centrally located over the head of the proximal phalanx. There should be no pivoting of the joint about one of the collateral ligaments as it goes into flexion. Should this occur, additional mobilization or release of this collateral ligament is required. If the extensor mechanism tends to shift in one direction, repair of the opposing transverse retinacular fibers to the lateral band can be performed to counteract this tendency.

At this point, the pneumatic tourniquet is released and additional wound hemostasis is achieved using electrocautery with or without topical hemostatic agents. Once tourniquet paresis has passed, the patient is allowed to flex and extend the PIP joint actively. If motion is inadequate, consideration must be given to the presence of additional pathology compromising tendon excursion. Extensor adhesions should be addressed in the same surgical setting by a more thorough tenolysis. Intrinsic tightness may require a more proximal mobilization, slide, or release of the intrinsic system. If the pathology exists in the flexor system, it is recommended that this be addressed in a second surgical setting, unless it is anticipated that the flexor adhesions can be released by a simple flexor traction tenolysis or limited surgical release.

Once full active motion is confirmed, the pneumatic tourniquet may be reinflated for closure if necessary. Skin-wound closure is accomplished with interrupted sutures of 5-0 nonabsorbable monofilament suture. Active and passive motion is checked a final time after wound closure if there is any concern regarding the influence of the soft tissues on joint motion. A bulky compressive dressing with a dorsal splint is applied while holding the fingers in a functional position of flexion.

Proximal Interphalangeal Palmar Capsulectomy

A Bruner incision is designed over the PIP joint (Fig. 23.7). A midlateral approach may be used if a flexor tenolysis is anticipated. Dissection is carried down sharply through the skin and subcutaneous tissues, with hemostasis achieved using electrocautery. Care is taken to avoid injury to the radial and ulnar digital neurovascular bundles. These structures are identified and retracted to the periphery of the wound. The digital artery is used as a guide for identifying the check-rein ligaments. The proximal

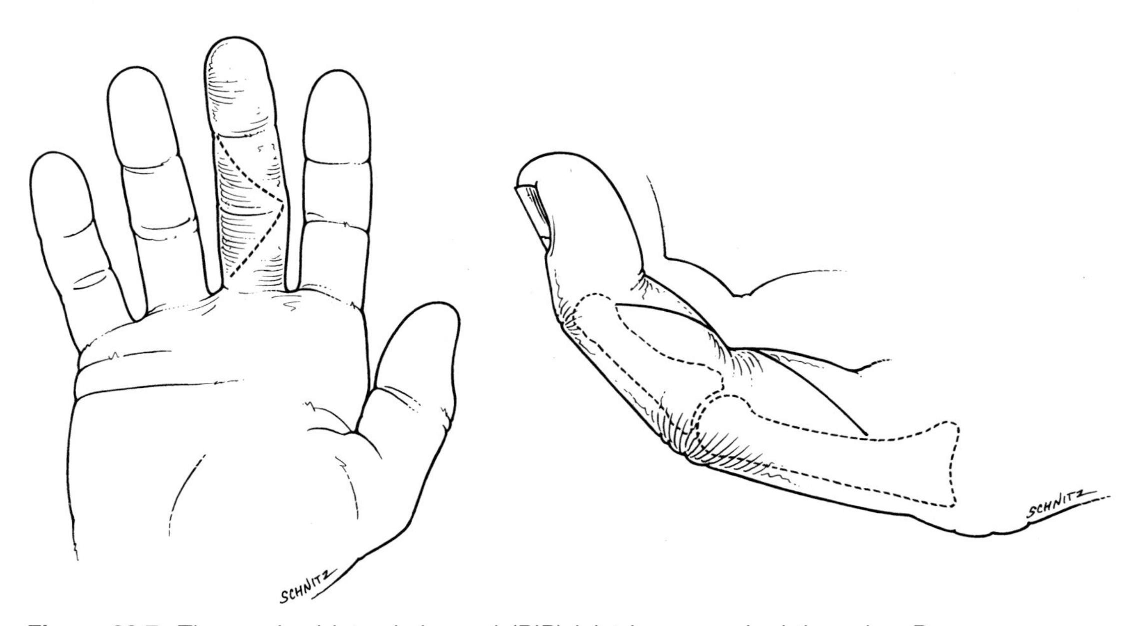

Figure 23.7. The proximal interphalangeal (PIP) joint is approached through a Bruner incision. The flexor sheath is exposed and the transverse digital vessels identified at this level.

transverse digital branches going to the vincular system supplying the vinculum brevis of the superficialis and vinculum longus of the profundus tendon, pass just distal and dorsal to the proximal insertions of the check-rein ligaments into the shaft of the proximal phalanx. After identifying this landmark, the C_1 portion of the flexor sheath is excised between the A_2 and A_3 pulleys (Fig. 23.8), exposing the flexor digitorum superficialis and profundus tendons. As needed, these are tenolysed in the exposed area of the flexor system. The check-rein ligaments are identified by passing a fine hemostat through the foramen of the transverse digital vessels, keeping the hemostat superficial to the vessels but deep to the check-rein ligament. Once the check rein is isolated, it is sharply divided. Both the radial and ulnar check rein ligaments must be released. At this point, an attempt is made to extend the PIP joint passively. If the joint cannot be fully extended or there is rebound that persists following extension, the palmar plate is released sharply from its attachments to the accessory collateral ligament on both sides of the joint up to the joint space. If there is persistent resistance to PIP extension, the collateral ligaments are recessed (Fig. 23.9) by passing a small, sharp scalpel blade into the collateral recess on each side of the joint and releasing the collateral ligaments from their insertion into the head of the proximal phalanx (Fig. 23.9). This procedure should be performed in a sequential manner beginning palmarly and progressing dorsally until full extension is achieved. If full passive extension of the PIP joint is still not possible, a careful search must be made for more proximal flexor adhesions or additional soft tissue or skin contractures that are preventing full PIP extension.

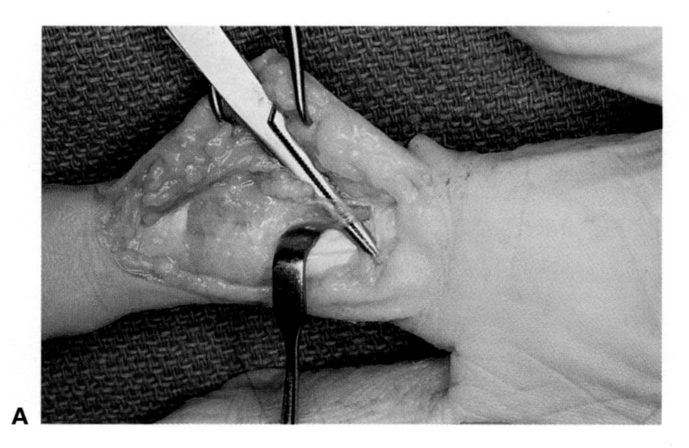

Figure 23.8. A, B: The flexor sheath is excised between the A_2 and A_3 pulleys. The check-rein ligaments are identified. The check-rein ligaments can be found passing over the transverse retinacular vessels as they enter the flexor sheath at this level.

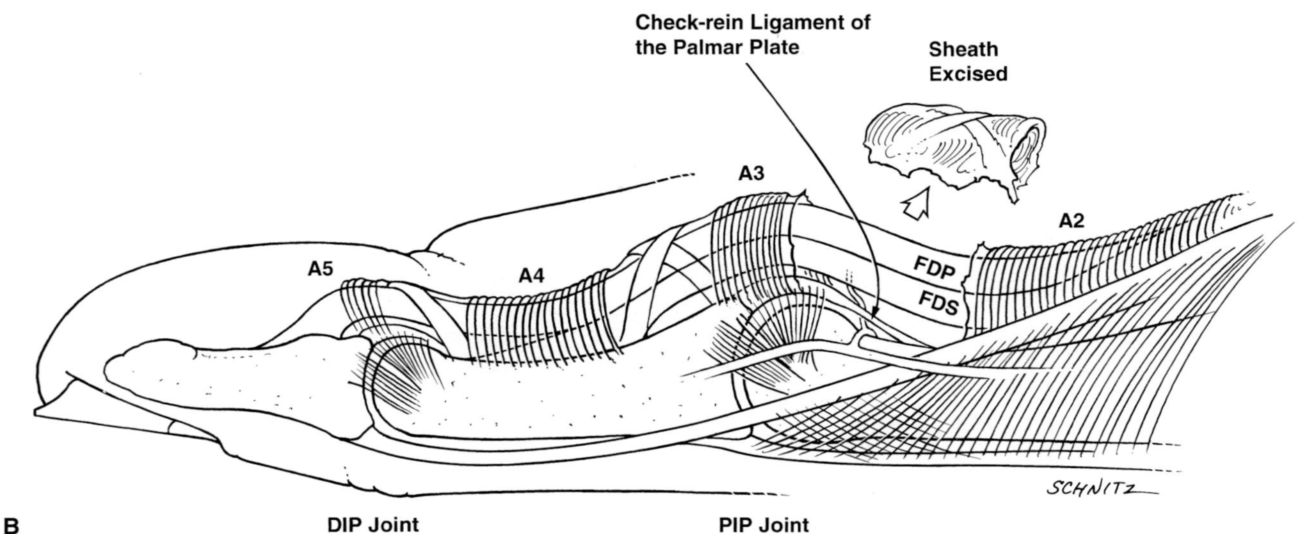

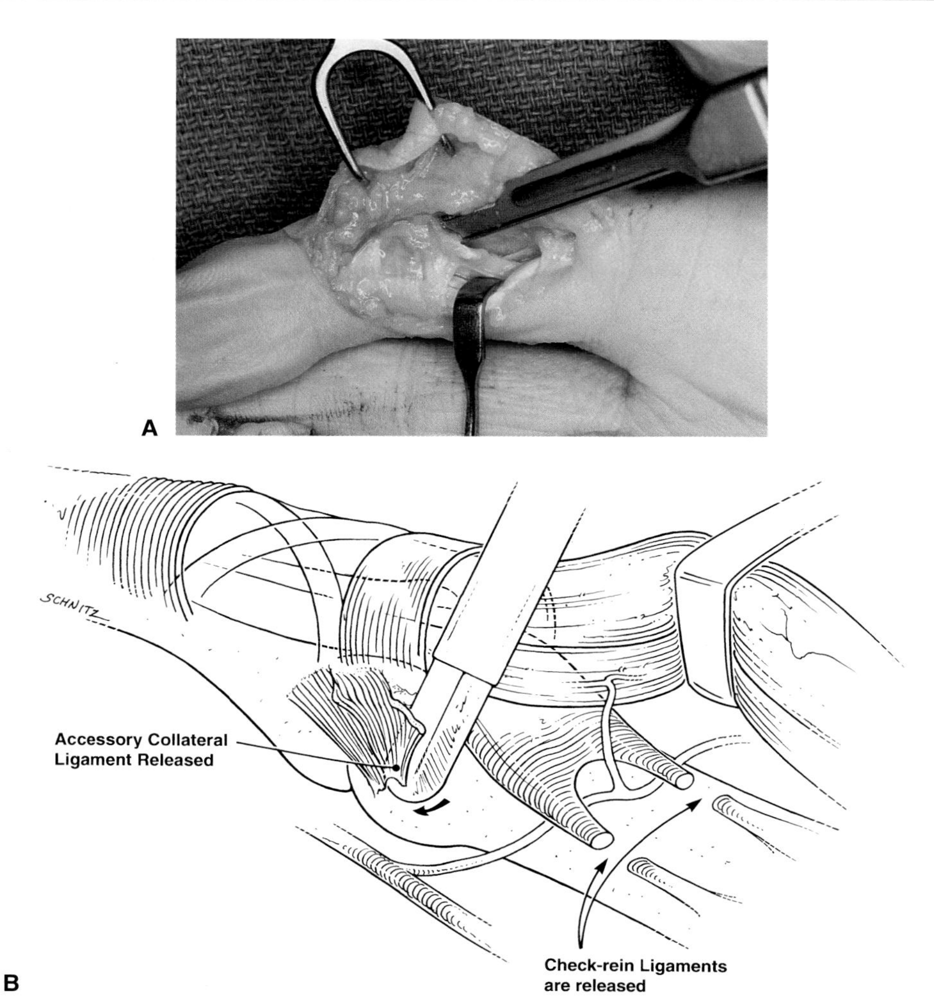

Figure 23.9. A, B: If full passive extension is not possible, the palmar plate is released from both accessory collateral ligaments. The collateral recess on either side of the proximal phalangeal head then may be probed with a small elevator. Persistent limitation in extension may require release in the collateral ligaments. If there continues to be limited extension of the joint, consideration should be given to more proximal tenolysis or other pathology.

After full passive extension is achieved, the pneumatic tourniquet is released. Additional wound hemostasis is achieved using electrocautery or topical hemostatic agents. Once tourniquet paresis passes, the patient is allowed to flex and extend the fingers actively. If the patient cannot actively achieve the full passive potential for joint motion, there may be problems with the excursion of either the flexor or extensor systems. Flexor adhesions may be addressed in the same surgical procedure with a more aggressive tenolysis. Pathology on the extensor side is best addressed in a second surgical procedure unless it is certain that only a limited extensor release is required.

At this point, the pneumatic tourniquet may be reinflated for wound closure if necessary. Skin-wound closure is accomplished with interrupted sutures of 5-0 nonabsorbable monofilament suture. Active and passive motion should be checked a final time if there is concern regarding the influence of these tissues on joint motion. A well-padded dressing is applied to the upper extremity, holding the MCP joints in a position of 40 to 60 degrees of flexion and the PIP joint fully extended. Once the dressing is in place, the pneumatic tourniquet is released.

POSTOPERATIVE MANAGEMENT AND REHABILITATION

In most instances, capsulectomy of the MCP or PIP joint is performed as an outpatient procedure. Consideration may be given to hospitalization of the patient in cases where the surgery has been extraordinarily involved and there is a need for parenteral administration of medications, such as antibiotics or analgesics. Immediately following surgery, arrangements are made for scheduling a postoperative therapy appointment for the patient. The therapist is contacted directly and given details about the operation, including the quality of the adjacent tendons, status of the articular surfaces, and documented active and passive range of motion measured intraoperatively. The therapist is given specific instructions regarding the types of exercises to be performed, their frequency, need for static or dynamic splinting, and modalities such as the use of transcutaneous electrical stimulation, continuous passive motion (CPM), or functional electrical stimulation.

Therapy usually is initiated within 24 to 48 hours of surgery. During that interval, the patient is instructed to continue elevation of the operated extremity above the heart level. The dressing is to be kept dry and intact until therapy is initiated. Bathing may be permitted with the use of a waterproof barrier over the dressing. Outpatients are provided with oral pain medication. A prophylactic dose of parenteral antibiotics may be administered before the initiation of surgery; however, patients are not routinely given postoperative antibiotics.

On initial presentation to the therapist, the surgical dressing is taken down. Wounds are inspected carefully for any evidence of erythema, drainage, hematoma formation, or postoperative swelling. The patient is instructed in performing active, active-assisted, and passive range-of-motion exercises to the released joint. When the joint release is performed at the PIP joint level, blocking of the MCP joint emphasizing motion at the PIP joint is frequently helpful. Initially, exercises are performed four to six times per day, depending on the patient's level of discomfort and postoperative swelling. If passive motion is acceptable but active motion deficient, functional electrical stimulation may be used. If problems are encountered maintaining passive motion, the use of taping, dynamic splinting, or CPM may be considered.

Patients are typically splinted between exercise sessions for comfort. In most instances, safe position splinting with the MCP joints in 60 to 80 degrees of flexion and the interphalangeal (IP) joints extended is the position of choice. As swelling and discomfort abate, light use of the hand may replace immobilization. Once functional use has been established for light activities, strengthening can be initiated. If at any time the patient shows evidence of redeveloping preoperative contracture, appropriate static or dynamic splinting is instituted immediately to counter this occurrence.

The initial frequency of formal therapy sessions is determined by the patient's progress in therapy. Daily sessions may be required if multiple digits have been released or if the patient performs poorly in the initial therapy sessions. It is stressed to the patient that he or she is responsible for maintaining the frequency of the therapy sessions when not in the attendance of a therapist. At each therapy session, careful measurements are made of the patient's active and passive range of motion at each operated joint, and appropriate adjustments in therapy are made based on these measurements. Assuming that the patient makes acceptable progress in therapy, the frequency of formal therapy sessions and daily exercises is tapered with incorporation of functional activities. It may be necessary, however, to continue with dynamic and static splinting for up to 6 to 12 weeks after surgery.

Patients can expect to reach a plateau in recovery by 3 months after surgery. In some situations, a quiescent state may not be reached until 6 months. Review of the literature and the author's personal experience reveal that results are inversely related to the number of structures that require manipulation to regain motion at the joint; that is, the simpler the procedure the better the result.

In discussing the outcomes of surgery with patients, several points must be made clear. As reflected in the results of the surgical literature, after release of the stiff digital joint, the patient cannot anticipate full restoration of motion but is likely to experience an improvement in motion. In some cases, there will be no improvement of motion; however, the arc of motion will be in a more functional position after surgery. The results of surgery will be highly dependent on the number of structures that require manipulation or release. In certain situations, such as post-traumatic arthritis or with postoperative complications, it is possible that joint motion will be worse following surgery. The patient must also understand that the results of surgery will be affected by the patient's willingness to participate in an aggressive therapy program to maintain the motion gained at surgery.

COMPLICATIONS

A number of complications specifically related to joint capsulectomy can occur, and both the surgeon and patient must be aware of these potential problems. As the loss of digital joint motion may be multifactorial, it is critically important after the capsulectomy that other causes of limited joint motion have been dealt with appropriately. To do so requires checking active and passive range of motion after capsulectomy and wound closure, most easily done in the situation where the patient has undergone only a local anesthetic and can actively move the joint intraoperatively. Performing this maneuver following capsulectomy is helpful in assessing the need for associated tenolysis. If the patient is not under local anesthesia, a tendon traction test should be performed, which involves exposing the tendon at a more proximal level outside the zone of pathology and applying traction on the flexor or extensor tendons to simulate active motion. If tenolysis is required, active motion or the tendon traction test should be repeated to determine its adequacy in improving active joint motion. Following release of the implicated tendon, its quality should be noted carefully for potential risk of rupture during postoperative therapy. Stability of the tendon about the released joint should also be evaluated. Decentralization of the extensor mechanism may occur dorsally at the PIP or MCP joint after surgical release. Likewise, bowstringing of the flexor tendon may occur across the PIP joint following flexor tenolysis. Either flexor or extensor tendon instability will compromise postoperative results. A final check of joint motion should be made after wound closure to ensure that noncompliant soft-tissue or skin contractures are not likely to compromise the final result. Typically, if these are anticipated to be a problem, they must be dealt with before proceeding with the joint release.

If, following joint release, full passive motion is restored but the patient is unable to generate comparable active motion through the opposing tendon system, consideration must be given to either incompetency or adhesion of that system. This scenario is encountered frequently in surgical intervention for joints that lack motion in both flexion and extension. Unless it is anticipated that active motion could be restored through a limited surgical or traction tenolysis, I recommend that surgery be confined to one side of the joint at a time to limit postoperative swelling and scarring; however, to do so requires changes in the postoperative therapy to substitute passive range of motion and dynamic splinting for the patient's absent active tendon excursion. If the patient is able to maintain the passive joint motion gained following the initial surgery, once soft-tissue equilibrium has been achieved, the joint is approached from the opposite side in a second procedure to attempt to restore active motion.

Depending on the extent of the surgical release and the quality of the periarticular tissues, considerable bleeding may occur after the surgical procedure. It is recommended that the tourniquet be let down following joint release and before wound closure. The use of thrombin, gelfoam, or other types of topical anticoagulants may be helpful in controlling intraoperative bleeding. If necessary, a drain may be placed in the wound to prevent hematoma formation. Should a postoperative hematoma develop, aspiration or surgical drainage is recommended.

Aggressive postoperative therapy may delay the process of wound healing. Therapy may also generate additional postoperative bleeding and edema. For this reason, the patient may be at increased risk of developing a wound infection and, therefore, must be monitored carefully. It is important that the therapist is experienced and knowledgeable about the early signs of infection so that these might be reported to the surgeon. In the case of a suspected postoperative wound infection, the patient should be treated with appropriate oral antibiotics, edema control, and immobilization until signs of infection have resolved. If such resolution does not occur within 48 hours after initiation of treatment for the presumed infection, more aggressive intervention in the form of parenteral antibiotics and wound exploration may be required.

In the setting of delayed wound healing, particularly in the event of an infection, wound dehiscence may occur. Minor wound breakdown may be addressed by temporarily decreasing the frequency and intensity of therapy until the wound stabilizes. More significant wound breakdown or exposure of tissues at risk of desiccation will require revision wound closure or coverage.

Radical release or excision of the collateral ligaments at either the MCP or PIP joint level may result in joint instability, which may present in the form of intraoperative or postoperative joint subluxation or dislocation. This complication is most likely to develop when secondary joint stabilizers also have been released or mobilized. Diao and Eaton reported no problems with instability following total collateral ligament excision at the PIP joint; however, my personal experience has not been as fortunate. Management may require temporary joint immobilization by splinting or percutaneous pin fixation for up to three weeks to regain joint stability. The usual consequence of this period of immobilization, however, is loss of joint motion. Chronic joint instability following capsulectomy may result in acceleration of post-traumatic arthritis. A painful unstable joint will require arthrodesis.

Long-standing contractures may have specific problems that present intraoperatively. Following release of a flexion contracture, the surgeon may encounter myostatic contracture of the flexor mechanism or arterial vasospasm, which limits the patient's potential for passive extension and postoperative immobilization. These problems are best addressed by immobilization of the MCP joint in maximum flexion and PIP joint extended as tolerated. Postoperatively, a program of interval dynamic extension splinting or graduated static extension splinting should be initiated as soon as possible.

RECOMMENDED READINGS

1. Curtis RM. Capsulectomy of the interphalangeal joints of the fingers. *J Bone Joint Surg* 36A:1219–1232, 1954.
2. Diao E, Eaton R. Total collateral ligament excision for contractures of the proximal interphalangeal joint. *J Hand Surg* 18A:395–402, 1993.
3. Gould JS, Nicholson BG. Capsulectomy of the metacarpophalangeal and proximal interphalangeal joints. *J Hand Surg* 4:482–486, 1979.
4. Harrison DH. The stiff proximal interphalangeal joint. *The Hand* 9:102–108, 1977.
5. Minamikawa Y, Horii E, Amadio PC, et al. Stability and constraint of the proximal interphalangeal joint. *J Hand Surg* 18A:198–204, 1993.
6. Sprague BL. Proximal interphalangeal joint contractures and their treatment. *J Trauma* 16:259–265, 1976.
7. Young VL, Wray C, Weeks PM. The surgical management of stiff joints in the hand. *Plast Reconstr Surg* 62: 835–841, 1978.

24

Treatment Options for Distal Tip Amputations

Raymond A. Wittstadt

INDICATIONS/CONTRAINDICATIONS

Tissue loss and amputations of the fingers are among the most common injuries encountered in the emergency room by those involved in care of the hand. These injuries have considerable social and economic impact and can lead to prolonged lost time from work. Unfortunately, treatment is often relegated to the least skilled or experienced providers. I feel that careful consideration and discussion of the treatment options can improve functional outcomes and minimize lost time from work.

By convention, the fingertip is that portion of the finger distal to the distal interphalangeal (DIP) joint and tendon insertions. It is a complex anatomic area with almost all appendicular tissue types represented and vulnerable to injury. The volar pulp consists of highly innervated glabrous skin and subcutaneous fat anchored by fibroseptae. The nail, nailbed, and germinal matrix are on the dorsal surface (Fig. 24.1).

Many techniques have been tried over the years to address tissue loss in the fingertip. There is no one best way to handle every injury, and treatment must be individualized. Each injury may have several solutions. The hand surgeon must fully evaluate each patient's occupation, hobbies, and emotional attitude regarding the injury. Only then can a rational choice be made regarding the treatment options.

Goals of treatment in fingertip injuries include preservation of adequate sensation (while avoiding or minimizing neuroma tenderness), provision of durable skin coverage, prevention of proximal joint contractures, maximizing finger length, and early return to work and other activities.

Absolute contraindications to any one technique cannot be given. However, some relative contraindications should be considered. Rotation or advancement flaps should be used with caution, or not at all, in patients with vascular disease (Raynaud's phenomenon, renal

Raymond A. Wittstadt, M.D., M.P.H.: Department of Orthopaedic Surgery, Johns Hopkins Hospital, Baltimore, MD, and The Curtis National Hand Center, Union Memorial Hospital, Baltimore, MD

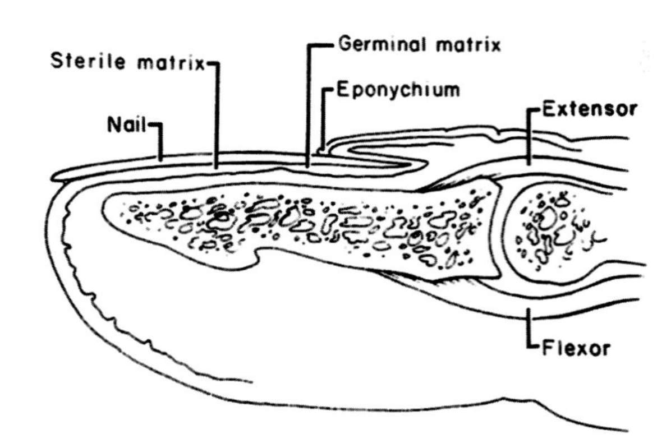

Figure 24.1. Fingertip anatomy. Note that the germinal and sterile matrix rests directly on the dorsal periosteum of the distal phalanx. Numerous fibrous septae anchor volar glaborus skin to the underlying bone.

failure, some connective tissue disorders, and inflammatory arthropathies). Coverage alternatives that require extremes of positioning or lengthy duration of immobilization must be weighed against potential joint contractures. Heroic efforts to salvage nearly unreconstructable injuries, including multistep operative plans requiring complex tissue transfers, must be balanced against ultimate functional and cosmetic concerns.

MECHANISMS OF INJURY

Causes of fingertip injuries fall into three main categories: crush, laceration, and avulsion. Crushing is caused by the application of pressure to the fingertip, crushing the structures or pinching with enough force to cause amputation. Catching the fingertip in a machine or door is typical of this mechanism.

Lacerations occur with sharp objects such as a knife or a saw. Laceration is a common component of essentially all open distal tip injuries. The amount of tissue trauma, contamination, and orientation of the laceration will determine the reconstructive options.

Avulsion occurs when tissue is removed by tangentially applied forces or distraction; "roller injuries" are typical examples of avulsion trauma. By definition, avulsion injuries involve a traction force on the tissues. This mechanism may present a greater zone of injury than is initially apparent because of traction injury to vessels and nerves.

Cleanly amputated fingers at or proximal to the DIP joint can be considered for replantation. Crushed or avulsed tissue is rarely suitable for replantation but can occasionally be used as a skin graft or composite graft when multiple adjacent digits have been traumatized.

PREOPERATIVE PLANNING

Operative planning begins with the patient's initial presentation in the emergency room. It is appropriate to perform and document an evaluation of the entire patient, particularly health status related to diabetes, vascular disease, and smoking. An expanded history should include mechanism and time of injury, whether the hand was caught in a machine and if so for how long, appropriate past medical and hand injury history, medications, and allergies. Hand dominance, occupation, and nonoccupational activities should be noted as well. Tetanus status is important in any open injury.

Examination requires complete careful removal of dressings. This can be painful, but sensation in the injured area must be determined before any local anesthesia is administered. Once sensation has been evaluated and documented (two-point discrimination may be the most available and logical objective data to record), local anesthesia can be given to provide pain relief and facilitate further evaluation of the injury. Examination of amputated tissue, if available, should also be performed. Factors such as angle of tissue loss, function of adjacent joints (tendon status), nail involvement, and amount of exposed bone should be noted.

RADIOLOGIC EVALUATION

Standard x-ray views are mandatory for all fingertip injuries. The amputated tissue should also be imaged in cases in which replantation or use of the amputated part for graft purposes is contemplated. Because a crushing mechanism is the cause of many distal tip injuries, it is important to check for fracture lines that may extend proximally into the joint and evaluate the degree of comminution of the involved segment. The bony injury often limits or influences the ultimate treatment choice.

SURGERY

Choosing among the various techniques available for repair can be daunting, and patient expectations demand that surgeons do not develop unidimensional approaches to the care of distal tip injuries. Often, more than one technique can be utilized; thus, the surgeon must maintain an expanded and current portfolio of treatment options. The final choice of treatment should take into consideration the total needs of the patient as well as the surgeon's experience and comfort level with various techniques.

Before describing the surgical alternatives, some consideration should be given to the venue and circumstances in which many of these procedures are performed. As noted previously, care for tip injury should not be assigned to trainees or less experienced physicians. The permanency and importance of the results requires greater attention and involvement of the hand surgeon. Many of these procedures can be safely, effectively, and efficiently performed in a well-stocked emergency department. Appropriate equipment, lighting, anesthetic capability, and manpower are the most important of the variables that determine whether this is feasible. It is never wrong to take a distal tip injury to a formal operating room, especially when multiple digits are involved or the flexor side is significantly traumatized. If there is any doubt about the level of care that can be rendered in a particular venue, then defaulting to the safest, most controlled environment will yield optimal results.

General Considerations

Unless there are exposed joint surfaces, tendons, or neurovascular structures, definitive treatment can usually be delayed by initial mechanical debridement and irrigation, followed by the application of a Xeroform Petrolatum dressing (Sherwood Medical, St. Louis, MO) or similar ointment dressing. There may be a benefit to delaying definitive treatment to assess the viability of traumatized tissue. In many cases, amputation may be the favored treatment after an initial assessment. However, if the digit is cleaned and dressed in the emergency department, later evaluation by the surgeon, consideration by the patient, and the "test of viability" afforded by reflection of 24 to 72 hours may alter that decision in favor of a reconstructive option over ablation.

Although this chapter focuses on local flaps for fingertip coverage, all techniques should be considered. Factors influencing the choice of technique include the angle of tissue loss, amount of exposed bone, condition of amputated part (if available), injuries to adjacent fingers, digit involved, size and location of defect, and patient wishes. Treatment principles should include preservation of all viable tissue and utilization of amputated parts. In general, it is best to choose the simplest procedure consistent with individual factors and the goals of treatment.

A reconstructive ladder is a consistent image to maintain when considering the options available to treat distal tip amputation. The steps up the ladder reflect increasing complexity of the reconstructive effort. The portfolio of treatment alternatives includes healing by secondary intention, shortening and primary closure, skin grafting (split or full thickness), and replacement of the amputated part (replantation with microsurgical techniques or a nonvascularized composite graft). Flaps that are attractive and useful for treating the tip injury include local flaps, regional flaps, and distant flaps.

Healing by Secondary Intention

Open treatment, or healing by secondary intention, results in healing by the re-epithelialization of granulation tissue and wound contracture. It is most useful in children and for defects of modest size (1 cm or less) or tangential injuries of variable levels of tissue loss. This treatment is simple to perform, burns no bridges because any reconstructive option can still be elected after an initial period of observation, and provides the best sensation. Complications are rare, including an almost nonexistent infection rate, and healing time is comparable to that of other methods. Like all tip injuries in which the distal phalanx is involved, if there is any unsupported nail bed, a hook nail deformity may result.

Primary Closure after Digital Shortening

Primary closure, when possible, is simple and provides good sensation, rapid healing, and early mobilization. The nail bed, or sterile matrix, should be trimmed to the level of the bony injury and should not be relied upon to cover exposed bone, which would inevitably lead to hook nail deformities. Bone should be trimmed to achieve a tension-free closure. Preservation of tendon insertions is helpful to maintain motion and strength.

Skin Grafting

Although favored by some surgeons involved in care of the hand, skin grafting is rarely used at our institution for reconstruction. It is inferior in the key parameters that are of greatest consideration in this common injury.

Skin grafts are associated with lack of durability, no sensibility, hyperpigmentation, asymmetric contraction, and donor morbidity. Almost any of the other options discussed will yield superior results to even a well-performed skin grafting procedure.

However, split- or full-thickness skin grafts can be used to cover defects considered too large to heal by secondary intention or those not felt to be candidates for the other coverage alternatives. Survival of a skin graft requires that the area on which it is placed has sufficient blood supply to support the transplanted skin. Exposed bone, cartilage, or tendon typically does not meet this requirement.

Skin texture and color match should be considered. When possible, glabrous skin from the hypothenar area or foot should be used. If primary closure of the donor site is not possible, it too can be skin grafted. If nonglabrous skin is used, avoid donor areas that are hair bearing. Glabrous skin from the amputated part, if available and not too damaged, can be used as well. When glabrous skin is used, the appearance can be quite satisfactory, but sensation is inferior to healing by secondary intention or primary closure.

Composite Grafting

Replacement of the amputated part as a nonvascularized composite graft works best in children younger than 2 years, but results are unpredictable as the child approaches 8 years, and this appealing technique has little chance of success in older children or adults. Failure may delay recovery, but the tissue often serves as a biologic dressing as the tip re-epithelializes. Microvascular replantation at this level may provide the best appearance, but it is technically demanding. Nerve recovery and sensation are variable, and joint stiffness often accompanies replantation, limiting functional recovery.

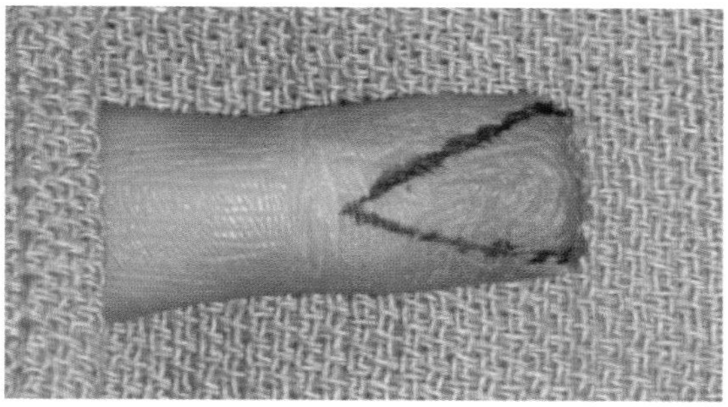

Figure 24.2. Volar V-Y flap. Preoperative outline of the skin incision used to create a volar skin flap in preparation for distal advancement. The tip of the V incision should be at the DIP joint flexion crease.

Regional flaps that will not reach to the fingertip, distant random flaps, and microvascular free flaps will not be discussed further, but they should be considered when appropriate.

Local Flaps for Fingertip Coverage

By definition, a flap consists of skin with a varying amount of underlying tissue. Unlike skin grafts, this tissue receives its blood supply from a source other than the tissue on which it is placed. Flaps that receive their blood supply from many minute vessels in the subdermal or subcutaneous plexus are termed "random" flaps. Flaps that receive blood via a single vessel are termed "axial." Local flaps available for fingertip coverage include both types.

Digital tip amputations with exposed bone can be treated by several methods already described, but local flaps are attractive because of their proximity, tissue match, possibility of enhanced function, and acceptable complication profile. Typically, if bone length has been preserved, then the use of local flaps is appropriate. Flaps to be discussed in detail include volar V-Y advancement, lateral V-Y advancement, volar flap advancement, thenar flap, and cross-finger flap.

Volar V-Y Advancement Flap. The volar V-Y advancement flap was first described in 1970, by Atasoy and Kleinert, for most tip amputations with exposed bone, especially transverse or dorsal oblique amputations. Volar oblique amputations may not have adequate skin for this technique. As a general rule, in order to be a candidate for a V-Y advancement, 50% of the skin of the distal tip must remain, as measured by assessing the distance between the proximal-most aspect of the wound to the DIP joint flexion crease.

This procedure can be done in the emergency room setting if all of the necessary equipment is available. Digital block anesthesia is used; I prefer Marcaine 0.5% administered via

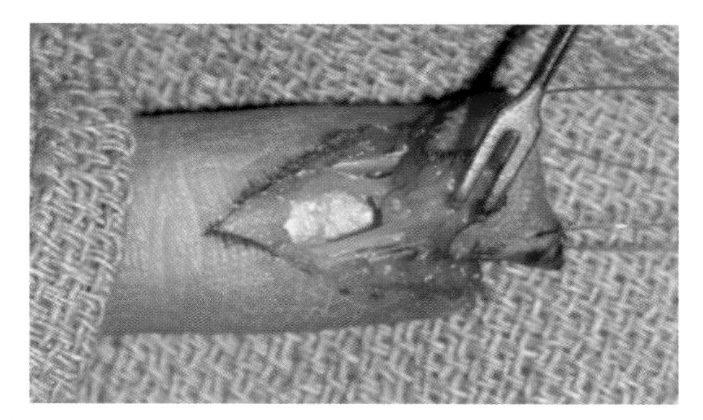

Figure 24.3. Volar V-Y flap. Skin and subcutaneous tissue have been incised. Great care must be taken to avoid injury to the radial and ulnar neurovascular bundles. Fibrous septae between the flap and the underlying bone must be carefully cut to permit distal translation of the flap.

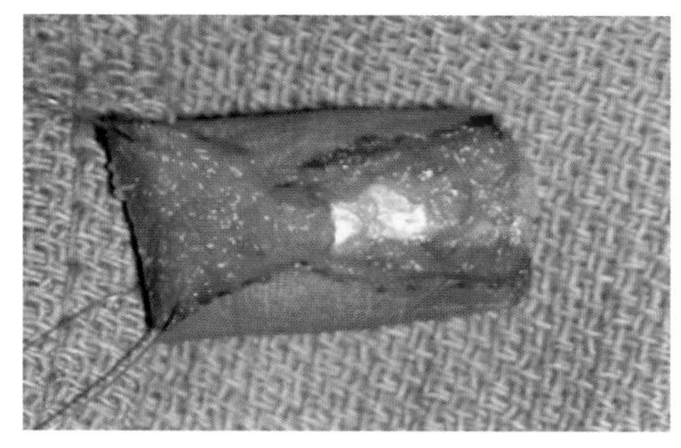

Figure 24.4. Volar V-Y flap. The flap has been mobilized and reflected proximally. Placement of stay sutures at the distal corners of the flap allows manipulation without the use of forceps that can traumatize the flap.

a single midline injection into the subcutaneous tissue at the base of the finger, although a metacarpal-level block at the digital nerve bifurcation can be administered from the dorsum of the hand. The hand is then prepped with Betadine and draped with sterile towels.

After verifying adequate anesthesia, a penrose drain is placed around the base of the finger and secured with a clamp. The size of the defect at the tip is measured or a pattern from the inner sterile glove wrapping is made. This is then transferred to the volar distal pulp that is to be advanced. A distally based triangle is drawn around the pattern. The apex of the triangle should be at the DIP joint flexion crease (Fig. 24.2). The skin is then incised.

Blunt dissection with sharp scissors is done to isolate the radial and ulnar digital neurovascular bundles (Fig. 24.3). All subcutaneous tissue except the bundles must be divided to allow tissue advancement. The deep fibrous septae between the flap and the underlying distal phalanx must be cut as well. This should free up the flap completely so that only the bundles remain as attachments (Fig. 24.4). At this point, the penrose tourniquet is released to check flap viability.

An alternative to raising the flap is to first mobilize the deep portion from the distal phalanx and flexor sheath by dividing the fibrous septae; the importance of this step, regardless of ultimate technique, cannot be overestimated. By then controlling the injured edge of the volar skin with two skin hooks and providing longitudinal traction, sharp dissection of the skin and underlying tissue mobilizes the flap. In this version, the terminal branches of the nerve and vessel are not directly isolated or even visualized consistently; the contact of the knife blade to the fibrous tissue under tension must be trusted to divide the correct tissue and spare the other vital ones. The more experienced the surgeon becomes at raising this flap, the more appeal that this option may present; the flap is not further traumatized by excessive spreading or jeopardized by skeletonizing the neurovascular bundles.

The flap is then carefully advanced distally and the base of the triangle is sutured to the remaining nail bed. I prefer 4-0 or 5-0 chromic suture. Care should be taken that the nail bed has adequate bony support to prevent hook nail deformities. Some defatting of the skin adjacent to the flap may be helpful for tension-free closure. Defatting of the flap itself is risky. The proximal V defect left by flap advancement is closed, converting the V to a Y, in the usual fashion (Fig. 24.5).

A sterile dressing with a petroleum gauze, dry gauze, or eye pad, followed by additional padding and overwrap, is applied. Splinting is usually not necessary. Early active motion is encouraged. Initial follow-up is at 3 to 5 days. A light dressing to protect the sutures is used until they are removed or dissolve in the case of chromic suture.

One report noted normal sensibility and motion in 91% of 61 patients, but other investigators have reported hypoesthesia, dysesthesia, hypersensitivity, or cold intolerance in 57% to 70% of cases.

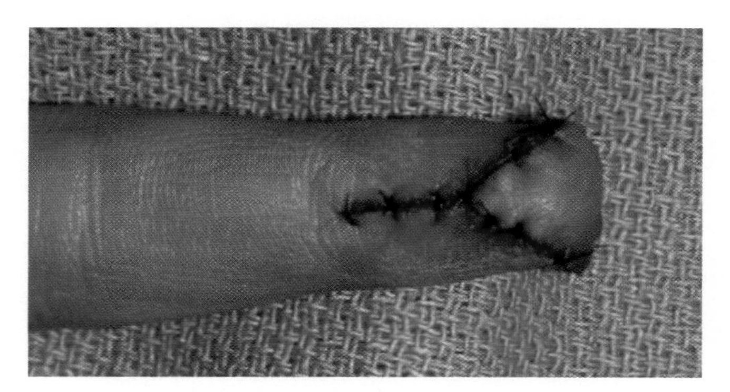

Figure 24.5. Volar V-Y flap. The flap has been advanced distally to cover the tip defect. The resultant defect has been closed, converting the V defect to a Y.

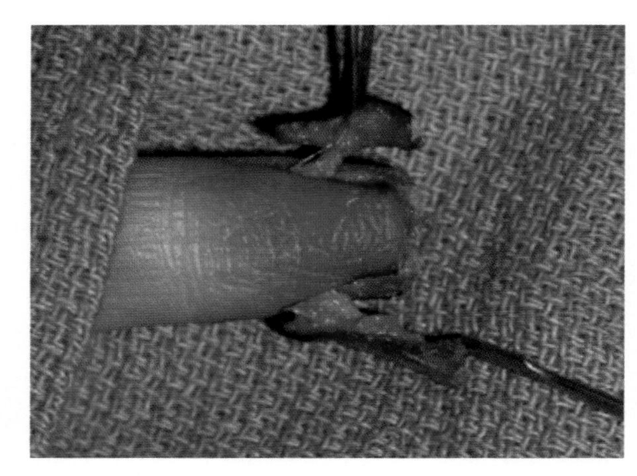

Figure 24.6. Lateral V flaps have been created. The proximal tip of the V is at the DIP flexion crease. Flaps have been raised, preserving the neurovascular bundles. Careful division of the underlying fibrous septae is necessary to allow flap advancement.

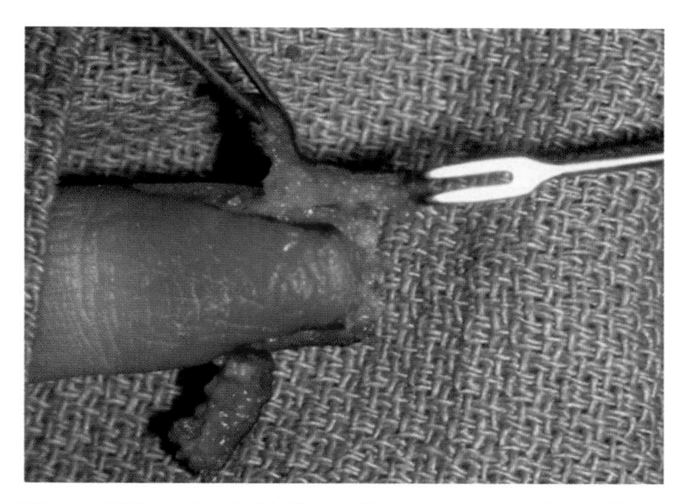

Figure 24.7. Lateral V-Y flaps. Complete separation of flaps from the underlying distal phalanx and proximal extent of the flaps.

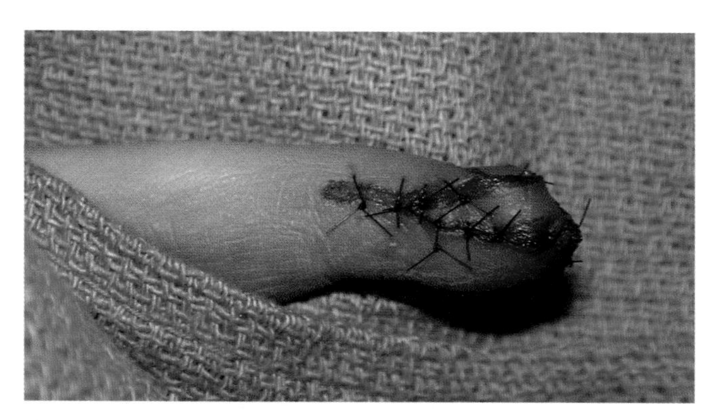

Figure 24.8. Lateral V-Y flaps. Flaps have been sutured together in the midline covering the defect. The resultant defect is closed primarily, converting the V defect to a Y incision.

Lateral V-Y Advancement Flaps. Kutler is credited with the first description of the bilateral, lateral V-Y flaps for fingertip coverage. He described two lateral triangular flaps, again based on the neurovascular pedicles, which are advanced over the fingertip. This is theoretically most useful in palmar oblique and transverse tip amputations. This procedure is rarely used because the amount of dissection, expectations placed on the traumatized bundles, creation of gracile flaps, and potential for excessive scarring limit its appeal compared with more robust alternatives.

Preparation of the digit, anesthesia, and tourniquet use is as described previously. Two distally based triangular flaps are drawn out on lateral sides of the finger. The apex is proximal and can extend to the DIP flexion crease (Fig. 24.6). The skin is carefully incised and blunt dissection is used to identify the neurovascular bundle, which will be entering on the volar side of the triangular flap at the midlateral line. The full thickness of the flap is elevated off the underlying bone. The flaps are completely freed up on their pedicles (Fig. 24.7). The tourniquet is released, flap vascularity is checked, and the flaps are advanced distally and sutured to each other in the midline. Suturing to the nail bed and remaining volar skin is continued. Again, defatting of the volar skin may help with tension-free skin closure. The proximal apex of the triangle is closed, converting the V to a Y (Fig. 24.8). Care must be taken to avoid strangulating the tenuous pedicle to this fragile flap. Postoperative care is similar to that of the volar flap.

One study found outcomes to be similar to those for volar flaps. Again, this technique is infrequently used at our institution.

Moberg Volar Advancement Flap. Moberg is generally credited with the technique of advancement of the entire volar skin for coverage of the fingertip. Creating a flap of the entire volar skin based on both neurovascular pedicles can provide sensate skin and subcutaneous tissue for tip amputations. Although more commonly applied to the thumb because of its more mobile skin and less tendency for flexion contractures, it has been utilized in all fingers.

Extreme caution should be exercised in using the Moberg concept in the triphalangeal digits. This is primarily due to the fact that the thumb alone has a generous dorsal blood supply that is largely independent of the more central, volar digital vessels. The remaining digits do not have that anatomic benefit, so the same type of surgical approach may significantly jeopardize the viability of the digits. Although not well reported, no other center has been able to duplicate Moberg's results with the volar advancement flap when used in digits other than the thumb. The basic anatomy is the likely reason for the inferior results and high complication rates accompanying this extreme tissue mobilization in the fingers.

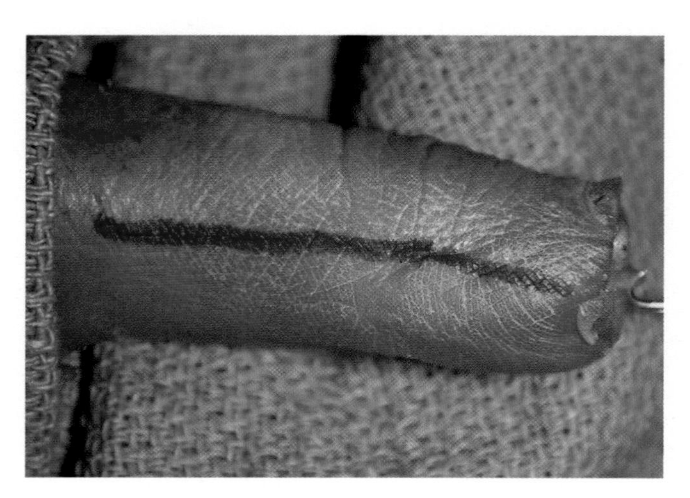

Figure 24.9. Moberg flap. Preoperative midlateral incision was utilized on both the radial and ulnar sides of the thumb.

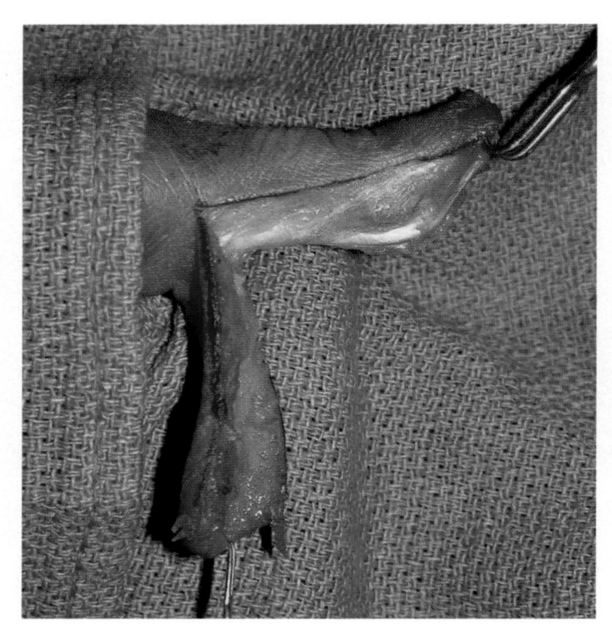

Figure 24.10. Moberg flap. An entire volar skin flap has been raised. The skin flap includes both neurovascular bundles. Flexor tendon sheath should not be injured or incised.

This procedure should be performed in the operating room after discussing all options with the patient. Regional or general anesthesia is used, the limb is exsanguinated, and an arm tourniquet is inflated. Midaxial incisions are outlined on both sides of the involved digit (Fig. 24.9). The incisions are deepened with care. Sharp and blunt dissection are used to completely separate the volar skin from the flexor tendon sheath (Fig. 24.10). Injury to the neurovascular bundles must be avoided. Particularly in the fingers, care must be taken to protect the takeoff of the dorsal branch of the sensory nerve.

Sectioning of the skin at the base of the finger, preserving the bundles, may help to gain additional advancement. One report noted that an additional 0.5 to 1.0 cm of advancement can be obtained. The defect created receives a skin graft if the advancement has required the transverse skin division. Typically, 1 cm of advancement can be achieved (Fig. 24.11). The tip may need to be contoured to fit the defect.

A postoperative dressing of petroleum gauze or dry gauze, followed by tube gauze or other bulky hand dressing, is applied. Dorsal splinting is used for 1 to 2 weeks, and then therapy to promote range of motion is begun. Complications include flexion deformity and flap necrosis.

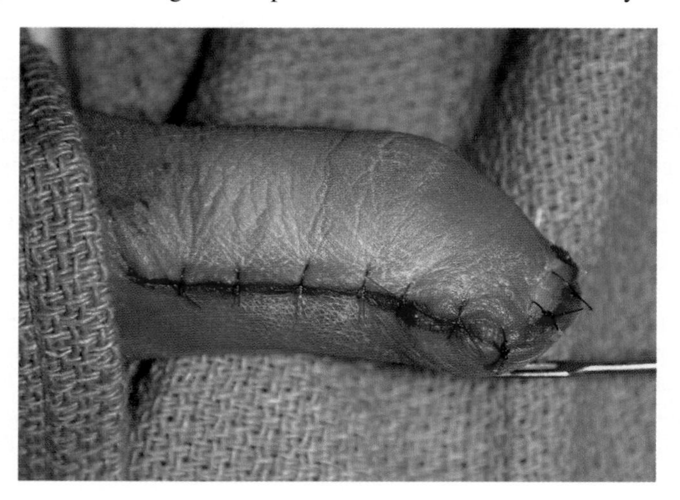

Figure 24.11. Moberg flap. The flap has been advanced distally to cover the defect and sutured in place. Note the slight flexion of the interphalangeal joint.

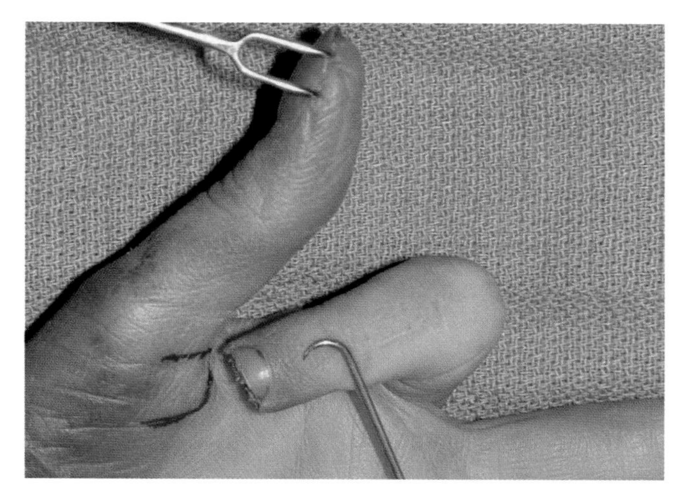

Figure 24.12. Thenar flap. The defect is on the flexed index finger, with outline of the thenar flap to cover the tip.

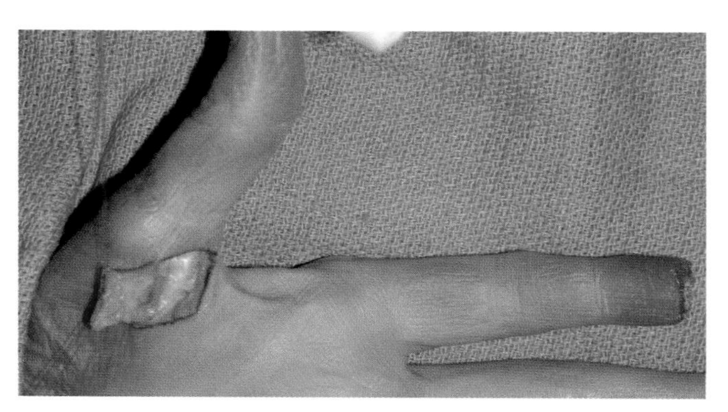

Figure 24.13. Thenar flap. The flap has been raised. The skin has full-thickness subcutaneous tissue elevated off deep fascia. Care must be taken not to injure the thenar neurovascular bundles or flexor tendon sheath.

Thenar Flap. When skin loss is mostly volar on the index and middle fingers, a thenar flap can be considered. This is indicated in younger individuals with no arthritis or trauma involving the finger joints. Use in the small finger is practically contraindicated because of the excessive opposition required of the thumb ray.

The thenar flap was first described in 1926 and has undergone subsequent modifications by Flatt, Smith and Albin, and others. This flap is indicated for amputations involving oblique volar tissue loss when length preservation is important. The potential for joint stiffness and palmar scarring needs to be discussed with the patient, or more often the parents, as this flap is almost exclusively utilized in a younger population.

This procedure should be done in the formal operating room under regional or general anesthesia. The size of the defect is measured. The flap should be approximately 20% to 30% larger in both length and width. The flap is usually proximally based, but it can be radially or ulnarly based depending on the orientation of the defect (Fig. 24.12).

The flap should be located over the volar aspect of the thumb at the level of the MP joint. Flaps that are based too low over the thenar eminence tend to have more painful scars. The flap should be elevated along with underlying subcutaneous tissue (Fig. 24.13). Care must be taken to protect the neurovascular bundles to the thumb. The donor defect can often be closed primarily or can be skin grafted (Figs. 24.14 and 24.15). Smith

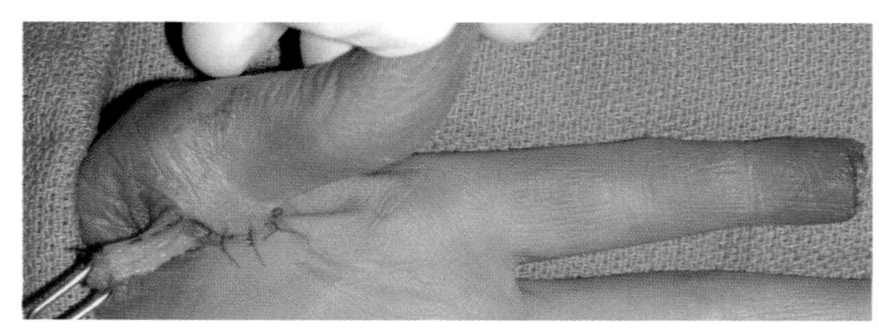

Figure 24.14. Thenar flap. A defect created by elevation of the thenar flap can usually be closed primarily, as shown here. Alternatively, a full-thickness skin graft can be applied to close the defect.

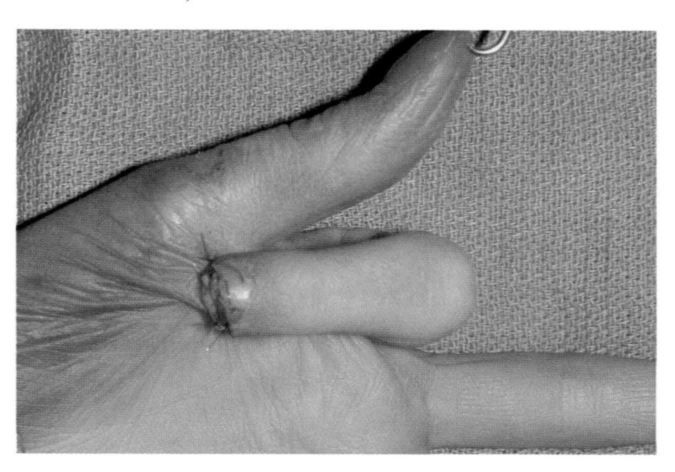

Figure 24.15. Thenar flap. The flap has been sutured in position to cover the defect. Note the amount of finger flexion.

and Albin described the thenar "H-flap" for more transverse amputations. The donor defect is closed at the time of flap sectioning between 2 and 3 weeks later. This can often be done under local anesthesia, usually in the operating room. Some contouring of the flap is often necessary at the time of sectioning. Postoperative therapy to regain finger motion is usually recommended.

Patients older than 30 years have a higher risk of joint stiffness, as do patients with any type of connective tissue disorder, arthritis, or adjacent finger injury requiring early motion. Flap loss is uncommon, as is traumatic premature separation of the flap. Pinning of any joint to help maintain the position of the finger is contraindicated.

Cross-Finger Flap. The cross-finger flap technique was initially described in 1950. This flap is useful when length needs to be maintained and the tissue loss is mostly volar. Careful consideration of its use is necessary because an adjacent finger provides the donor tissue and the skin-grafted defect is on the dorsum of the finger. Curtis was an early advocate of this flap and reported on its advantages.

This procedure is done under regional or general anesthesia. The size of the defect is transferred to the dorsum of the finger over the middle phalanx (Fig. 24.16). The flap is based on the side closest to the injured finger. In general, the flap is made about 2 mm larger on its three sides. Usually, the far edge of the flap should be at or dorsal to the midlateral line. The proximal and distal extent of the flap should not extend beyond the midlines of the DIP or proximal interphalangeal joints, but taking the flap to these levels is almost always the best option, because undersizing the donor is a distinct issue that must be avoided.

The flap is carefully incised on the three sides and elevated gently (Fig. 24.17). Retraction sutures at the corners can help minimize the use of forceps on the flap. The skin and subcutaneous tissue is elevated off the paratenon of the extensor tendon. As the flap depends on the subdermal plexus for its blood supply, care must be taken to prevent cutting into the subcutaneous tissue at the lateral base of the flap. The flap is reflected and the

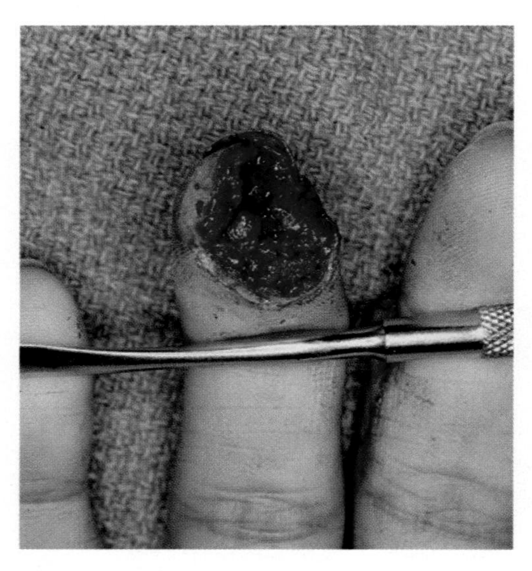

Figure 24.16. Cross-finger flap. A volar soft-tissue defect with no bone loss. The dorsal nail is uninjured.

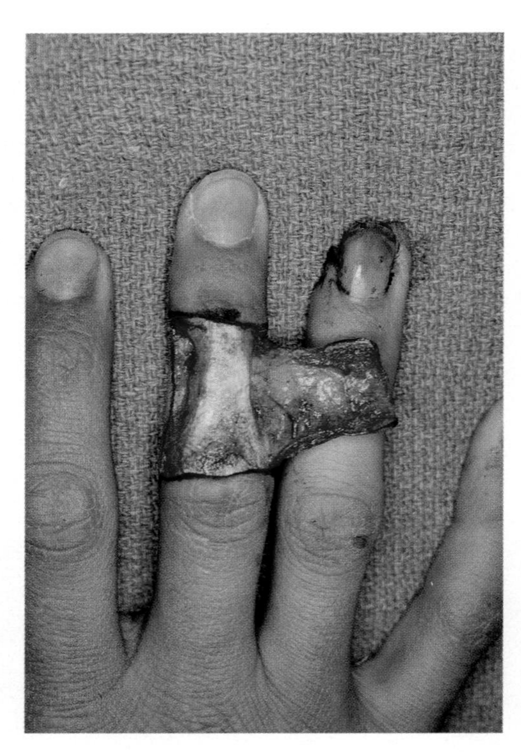

Figure 24.17. Cross-finger flap. Dorsal view of a cross-finger flap raised to cover a volar defect on an adjacent finger. Note the full thickness of tissue elevated and the preservation of paratenon on the extensor tendon.

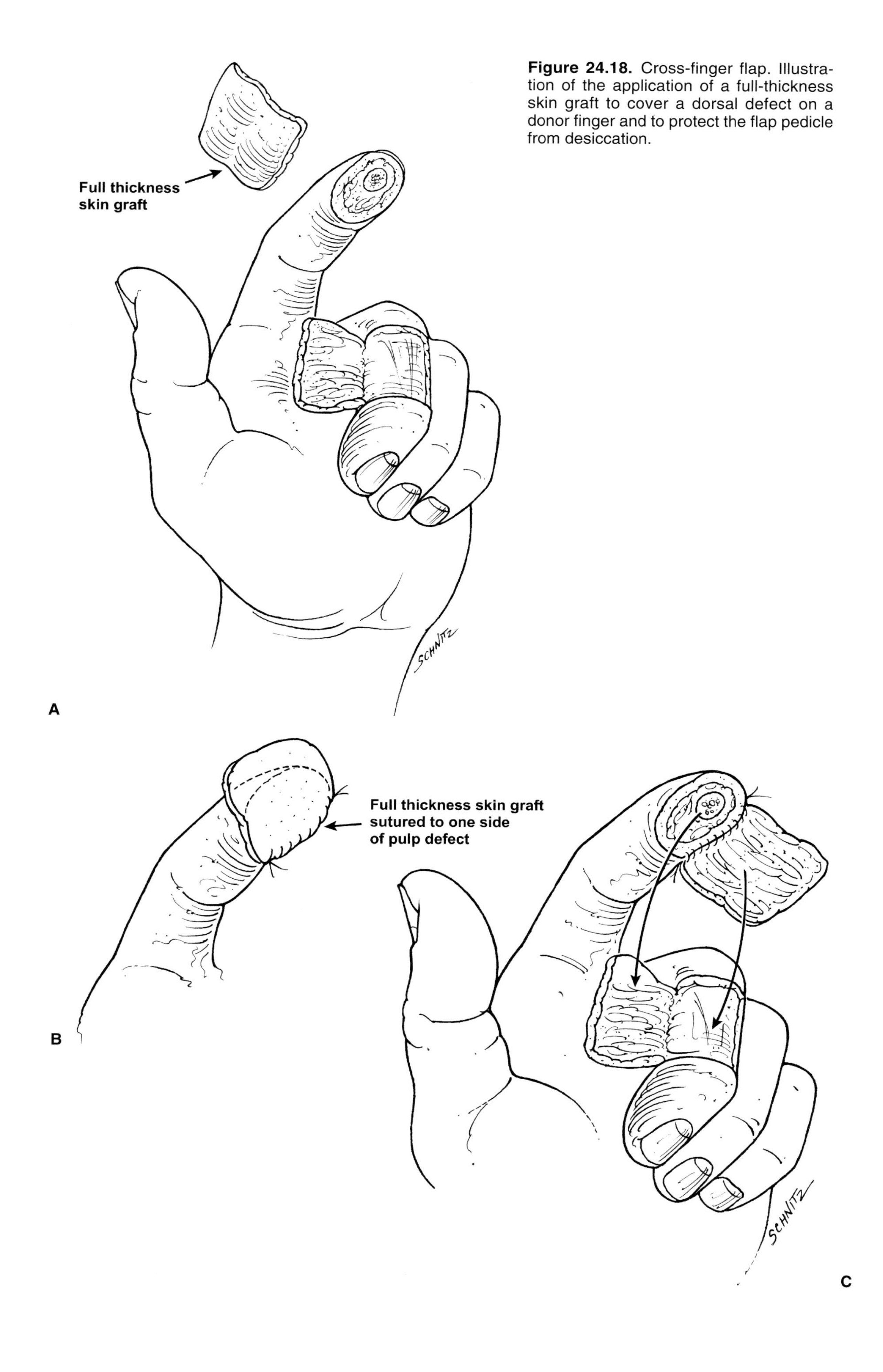

Figure 24.18. Cross-finger flap. Illustration of the application of a full-thickness skin graft to cover a dorsal defect on a donor finger and to protect the flap pedicle from desiccation.

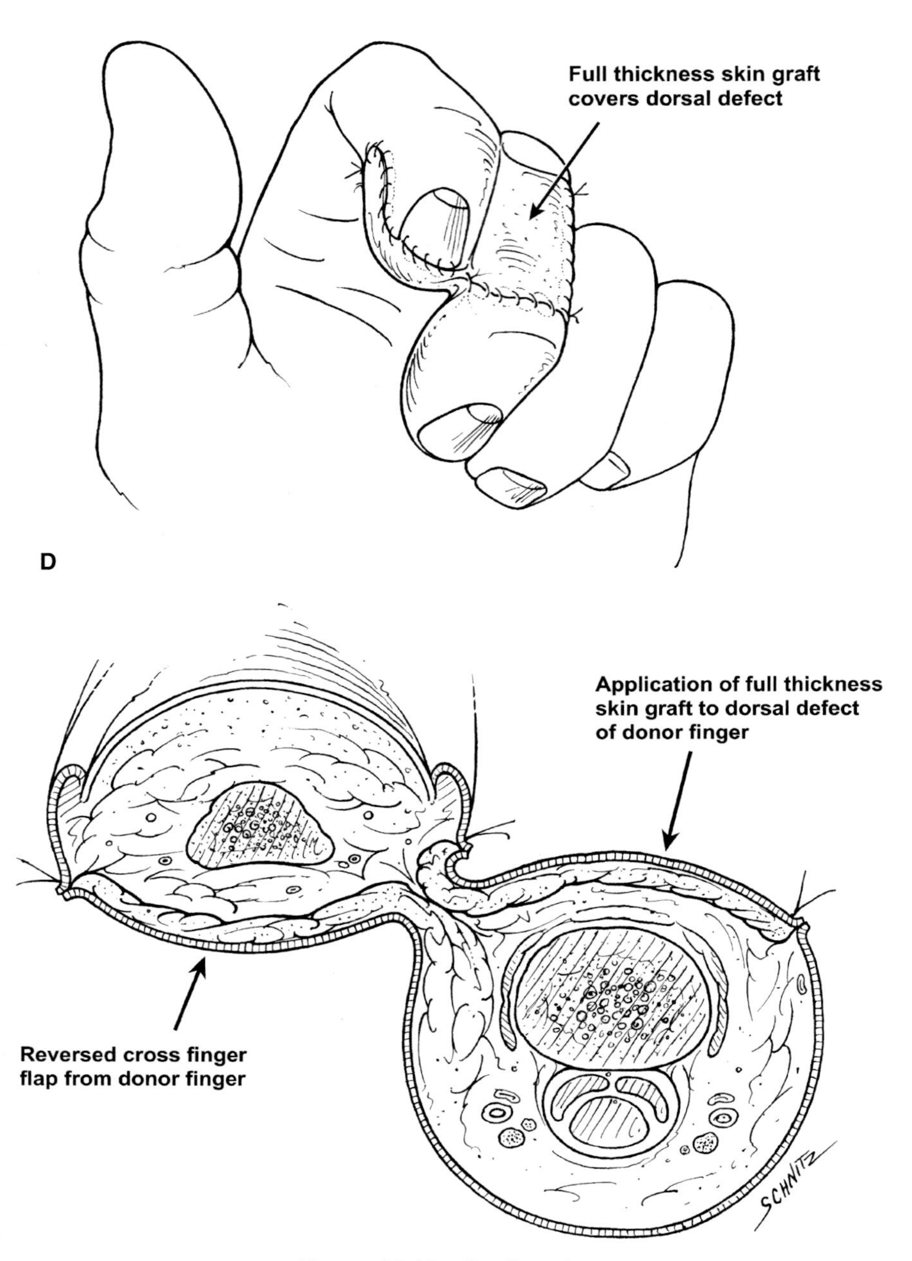

Figure 24.18. *Continued.*

tourniquet is released to check the flap's vascularity. The flap is then sutured in place on the injured finger. A full-thickness skin graft is then usually harvested from the groin to cover the donor defect on the dorsum of the finger (Fig. 24.18). The graft should be large enough to cover the portion of the flap between the two fingers. This is important to prevent desiccation of the base of the flap. Generally, suture repair and careful dressing of the flap are sufficient to maintain the position of the joined fingers. Avoid the temptation to pin the digits in the associated position; the chances of injuring the bundles and pin-associated complications are simply too great.

A soft bulky dressing incorporating a plaster splint is applied. I generally change the dressing at 1 week to check both the skin graft and the flap. The flap is divided at 2 to 3

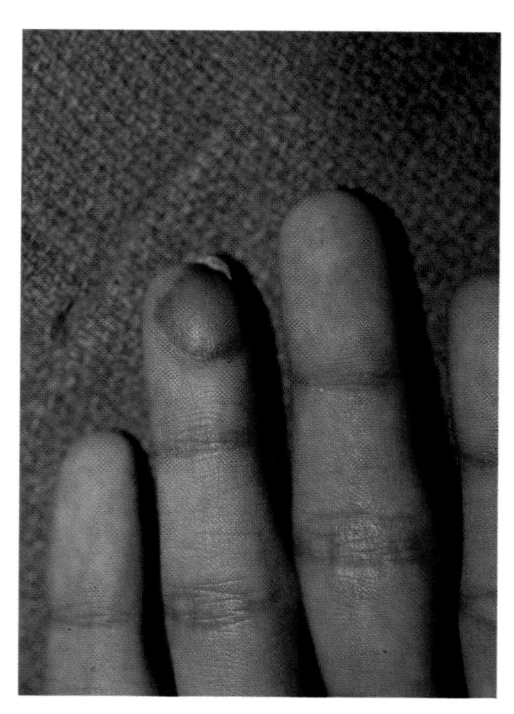

Figure 24.19. Cross-finger flap. Final result after division and inset of the flap.

weeks in the operating room. This can be done under local anesthesia. Both the flap and the skin-grafted area will need to be contoured, trimmed, and inset (Fig. 24.19). Hand therapy is recommended to facilitate the recovery of finger motion. Protective sensation returns in 3 to 6 months. Two-point discrimination of 5 to 10 mm can be expected in 1 to 2 years; careful inclusion of a dorsal sensory nerve near the proximal, volar aspect of the flap can improve those results.

POSTOPERATIVE MANAGEMENT AND REHABILITATION

Most patients are seen at 5 to 7 days postoperatively. Those with skin grafts and flaps are seen at 1 week for a dressing change. Early hand therapy is encouraged to maximize recovery of motion when flap viability is not at risk.

Time off work is quite variable and difficult to predict. The type of treatment seems to have little effect on return to work unless a complication, such as flap necrosis or infection, prolongs recovery. Bojsen-Moller found that recovery was similar for patients treated surgically or conservatively.

In my experience with cross-finger flaps, the final appearance of recipient and donor areas is well accepted and loss of motion is uncommon. The use of volar and lateral advancement flaps eliminates the need for a second procedure, but care must be taken to not try and cover too large a defect. The more tension that is needed to cover the tip with the advancement flaps, the higher the tendency toward hypersensitivity. The return to heavy manual labor is usually in the range of 4 to 8 weeks.

RESULTS

Although more conservative treatments should always be carefully considered for all fingertip injuries, skillful use of the flaps discussed here can lead to excellent functional recovery. Transverse amputations can be treated by many methods. Injuries with oblique tissue loss in which length should be preserved lend themselves to the various flaps reviewed (Fig. 24.20).

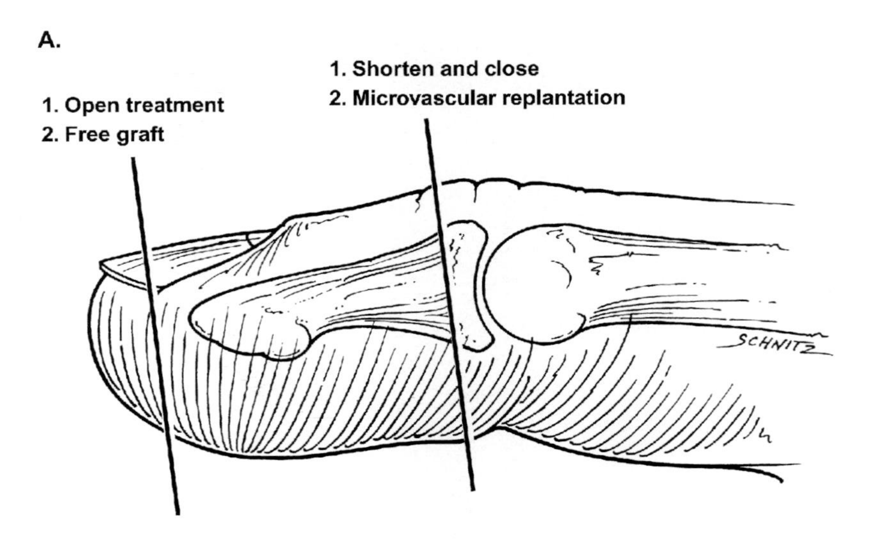

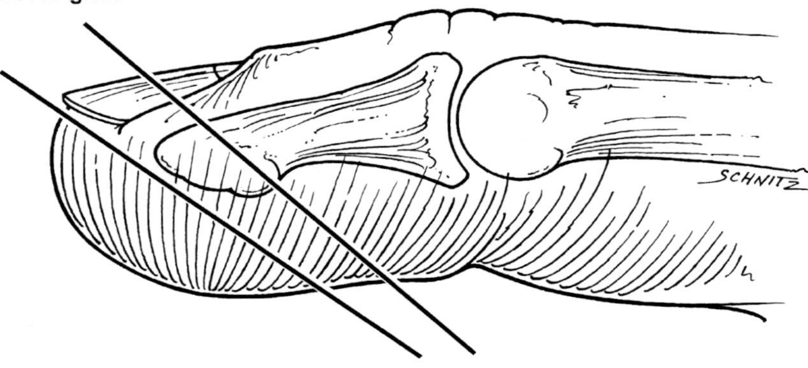

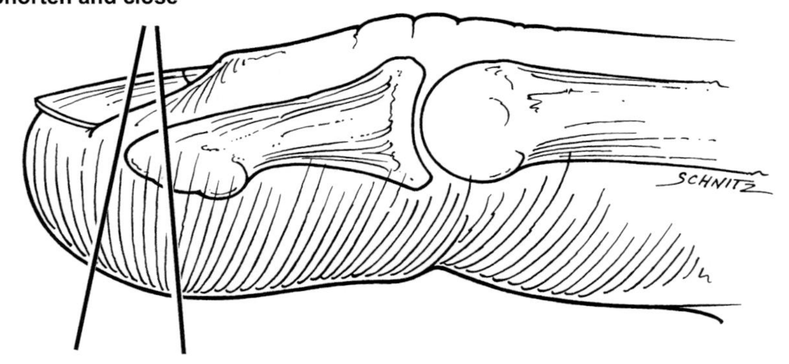

Figure 24.20. Summary of treatment options based on the level of amputation and the angle of tissue loss.

Results specific to each flap are typically good but may reflect the fact that more extensive coverage procedures are typically chosen for more extensive or complex wounds. Complications rates are low when experienced surgeons choose reasonable coverage alternatives for appropriate patients and injuries.

Although the cross-finger flap may appear to be a procedure fraught with technical demands and potential pitfalls, my extensive experience with it suggests otherwise. The thickness of tissue transferred from the dorsum of the adjacent digit to the amputated tip is adequate with a good color match. The appearance of the dorsal defect and skin graft is often quite good as well. However, skin color mismatch with transfer of dorsal skin to the volar aspect in patients of color should be considered. Recovery after flap division is about 3 weeks for lighter work and 6 weeks for more manual work. Nicolai and Hentenaar report that 75% of patients at 4 years have two-point discrimination within 2 mm of their opposite side. However, only those younger than 21 years had consistent return of sensation. Kleinert et al. reported results by age. In patients younger than 12 years, more than 90% had 6 mm or less two-point discrimination; by 40 years, this declines to only 40%.

For all of these reasons, the cross-finger flap, as with all of these reconstructive alternatives, falls within the purview of the surgeon interested and experienced in the care of the hand.

COMPLICATIONS

Outcome studies on fingertip injuries are complicated by the difficulty of separating results by the injury itself from those for different types of treatment. Complications include infection, hook nail deformity, flexion contracture, cold intolerance, altered sensibility, and graft or flap failure. Infection can be minimized by adequate debridement. Routine use of antibiotics beyond the usual prophylactic recommendations is usually not helpful. Injuries that occur in a marine or farm environment may need the usual special considerations.

Trimming the nailbed back to the same level as the bone can prevent hook nail deformity. Unsupported nailbed that is allowed to heal by secondary intention can result in hook nail deformity.

Flexion contractures can be related to the flexed posture of the finger when thenar, Moberg, or cross-finger flaps are utilized. This needs to be discussed with the patient before surgery. Careful patient selection is necessary. Use of the thenar or cross-finger flap in patients older than 30 years increases the risk of contractures. Distal interphalangeal joint contractures in the thumb with use of the Moberg flap are less problematic with little functional loss. Flap division between 2 and 3 weeks along with early hand therapy help to minimize this uncommon problem.

Cold intolerance is a common problem occurring in 30% to 70% of fingertip injuries. While this seems to be largely related to the injury itself, some authors feel that the incidence is higher in those treated by surgical methods. Louis, Jebson, and Graham reviewed several follow-up studies and concluded that fingertip injuries in adults with pulp loss have a 30% to 50% chance of cold intolerance and a 30% chance of altered sensibility regardless of the technique used. They feel that these problems are a consequence of the injury and not the treatment.

Altered sensibility also can be a function of either the injury or the treatment. Overstretching the neurovascular bundles not only risks flap failure due to ischemia but also can increase hypersensitivity at the fingertip. Sensory recovery is best when wounds are allowed to heal by secondary intention. Moberg flaps tend to have good sensibility, followed by the local V-Y flaps. Cross-finger flaps do not recover sensation to the same degree as other flaps, but sensation improves with time.

RECOMMENDED READING

1. Atasoy E, Kleinert HE, et al. Reconstruction of the amputated fingertip with a triangular volar flap: a new surgical procedure. *J Bone Joint Surg* 52A:921–936, 1970.
2. Bojsen-Moller J, Pers M, Schmidt A. Fingertip injuries: late results. *Acta Chir Scand* 122:177–183, 1961.
3. Curtis RM. Cross finger pedicle flap and hand surgery. *Ann Surg* 145:650–655, 1957.

4. Douglas BS. Conservative management of guillotine amputation of the finger in children. *Aust Paediatr J* 8:86, 1972.
5. Flatt AE. The thenar flap. *J Bone Joint Surg* 39B:80–85, 1957.
6. Holm E, Zachariae L. Fingertip lesions: an evaluation of conservative treatment versus free skin grafting. *Acta Orthop Scand* 45:382, 1974.
7. Kleinert HE, McAlister CG, MacDonald CJ, et al. A critical evaluation of cross finger flaps. *J Trauma* 14:756–763, 1974.
8. Kutler W. A method for repair of finger amputation. *Ohio State Med J* 40:126, 1944.
9. Louis DS, Jebson PJL, Graham TJ. Amputations. In Green DP, Hotchkiss RN, Pederson WC, eds. *Green's Operative Hand Surgery*. 4th ed, vol. 1. Philadelphia: Churchill Livingstone, 1999:48–94.
10. Nicolai JPA, Hentenaar G. Sensation in cross-finger flaps. *Hand* 13:12–16, 1981.
11. Nystrom A, Backman C, et al. Digital amputation, replantation, and cold intolerance. *J Reconstr Microsurg* 7:175–178, 1991.
12. Smith RJ, Albin R. Thenar "H-flap" for fingertip injuries. *J Trauma* 16:778–781, 1976.

25

Microsurgical Repair of Soft-Tissue Deficits of the Upper Extremity: Use of the Lateral Arm Flap and the Latissimus Dorsi Free Flap

Michael A. McClinton

INDICATIONS/CONTRAINDICATIONS

The upper extremity surgeon will encounter soft-tissue deficits requiring complex closure that are best treated by the transfer of tissue from another site. These injuries most commonly occur from trauma but also follow tumor resection, extensive infection, vascular insufficiency, and postoperative complication. If transferred tissue must bring its own blood supply, the surgeon will use a tissue flap rather than a skin graft. This flap will be either continuously attached to its blood supply during the transfer (pedicle flap) or temporarily separated and reconnected microsurgically to its eventual blood supply (free flap).

Multiple factors determine whether or not microsurgical techniques will be necessary to cover a wound. These include the size and location of the defect, the adequacy of the local tissue support, and the availability of alternative coverage. If the recipient region can support nonmicrosurgical coverage options, the surgeon chooses among a tissue flap, skin graft, primary closure, or healing by secondary intention. The treatment algorithm that once proceeded from simple to complex for selecting methods of wound closure now is based on selecting the best method of wound closure for the patient, even if the chosen technique requires microsurgery.

Michael A. McClinton, M.D.: Division of Plastic Surgery, Johns Hopkins Hospital, Baltimore, MD, and Curtis National Hand Center, Union Memorial Hospital, Baltimore, MD

Advantages of Free Flaps

Free flaps have several advantages compared with pedicle flaps. There is no local or distant pedicle to restrict the transfer process, so virtually the entire flap is used to close the defect. In contrast, during groin flap transfer, the injured extremity is attached to the trunk for 3 weeks, usually in a dependent position that fosters edema and precludes hand therapy.

Often, part of a local flap is used as a pedicle, reducing the amount of tissue available for wound coverage. Local flaps and their pedicles impair the function and appearance of the upper limb. In the case of the radial forearm flap, a common alternative to free flaps for the upper limb, the radial artery is interrupted. Free flaps can be customized to meet the requirements of an injured extremity.

Small skin defects are handled by free muscle flaps, such as the gracilis or extensor digitorum brevis of the foot, and fasciocutaneous flaps, including lateral arm or dorsalis pedis. Medium and large wounds can be closed by the latissimus dorsi and rectus abdominis muscle flaps or scapular and parascapular fasciocutaneous flaps.

Perhaps the most important contribution of the microsurgical age is the flexibility with which complex wound problems can be approached. This flexibility can be seen in the timing, sizing, types of tissues available for transfer, and functional outcomes that are offered to the patient.

One-stage repair of complex injuries is also possible because free flaps can carry vascularized bone, tendon, nerve, arterial grafts, and functioning muscle. Critical sensibility can be restored to important contact areas of the thumb and index finger pads, for example, by transfer of free toe web-space or pulp flaps. Similarly, sizable wounds created by high-energy trauma can be aggressively debrided and covered early to promote healing, diminish complications, and enhance eventual outcomes.

Disadvantages of Free Flaps

Contraindications to free flap transfer may be relative or absolute. Microsurgical expertise and proper equipment are mandatory. Recipient arteries and veins must be suitable for repair to the flap vessels, which may not be the case in patients with peripheral vascular disease or local irradiation. Microsurgical operations are often lengthy, require general anesthesia, and may necessitate a change in position during the procedure. These procedures may put additional physiological stress on ill patients.

Choices of Free Flaps for the Upper Extremity

A majority of free flaps fall conveniently into one of three categories: skin flaps, fascial flaps, or muscle flaps. This does not diminish the fact that bone and nerve can also be transferred with microsurgical techniques, either independently or with a composite flap of the tissues described previously.

Both muscle and fascial flaps provide a vascularized bed for skin grafts. Specific flaps can be used to match unique qualities of various areas of the hand, such as the palmar and dorsal surfaces of the hand and the digital tips. For example, dorsal hand skin is thin, moves freely with the extensor tendons during digital flexion and extension, and does not require critical sensibility. Good choices for this area are the lateral arm flap with or without skin (skin flaps can be bulky and may have to be thinned), the temporoparietal fascial flap, and the serratus anterior muscle flap. Conversely, the palmar surface of the hand has thick skin with a limited subcutaneous layer to allow free movement with digital motion. In addition, septal attachments to the skin prevent slipping or shearing over the underlying tissues during strong gripping. Skin flaps do not serve as well here.

Fascial and muscle flaps are excellent solutions for the palmar surface; choices include lateral arm, temporoparietal, serratus anterior, and for small defects the extensor digitorum brevis muscle. Coverage of digital pads, especially on the radial side of the hand, demands

Table 25.1. *Coverage for Dorsal/Palmar Hand and Digits*

Flap	Size	Arterial diameter	Pedicle length	Transfer location	Sensation	Modification
Lateral Arm	Skin 6 × 30 Fascia 14 × 20	1.3–2.0mm	5 × 7cm	Dorsal/Palmar Hand	Skin (protective)	Split, extended, with tendon, bone, nerve
Temporoparietal	14 × 17cm	1.5–2.4mm	2.5–5mm	Dorsal/Palmar Hand	No	Double fascial layer
Extensor digitorum brevis	5 × 6cm	2–3mm (Dorsalis pedis)	20cm (Anterior Tibial)	Dorsal/Palmar Hand (small defect)	No	Functional muscle
Serratus Anterior (lower 3–4 slips)	4 × 10cm	1.5–3mm (thoracodorsal)	10–15cm	Dorsal/PalmarHand	No	Split muscle slips, functional
Toe Pulp and Webspace	7 × 8cm	2–3mm (Dorsalis pedis)	6–11cm	Digits	Critical sensibility	Wrap-around flap

critical sensibility for discrimination and pinch function. Innervated skin flaps from the foot are good choices for digital tip coverage and include great and second toe pulp transfer and vascularized transfer of the web space between the great and second toes.

Dorsal and volar forearm injuries are often extensive and may require large flaps. If wound contamination is suspected and the defect is large, choose muscle flaps such as the latissimus dorsi or rectus abdominis. Clean wounds requiring closure, especially if later reconstructive procedures are planned, can be handled with skin flaps such as scapular and parascapular flaps, anteriolateral thigh flaps, or microsurgical groin flaps. For smaller forearm wounds, I like the gracilis muscle, which has a concealed donor scar and is harvested conveniently while the recipient site is prepared. The radial forearm flap can be taken from the contralateral arm as a free flap, although patients with major trauma are reluctant to jeopardize the opposite extremity, however small the risk.

Table 25.1 lists the flaps for the hand and digits that have demonstrated reliability and usefulness to the upper extremity surgeon. Table 25.2 lists flaps for the forearm.

PREOPERATIVE PLANNING

I cannot stress too much the importance of careful preoperative planning for free flap transfers. Evaluate the patient medically to determine tolerance for the anesthetic demands of the procedure. Detailed assessment of the suitability of the recipient vessels will prevent unpleasant surprises intraoperatively. I generally use arteriography to demonstrate the arterial anatomy of the recipient area. Noninvasive studies, including magnetic resonance angiography, duplex imaging, and Doppler evaluation, may be sufficient, but they do not truly provide the "road map" usually necessary for complex microsurgical dissection and transfer. Noninvasive demonstration of venous flow is warranted when the status of proximal veins is in question.

Table 25.2. *Coverage for Forearm*

Flap	Size	Arterial diameter	Pedicle length	Transfer location	Sensation	Modification
Latissimus dorsi	20 × 38cm	1.5–3mm	8–11cm	Hand/Forearm (large defect)	No	Functional, Split, with bone
Rectus Abdominis	6–8 × 30cm	2 × 3.5mm	7 × 14cm	Forearm	No	
Parascapular	10–12 × 30cm	2.5 × 3.5mm	7 × 10cm	Forearm/ Hand(dorsum)	No	Fascia only
Gracilis	4.5 × 25cm	1.2 × 1.8mm	6cm	Hand/Forearm	No	Functional
Anterolateral Thigh flap	10–15 × 20cm	2mm	8cm	Forearm	Protective	Fascia only

The surgeon next evaluates the soft-tissue defect for repair. The three-dimensional size, shape, and depth of the wound, nearest recipient vessels, and need for additional reconstructive procedures will often point the surgeon to a limited number of preferred flaps. Often, the complex wound overlies a fracture or prosthesis. In these cases, it is critical to consider the type of skeletal stabilization or communication with the surgeon treating the bone.

Specific issues taken up during preoperative planning are level of bacterial contamination, timing of flap transfer, single versus multiple stages, and location of the vascular anastomoses. Godina and Lister advocated closing wounds as soon as possible, even emergently. Certainly, the recipient vessels are never better than at the initial operation. Most facilities do not have the manpower to carry out flap procedures 24 hours a day, so wounds are generally closed within 2 to 5 days.

It may be helpful even for an experienced hand surgeon to list the reconstructive needs, such as bone, tendon, and nerve repair. Historically, reconstruction of complex injuries occurred in multiple stages. Scheker has shown with dorsal hand injuries that single-stage reconstruction of bone, tendon, and skin, aided by microsurgery, limits recovery time and may improve the outcome. Unplanned vein grafts reduce the survival of free flaps. This situation nearly always results from a failure to determine the course and location of the donor vessel to recipient vessel connection.

Early free tissue transfers to the upper limb, especially to the hand and wrist, resulted in thick mounds of tissue that were cosmetically unappealing. Microsurgeons now have a plethora of free flaps to choose from to match the ideal flap thickness with a defect. Most muscle flaps are not transferred with overlying skin but simply transferred as muscle-only flaps, and skin is grafted to maintain a low contour on the hand. I have found that secondary tendon reconstruction beneath a muscle flap for dorsal hand coverage can be problematic. If the wound is closed with a skin flap, subsequent tendon grafts can be passed through the subcutaneous fat. Hunter rods can be placed beneath a muscle flap and later replaced with tendon grafts.

Two of the most commonly used and versatile flaps for upper extremity reconstruction will be reviewed in detail. The lateral arm flap is appealing because of its size, contour, and ready availability in the ipsilateral arm to the site of required coverage. The latissimus dorsi flap can be used to cover extremely large defects and can be utilized as a functioning transfer.

SURGERY

Preoperative planning is completed and the patient is in the operating room for a potentially long free flap procedure. Your anesthesiologists should address the following issues: adequate hydration to maximize the pressure head across the anastomoses, maintenance of core temperature to reduce peripheral cooling and vasospasm, and avoidance of pressure areas on the heals, the back of the head, and the contralateral arm.

Lateral Arm Flap

The lateral arm flap now has a 20-year track record of reliability and usefulness for coverage of hand wounds. Usually taken as a fasciocutaneous flap from the upper arm, it can be taken as a fascial flap if larger dimensions or a very thin flap is needed. Patients are attracted to the idea that the flap and defect are kept on the same limb. Keep the width of the fasciocutaneous flap to 6 cm or less so that primary closure of the donor site is possible.

The flap is based on the posterior radial collateral artery that is one of two terminal branches of the profunda brachii artery after it passes posterior to the humerus next to the radial nerve. It then proceeds inferiorly next to the humerus in the lateral intermuscular septum of the upper arm (Fig. 25.1). A pedicle length of 5 to 7 cm and an arterial diameter of 1.0 to 2.3 mm are expected with the standard flap location.

Two nerves run in the flap. The posterior cutaneous nerve of the arm innervates the flap and may be taken to create a sensate flap. The posterior cutaneous nerve of the forearm

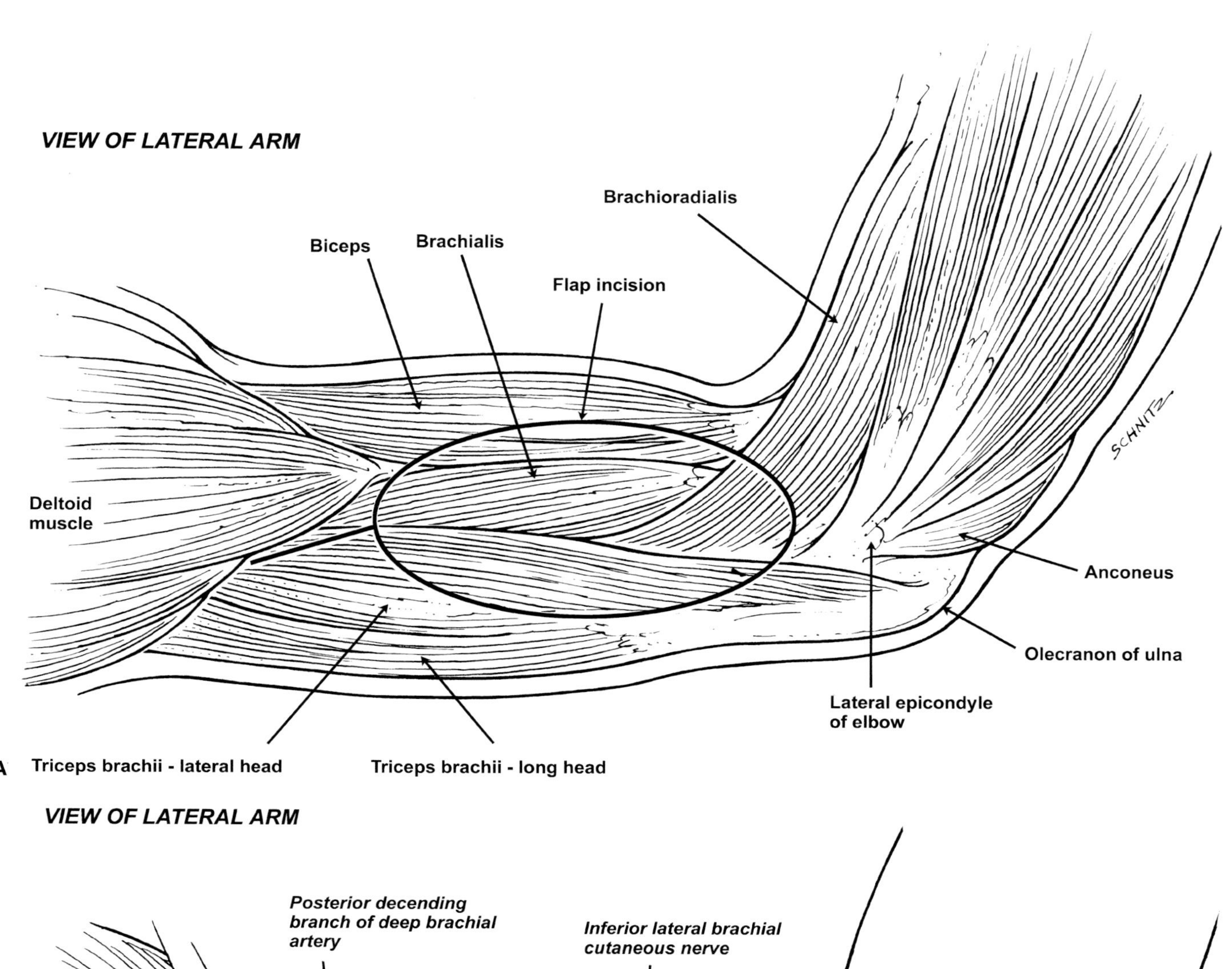

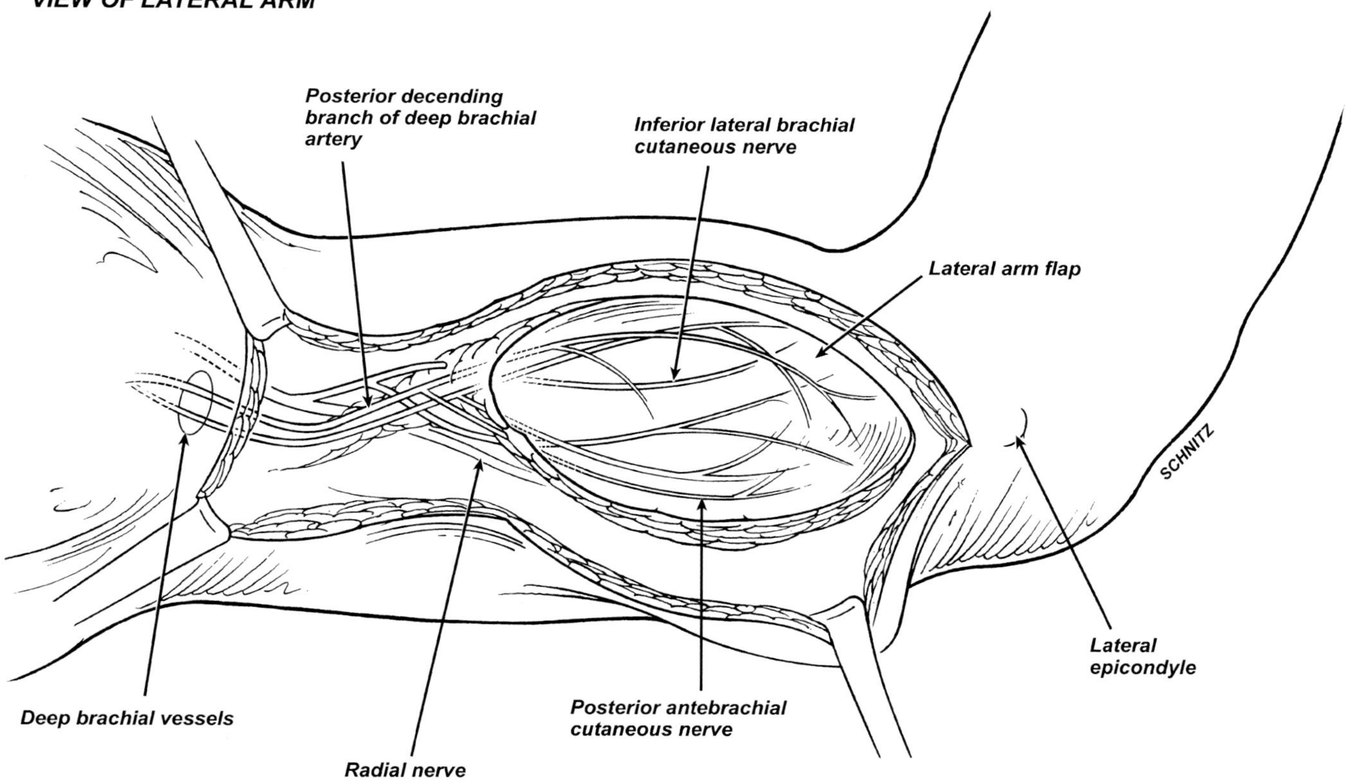

Figure 25.1. Arterial and nerve anatomy of the lateral arm flap.

passes with the vascular pedicle to innervate the skin of the lateral forearm. This nerve is usually divided when raising the flap to avoid endangering the vascular pedicle. It can be kept in the flap and used as a vascularized nerve graft. Vascularized tendon and bone (a 1-cm-wide segment of humerus of variable length) may be transported in the flap. For dorsal hand coverage, the flap is split transversely and folded to change a long, narrow flap to one of circular or rectangular dimensions.

The following case illustrates the technique of flap elevation. A 35-year-old man with Hodgkin's disease received adriamycin through an intravenous line placed in the dorsum of his left hand. Infiltration of this medication into the hand resulted in a chronic ulcer and surrounding indurated tissue that persisted for a year despite local wound treatment (Fig. 25.2).

The patient is placed supine with the arm on a hand table if the flap is to be transferred to the ipsilateral hand. With some maneuvering, two teams can work simultaneously to prepare the defect (Fig. 25.3) and raise the flap. After establishing the shape and dimensions necessary for the flap to cover the defect, first establish the vascular axis of the flap, which is in the fascial septum between the biceps and triceps muscles located on a line between the deltoid insertion and the lateral epicondyle (Fig. 25.4). A Doppler examination of this area will identify the flap artery more precisely. It may be helpful to lay a pattern of the defect on the vascular axis to draw the flap margin (Fig. 25.5).

I have followed others who have moved the standard flap location more distally on the arm, extending as far as 12 cm past the lateral epicondyle. This results in a thinner flap with a longer pedicle. Once the flap dimensions are drawn, incise its posterior border, carrying the incision through the fascial layer over the triceps muscle, down to the muscle fibers (Fig. 25.6). The fascial layer includes the arterial perforators and must be included for flap survival. Flap elevation in an anterior direction is virtually bloodless until muscular branches to the triceps are encountered. A common mistake when first elevating this flap is to continue the plane of dissection in a horizontal direction when the edge of the muscle is reached. Be sure to retract the triceps muscle gently toward you and follow its anterior border as it curves deep toward the humerus. Damage to the vascular pedicle may occur if the dissection continues in a horizontal direction and enters the lateral intermuscular septum. As you sweep the triceps muscle from the septum, divide muscle branches until you arrive at the periosteum of the humerus. You are now deep to the flap pedicle. You can continue in this plane to elevate the septum from the humerus or move to the anterior border

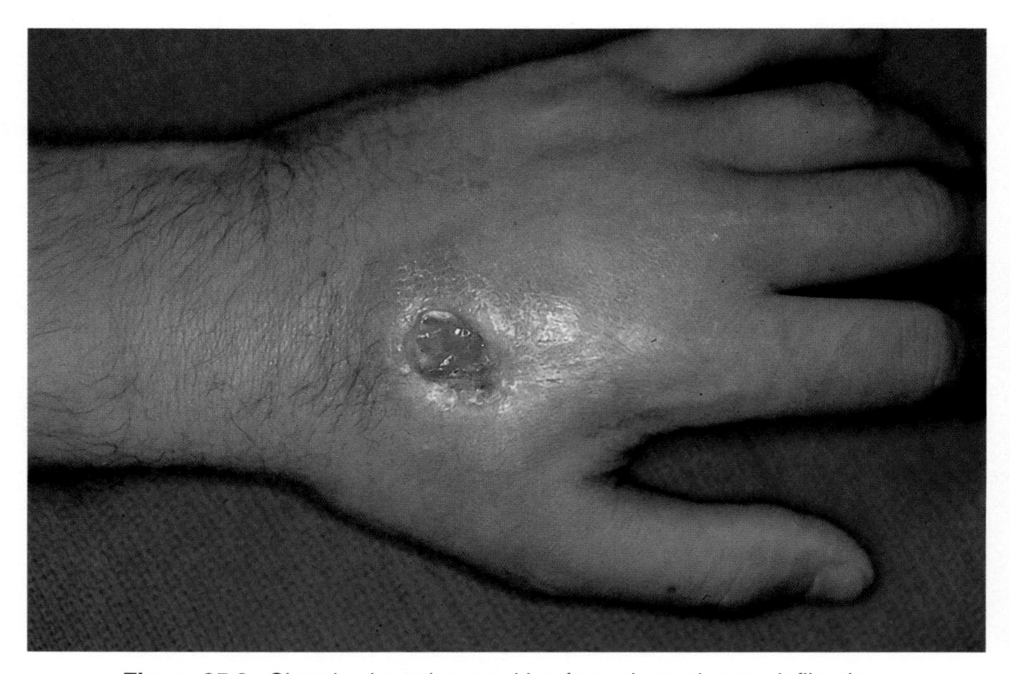

Figure 25.2. Chronic ulceration resulting from chemotherapy infiltration.

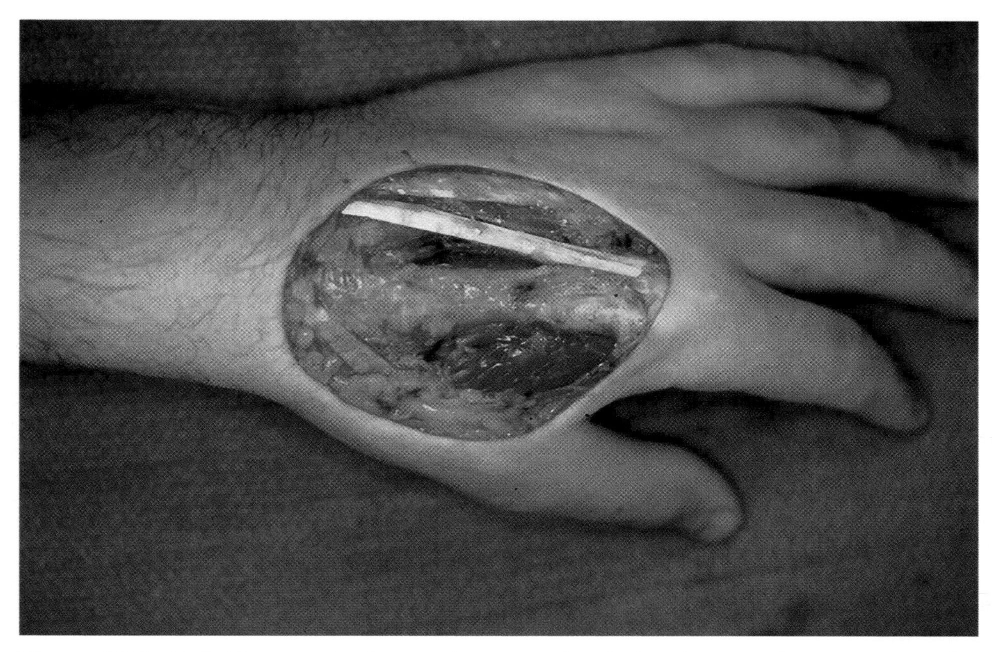

Figure 25.3. Debridement of ulcer and surrounding induration creating exposure of a metacarpal and extensor tendon.

of the flap. The anterior flap border is also elevated beneath the investing fascia of the upper arm on the brachialis and brachioradialis muscles.

The surgical caveat here is to avoid injury to the radial nerve. This nerve passes around the humerus at its upper level, runs with the profunda brachii artery beneath the lateral arm flap, and passes anteriorily through the interval between the biceps and brachioradialis muscles. Continue elevating the anterior flap border in a posterior direction, again following the

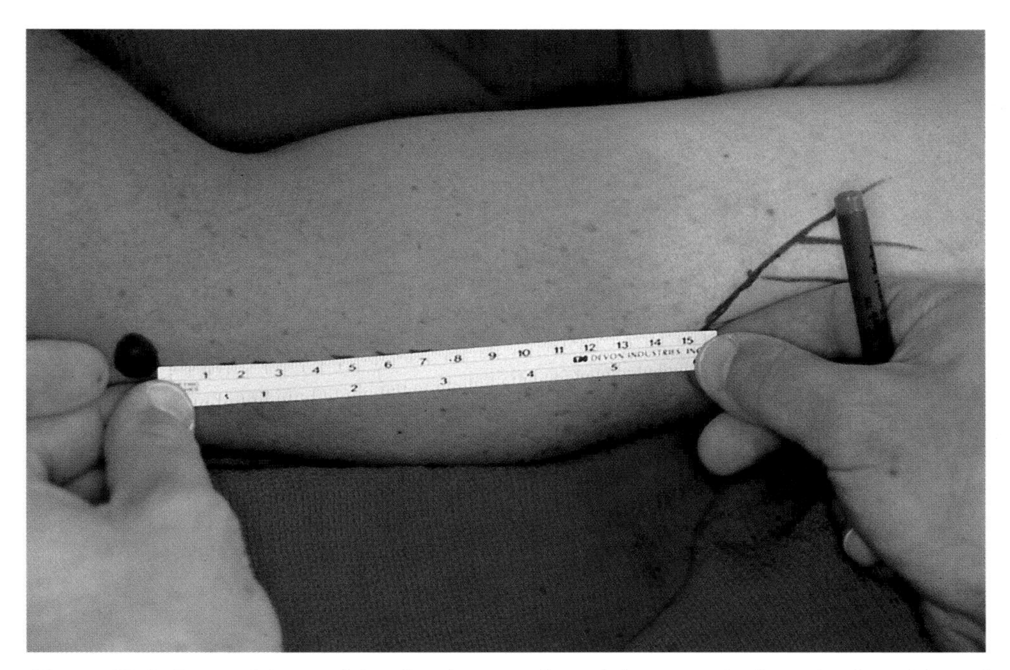

Figure 25.4. Determining and drawing the vascular axis between the lateral epicondyle and the deltoid insertion.

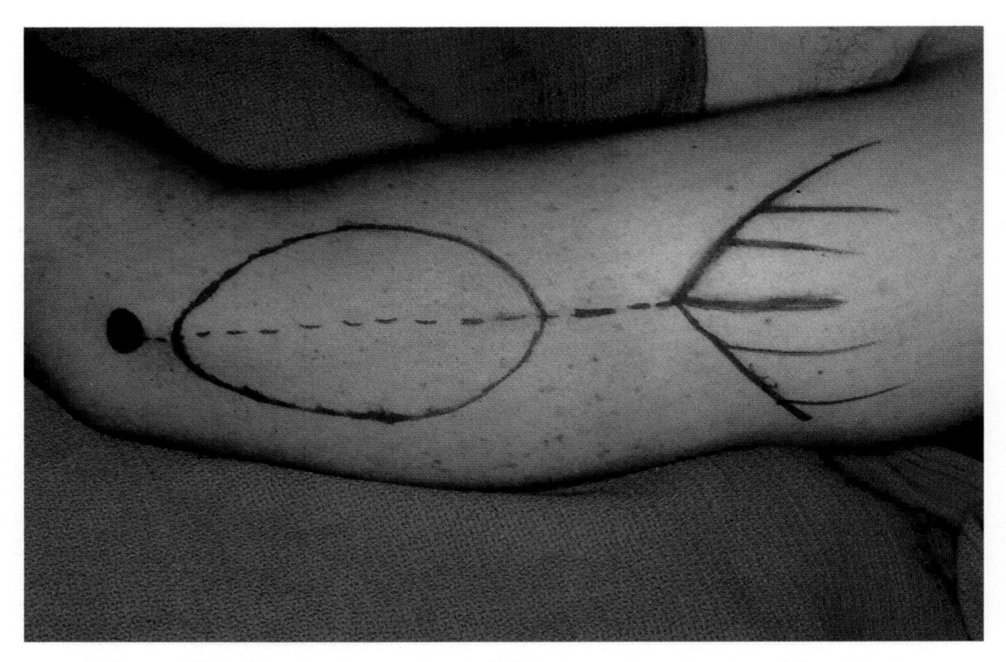

Figure 25.5. Flap borders outlined slightly larger than the size of the defect.

curve of underlying muscle belly, until you reach the humerus. Dissection continued over the humerus and beneath the vascular pedicle will meet the completed dissection from the posterior flap elevation. Now the flap elevation proceeds from its distal extent, at or distal to the lateral epicondyle, in a proximal direction on the humerus periosteum. Carefully protect the radial nerve, sacrifice the posterior cutaneous nerve of the forearm if necessary, and continue proximally to the junction of the deltoid and triceps muscles (Fig. 25.7).

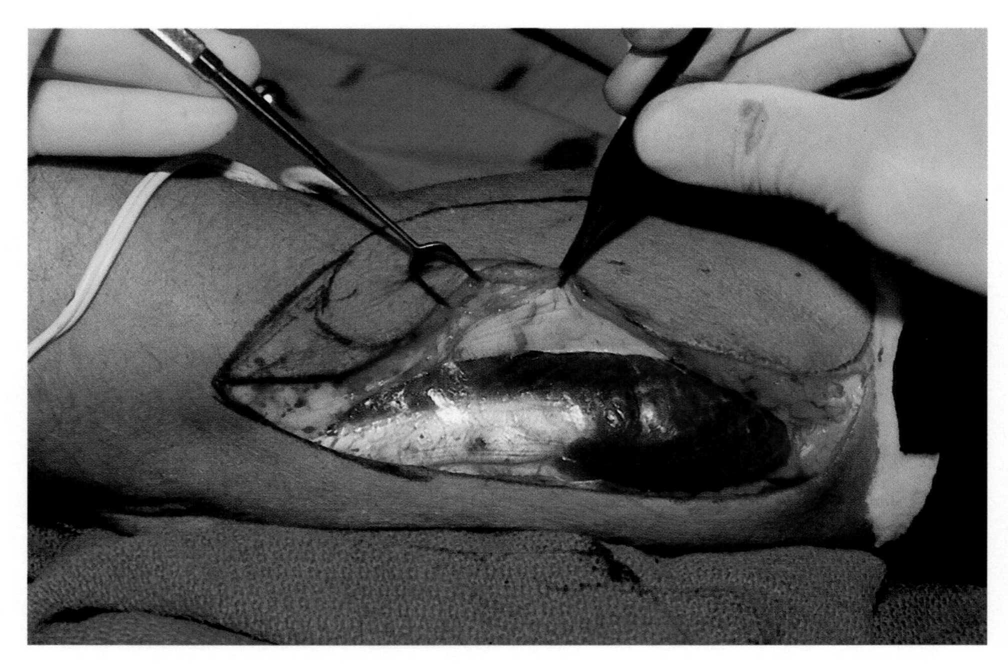

Figure 25.6. Elevation of the posterior lateral arm flap beneath the fascial layer. Note the perforator visible through the fascia.

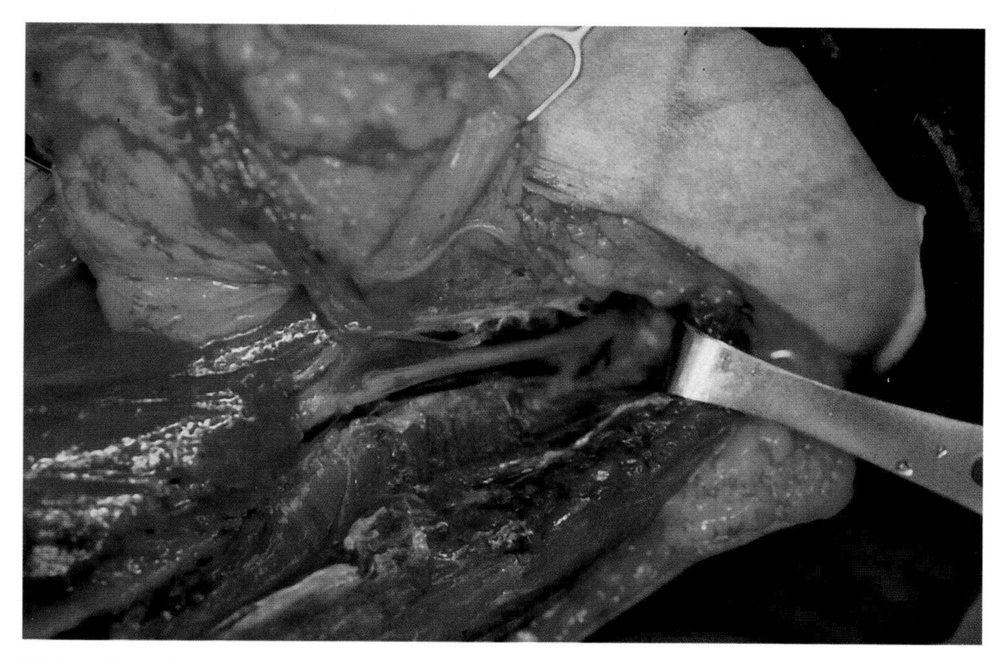

Figure 25.7. Vascular pedicle and radial nerve exposed as dissection proceeds in the proximal direction.

Here, the pedicle passes deep around the posterior border of the humerus and becomes difficult to follow. I generally elevate this flap with a very proximally applied arm tourniquet, and at this juncture of flap elevation the tourniquet begins to get in the way and may have to be removed (Fig. 25.8). Persistence in following the vascular pedicle will be rewarded with a longer and larger flap pedicle (Fig. 25.9). Temporarily fix the flap to the anterior skin edge so that inadvertent flap traction does not damage the pedicle until you are

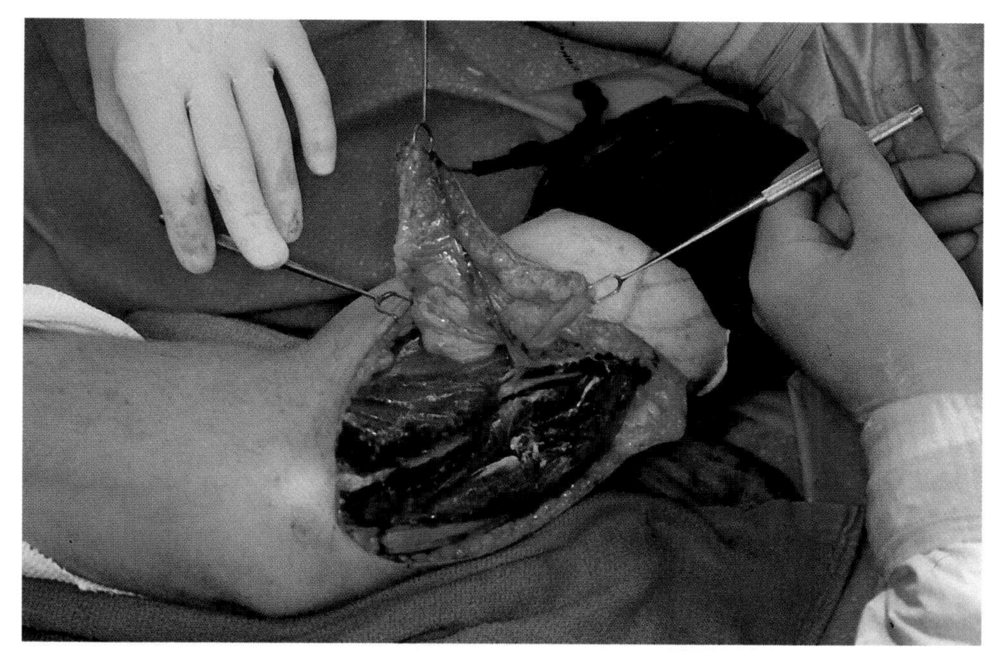

Figure 25.8. Flap freed from underlying muscle. Dissection of the vascular pedicle can begin between the deltoid and triceps muscles.

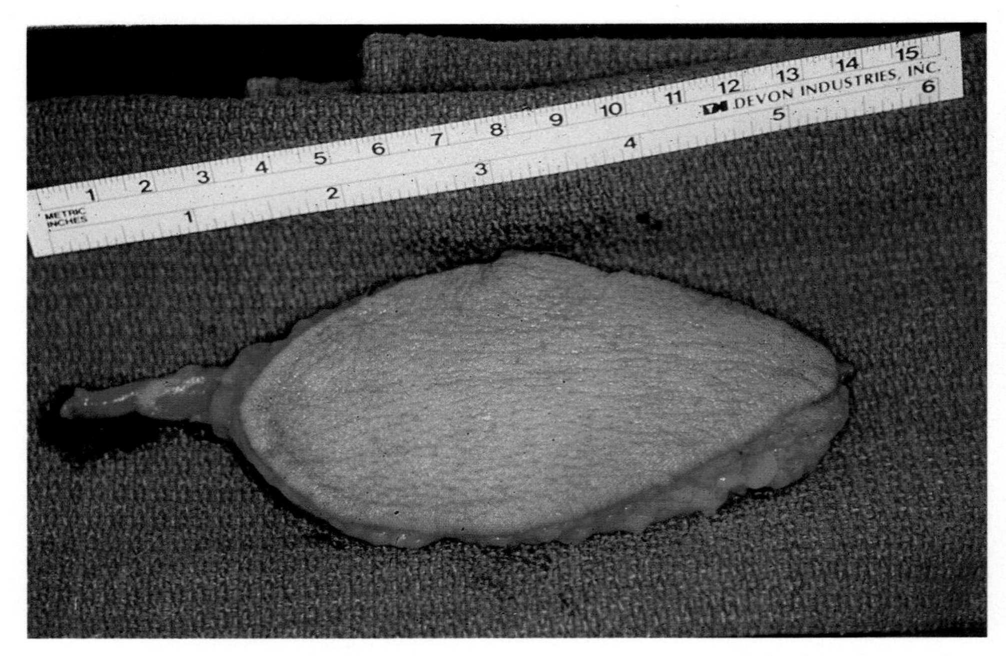

Figure 25.9. Lateral arm flap detached and vascular pedicle divided.

ready to move the flap to the defect. As long as the flap is not wider than 6 cm, it can be closed primarily with a resultant longitudinal scar that usually widens with time.

For defects of the hand dorsum, I generally use the radial artery or its dorsal branch as the recipient vessel (Fig. 25.10). If the radial artery is in continuity, consider an end-to-side arterial hookup. On the palmar side of the hand, common digital arteries are an excellent size match for the artery of the lateral arm flap. Often the flap is not wide enough for dorsal hand avulsion injuries. In this case, take advantage of the fact that the lateral arm flap is a fascia-based flap. The skin of the flap can be divided into two segments by incising the

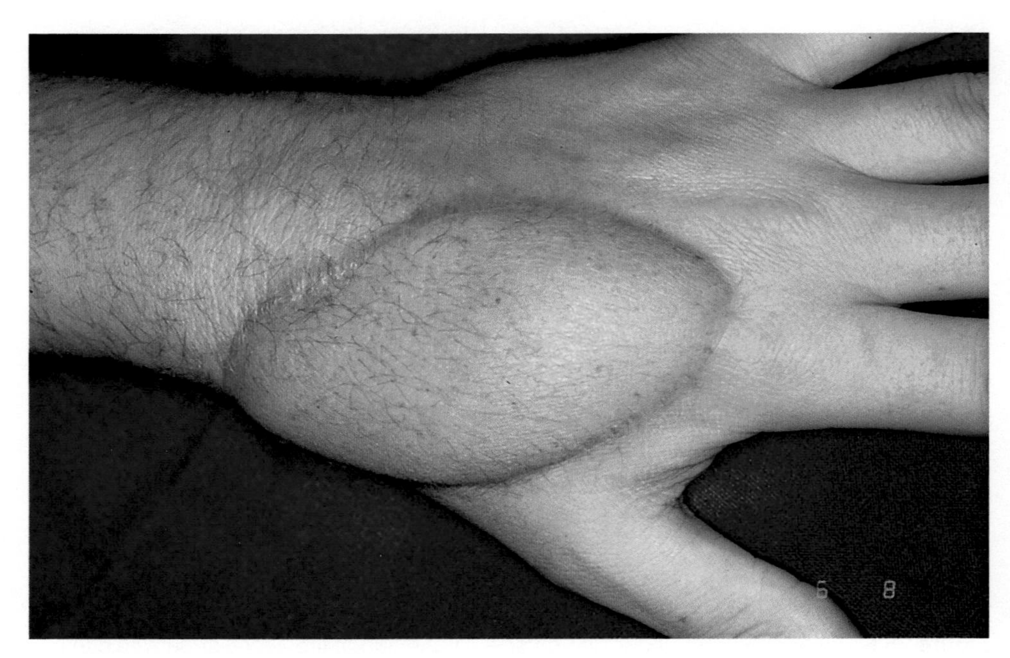

Figure 25.10. Flap in place 6 months after operation, before final defatting procedure.

skin and subcutaneous tissues as long as the fascia is kept intact. Using this trick, you can raise a 6-cm-wide and 20-cm-long flap and convert this to a flap 12 cm wide and 10 cm long, a better match for the dimensions of the dorsal hand.

Obese patients are not good candidates for this flap on the dorsum of the hand, and women may object to the donor scar. For obese patients with defects of the palm of the hand, consider harvesting this flap as a fascia-only flap, then consider a full-thickness skin graft for ultimate coverage.

Specific complications with this flap include injury to the radial nerve, hypertrophied and unsightly donor scar, and inability to primarily close the donor site. Although not a complication, patients should be warned that an area of numbness of the dorsal radial aspect of the forearm will generally result. Postoperative management, rehabilitation, and results will be similar for lateral arm and latissimus dorsi flaps once they have been transferred to the donor site, so I will cover these areas after reviewing the latissimus dorsi muscle.

Latissimus Dorsi Flap

The hand surgeon who deals with major upper extremity trauma must have access to this large, versatile flap (Fig. 25.11). Originally used and reported as a musculocutaneous flap, it is now usually used as a muscle flap covered with split-thickness skin grafts. This allows the thickness of the flap to better match the thickness of hand and forearm skin. The latissimus muscle has the largest surface area of any muscle in the body (25 × 35 cm) and after nerve division for free tissue transfer is only 1 cm thick. It can easily contour to surface irregularities, and studies by Mathes and others have demonstrated superior bacteria-killing ability compared with skin flaps (Fig. 25.12). As if this were not enough, the vascular pedicle is large (1.5–2.5 cm diameter), long (8–12 cm), and highly predictable (Fig. 25.13).

The major drawback of this flap is its location on the posterior thorax, which means that the flap is usually taken from the contralateral side with the patient in the decubitus position and the injured hand in the down position. No study has convincingly demonstrated a functional deficit from latissimus harvest, but its use in someone who needs crutches or a

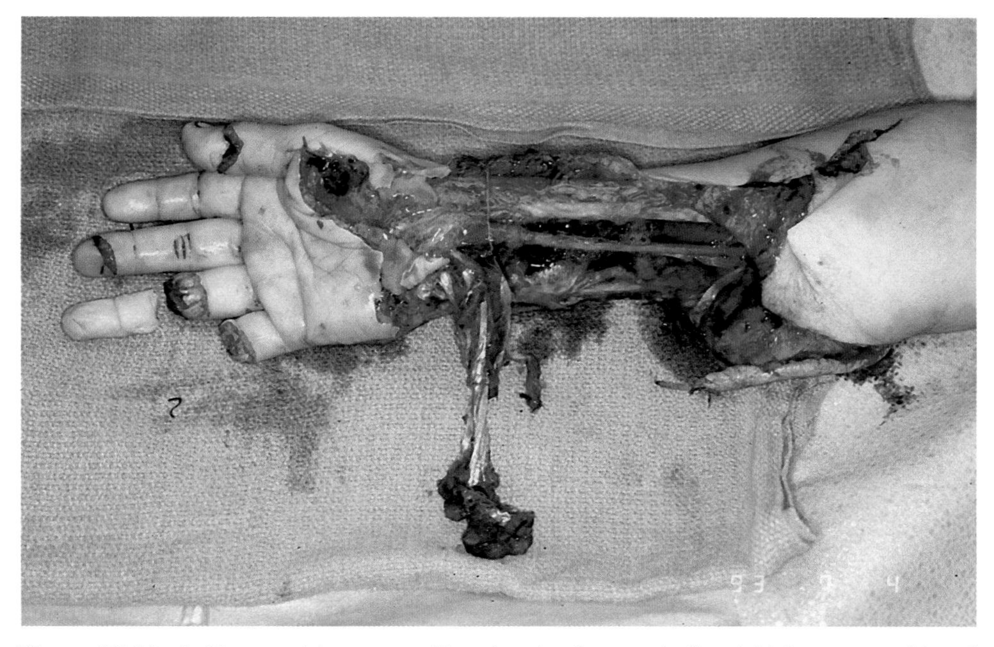

Figure 25.11. A 42-year-old woman with extensive trauma to the right forearm and hand following riding lawnmower injury.

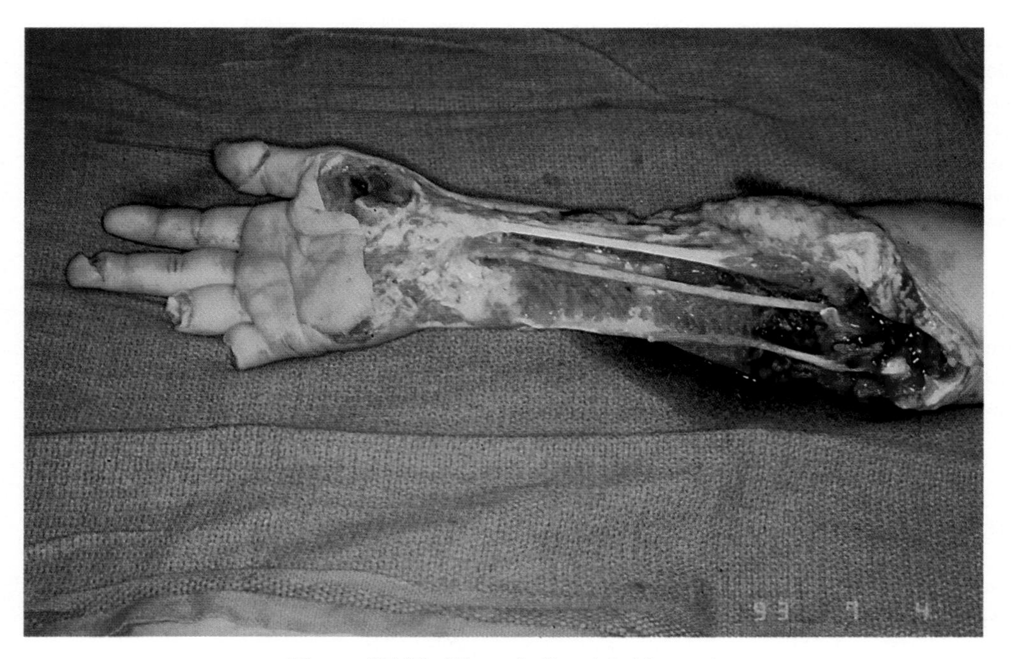

Figure 25.12. Wound after debridement.

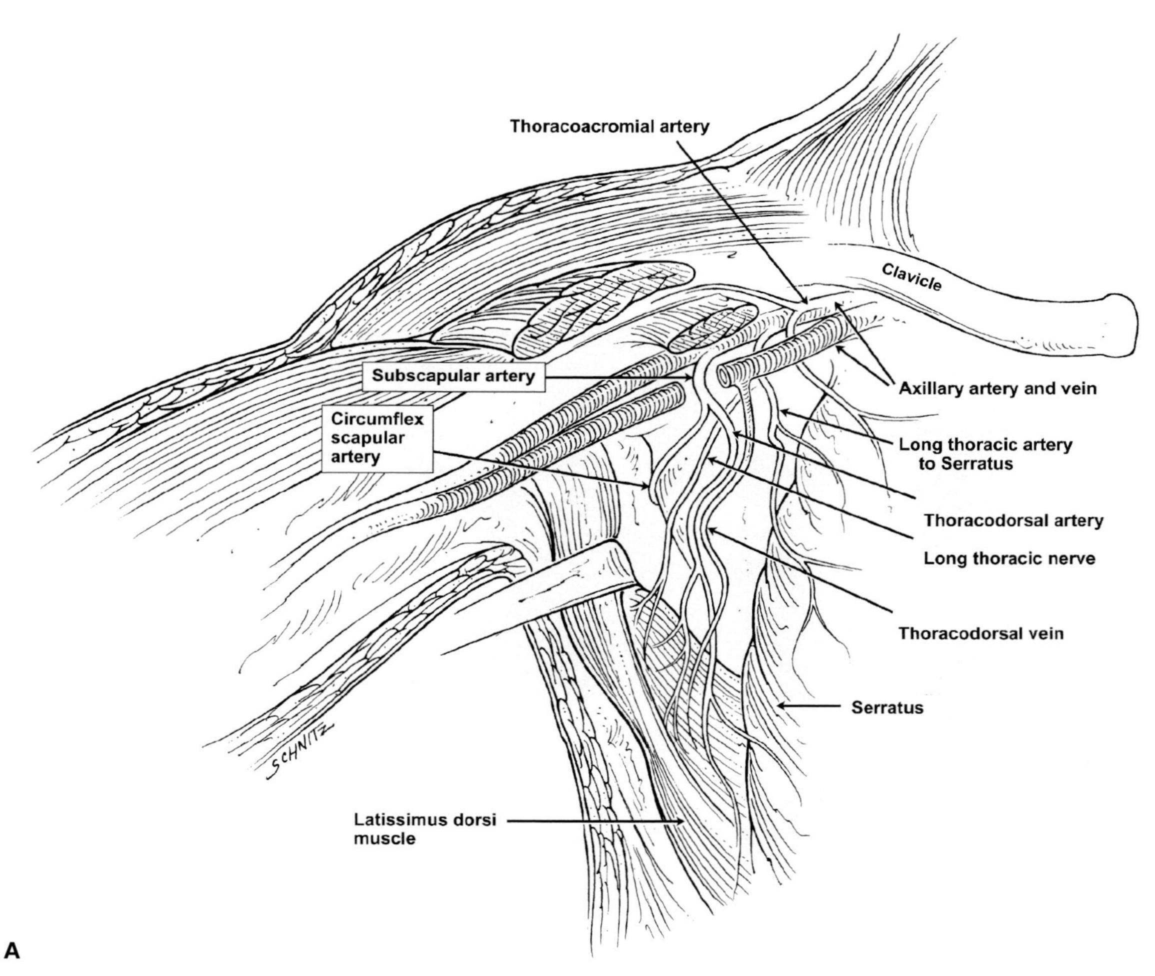

Figure 25.13. Neurovascular anatomy of the latissimus dorsi muscle flap.

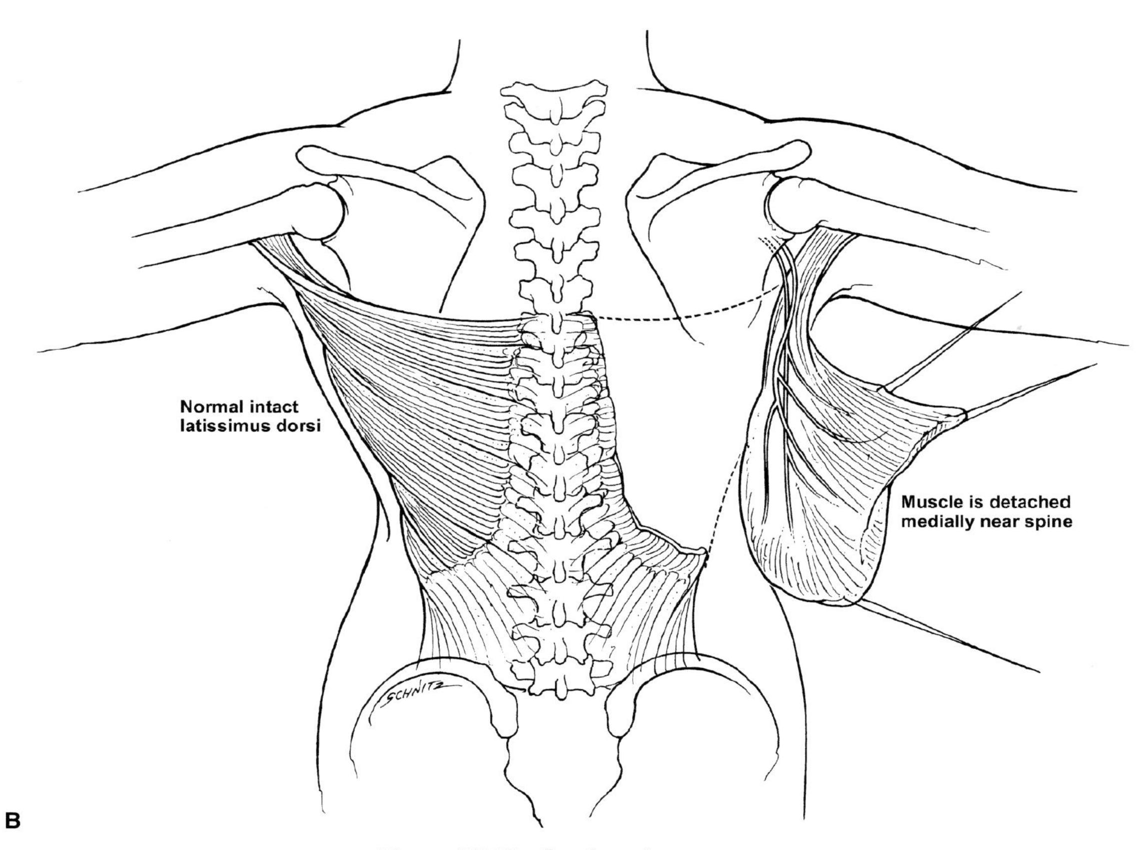

Figure 25.13. *Continued.*

wheelchair should be considered carefully. After induction of general anesthesia, the patient is positioned with the contralateral arm draped free or placed on an arm holder with the arm abducted for exposure of the axilla (Fig. 25.14). The patient position will sometimes encroach upon the surgeon preparing the defect and vessels, especially if the defect is in the proximal forearm or elbow.

Preoperative planning involves determining the size and geometry of the required flap and the course and length of vascular pedicle required. No Doppler study is required. Once the patient is properly positioned, two surgical teams may begin simultaneous work.

The muscle can be approached through a variety of incisions, but for harvest of the entire muscle an oblique or S-shaped incision works well (Fig. 25.15). It is helpful to mark the posterior axillary fold, which is the anterior border of the latissimus muscle, the inferior tip of the scapula, spinous processes, and iliac crest, to properly locate the skin incision. The incision is made to the level of the muscle passing through the overlying fascia (muscle is a better bed than fascia for skin grafts).

Skin flaps are elevated anteriorly to the lateral muscle border and posteriorly to the fascial origin from the lateral spine. The distal 2 to 3 cm of the flap at the muscle origin may not be reliable to support skin grafts. If you have an idea of the length of muscle needed, elevate skin from the muscle just distal to this level. Most authorities recommend beginning elevation of the flap from lateral to medial (i.e., at the anterior border). The vascular pedicle begins as the subscapular artery in the axilla and divides into the circumflex scapular and thoracodorsal arteries. The thoracodorsal artery enters the muscle and splits into two intermuscular branches, one transverse and one longitudinal, paralleling and 3 cm posterior to the anterior muscle border.

The surgeon elevates the muscle from the underlying ribs with care not to simultaneously raise the serratus anterior muscle. I often prefer to begin the flap elevation medially along the posterior border between the teres major and the latissimus dorsi. This bloodless plane

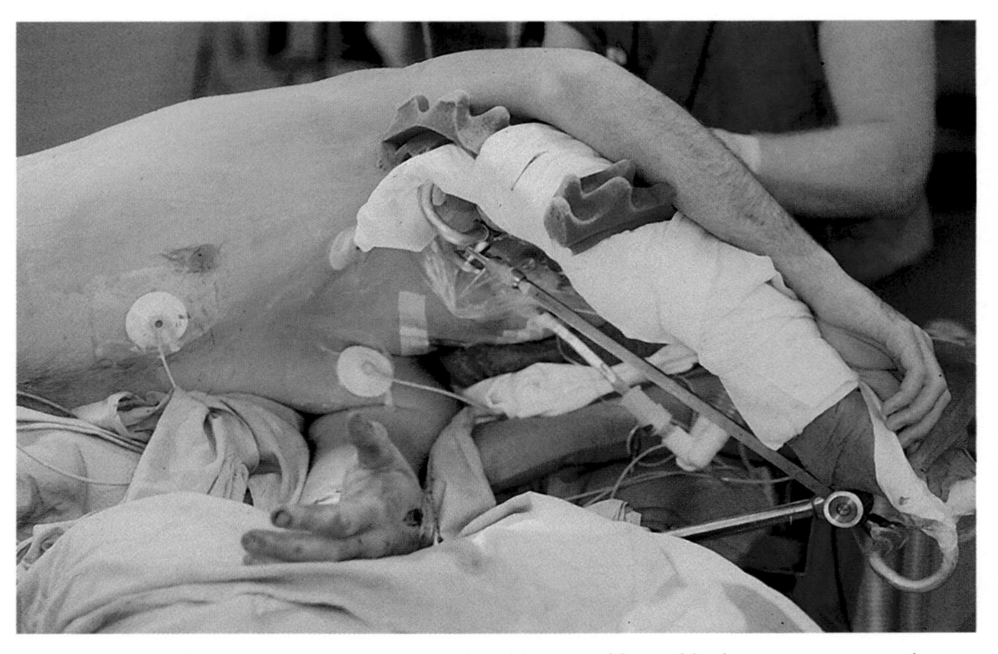

Figure 25.14. Patient positioned in the decubitus position with the arm supported on a padded arm holder.

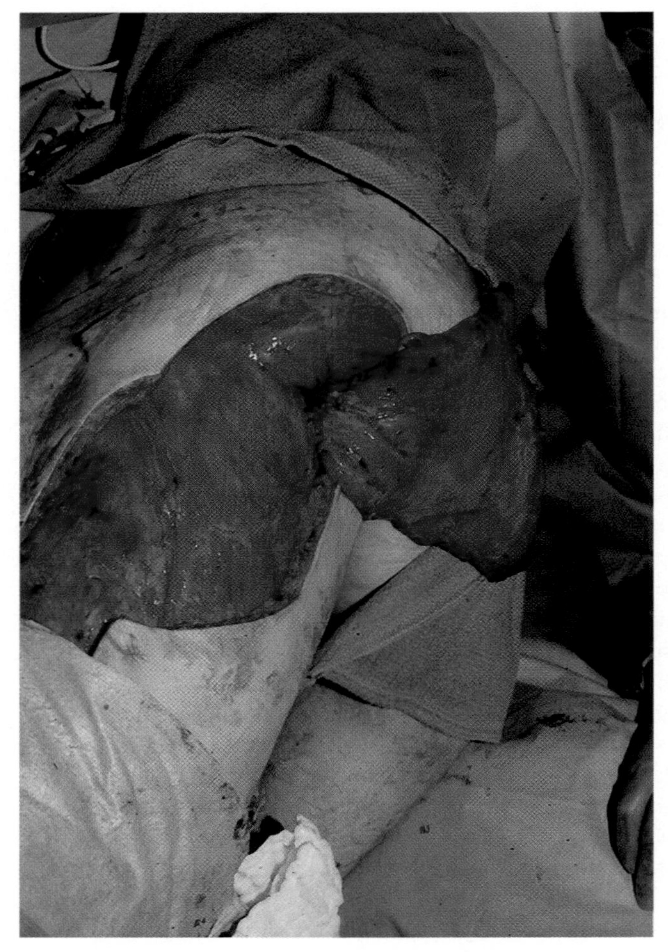

Figure 25.15. S-shaped incision on the posterior thorax and the latissimus muscle partially elevated.

keeps the surgeon above the serratus anterior muscle. Once the middle third of the muscle is raised, the muscle is freed from its distal attachments, watching for some large perforators passing to the muscle from the underlying intercostal arteries. It is helpful for the surgeon's hand to support the muscle from beneath and to divide the muscle at the level where it becomes difficult to separate muscle fibers from the underlying ribs. Flap elevation now turns north and toward the axilla as the proximal third of the muscle is freed from deep tissue (Fig. 25.16). One to three branches of the thoracodorsal artery pass to the serratus anterior and must be divided.

Initially deep to the proximal muscle, the vascular pedicle passes anterior to the tendon of origin into the axilla. As the pedicle is followed proximally, branches to the scapula and the circumflex scapular artery are noted and divided if the full length of the vascular pedicle is required. The dissection generally ends at the subscapular artery formed by the union of the thoracodorsal and circumflex scapular arteries. It may be helpful to divide the tendon of origin of the latissimus dorsi muscle to improve access, but remember that the flap is only attached by the vascular pedicle and that the weight of the muscle can easily apply harmful traction on the pedicle if unsupported, especially in the decubitus position.

Again, as with the lateral arm flap, temporarily attach the latissimus muscle to chest skin until ready for transfer. The skin incision may be partially closed from its inferior extent to save incision closure time after the muscle is detached. The donor incision is closed primarily, and we use two large suction drains to prevent the postoperative seroma formation so common with this flap.

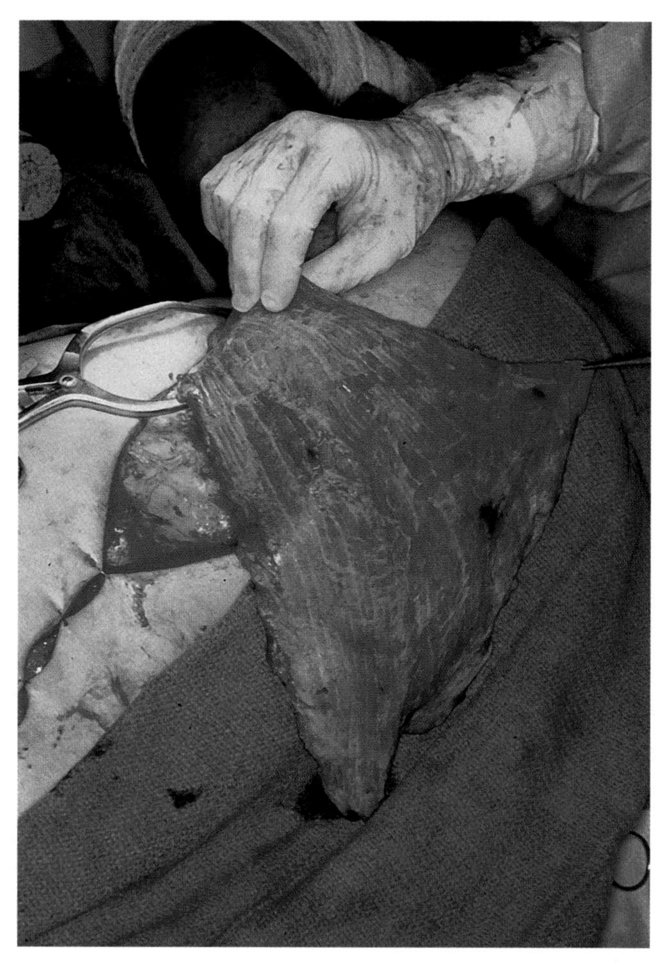

Figure 25.16. Muscle elevated to tendon insertion and final pedicle identification commencing.

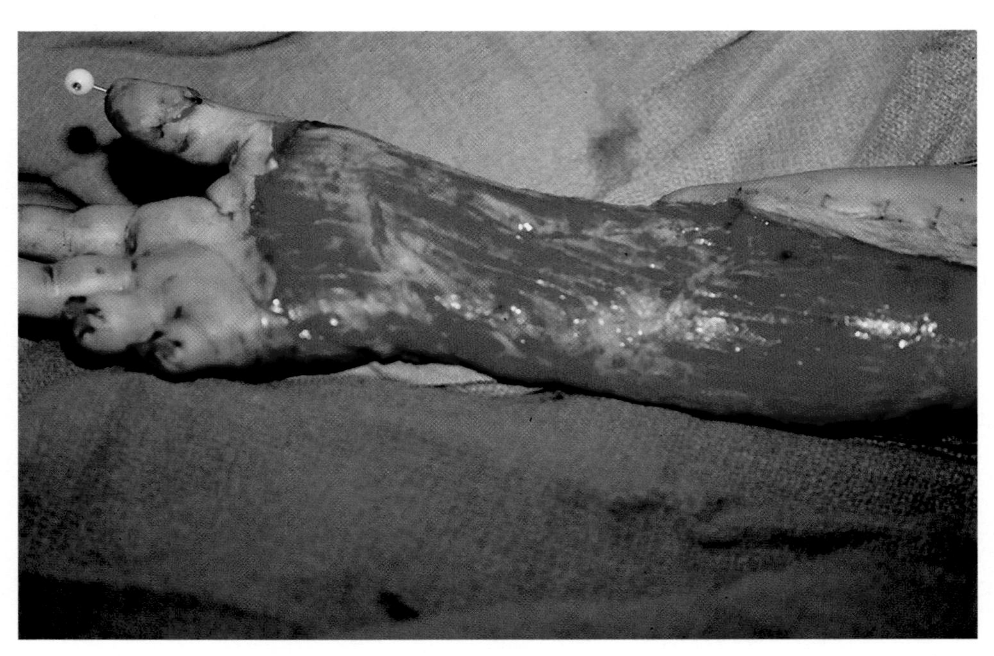

Figure 25.17. Muscle flap applied to the upper limb, vascular hookup performed, and muscle trimming and insertion completed.

I encourage the use of suction drains as long as there is any wound drainage of substance until the amount collected over a 24-hour period diminishes to the level of 30 mL per day. Often, nearly the entire muscle is raised and trimmed to fit the defect after the vessels are repaired (Fig. 25.17). Figure 25.18 shows one-year follow-up in a patient with lawnmower injury to the forearm and hand and early wound coverage with latissimus dorsi muscle flap and skin graft.

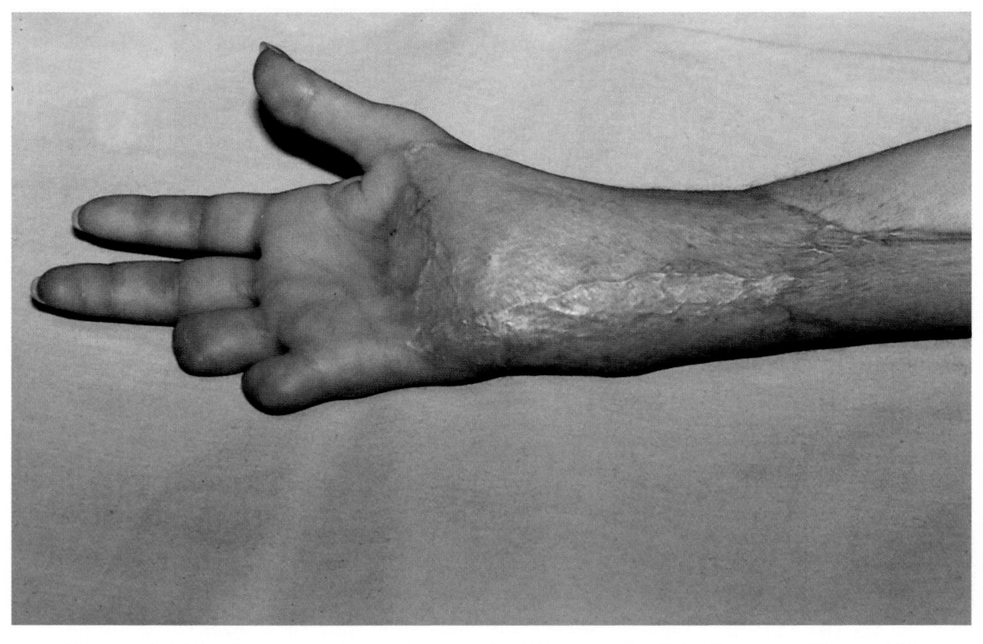

A

Figure 25.18. One year after microsurgical flap repair of the forearm. Finger (**A**)

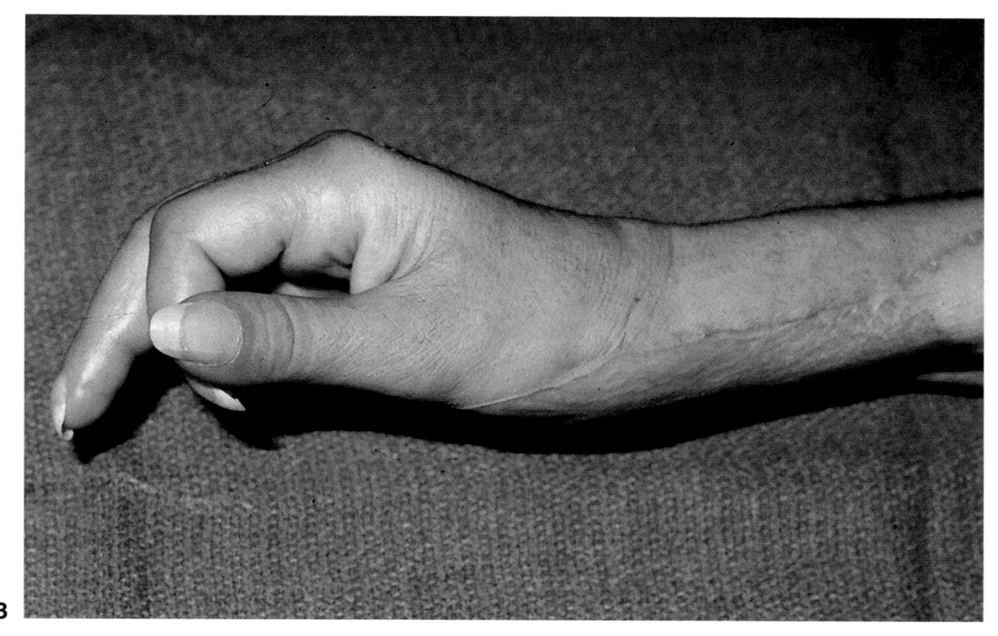

B

Figure 25.18. *Continued.* and thumb (**B**) motion are demonstrated.

This flap, which is such a friend to the upper and lower extremity microsurgeon, has few specific complications. This versatile flap has proven its usefulness in a variety of situations. Despite the size of the harvest, there are few complications that should deter the experienced microsurgeon from considering the latissimus dorsi flap as the primary alternative in complex coverage situations. The anesthetized patient has no muscle protection of the nerves passing through the axilla. These nerves can be damaged by stretch from hyperabduction and hyperextension of the arm. Seroma formation has been mentioned, and the scar, although somewhat hidden by its location, can hypertrophy.

POSTOPERATIVE MANAGEMENT

Microsurgical vessel repairs need postoperative monitoring to have any hope of salvaging the ischemic or congested flap. Skin flaps are the easiest flaps in which to visually detect vascular problems, and temperature monitoring is feasible. Surface Doppler monitoring for arterial and venous signals is helpful but requires some skill and experience with the technique. Implantable Doppler sensors are highly reliable and can be removed when no longer needed. We generally heat the room to 80°F postoperatively and withhold caffeine and tobacco.

Much debate has centered on the use of anticoagulation in these patients after surgery. I generally use one aspirin per day and dextran at 25 mL per hour in adults. There are excellent microsurgeons who do not use anticoagulation. If loss of arterial or venous flow is detected after surgery, then a rapid return to the operating room is indicated. The anastomoses are examined, and occasionally the vascular pedicle needs to be unkinked. More commonly, a revision of the anastomosis is needed. Fifty percent survival of these flaps returned to the operating room is expected.

REHABILITATION

Generally, the underlying repairs of bone, tendon, and nerve will determine the specifics of formal rehabilitation. Once the acute phase of recovery has passed, and with it the risk of vessel thrombosis and infection, the surgeon can look at making the flap as aesthetically acceptable as possible. Light compression of flaps, particularly muscle, seems to aid in atrophy of the flap, which is desirable. Flap revision by open defatting and flap reduction or liposuction may be required for optimum appearance.

RESULTS

Microsurgical flap transfer is now definitely in the upper extremity trauma, oncologic, and even pediatric surgeon's toolbox. Studies reviewing free flap survival to all areas of the body indicate that microsurgeons expect at least 95% flap survival. This figure may be slightly higher for flaps to the upper extremity. Success is not achieved with flap survival but is now determined by the reconstructive outcome: functionally, aesthetically, and with acceptable donor site morbidity. The ability to reliably cover large and complex wounds in a single stage while carrying vascularized bone, tendon, and nerve has fostered the concept of single-stage reconstruction. This reduces the risk of infection, limits joint stiffness, and significantly shortens the recovery period of major injuries and resections.

COMPLICATIONS

I have pointed out the specific complications of the two illustrative flaps in the surgery section. The dreaded complication of free flap transfer is vessel occlusion and flap loss. Careful microsurgical technique is important, but the origin of problems is often traced to a poor preoperative plan, including the choice of an unsuitable flap, disregard for patient positioning, and limited and inadequate surgical exposure of recipient vessels and the donor site. The most common intraoperative error in trauma reconstruction is attempting vessel repairs in the zone of injury. Stretching or compression of the vascular repairs is often the result of an unplanned disparity between the defect dimensions and the elevated flap size. The surgeon may be tempted to forcibly pull the wound and flap edges together when a small skin graft will close the wound without increasing wound tension.

Once feared as arduous and unpredictable surgical procedures, microsurgical flap reconstruction of the upper limb is now widespread and often routine, with results unmatched by other techniques.

RECOMMENDED READING

1. Acland RD, Clapson JB. The Lateral Arm Flap. In: Buncke HJ, ed. *Microsurgery: Transplantation and Replantation*. Philadelphia: Lea & Febiger, 1991:187–204.
2. Buncke HJ. Latissimus Dorsi Muscle Transplantation. In: Buncke HJ, ed. *Microsurgery: Transplantation and Replantation*. Philadelphia: Lea & Febiger, 1991:394–433.
3. Jones NF, Lister GD. Free Skin and Composite Flaps. In: Green DP, Hotchkiss RN, Pederson WC, eds. *Green's Operative Hand Surgery*. Philadelphia: Churchill Livingstone, 1999:1159–1200.
4. Katsaros J. The Lateral Arm Free Flap. In: Evans DM, ed. *Skin Cover in the Injured Hand*. Edinburgh: Churchill Livingstone, 1992:89–102.
5. Mathes SJ, Nahai F. Latissimus Dorsi Flap. In: Mathes SJ, Nahai F, eds. *Reconstructive Surgery: Principles, Anatomy, & Technique*. New York: Churchill Livingstone, 1997:565–616.
6. Mathes SJ, Nahai F. Lateral Arm Flap. In: Mathes SJ, Nahai F, eds. *Reconstructive Surgery: Principles, Anatomy, & Technique*. New York: Churchill Livingstone, 1997:729–746.
7. Scheker LR, Langley SJ, Martin DL, et al. Primary extensor tendon reconstruction in dorsal hand defects requiring free flaps. *J Hand Surg* 18B:568–575, 1993.
8. Swartz WM. Free Flaps. In: Achauer BM, Eriksson O, Quyuron B, et al., eds. *Plastic Surgery Indications, Operations, and Outcomes*. St. Louis: Mosby, 2000:2149–2164.

26

The Reversed Radial Forearm Flap

Matthew M. Tomaino

INDICATIONS/CONTRAINDICATIONS

The reverse radial forearm flap (RRFF), initially described by Chinese authors in 1978, is tremendously versatile as a distally based flap in complex cases where skin-coverage needs may be accompanied by defects in nerve and tendon. Arterial perfusion of this distally based flap is retrograde, via the normal communication between deep and superficial palmar arches, and its venous drainage occurs through the accompanying vena comitantes. This flap is indicated for defects, which involve the dorsum of the hand, the palm, and the thumb-index web space. When ligated proximally, the radial artery is capable of an arc of rotation that allows coverage of any of these recipient sites.

Preoperative vascular assessment must include an Allen's test to ensure that ligation of the radial artery in the proximal forearm will not result in ischemia of the hand and fingers, as might be expected when a clinically incomplete superficial arch exists. Accordingly, an abnormal Allen's test or previous injuries to either the radial artery or its vena comitantes contraindicate the use of this flap. Although primary closure of the donor site may be possible, it typically requires reconstruction with a split-thickness skin graft; thus, concern regarding the appearance of the forearm postoperatively might prompt the use of a free flap as an alternative.

PREOPERATIVE PLANNING

Levine has referred to the list of alternatives for soft-tissue replacement as "the reconstructive ladder," in light of increasing complexity from simple skin grafting, for example, to more complex free tissue transfers. Skin grafting may be feasible in many settings if a healthy vascularized tissue bed exists, but in cases of composite loss when tendon repair or reconstruction is necessary it is contraindicated. While alternative regional

Matthew M. Tomaino, M.D., M.B.A.: Division of Hand, Shoulder, and Elbow Surgery, University of Rochester Medical Center, Rochester, NY

pedicled tissue transfers, such as the posterior interosseous and ulnar forearm flaps, provide vascularized tissue without requiring microvascular anastomoses, defect size is often a limiting factor for the former, and the latter option is less attractive because of the normal dominance of the superficial arch.

It must be emphasized that composite tissue loss from the dorsum of the hand need not be treated in the majority of cases with "composite" tissue transfers. Although tissue transfers can be selected to provide simultaneous replacement of skin, tendon, and bone using a single donor source, these techniques may result in unsatisfactory donor site morbidity and less optimal functional return. Similarly, the radial forearm flap can be elevated with palmaris longus tendon and a portion of the radius, but in the final analysis, it has not been shown that vascularized tendon grafts function better than tendon transfers or grafts placed in a suitable soft-tissue bed. Indeed, composite tissue transfers are often more intriguing in concept than in practice because of the difficulty in matching the unique requirements of the individual tendon, bone, and skin defects with available donor tissue.

It is for that reason that the RRFF is most attractive as a generous soft-tissue replacement, alone, when confronted with a complex injury to the dorsum of the hand. Subsequent tendon transfers and grafting of one defect can follow this fairly straightforward and quick, single-stage reconstruction with its advantages of proximity, tissue match, and avoidance of microsurgery.

Ideally, fracture fixation should be performed at the initial surgical setting. Although external fixation has traditionally been recommended for severe Grade III open fractures, the upper extremity is relatively privileged because of its blood supply, and can be safely managed stable internal fixation in many cases, after adequate debridement. For cases in which small bone defects are present, Freeland et al. have convincingly shown the advantages of early bone grafting within the first 10 days as long as debridement has created a clean wound. The choice of implant will be dictated by fracture location, pattern complexity, and the surgeon's experience and level of comfort.

When tendons are damaged, tension-free repair of good quality tissue is required. If debridement results in tendon loss, intercalary grafts can be used, but if the proximal motor is damaged, or if lengthy tendon defects have resulted, tendon transfer is the logical solution. In each of these cases, acceptable function rests on tendon excursion. Tendon excursion requires a favorable soft-tissue environment as well.

Scheker et al. have shown that primary extensor-tendon reconstruction resulted in satisfactory functional restoration for complex dorsal hand wounds with associated fractures in which free flaps were selected for coverage. They used free lateral arm or groin flaps and tunneled extensor tendon grafts, either extensor digitorum longus or plantaris, through the subcutaneous fat of the flap. Iliac crest bone grafting of metacarpal fractures along with either plate and screw or Kirschner-wire fixation was used and dynamic extensor splinting began within 48 hours. Arguably, the RRFF can achieve the same outcome, but without the need for microsurgical anastomoses.

Although the established traditional method of extensor reconstruction utilizes a staged approach, allowing for soft-tissue replacement before bone and tendon reconstruction, Sundine and Scheker showed that immediate, single-stage reconstruction of composite loss resulted in significantly faster restoration of maximum range of motion, fewer operations, and a greater chance of returning to work. These authors deserve credit for questioning the role, if any, of composite tissue transfers, demonstrating that nonvascularized tendon grafts passed through free skin flaps are not complicated by postoperative adhesions. The author's favorable experience passing tendon grafts and transfers beneath thin, pedicled radial forearm flaps has caused the author to question the absolute necessity for subcutaneous fat when dynamic extension splinting is initiated early.

SURGERY

The technical execution of the RRFF is relatively straight-forward for those engaged in sophisticated surgery about the hand and forearm. The initial wound should be debrided, and tissue inventory should be conducted to assess the presence and viability of the ten-

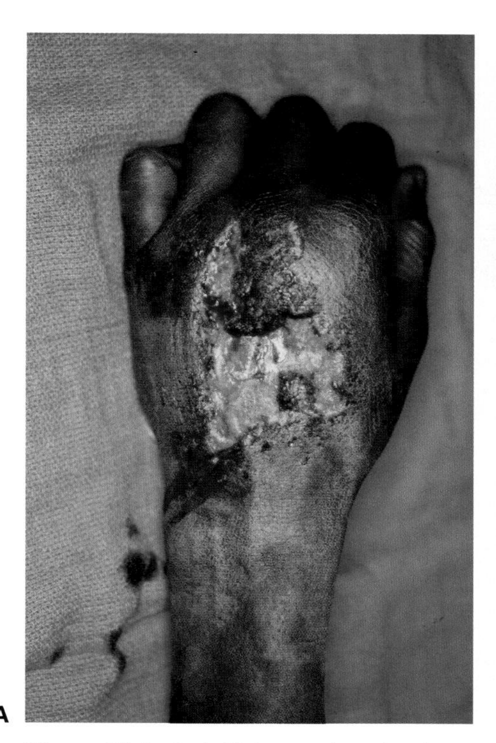

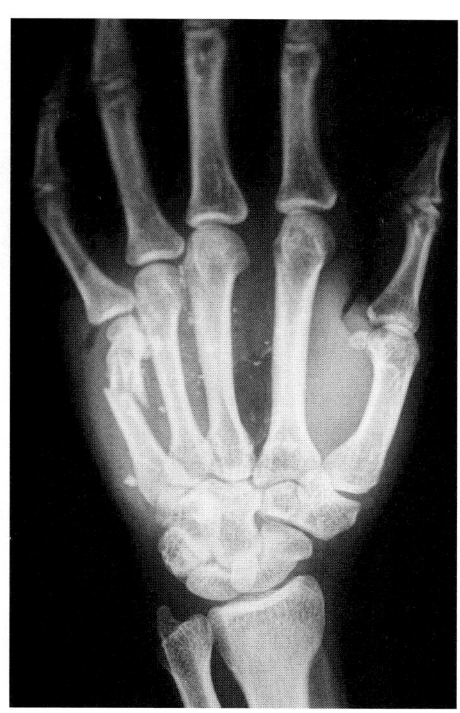

Figure 26.1. A: Initial wound on the dorsum of the left hand following a motor vehicle accident. **B:** PA x-ray shows a fracture of the 5th metacarpal. This was fixed with two crossed Kirschner wires rather than a plate because of distal comminution.

dons, bone, nerves, and vessels. In other words, if fracture or extensor injuries need to be addressed, this should be performed prior to flap elevation (Figs. 26.1 and 26.2). The temporal concerns or reconstruction, not just the tissue concerns, should be optimized.

A line is drawn from a point 1 cm below the center of the antecubital fossa to the scaphoid tuberosity—to represent the axis of the radial artery and the intermuscular

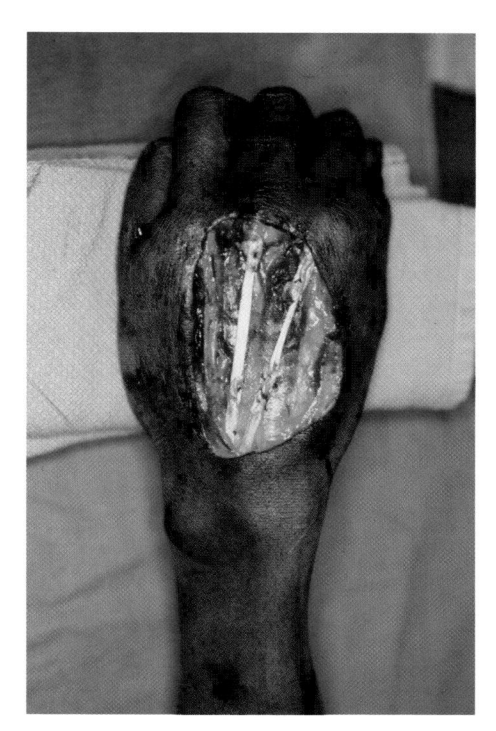

Figure 26.2. The wound has been debrided, and intercalary extensor tendon grafting has been performed to restore the continuity of the index and long finger extensor communis tendons using palmaris longus as donor tendon.

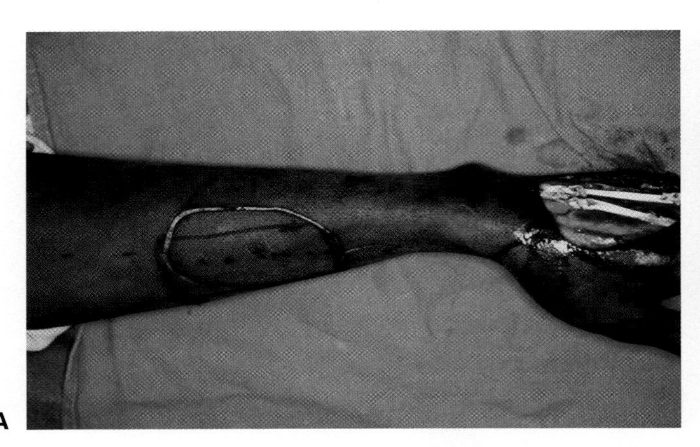
A

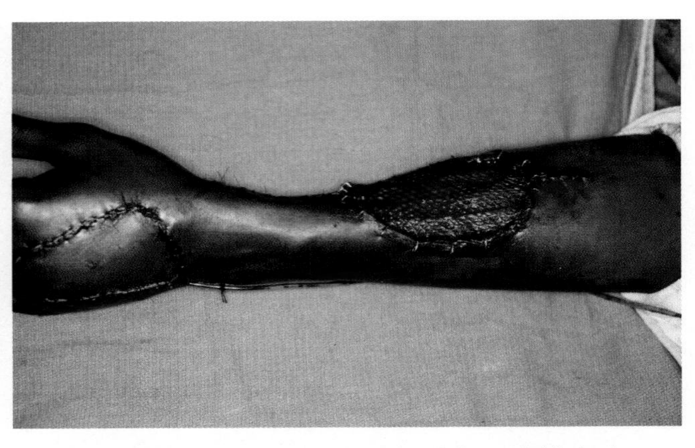
B

Figure 26.3. A: A template of the dorsal hand wound is made using felt, and this is then used to draw the shape and size of the tissue defect on the volar forearm. The "rotation axis" selected was at the distal volar wrist in this case. The template is drawn on the forearm at a distance from this "axis point" equal to 1 cm more than the distance between the defect on the hand and the "axis point." **B:** After the proximal radial vascular bundle is divided and ligated, the skin flap is elevated with the forearm fascia as well. Distal to the flap, the radial artery and its vena comitantes are carefully dissected to the axis point or even a bit beyond, if needed, to ensure a smooth arc for the vascular bundle before insetting the flap into the wound defect. The proximal donor site is covered with a split-thickness skin graft, and a small suction drain is placed beneath the flap for 2 days.

septum, through which small branches from the artery make their way to the forearm fascia and overlying skin. A template of the dorsal hand wound is made using felt or a piece of the esmarch bandage, and this is then used to draw the shape and size of the tissue defect on the volar forearm—centered along this arterial axis. The "rotation axis point" is selected distally, and may vary depending on the location of the defect, but typically the palpable radial pulse at the distal wrist suffices. The template is drawn on the forearm at a distance from this "axis point" equal to 1 cm more than the distance between the defect on the hand and the "axis point." This allows a gentle arc for the vascular bundle once it is time to transpose the flap to the defect. It is also wise to make the dimensions of the flap slightly larger than the actual defect, to allow for slight "shrinkage" after elevation (Fig. 26.3).

The arm is then exsanguinated, and a pneumatic tourniquet is elevated. The proximal radial neurovascular vascular bundle is exposed, divided, and ligated at the outset. At the distal border of the flap, the radial vascular bundle is identified at the lateral edge of the flexor carpi radialis (FCR) tendon and carefully dissected. Next, the skin flap is elevated along with the underlying forearm fascia, working first from radial to the axis of the artery, and then ulnar (or vice versa).

Proximally and distally large-caliber subcutaneous veins should be ligated. Smaller vessels can be coagulated with bipolar cautery. During flap elevation, special attention should be paid to preserve the paratenon on all the tendons. Once the vessel is neared, the dissection deepens in order to include the radial artery and its vena comitantes. Distal to the flap, the radial artery and its vena comitantes are carefully elevated to the axis point or even a bit beyond, if needed, to ensure a smooth arc for the vascular bundle before insetting the flap into the wound defect. The radial sensory nerve should be identified in the subcutaneous tissue distal to its exit point between the brachioradialis and extensor carpi radialis longus tendons, but the lateral antebrachial cutaneous nerve of the forearm will typically need to be divided. The tourniquet is deflated so that perfusion can be checked, hemostasis obtained, and the arc of the vascular pedicle examined.

The flap is carefully inset with 4-0 suture, over a suction drain (positioned in such a way that removal will not injure the pedicle). A split-thickness skin graft (18/1000 inch) is harvested from the thigh. Although the author has meshed these in the past (1:1.5), the current practice is to apply unmeshed graft except for a couple of small openings to allow drainage of hematoma. A compressive dressing is placed consisting of a single layer of bacitracin-impregnated adaptic followed by saline-moistened four-by-eight sponges.

POSTOPERATIVE MANAGEMENT

A wrist splint is placed for 5 days, and then the dressing is changed and the donor site examined. The drain is typically removed from the recipient site on the second postoperative day. The flap is monitored daily based on appearance as well as by using a Doppler probe to listen to the arterial signal. The skin-graft donor site (thigh) is covered at the end of surgery with a large plastic dressing. This is typically left in place until a week or so after surgery, when it can easily be removed in the shower. Thereafter, for a month or two, the thigh is kept moist with a thin coating of antibiotic ointment until sweat glands regenerate. Allow the patient to gently wash the flap and the forearm at 10 days—once the sutures have been removed.

REHABILITATION

When extensor-tendon repair or reconstruction has been necessary, begin dynamic extensor splinting at 1 week postoperatively (Fig. 26.4). The author emphasizes the importance of hand elevation for the first few weeks to decrease swelling, and, generally, do not rely on any type of custom-made anti-edema glove.

RESULTS

If the basic tenets described in the Preoperative Planning and Surgery sections are closely followed, the RRFF is exceedingly reliable (Fig. 26.5). In the author's experience, they have never had a pedicled flap fail, and when either marginal necrosis at the recipient site or incomplete healing of a skin graft at the donor site occur, dressing changes have sufficed. Of course, functional outcome is critical; thus, any accompanying procedures in the hand require their own special rehabilitation considerations. Skeletal injury may include metacarpals and/or the wrist, and construct rigidity should be sufficient enough to allow dynamic extension splinting postoperatively, when extensor-tendon repair or reconstruction have been required. The author allows passive digital extension and active

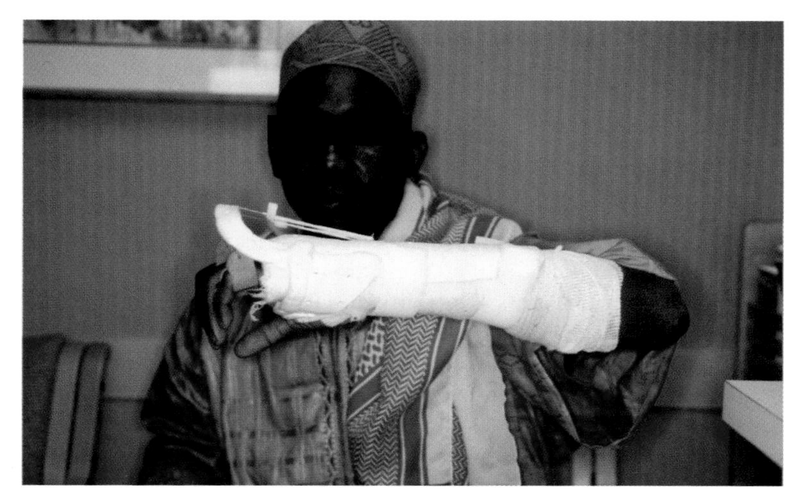

Figure 26.4. Dynamic extension splinting is started at 1 week.

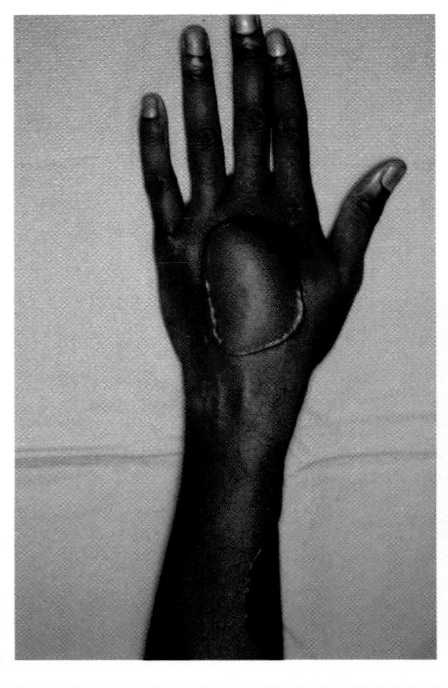
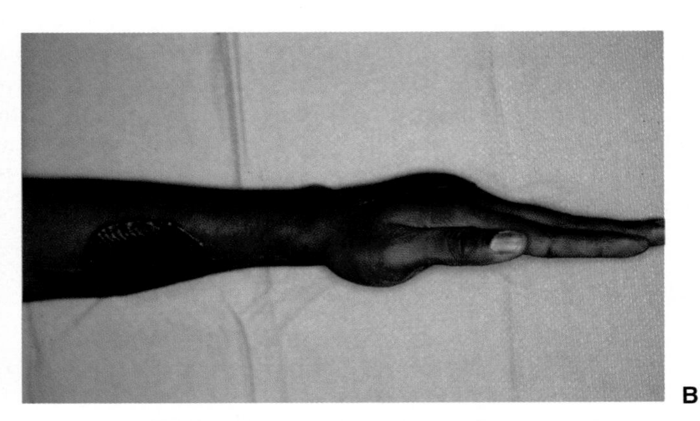
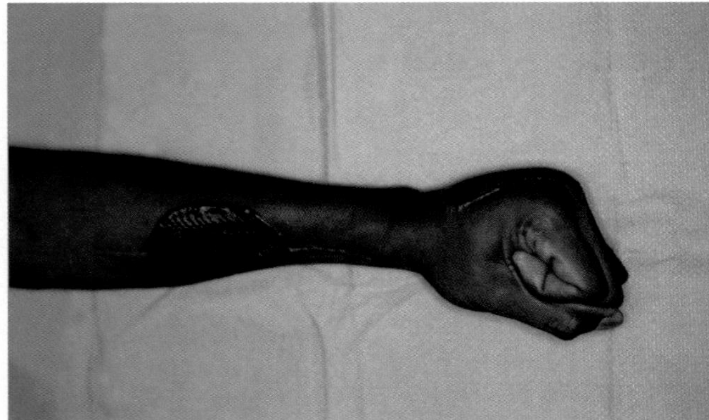
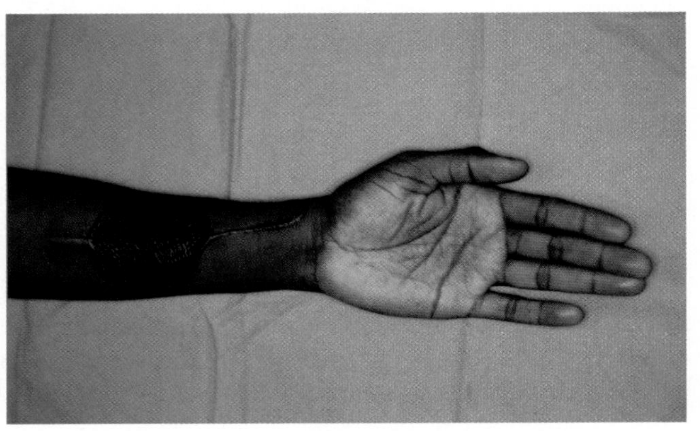

Figure 26.5. Appearance of the hand eight weeks following surgery. **A:** Thin tissue contour. **B:** Full digital extension. **C:** Full digital flexion. **D:** Well-healed donor site.

flexion within the first week, since as little as 30 degrees of motion at the metacarpal (MP) joint results in 5 mm of tendon excursion, and will minimize postoperative adhesions.

COMPLICATIONS

Complications such as flap failure, incomplete healing at the wound margins, and infection are uncommon. Donor-site complications are most problematic, but can be minimized by careful split-thickness skin grafting (STSG) technique and the use of a compressive dressing. Suprafascial elevation of the RRFF has been suggested to improve the success of donor-site skin grafting, but careful skin grafting of the donor site has been satisfactory in my experience. Other options for addressing the donor site following RRFF include techniques for direct wound closure, the use of skin stretching devices, and the use of full-thickness skin graft. Split-thickness skin grafts have been more securely attached to the recipient bed with the use of vacuum-assisted closure, and unsightly skin-grafted wounds have been removed following secondary skin expansion to allow more aesthetic wound closure. In conclusion, the RRFF is a time-honored alternative to a pedicled groin flap or free tissue transfer when dealing with either simple or complex soft-tissue defects in the hand.

RECOMMENDED READING

1. Chang TS, Wang W. Application of microsurgery in plastic and reconstructive surgery. *Journal of Reconstructive Microsurgery* 1: 55–63, 1984.
2. Evans RB, Burkhalter WE. A study of the dynamic anatomy of extensor tendons and implications for treatment. *J Hand Surg* 11:774–779, 1986.
3. Levin LS. The reconstruction ladder, an orthoplastic approach. *Ortho Clinics of North America* 24:393, 1993.
4. Lutz BS, Wei F, Chang SCN, et al. Donor-site morbidity after suprafascial elevation of the radial forearm flap: a prospective study in 95 consecutive cases. *Plastic and Reconstructive Surgery* 103:132–137, 1999.
5. McGregor AD. The free radial forearm flap–the management of the secondary defect. *British Journal of Plastic Surgery* 40:83–85, 1987.
6. Scheker LR, Langley SJ, Martin DL, et al. Primary extensor tendon reconstruction in dorsal hand defects requiring free flaps. *Br J Hand Surg* 18B:568–575, 1993.
7. Soutar DS, Tanner NS. The radial forearm flap in the management of soft-tissue injuries of the hand. *British Journal of Plastic Surgery* 37:18–26, 1984.
8. Sundine M, Scheker LR. A comparison of immediate and staged reconstruction of the dorsum of the hand. *J Hand Surg* 21B:216–221, 1996.
9. Timmons MJ, Missotten FE, Poole MD, et al. Complications of radial forearm flap donor sites. *British Journal of Plastic Surgery* 39:176–178, 1986.

27

Ray Amputation With and Without Digital Transposition

Peter J.L. Jebson and Dean S. Louis

INDICATIONS/CONTRAINDICATIONS

Ablation of all digital elements at or just distal to the carpometacarpal joint of the digital ray (ray amputation) is not a commonly performed procedure. However, when performed correctly it can dramatically improve hand function and cosmesis. In general, a ray amputation is most commonly indicated following a traumatic injury such as a ring-avulsion injury in which all the skin, tendons, and neurovascular structures have been avulsed. It may also be performed following a partial digit amputation or replantation where the residual digit is essentially functionless and is stiff and/or insensate. Ray resection may also be performed as part of the salvage of a malignant tumor of the digit or hand, such as the resection of an epithelioid sarcoma or malignant fibrous histiocytoma.

Ray amputation may also be indicated in the patient with a gangrenous digit secondary to profound occlusive vascular disease. A relative contraindication to ray amputation exists when an alternative procedure could preserve better function.

PREOPERATIVE PLANNING

The preoperative evaluation of the patient who is going to undergo a ray resection includes the standard clinical history and physical examination supplemented with appropriate imaging techniques. For the majority of patients, plain radiographs are sufficient. If a ray resection is being performed for excision of a malignant tumor, the magnetic resonance (MRI) and/or CT scan images should be carefully studied to help guide incision placement and surgical dissection to ensure negative residual tumor margins. The patient should be counseled preoperatively with respect to the anticipated appearance of the hand. Showing photographs of other patients who have had a ray resection is particularly helpful. Although

Peter J. L. Jebson, M.D., Department of Orthopaedic Surgery, University of Michigan Medical Center, Ann Arbor, MI

Dean S. Louis, M.D.: Department of Orthopaedic Surgery, University of Michigan Medical Center, Ann Arbor, MI

most ray resections are performed electively, the specific timing of the procedure is largely related to the condition for which it is being performed. In the case of a malignant tumor, for example, the procedure should be carried out as soon as possible. If a transposition is going to be performed in conjunction with an osteotomy and skeletal fixation, the absence of any metal allergy must be confirmed.

SURGERY

The patient is positioned supine on the operating room table with the arm extended over a hand-surgery table. For most ray amputations, it is preferable for the surgeon to be sitting on the side of the table above the shoulder. This permits the surgeon to view the dorsum of the hand, where most of the major dissection is performed. The anesthetic technique used is somewhat dependent on the clinical condition for which the amputation is being performed. Tumors and infections are considered a contraindication to exsanguination with an Esmarch bandage; therefore, intravenous regional anesthesia cannot be used in these circumstances. An axillary block or general anesthesia is used in most patients. The final decision is made jointly by the patient, surgeon, and anesthesiologist. A bloodless field is ideal, and a pneumatic tourniquet is always used. If compressive exsanguination cannot be used, the tourniquet is inflated following five minutes of gravity exsanguination. Loupe magnification is also preferred.

In any ray resection, the surgical steps are replicable from digit to digit:

1. Skin incision and subcutaneous division
2. Incision of the extensor tendon
3. Subperiosteal stripping of the metacarpal
4. Carpometacarpal disarticulation or metacarpal osteotomy
5. Release of the intrinsic muscles
6. Correct identification and division of the neurovascular structures
7. Division of the deep intermetacarpal ligaments
8. Division of the flexor tendons
9. Release of all remaining fascial structures
10. Ray removal
11. Positioning of nerve ends
12. Transposition or approximation of adjacent remaining rays
13. Skin-flap contouring and closure
14. Application of dressings

A racket-shaped incision is drawn around the digit to be amputated (Fig. 27.1). If possible, a commissure on one side or the other of the digit to be amputated may be preserved and then used to recreate a new commissure at the time of wound closure. The skin incision should be placed to leave more skin with the remaining part of the hand, which can then be shaped at the time of final closure. The racket incision is extended proximally directly over the metacarpal shaft. The incision may need to be carefully modified in the patient with a malignant tumor to permit complete tumor excision and negative residual tumor margins. Hemostasis is obtained with electrocautery. The extensor tendon(s) to the amputated ray is divided proximally at the level of the base of the metacarpal and reflected distally (Fig. 27.2). The junctura tendini are divided such that the extensor tendon can be reflected out to the distal wound margin over the proximal phalanx (Fig. 27.3). The periosteum is incised, and subperiosteal stripping is performed around the base of the metacarpal. The intermetacarpal and carpometacarpal ligaments are incised, permitting distal reflection of the metacarpal. In the case of a ring-finger ray amputation, there are no tendinous attachments to the ring metacarpal, therefore, the entire fourth metacarpal is removed. In the case of the index, long, and small metacarpals, the base of the metacarpal and the insertion sites of the wrist

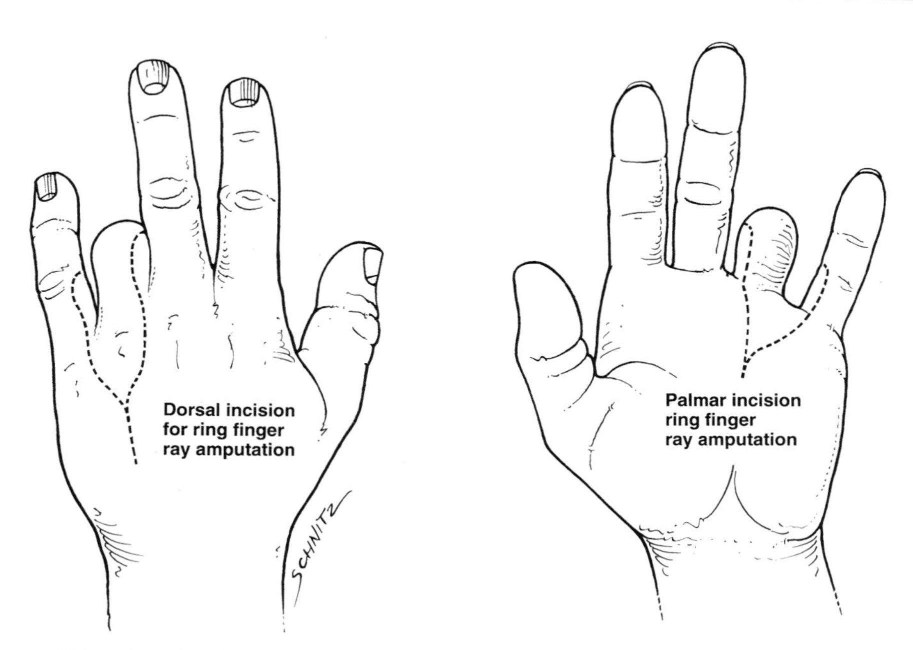

Figure 27.1. A racket incision is made as far distally as possible on the proximal phalanx, which preserves the adjacent commissures to allow reconstruction of the web between the adjacent fingers at the completion of the procedure.

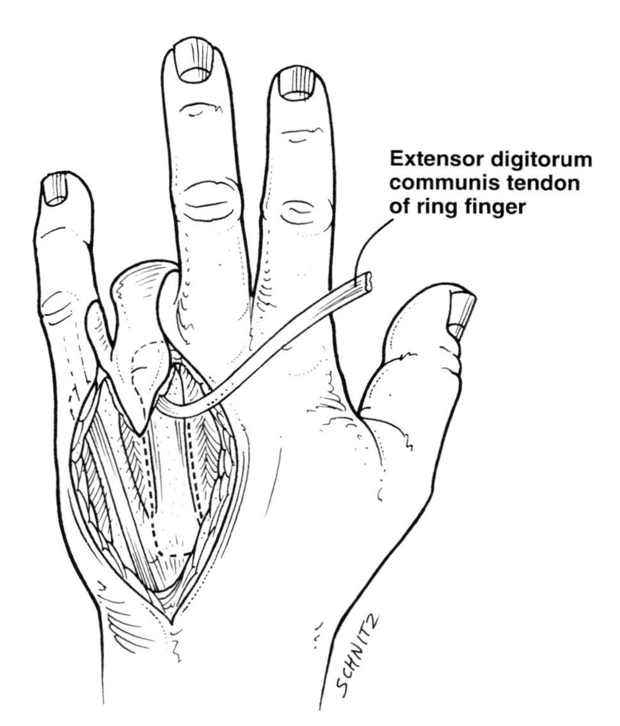

Figure 27.2. The extensor apparatus is reflected distally, and the metacarpal is subperiosteally stripped.

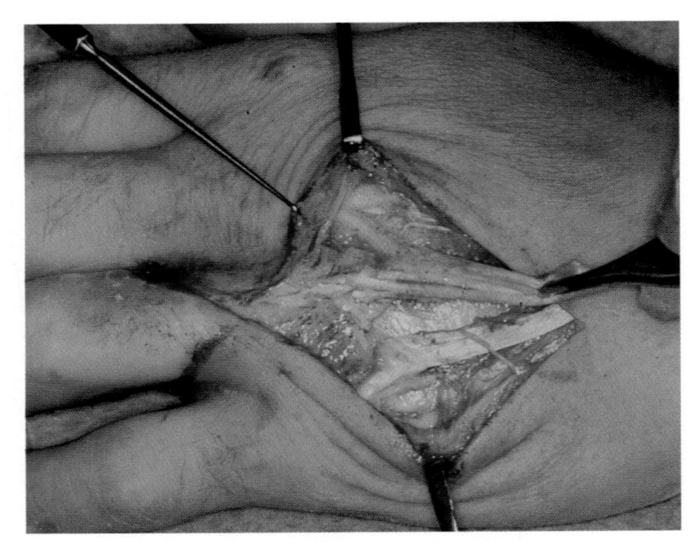

Figure 27.3. The tendinous interconnections between the small, ring, and long fingers are severed, and the proximal aspect of the extensor digitorum communis tendon to the ring finger is divided and reflected distally.

extensors can be preserved by osteotomizing the base of the metacarpal just distal to their insertion. A power saw is preferred to complete the osteotomy. Alternatively, the tendinous insertion may be released and the tendon transferred and reattached to the carpus more proximally. Once the metacarpal is reflected, the dorsal and volar interossous tendons and radial sided lumbrical tendons are transected. The deep intermetacarpal ligaments are then exposed and released from the volar plate. The forearm is supinated, and the volar portion of the hand incision is completed (Fig. 27.4). The neurovascular structures are carefully identified. The digital nerves are divided as far distally as possible through this wound, and they are ligated with absorbable suture and preserved for later positioning. The digital arteries are cauterized. The flexor tendons are retracted distally and sharply divided as far proximally as possible, permitting them

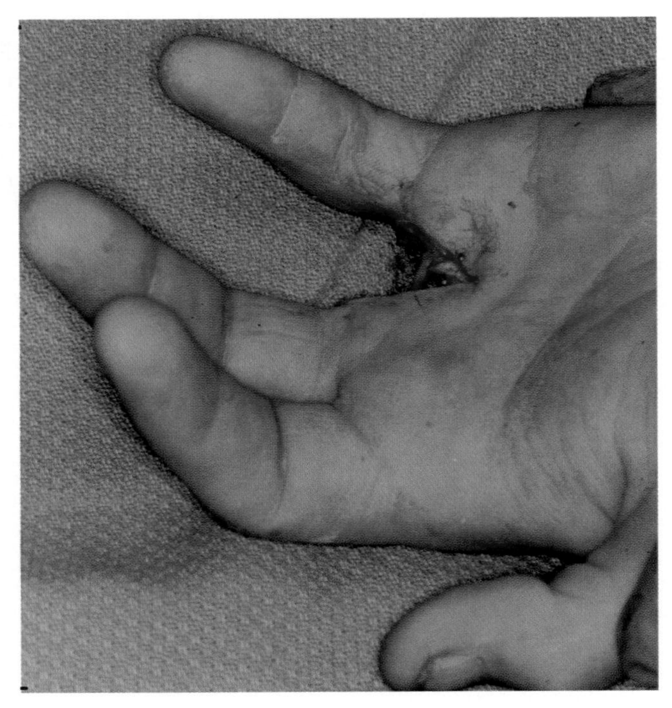

Figure 27.4. On the volar surface, the skin is likewise fashioned.

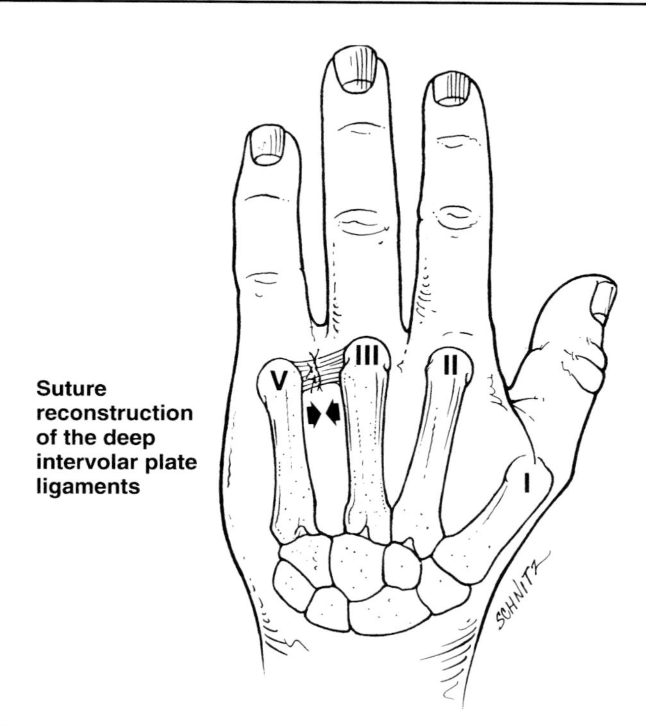

Figure 27.5. The deep intermetacarpal ligaments are approximated. The skin of the commissure is carefully fashioned to create the new web between the adjacent fingers.

to retract proximally. The remaining attachments of the palmar fascia are released from the metacarpal shaft. The ray to be deleted is then delivered. The tourniquet is released and hemostasis obtained. The residual digital nerve ends are then transposed into the intersosseous space vacated by the metacarpal, and the periosteal sleeve is closed around them in an attempt to prevent symptomatic neuroma formation. If approximation of the remaining metacarpal shafts is selected, the deep intermetacarpal ligaments are approximated and sutured together with nonabsorbable suture to draw the metacarpals together (Figs. 27.5 and 27.6). The use of transmetacarpal pinning to se-

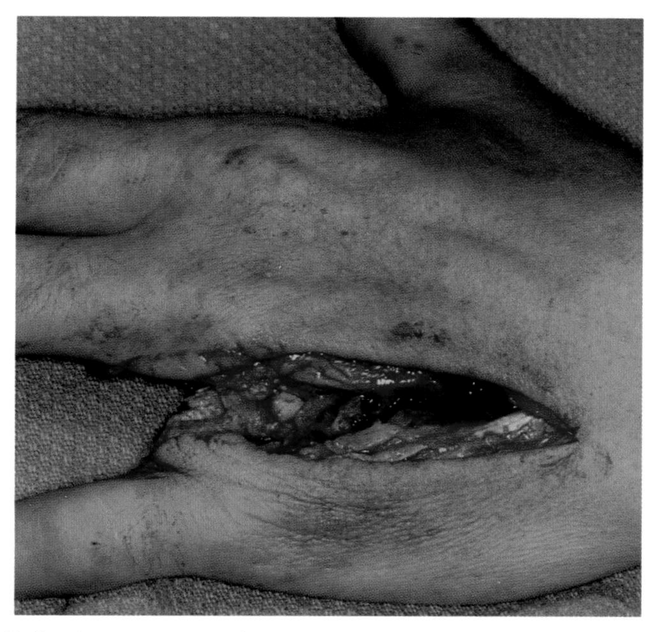

Figure 27.6. Following removal of the ray, the deep intermetacarpal ligaments are approximated.

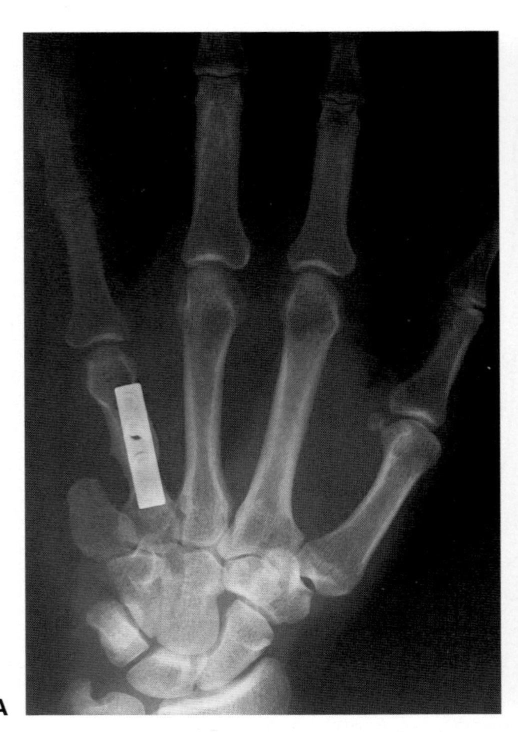

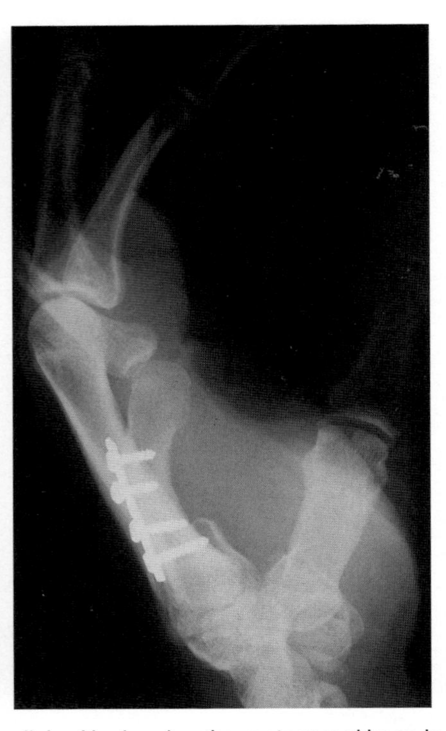

Figure 27.7. A: Ray transposition may be accomplished by leaving the metacarpal base intact with the tendinous insertion and transferring an osteotomized adjacent ray. In this patient the base of the ring metacarpal was preserved following ray resection. The small finger metacarpal was osteotomized and transferred to the ring metacarpal. Fixation was achieved with plate and screw fixation. This technique is technically demanding and if not performed correctly can result in significant problems. **B:** This is the lateral view of the patient seen in the subsequent angular malunion and shortening resulted in a prominent metacarpal head within the palm, pain with gripping, and hyperextension at the metacarpophalangeal joint.

cure the desired position depends upon the preference of the surgeon. If ray transposition is preferred, the technique used is dependent upon which particular ray has been amputated. In the case of a ring-finger ray amputation, the small metacarpal may be transposed radialward. There are two alternative methods to achieve this: The first is to release the fifth carpometacarpal joint and preserve the insertion of the extensor carpi ulnaris (ECU) during transposition of the entire small metacarpal. This necessitates "seating" and stabilizing the small finger metacarpal base upon the radial articular facet of the hamate and the ulnar articular facet of the capitate. This is often difficult because of the variable nonreciprocating anatomy of these articulations. The alternative technique involves an osteotomy of the ring metacarpal just distal to the metacarpal flare, and a similar osteotomy of the small metacarpal distal to the ECU insertion with transposition of the remaining small metacarpal shaft onto the ring metacarpal base (Fig. 27.7). This technique requires skeletal fixation with plates and screws, interosseous wires, or crossed Kirschner wires. With either method of transposition it is essential that digital rotation and angulation be carefully checked to avoid iatrogenic scissoring or divergence (Fig. 27.8). The wound is copiously irrigated with saline prior to closure (Figs. 27.9 and 27.10). A nonadherent dressing, such as Vaseline gauze, is placed over the incisions, and a bulky, soft dressing is applied, incorporating a volar plaster splint.

Long-Finger Ray Amputation

Amputation of the long- or ring-finger ray will leave a space in the hand if specific measures are not taken to approximate the remaining rays, that is, the index and ring in the case of a long-finger ray amputation, and the small and long in the case of a ring-finger ray am-

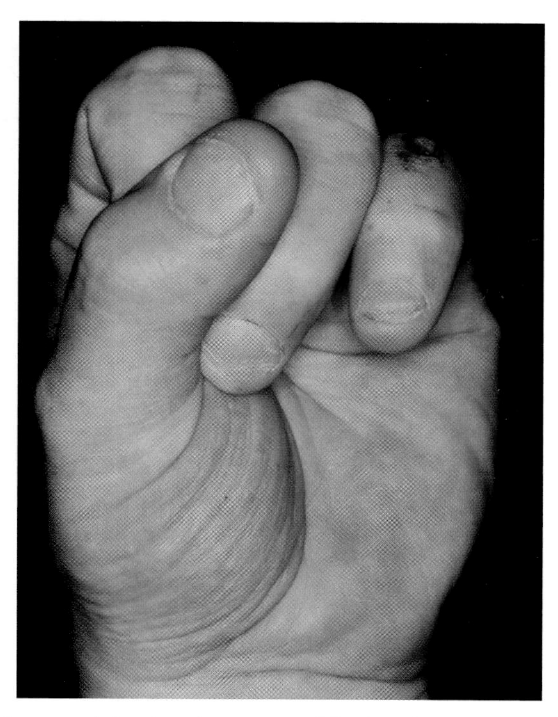

Figure 27.8. Full closure of the hand was possible despite malrotation between the long and small fingers.

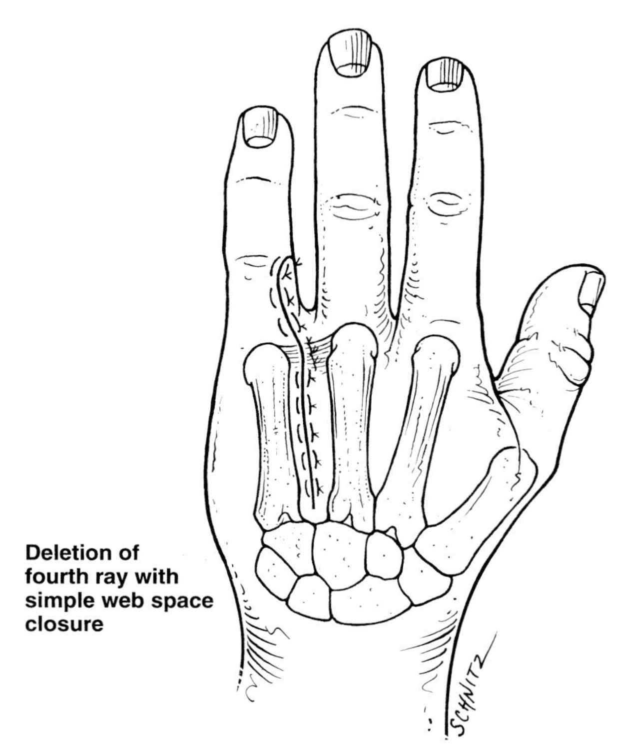

Figure 27.9. The skin is closed on both the dorsal and volar surfaces after appropriate contouring.

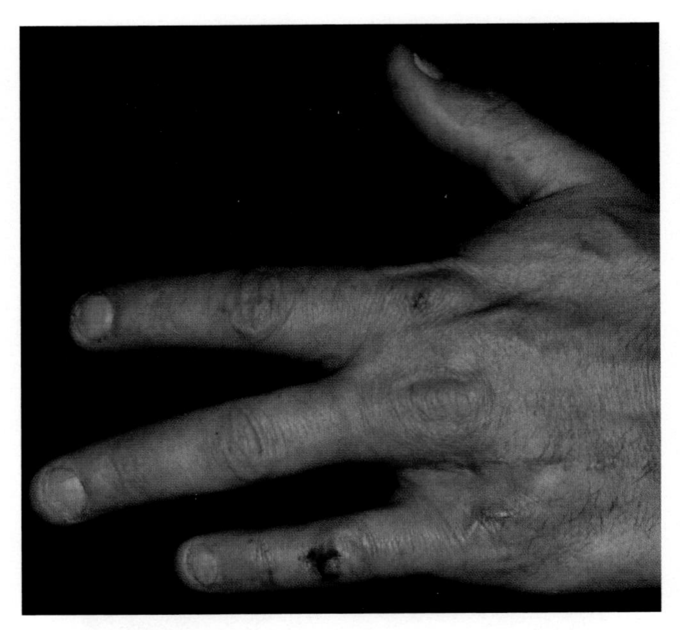

Figure 27.10. Five-and-a-half months following a ring-ray amputation, the web between the small and long fingers has been appropriately fashioned by intermetacarpal ligament reapproximation and closure.

putation. The techniques that have proven most satisfactory have been the transfer of a border digit, that is, the index or the small finger, to the base of the remaining ray that has been amputated. The transposed metacarpal is secured following an osteotomy with pins, bone pegs, or a plate and screws. Alternatively, the intermetacarpal ligaments may be imbricated to each other to approximate the adjacent rays and close the space distally.

The technique for a ring- or long-finger ray amputation is identical (Figs. 27.10–27.17), except that when amputating the long-finger ray, the second and third dorsal interosseous, lumbrical, and intrinsic muscles are released. In addition, if intermetacarpal ligament approximation is selected, the base of the long-finger metacarpal is usually not removed com-

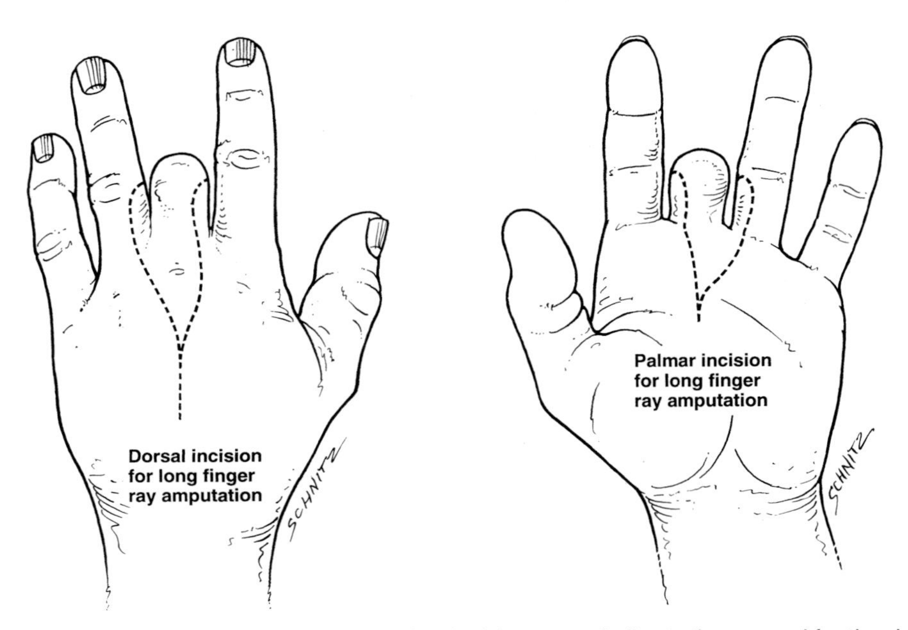

Figure 27.11. The dorsal and palmar racket incisions are similar to those used for the ring-finger amputation.

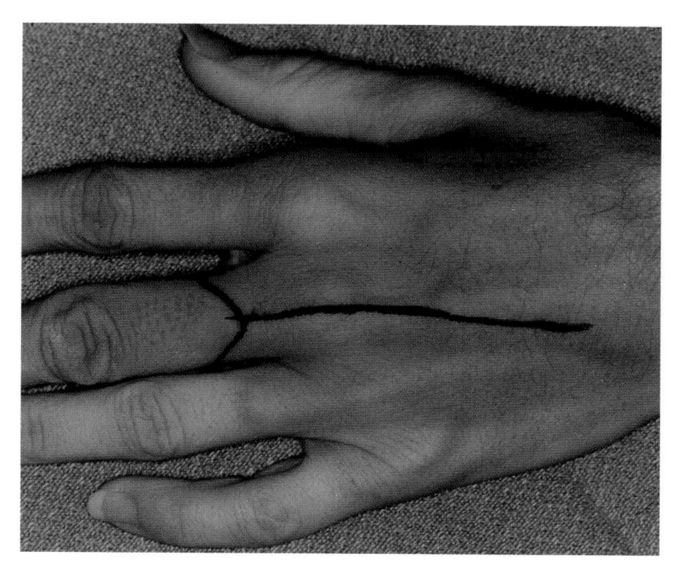

Figure 27.12. This patient has digital ischemia of the nondominant left long finger secondary to a vascular malformation. While the dorsal-racket incision is similar to what has been depicted in the preceding illustrations, the volar extent of the incision was greater.

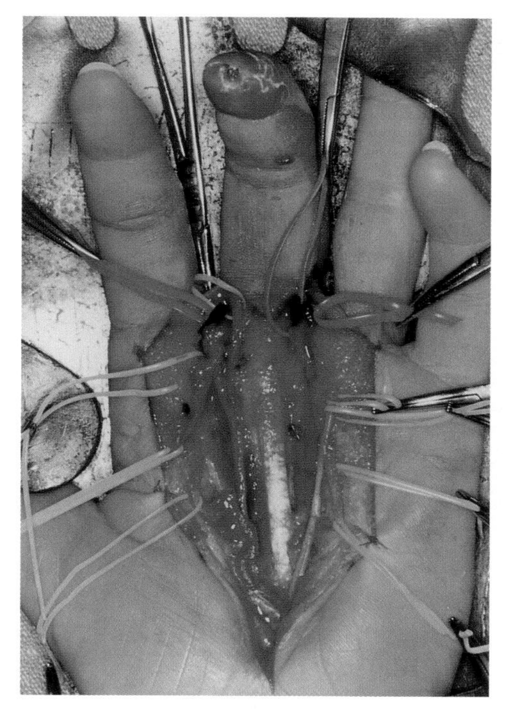

Figure 27.13. The neurovascular structures have been carefully identified, individually retracted, and the flexor tendon apparatus exposed.

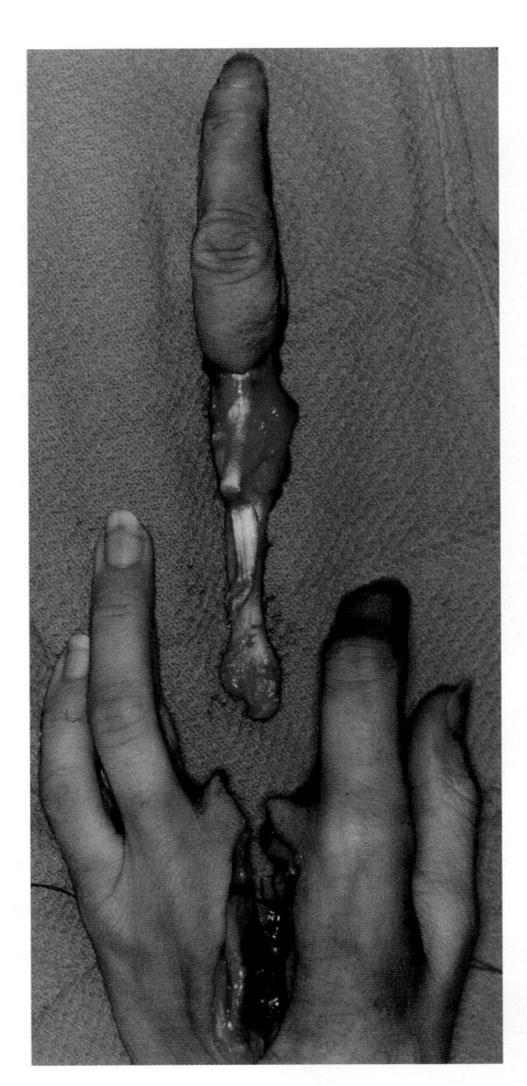

Figure 27.14. The ray has been deleted completely at the base in this situation. The extensor carpi radialis brevis (ECRB) tendon was transferred to a new insertion on the carpus.

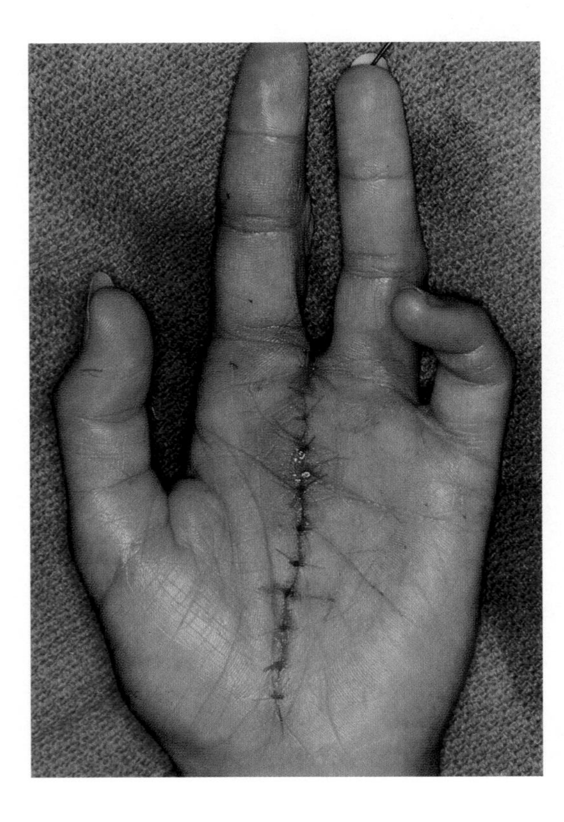

Figure 27.15. The commissures have been approximated, thus preserving a semblance of the normal web.

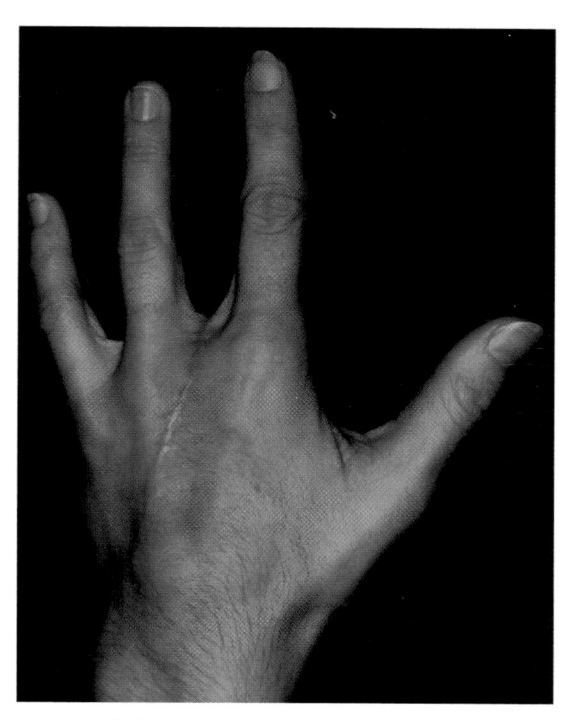

Figure 27.16. Six months following the procedure, the dorsal commissure is nicely preserved, with a satisfactory cosmetic appearance.

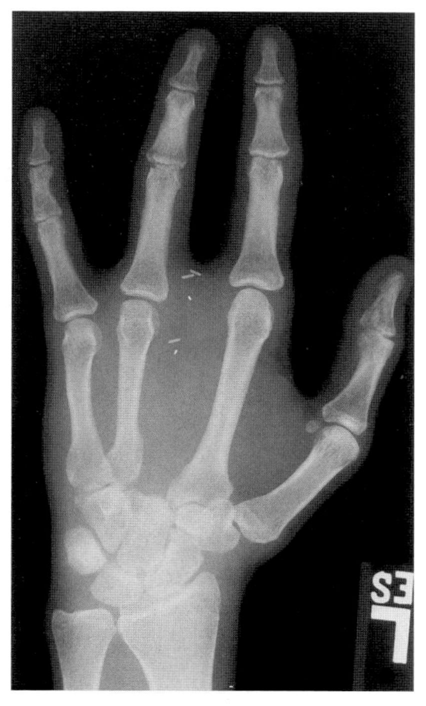

Figure 27.17. The radiographic appearance of the hand in Figure 27.16. The third metacarpal was completely ablated, with distal approximation of the deep intermetacarpal ligaments.

pletely because of the attachment of the extensor carpi radialis brevis (ECRB). The metacarpal base may be osteotomized as previously discussed, or the tendon transferred to the carpus and reinserted (Fig. 27.14). If ray transposition is chosen, the index ray is osteotomized at its metaphyseal flare distal to the insertion of the extensor carpi radialis longus (ECRL) and transposed and secured onto the long metacarpal base.

POSTOPERATIVE MANAGEMENT

The operated extremity is elevated continuously for a minimum of 48–72 hours postoperatively and as much as necessary during the first postoperative week. Active and passive flexion and extension of the digits is initiated immediately. Adequate analgesia is essential. Sutures are removed 10–14 days postoperatively, and a home program of scar massage and desensitization is encouraged. If swelling is pronounced, a compressive glove is provided. A supportive forearm orthosis is used until sufficient soft tissue and osseous union has occurred. When closure of the central defect is accomplished by approximation of the intermetacarpal ligaments, external support is used for 4 to 6 weeks. When ray transposition is carried out, protection is maintained for at least two months and occasionally longer if clinical and radiographic evidence of osseous union is not present. If transmetacarpal pinning was used following transposition, the wires are removed no earlier than 8 weeks postoperatively. Following discontinuation of splinting, a strengthening and work hardening program is utilized to optimize the final functional outcome. In general, full activity can be expected 3 months postoperatively.

RESULTS

Ray amputation is usually a very gratifying operation. Patients are typically subjectively satisfied with the improvement in function, and are pleasantly surprised at the cosmetic appearance and social acceptance (Figure 27.18). The majority of patients return to their preinjury occupation. The patients usually adjust well to their new functional pattern, and

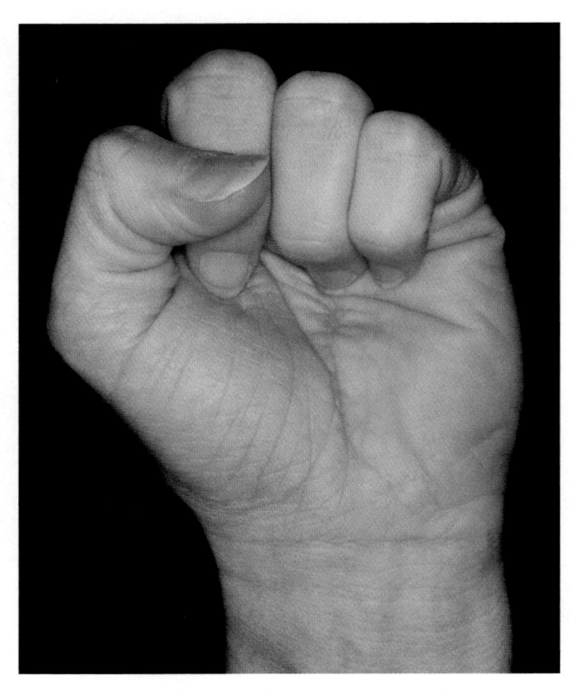

Figure 27.18. Full grasp was achieved.

eventually most achieve grip strength of approximately 70% of the opposite extremity, although a diminution in digital dexterity is the norm. Some of our patients have experienced difficulties, such as post-traumatic stress, depression, and sleep disorders, in adjusting to the loss of a finger prior to the ray amputation. These patients need to be carefully counseled preoperatively, and some have required the assistance of a psychologist or psychiatrist. We have found that of those patients who are unsatisfied or do not do well following ray amputation, the majority are involved in non-settled litigation or worker's compensation claims. However, we still offer the procedure in such patients. We prefer to leave the insertions of the ECRB, ECRL, and ECU intact on the osteotomized metacarpal base, and we avoid transposition with skeletal fixation if possible because of the technical challenges and risk of nonunion and malunion.

COMPLICATIONS

Aside from the general operative complications of infection and wound dehiscence, a few specific complications may develop following ray amputation.

Nonunion

If digital ray transposition is performed in conjunction with a metacarpal osteotomy, a nonunion is always a possibility. The risk of a nonunion is higher in those patients who are smokers. Such patients are discouraged from smoking for the 6 weeks prior to surgery and for 3 months postoperatively. A nonunion may also occur if a fixation technique is utilized but lacks rigid stabilization. We prefer compression plate and screw fixation to minimize the possibility of nonunion. Supplementing the osteotomy site with autogenous cancellous bone graft from the amputated ray or from a local site, such as the distal radius, may stimulate bony union and prevent a nonunion from developing. If an established nonunion occurs, the nonunion site must be taken down and reconstructed with bone grafting and plate fixation. The presence of infection should always be ruled out in the patient with a nonunion.

Malunion

Malunion following ray transposition may result in an angular or rotational deformity, particularly if digital rotation was not carefully assessed intraoperatively. The functional consequence of a rotational malunion is digital scissoring or divergence (Fig. 27.8). Following temporary skeletal fixation, passive motion of the fingers should be assessed and normal rotation confirmed prior to definitive skeletal fixation. An angular malunion affects metacarpophalangeal (MP) joint motion. If a malunion compromises hand function, it should be taken down and realigned appropriately.

Postoperative Stiffness

Postoperative stiffness may occur if the patient is not encouraged to move the fingers or if the patient fails to move them. Stiffness can be avoided with good edema control and the early initiation of range-of-motion exercises. The assistance of a hand therapist can be particularly helpful.

Neuroma Formation

Occasionally, a symptomatic neuroma may occur even when great care has been taken to transfer the digital nerve end into the interosseous space and when the dorsal cutaneous branches of the ulnar or radial nerves become entrapped in scar. Exploring the hand and translocating the neuroma to a protected noncontact area without transection of the nerve is the most appropriate management.

Skin Problems

Wound problems may occur if too much skin is inadvertently excised, if the web space is closed too tight, or when too much skin is left, resulting in an overly wide space between the adjacent approximated digits. Thus, the skin incisions and fashioning of the web should be performed carefully and meticulously adjusted at the time of the original amputation. If too much skin was removed, a secondary procedure with additional skin grafting will be necessary to remove the cutaneous tether. If too little skin was removed, a secondary procedure to close the web must be performed.

Flexor and Extensor Tendon Adherence

If early range of motion is not initiated, the flexor and/or extensor tendons may become adherent, potentially resulting in a loss of motion in the adjacent fingers. If the problem is correctly identified early in the postoperative course, careful passive manipulation under regional anesthesia may be effective in breaking up any early adhesions. If it becomes evident later, surgical tenolysis may be necessary.

RECOMMENDED READING

1. Carroll RE. Transposition of the index finger to replace the middle finger. *Clin Orthop* 15:27–34, 1959.
2. Carroll RE. The level of amputation in the third finger. *Am. J Surg* 97:477–483, 1959.
3. Colen L, Bunkis J, Gordon L, et al. Functional assessment of ray transfer for central digital loss. *J Hand Surg* 10A:232–237, 1985.
4. Hanel DP, Lederman ES. Index transposition after resection of the long finger ray. *J Hand Surg* 18A: 271–277, 1993.
5. Hyroop GL. Transfer of a metacarpal, with or without its digit, for improving the function of the crippled hand. *Plast Reconstr Surg* 4:45–58, 1949.
6. Iselin F, Peze W. Ray centralization without bone fixation for amputation of the middle finger. *J Hand Surg* 13B:97–99, 1988.
7. Louis DS, Jebson PJL, Graham TJ. Amputations. In: Green DP, ed. *Operative Hand Surgery*, 4th ed. New York: Churchill-Livingstone, 1998.
8. Peacock EE. Metacarpal transfer following amputation of a central digit. *Plast Reconstr Surg* 29:345–355, 1962.
9. Peimer CE, Wheeler DR, Barrett A, et al. Hand function following single ray amputation. *J Hand Surg* 24A:1245–1248, 1999.
10. Plasschaert MJJT, Hage JJ. A web-saving incision for the amputation of the third or fourth ray of the hand. *J Hand Surg* 13B:340–341, 1988.
11. Posner MA. Ray transposition for central digital loss. *J Hand Surg* 4:242–257, 1979.
12. Steichen JB, Idler RS. Results of central ray resection without bony transposition. *J Hand Surg* 11A: 466–474, 1986.

28

Reconstruction of the Partially Amputated Thumb with Metacarpal Lengthening

Todd M. Guyette and Thomas J. Graham

INDICATIONS/CONTRAINDICATIONS

The thumb provides a stable pinch post for dexterous activity and a radial bracket for cylindrical grasp. Because of the thumb's pivotal role in hand function, it is critical that thumb trauma and post-traumatic sequelae be approached with a full portfolio of treatment alternatives. The reconstructive ladder of surgical options incorporates increasingly complex concepts of skeletal handling, soft-tissue management, and microsurgical techniques.

The options for the partially amputated thumb, including phalangealization, pollicization, osteoplastic reconstruction, free-tissue transfer, and metacarpal lengthening, are intellectually and technically challenging. The reconstructive algorithm incorporates the level of the amputation, adequacy of the soft-tissue envelope, the functional capacity of the remaining digits, and the patient's vocational and avocational requirements. One of the most attractive tools in the reconstructive armamentarium is metacarpal lengthening and web-space deepening.

Although applicable to thumb amputations at any level, metacarpal lengthening is best indicated for amputations at or near the metacarpophalangeal (MCP) joint (Fig. 28.1). At least two-thirds of the metacarpal should be present. Additionally, there must be a generous and compliant soft-tissue envelope with sensibility to accommodate the lengthening process. If necessary, this requirement can be met with local or distant flaps at the time of osteotomy or in a staged fashion.

Todd M. Guyette, M.D.: The Curtis National Hand Center, Union Memorial Hospital, Baltimore, MD

Thomas J. Graham, M.D.: Department of Orthopaedic Surgury, The Curtis National Hand Center, Union Memorial Hospital, Baltimore, MD, and Departments of Orthopaedics and Plastic Surgery, Johns Hopkins University Hospital, Baltimore, MD

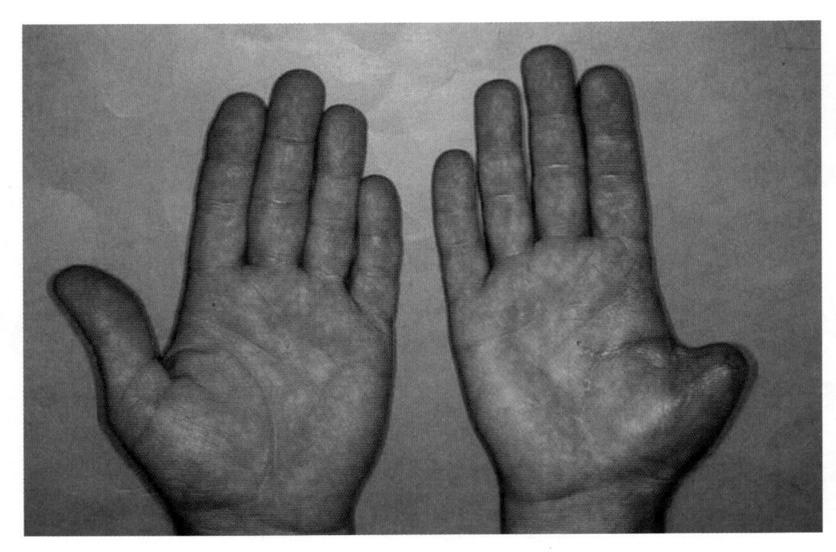

Figure 28.1. Preoperative clinical exam noting status of soft-tissue envelope.

Furthermore, for metacarpal lengthening to increase the hand breadth for grasp, the first web space must be adequate. Z-plasty with or without skin grafting should accompany the course of thumb metacarpal lengthening.

Lengthening of up to 3.0–3.5 cm has been routinely attained, with a maximum length of 4.0 cm as a clinical reality. This can be reliably achieved without associated neurovascular complications. Thumb metacarpal lengthening does not increase mobility, sensibility, or stability, yet functional improvements resulting from lengthening can be satisfying.

Matching the patient's individual needs and the soft-tissue envelope with the surgeon's skill and experience typically directs the reconstructive ladder. Metacarpal lengthening remains one of the most attractive nonmicrosurgical alternatives.

PREOPERATIVE PLANNING

Beyond assessment of thumb length, a comprehensive examination of the hand is performed to evaluate the current status and potential impact of lengthening. This includes examination of the soft tissue overlying the thumb stump, the suppleness of the first web space, and the stability of the carpometacarpal joint.

Plain radiographs assist in evaluating the status of the carpometacarpal articulation and the length of metacarpal available for lengthening. Presence of a proximal phalanx remnant should be noted and taken into surgical consideration because the potential of progressive interphalangeal contracture during lengthening.

There are several commercial metacarpal distraction devices available; common to them is the application of threaded or smooth pins proximal and distal to the osteotomy site with a distraction gear mechanism. The gear is usually turned by hand or screwdriver with a complete revolution distracting approximately 1 mm. The surgical principles for application of the fixator remain the same regardless of model.

In addition to the required understanding of the risks and benefits of any surgical reconstruction, the patient must become familiar with the operation of the device that he or she will be adjusting during the distraction phase. We have found it most useful to engage the patient as an active participant in his or her own care by introducing the device long before the initial surgery. Furthermore, this early education may identify a patient who is intellectually or technically incapable of participating in this somewhat demanding surgical exercise.

SURGERY

Thumb metacarpal lengthening is a temporally protracted, methodical process that is best approached as three separate stages.

Stage One: Frame Application and Corticotomy

The goal of the first stage is to apply the frame and ensure complete bone separation through which the eventual distraction will be completed. Although this seems to be the least technically demanding of the stages, meticulous tissue-handling, exact placement of hardware, and seemingly simple checks of thoroughness cannot be overemphasized. If mistakes or suboptimal performance of steps is perpetrated at the outset, the entire process is doomed to failure or suboptimal result.

The procedure is performed with the extremity abducted on a hand table. It can be done under general or regional anesthesia, after exsanguination and application of a brachial tourniquet. The first step is to apply the frame to the metacarpal, minimizing soft tissue dissection while accomplishing the mechanical and surgical objectives of the surgery.

The authors advocate the use of four threaded 2.5-mm pins to secure the frame. These pins are applied through small stab incisions at the glabrous border of the thenar eminence. The optimal locations of pins can be thought of in three dimensions; they should be perpendicular to the long axis of the metacarpal, transverse through the midaxis of the bone, and reside in the proximal and distal metaphyses (Fig. 28.2). Each set of two pins, proximal and distal, should be placed as close to parallel as possible.

Obviously, the frame should be applied with the greatest capability for expansion. Only intimate familiarity with the device will ensure that the surgeon does not make these fundamental errors. Applying the frame with an abbreviated distraction capability will necessitate later reapplication and introduce numerous potential problems.

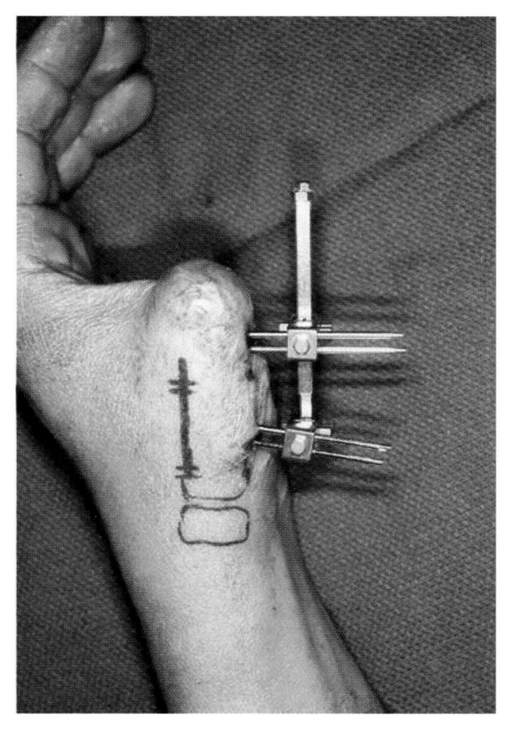

Figure 28.2. External fixator pins are applied through standard incisions at the glabrous border into the proximal and distal metacarpal metaphyses.

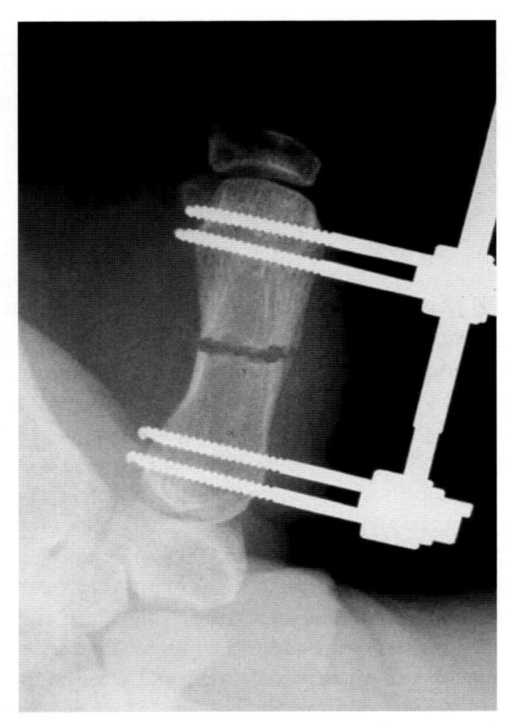

Figure 28.3. A radiograph demonstrating complete corticotomy prior to initial distraction.

A dorsal incision is then made over the thumb metacarpal at its midshaft. The extensors are retracted, or interval between them incised, while care is taken to avoid soft-tissue and periosteal disruption around the eventual corticotomy/osteotomy site.

A 0.045- or 0.062-inch smooth wire is used to create multiple transverse and oblique perforations around the minimallyexposed midshaft osteotomy site (Fig. 28.3). A small, straight osteotome then completes the cortical disruption. This "low energy" corticotomy method is necessary to minimize soft-tissue and vascular damage at the osteotomy site.

The frame is then distracted to confirm that circumferential corticotomy has been achieved. The osteotomy site is then again closed down via the frame so that the amount of initial separation is roughly 1 to 2 mm. The wound is closed per routine. Relaxing incisions are made around the metacarpal pins if there is skin tension.

When a proximal phalanx remnant is present, a 0.62-inch K-wire can be placed axially across the extended MCP joint to avoid progressive flexion during lengthening from soft-tissue tethering and myodesis. Infrequently, we have performed a formal flexor tenotomy or even removal of a small phalangeal remnant that compromises the overlying skin.

Recent investigations have suggested that proximal metaphyseal osteotomies have shorter ossification times, but in our experience mid-diaphyseal osteotomies heal reliably with bone grafting, a must in the adult. Thus, for ease and stability of pin placement, we use a mid-diaphyseal corticotomy.

A volar thumb spica splint or bulky dressing is applied for patient comfort until lengthening is begun, approximately postoperative day five.

Stage Two: Distraction

Dynamic lengthening commences postoperative day five. Lengthening is started at 0.5–1.0 mm a day, equally divided into four sessions. In our experience, lengthening of greater than 1.5 mm a day is associated with increased patient discomfort and higher pseudoarthrosis rates. Pin care is initiated with half-strength hydrogen peroxide twice daily, and skin sutures are removed as per routine at 10 to 14 days. Radiographs are obtained at weekly intervals to inspect the distraction, potential angulation, and evaluate osteogenesis at the osteotomy site. Distraction is continued for 25 to 40 days, or until the desired length is achieved or further distraction is technically impossible.

Stage Three: Thumb Web Z-plasty and Bone Grafting

Metacarpal lengthening of 2.5 to 3.0 cm can usually be obtained without complication, although several authors have arbitrarily established 4 cm as the maximum amount (Fig. 28.4). In patients younger than 15 years old, the gap undergoes intramembranous ossification rapidly within two to three months and may not require grafting. For patients older than 15, the time to ossification can be longer than three months and, therefore, the authors recommend immediate intercalary grafting with corticocancellous iliac crest graft in essentially all adult patients. Admittedly, the authors' experience with this procedure is almost completely limited to the skeletally mature, so bone grafting at a second-stage operation is the rule rather than the exception. It is tempting, however, to await the ossification of what appears to be regenerate callus in the interval; the authors would suggest against that.

At the time of second-stage bone grafting, one routinely notes the presence of a thick periosteal tube in continuity with the proximal and distal metacarpal fragments. This tube is filled with a xanthochromic fluid that is evacuated through a dorsal longitudinal incision in the tube in preparation of inlaying the graft. This provides an ideal framework in which to pack cancellous graft around a cortical strut.

The corticocancellous graft, usually harvested from the ipsalateral iliac crest, is placed in the void after slight overdistraction of the frame for a final time. The frame is then collapsed to create coaptation and compression at the proximal and distal sites before stabilization.

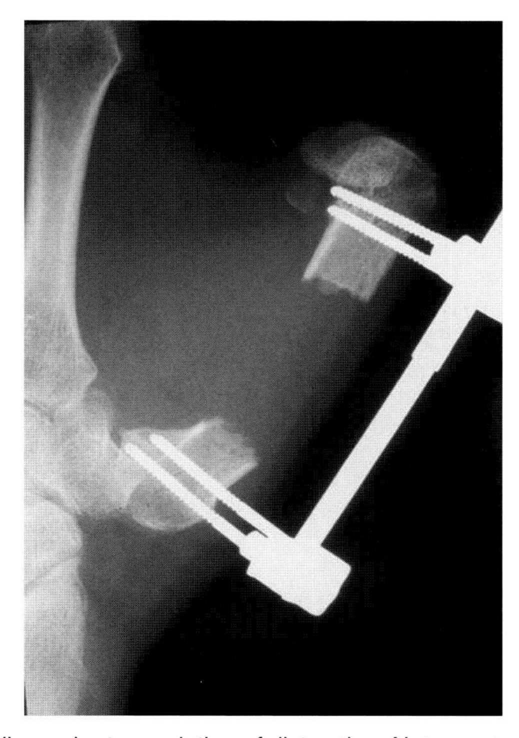

Figure 28.4. AP radiograph at completion of distraction. Note presence of periosteal tube.

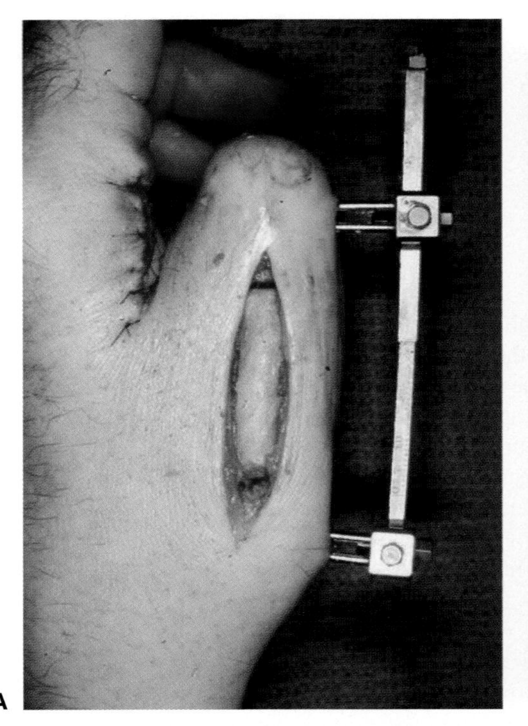
A

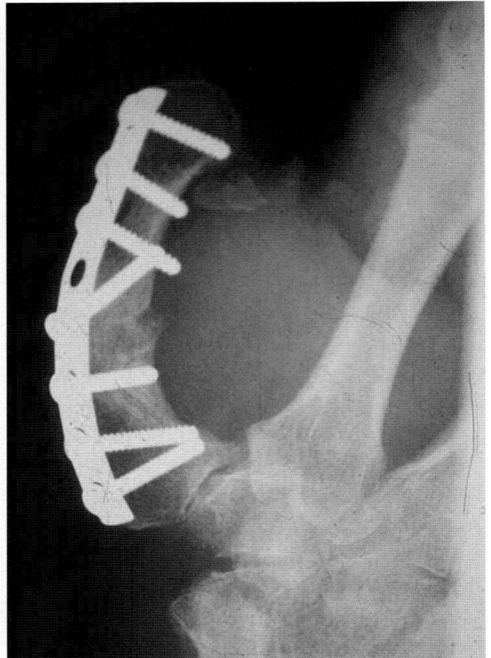
B

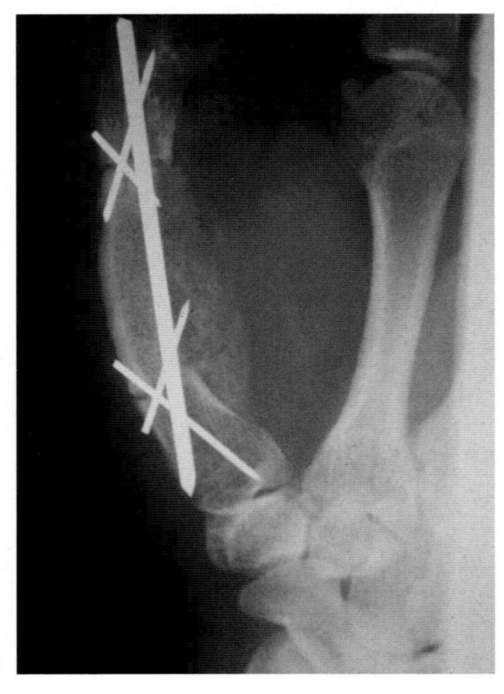
C

Figure 28.5. **A**: Intraoperative photograph demonstrating bone graft insertion prior to initial compression. Radiographs showing fixation of bone graft by plate (**B**) or smooth Kirschner wires (**C**).

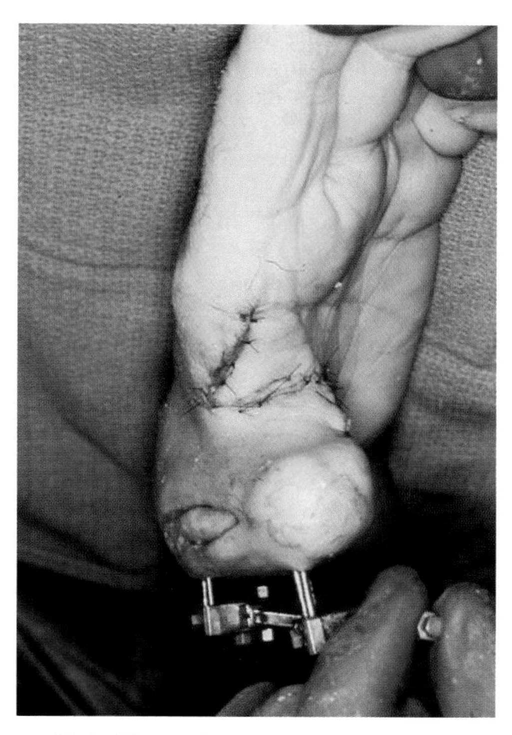

Figure 28.6. First web space deepening via Z-plasty.

Graft stabilization can be performed with K-wires, but rigid fixation with plate and screws allows compression across the graft site with earlier return to active motion (Fig. 28.5).

At the time of bone grafting, we also recommend first-web space deepening via Z-plasty or a dorsal rotational flap to increase the span of the thumb for grasping (Fig. 28.6). Contour is not as important as ultimate depth, so fewer limbs are preferred. Skin grafting is avoided because of additional donor morbidity, contraction, and hyperpigmentation. However, in the multiply operated thumb with inadequate skin coverage, harvest of a full-thickness graft from the same site as the iliac bone harvest is logical.

REHABILITATION

During the lengthening process, the authors do not employ any specific physical therapy protocols, but rather encourage the patient to move the thumb carpometacarpal joint as tolerated. After removal of the external fixator, active range of motion of all joints is encouraged within the limitations of any internal fixation stability. This is coupled with opposition retraining and sensory education of the thumb stump. With radiographic evidence of consolidation, strength training of the hand is initiated.

RESULTS

The patient who has lost any part of the hand, especially the thumb, has many physical and emotional challenges to which the surgeon must be sensitive. Just as important is our own intellectual honesty about what we can deliver.

Chances are that the patient has been introduced to several different options for thumb reconstruction and now has selected the metacarpal lengthening for a personal set of reasons. Our results in over 20 patients in whom this procedure has been performed have demonstrated some consistent observations. Patients are uniformly disappointed with the appearance initially (especially while the initial swelling persists). The other consistent comment has been the patients' observation that they anticipated that the thumb would be longer. That is why careful counseling and objective measurement and documentation are crucial.

What is observed between the second month and the sixth month after the entire process has been completed is an expansion of capabilities that usually mollifies the patient. One of the biggest issues by which the success of this operation will be judged is the circumference of the object that can be controlled in the reconstructed hand. For example, if the patient can stabilize a soda can, he or she will judge the procedure successful. Additionally, finer motor or dexterous activity can be restored (Fig. 28.7).

Be cognizant of the patient's individual vocational and avocational desires before embarking on this reconstructive path and consistently throughout the entire postoperative course–which may be for the rest of your career. Be prepared for the patient's second-guessing, as in saying, "Maybe I should have given up my toe." This will be especially true if you encourage your patients with similar problems to communicate with each other, a policy our group embraces.

Practical considerations in follow-up would be the potential need for hardware removal. We have had two patients with delayed union or nonunion of the graft (one proximal and one distal) that required bone graft to affect eventual healing. We have not experienced distal-wound complications. Creating tension in this scarred skin can certainly invite breakdown; this is combated by careful planning and vigilant observation throughout the lengthening process.

We have also encountered a peculiar phenomenon of uncertain etiology and clinical significance. In about one-quarter of our patients, the trapeziometacarpal joint has tended toward volar-radial subluxation. In two patients, the joint seemed to translate over 50%. The accompanying complaints were not of instability or even discomfort, but motion limitation. This has been observed as early as during the distraction period, but has also been noticed after everyday use of the thumb in pinching and grasping activities has been resumed.

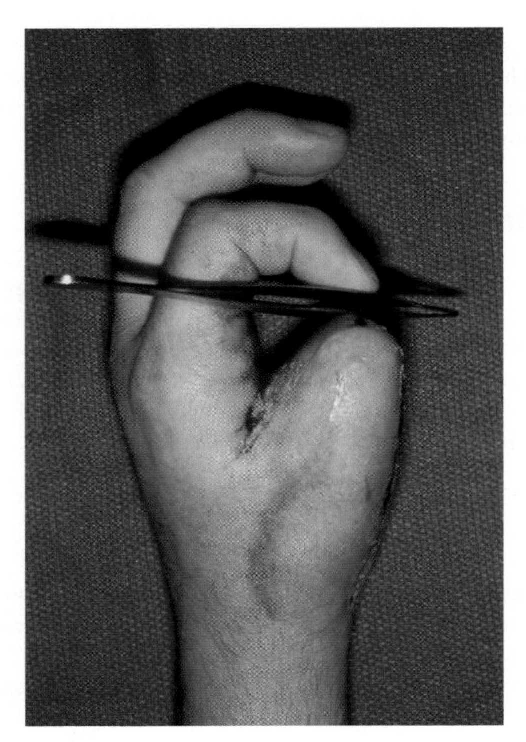

Figure 28.7. Clinical photo after completion of metacarpal lengthening, demonstrating fine-pinch activity.

We have never elected to reconstruct that joint through stabilization or fusion, and have not found a logical explanation of the finding of volar-radial subluxation. Many of our colleagues have held their own cases to scrutiny after this issue was related and have reported similar findings. Future cases or studies may elucidate this point further.

As always, the balance between the magnitudes of surgery and the desired outcome is dynamic. Several factors contribute to the ultimate decision regarding the path of reconstruction taken by the patient with thumb loss.

COMPLICATIONS

The most common complications are pin loosening and infection. Power drilling all pin sites with a sharp drill bit decreases local thermal injury and is less likely to propagate microfractures, both of which have been associated with late loosening. Closure of soft tissue and skin around the pin sites in a tension-free manner also assists in reducing the rate of pin infections.

Nonunions are rare if staged bone grafting is planned for patients older than 15 years of age and/or patients with defects greater than 3.0 cm. It has also been suggested that lengthening rates greater than 1 mm a day increase the risk of pseudoarthrosis, a problem than can be overcome with patient education and close physician follow-up.

There are no problems with vessel thrombosis or nerve traction injury with thumb metacarpal lengthenings reported in the literature. Meticulous surgical technique coupled with close follow-up decreases the risks of most complications and can provide a stable and sensate post to provide opposition and cylindrical grasp.

RECOMMENDED READING

1. Ilizarov GA. Clinical application of the tension-stress effect for limb lengthening. *Clin Orthop* 1990 Jan;(250):8–26. Review.
2. Kessler I, Hecht O, Baruch A. Distraction-lengthening of digital rays in the management of the injured hand. *J Bone Joint Surg Am* 61(1):83–87, 1979.
3. Lister G. The choice of procedure following thumb amputation. *Clin Orthop* 195:45, 1985.
4. Matev IB. Thumb reconstruction after amputation at the metacarpophalangeal joint by bone lengthening: A preliminary report of three cases. *J Bone Joint Surg Am* 52:957–965, 1970.
5. Moy OJ, Peimer CA, Sherwin FS. Reconstruction of traumatic or congenital amputation of the thumb by distraction-lengthening. *Hand Clinics* 8(1):57–62, 1992.
6. Matev I. Thumb reconstruction through metacarpal bone lengthening. *J Hand Surg* 5:482, 1980.
7. Mulliken JB, Curtis RM. Thumb lengthening by metacarpal distraction. *J Trauma* 20(3):250–5, 1980.
8. Toh S, Narita S, Arai K, et al. Distraction lengthening by callotasis in the hand. *J Bone Joint Surg* 84B;2:205–210, 2002.

PART VII

Arthritis, Dupuytren's Disease, and Infections

29

Silicone Metacarpophalangeal Joint Arthroplasty

Jennifer L. M. Manuel and Arnold-Peter C. Weiss

INTRODUCTION

Metacarpophalangeal (MCP) arthroplasty is performed to relieve joint pain, stiffness, and deformity in those joints with articular destruction. This condition arises most commonly in patients with rheumatoid arthritis. However, MCP arthroplasty may also occasionally be of benefit in the treatment of post-traumatic deformity and osteoarthritis.

Patients with rheumatoid arthritis typically present with pain and characteristic deformities (Fig. 29.1). Palmar translation of the proximal phalanx with ulnar subluxation of the extensor tendon results in a flexed attitude of the MCP joint that impairs overall hand function (Fig. 29.2). Ulnar deviation of the digit further impairs function by decreasing the overall power transmitted to the finger by the flexor and extensor tendons.

In the 1960s Swanson developed a silicone-based implant (Wright Medical, Memphis, TN) that contains a nonfixed flexible hinge that functions as a spacer to improve the stability of resection arthroplasty. Advantages in the use of silicone-based implants include a relatively short operative time and predictable function postoperatively. Disadvantages include the inability to obtain a postoperative range of motion similar to that of the normal hand and the possibility of fracture of the implant over time, secondary to the mechanics of the MCP joint and the quality of the material used (Fig. 29.3). Despite these factors, silicone-based implants remain the gold standard for the treatment of those patients with severe degenerative destruction of the joints. Newer designs mimic the normal arc of motion of the MCP joint, decrease the stress through the implant itself, and improve the functional arc of motion postoperatively (Fig. 29.4).

The NeuFlex metacarpophalangeal joint implant (DePuy, Warsaw, IN) has improved on the mechanics at the MCP joint, thereby decreasing the stress on the material itself and improving overall postoperative range of motion. Silicone implants with a 0° prebend lead to

Jennifer L. M. Manuel, M.D.: Department of Orthopaedics, Brown University/Rhode Island Hospital, Providence, RI

Arnold-Peter C. Weiss, M.D.: Department of Orthopaedic Surgery, Brown University, Providence, RI, and Department of Orthopaedics, Rhode Island Hospital, Providence, RI

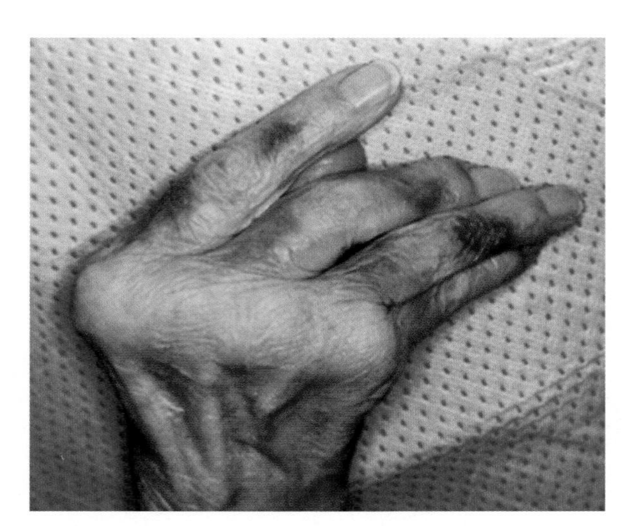

Figure 29.1. A typical-appearing hand of a patient with rheumatoid arthritis. Note the classic lack of full extension of the fingers at the MCP joint and the ulnar deviation.

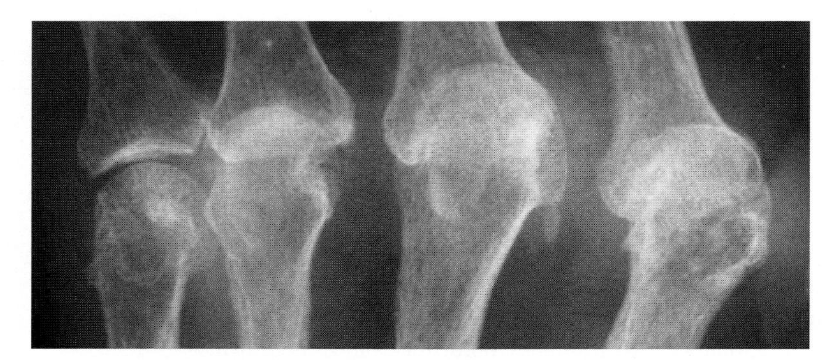

Figure 29.2. Radiographs of the MCP joints of a patient with rheumatoid arthritis demonstrate loss of joint space and some overlap of the metacarpal head on the proximal phalanx, indicating early palmar subluxation of the proximal phalanx. These findings are usually seen in a progressive fashion, with the radial side being worse.

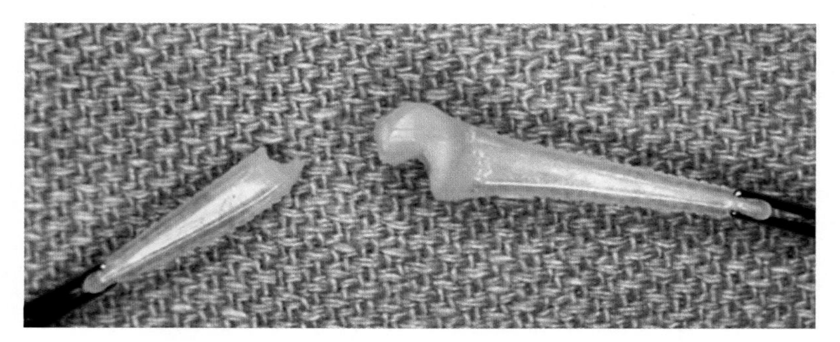

Figure 29.3. An example of a broken Swanson implant.

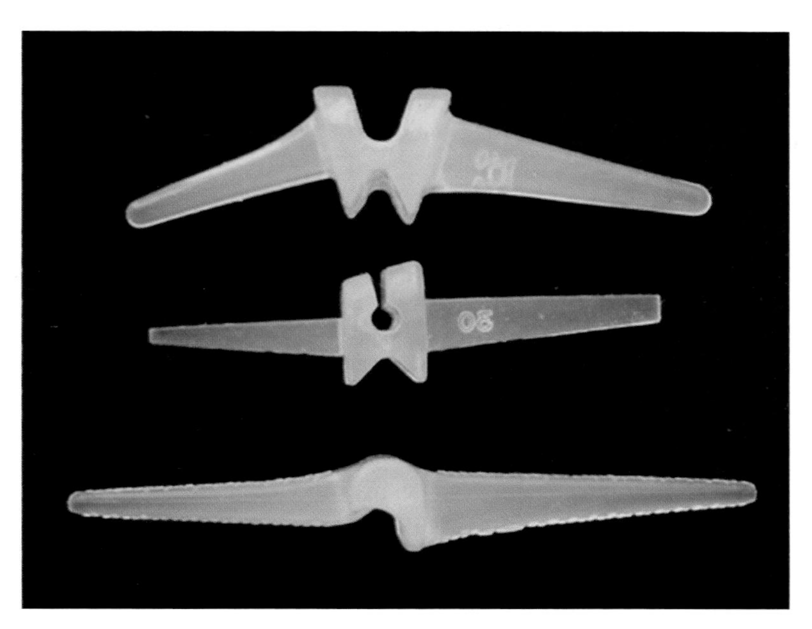

Figure 29.4. The lateral view of the three most common silicone-based implants; NeuFlex *(top)*, Avanta *(middle)*, Swanson *(bottom)*. Note that the Avanta and Swanson implants are of a zero-degree bend type.

higher stresses on the implant during flexion of the joint postoperatively, which can increase the risk of microfracture of the implant material and eventual failure. In addition, despite the design of 0° prebend, the joint typically has an extensor lag, which is likely due to a reduced moment arm of the extensor tendon and a change in the center of rotation of the joint following resection.

The NeuFlex implant has a 30° prebend in flexion, which mimics the anatomically neutral position of the digits at the MCP joint level (Fig. 29.5). This allows stresses on the silicone to be distributed between both extension and flexion from this position, decreasing the stress on the implant through a functional arc of motion. The shape and height of the implant has also been modified to more accurately imitate the anatomic center of rotation of the MCP joint, thereby improving the moment arm of both the flexor

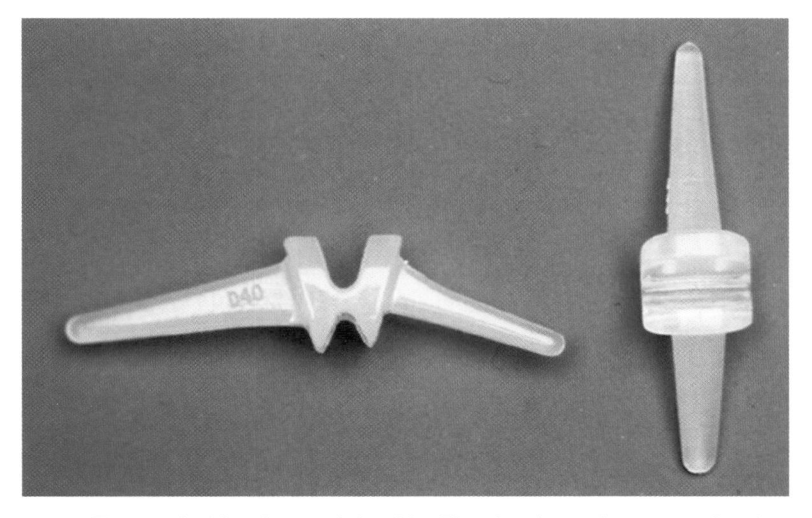

Figure 29.5. Top and side views of the NeuFlex implant, demonstrating its 30-degree anatomic bend and the block designed hinge, which improves extensor tendon moment arm.

and extensor tendons. Accordingly, the patient has more power and ability to move the finger effectively.

Biomechanical testing of the NeuFlex implant versus the Swanson and Avanta (Avanta, San Diego, CA) implants has confirmed that the NeuFlex implant optimizes center of rotation, implant pistoning, tendon excursion, and tendon moment arms.

INDICATIONS/CONTRAINDICATIONS

MCP joint arthroplasty is indicated in those patients with rheumatoid arthritis, or occasionally osteoarthritis, who experience pain and deformity of the MCP joint that affect hand function. Typically, patients with rheumatoid arthritis have significant destruction of the joints secondary to pannus erosion of both soft tissue and bone. In those patients without evidence of bony destruction, synovectomy and tendon-rebalancing procedures may improve function and decrease pain, although these are generally temporary measures. In general, alternative procedures, such as MCP arthrodesis, are less ideal, appear to be much more functionally limiting, and less well accepted by the patient.

Like any joint-replacement surgery, there are potential complications, such as implant failure, deep infection, and recurrent deformity, which must be considered in the decision to proceed with MCP implant arthroplasty. The younger patient will obviously have a higher risk of implant failure over time and recurrent deformity as compared to the older patient. The more active patient may also have greater risk of implant failure as the implant is placed through more vigorous and repetitive stress.

Candidates for MCP arthroplasty should have adequate bone stock for implant stability, as well as functioning extensor and flexor tendons to allow for proper range of motion of the joints. The patient with rheumatoid arthritis is unlikely to have isolated MCP pathology, and the remainder of the upper as well as lower extremities should be considered in any operative decision-making.

PREOPERATIVE PLANNING

When considering MCP arthroplasty, examination of the adjacent joints must be included. The function of the proximal interphalangeal (PIP) and distal interphalangeal (DIP) joints is essential to the success of a MCP arthroplasty. If a swan-neck deformity exists, PIP hyperextension will prevent full MCP extension. Similarly, deformity at the wrist may yield less than optimal results from an MCP arthroplasty. Radial deviation of the wrist may allow extrinsic flexors and extensors to create and/or worsen an ulnar deviation deformity of the fingers at the MCP joint. If the position of the wrist is not corrected, MCP arthroplasty will likely fail secondary to recurrence of ulnar deviation. Rheumatoid arthritis patients also commonly have abnormalities of the extensor hood, including radial hood attenuation and volar/ulnar subluxation of the extensor tendon. If these findings are not recognized preoperatively, optimal function is unlikely to be obtained from MCP arthroplasty alone. Tenosynovitis and restricted tendon excursion may also restrict MCP motion and, accordingly, should be addressed prior to, or concurrently with, MCP arthroplasty.

Soft-tissue abnormalities at the level of the joint should also be corrected to achieve satisfactory results. Typically, as the joint rests in an ulnar deviation from a loss of dorsoradial support, the ulnar aspect of the joint capsule and the ulnar extensor hood become contracted. Typically, this necessitates release of the ulnar extensor hood. Similarly, the attenuated-radial extensor hood often requires reconstruction via a reefing procedure. Alignment of the flexor tendons centrally over the MCP joint is essential in preventing a recurrence of ulnar deviation deformity. All of these forces must be balanced at the time of MCP arthroplasty to prevent recurrent deformity.

SURGERY

The MCP joints are approached via dorsal incisions utilizing either a single, transverse incision across all the joints or two longitudinal incisions (one between the index and middle finger MCP heads and the other between the ring and small finger MCP heads) (Fig. 29.6A, B). The dissection is carried down to the extensor hood, carefully protecting any sensory nerves encountered and trying to preserve as much of the dorsal venous system as possible. In the rheumatoid patient, the extensor hood is usually stretched out on the radial aspect, and the extensor tendon is usually subluxated ulnarward off the MCP head. Incise the extensor hood along the ulnar border of the extensor tendon in a longitudinal fashion, exposing the underlying capsule (Fig. 29.7). By releasing the tight ulnar extensor hood, the extensor tendon is easily subluxated radially, thereby exposing the MCP joint. Next, incise the capsule carefully so that repair can be performed if desired after the implants have been placed, then dissect the extensor hood and capsule from the underlying synovium. Perform a thorough synovectomy, using a rongeur.

The soft-tissue release needs to be generous enough to expose the base of the proximal phalanx as well as the neck and head of the metacarpal. Rheumatoid patients often have a pronation deformity at the index, and occasionally the middle finger, MCP joint. To correct this deformity, the radial collateral ligaments are reconstructed. Release the ulnar collateral ligament completely. Release the radial collateral ligament from the distal metacarpal and preserve it for later reconstruction.

The level of resection of the metacarpal head should be at the distal flare of the metacarpal shaft (Fig. 29.8). Once the level of resection is determined, use an oscillating saw to resect the metacarpal head at the level of the metaphyseal flare (Fig. 29.9). This allows enough resection of the bone to hold the hinge of the implant securely without impingement. Resections, either distal or proximal to the level of the flare, will create abnormal tightness or laxity, respectively. Using a rongeur, remove any osteophytes from the base of the proximal phalanx (Fig. 29.10). There is usually no need to resect the base of the proximal phalanx. However, if the patient has significant palmar subluxation of the proximal phalanx, there may be substantial erosion of the dorsal base of the proximal phalanx.

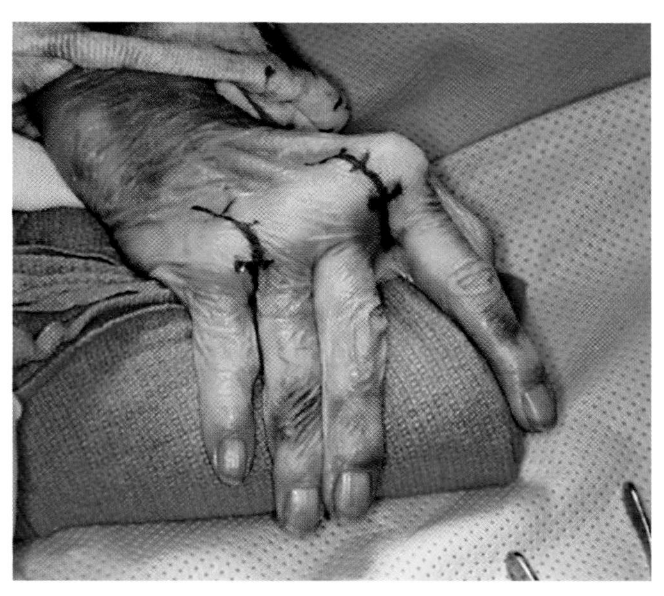
A

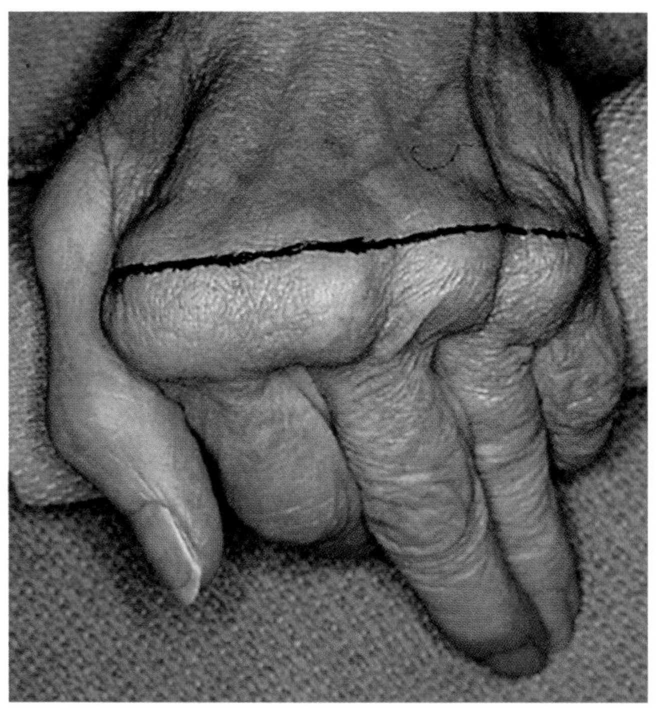
B

Figure 29.6. A: Double longitudinal or **(B)** transverse incisions may be used to expose the MCP joint.

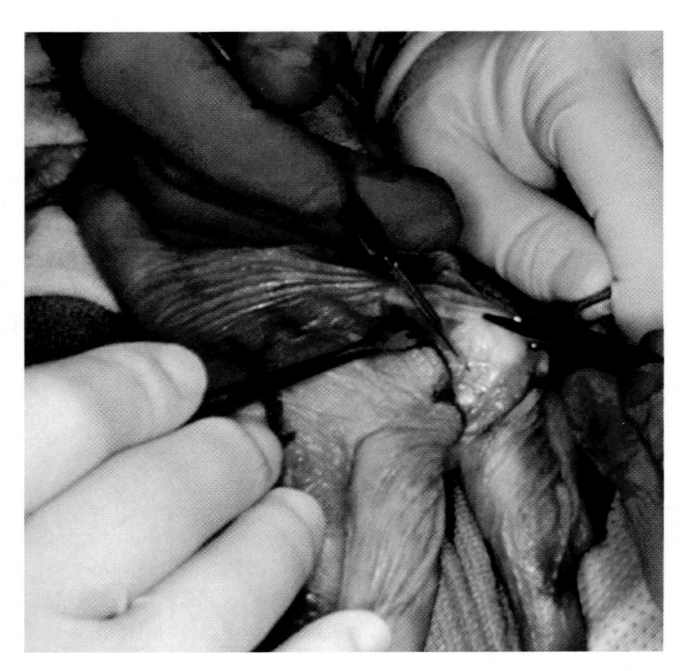

Figure 29.7. The tight ulnar extensor hood is released, allowing the entire extensor mechanism to be dislocated radially, exposing the MCP joint.

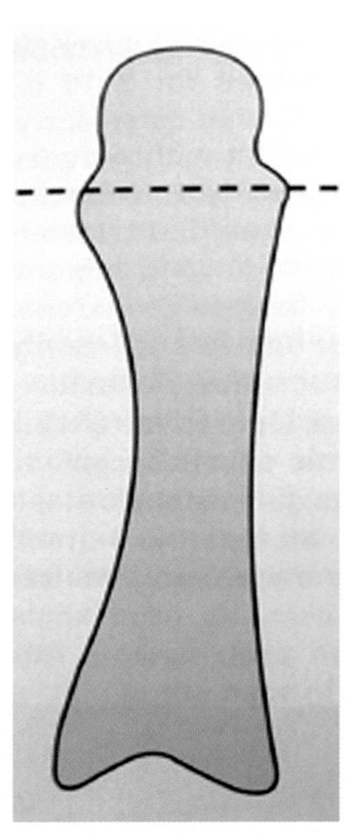

Figure 29.8. An illustration demonstrating the appropriate resection level for NeuFlex MCP arthroplasty.

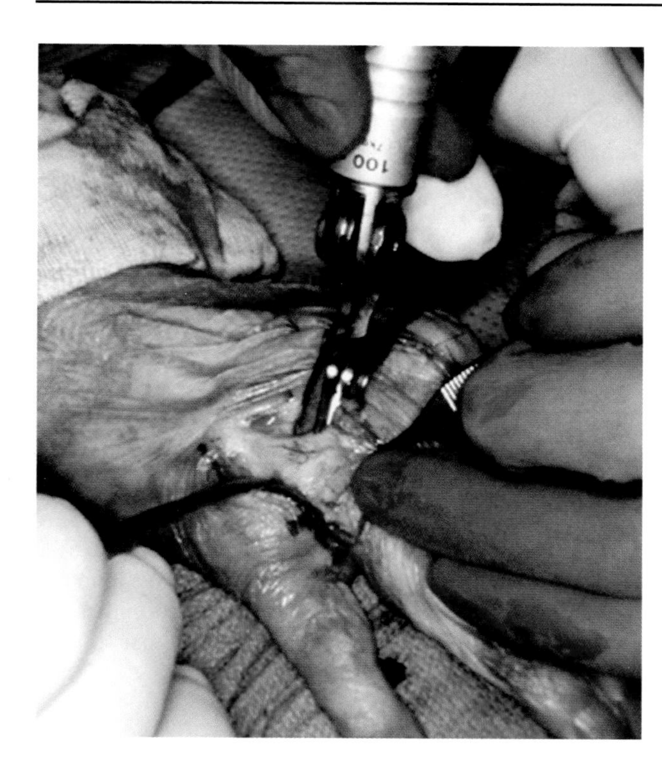

Figure 29.9. A sagittal saw is used to resect the MCP head.

In this case, resection of some (usually 2–4 mm) of the base of the proximal phalanx is warranted to improve resection gap, and will also provide a perpendicular base for the implant to seat properly into the bone.

Use a starter awl with a rasping motion to begin opening the intramedullary canal of the proximal phalanx and metacarpal (Fig. 29.11). Continue to prepare the intramedullary canal of the metacarpal using sequentially larger broaches, taking care not to violate the

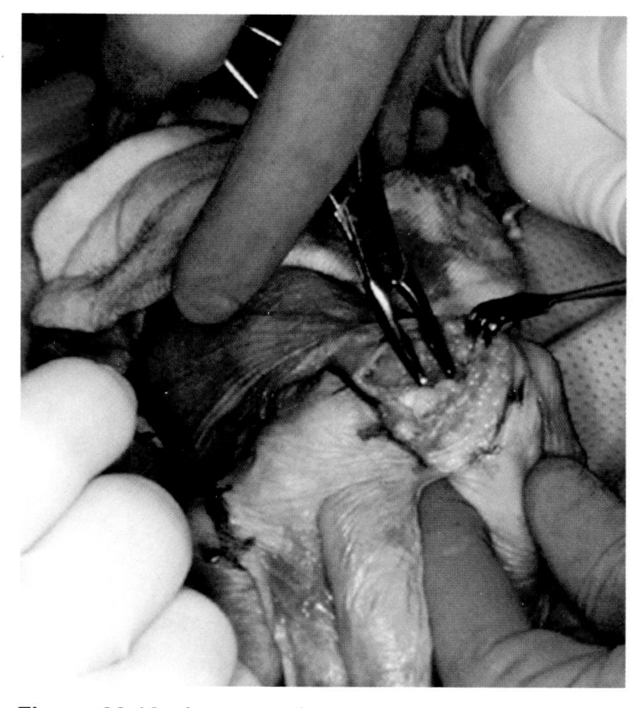

Figure 29.10. A rongeur is used to remove any osteophytes from the base of the proximal phalanx.

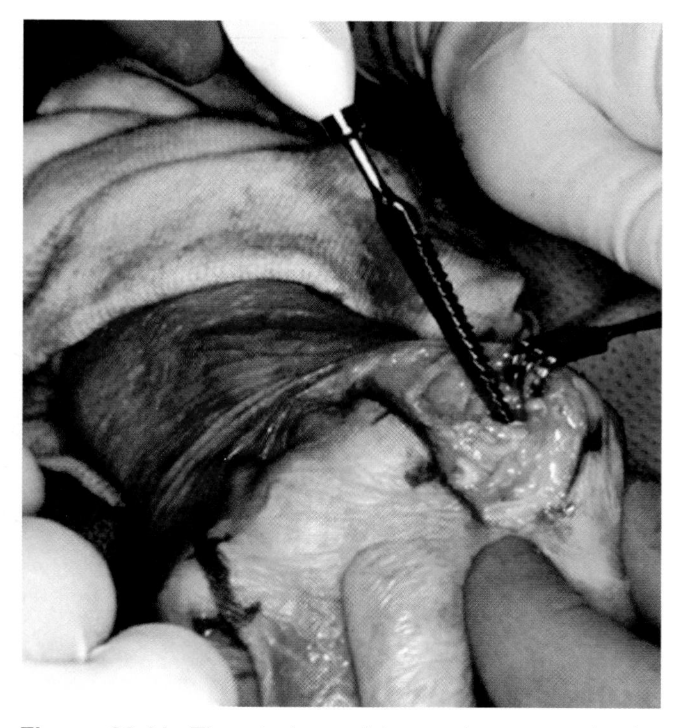

Figure 29.11. The starter awl is used to open the intramedullary canal for the broaches.

cortex (Fig. 29.12 A, B). The intermedullary canal of the ring finger metacarpal is relatively narrow, and aggressive reaming may perforate the cortex. The broaches are marked to indicate which side is dorsal, and contain a broach "stop" to avoid pushing the broach too deeply down the intramedullary canal. By using a rasp, smooth any rough edges or surfaces. Attention is then turned toward the proximal phalanx. Correction of a pronation or supination deformity may be partially achieved by choosing the site of reaming. Ream the proximal phalanx of the index finger in a rectangular fashion high on the ulnar-dorsal and low on the radial-volar sides. This position allows for an implant position of slight supination to compensate for the index finger tendency toward a pronation deformity. In the small finger, ream the medullary canal high on the radio-dorsal and low on the ulnar-volar aspects to create a slightly pronated position.

Use broaches of increasing size until the largest broach possible allows complete seating of the flanged stop. The size of the broach number is usually dictated by the metacarpal rather than the phalangeal side. If significant volar soft-tissue tightness is present, release of the volar plate, and occasionally intrinsic tendons, can be performed to balance the flexion and extension gaps prior to implant placement.

Trial implants are then placed. Use the trial corresponding to the largest broach size used (again, this is usually from the metacarpal side). Check the range of motion of the joint and confirm that full flexion and extension can be achieved without significant tightness. If there is a significant amount of tightness limiting full flexion and extension, either soft-tissue release or further resection of bone is warranted.

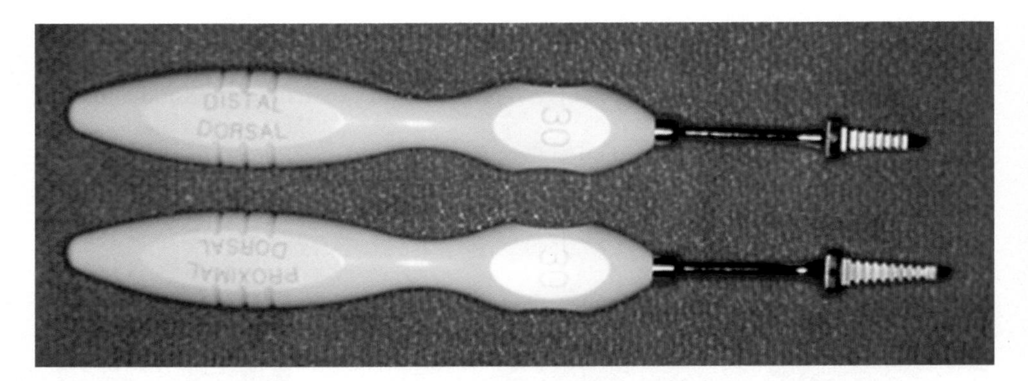

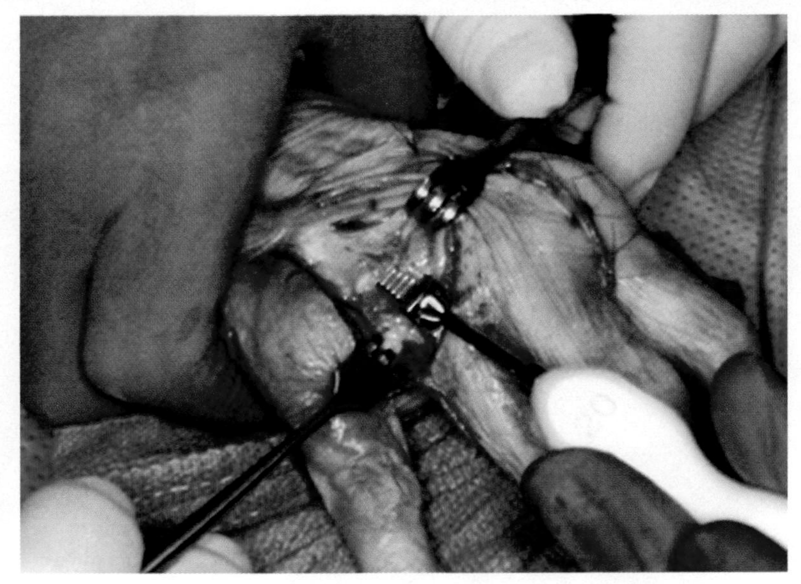

Figure 29.12. Broaches are available for both the metacarpal and phalangeal sides; broaching is undertaken to the largest size possible while still getting the stop flange on the broach to seat fully.

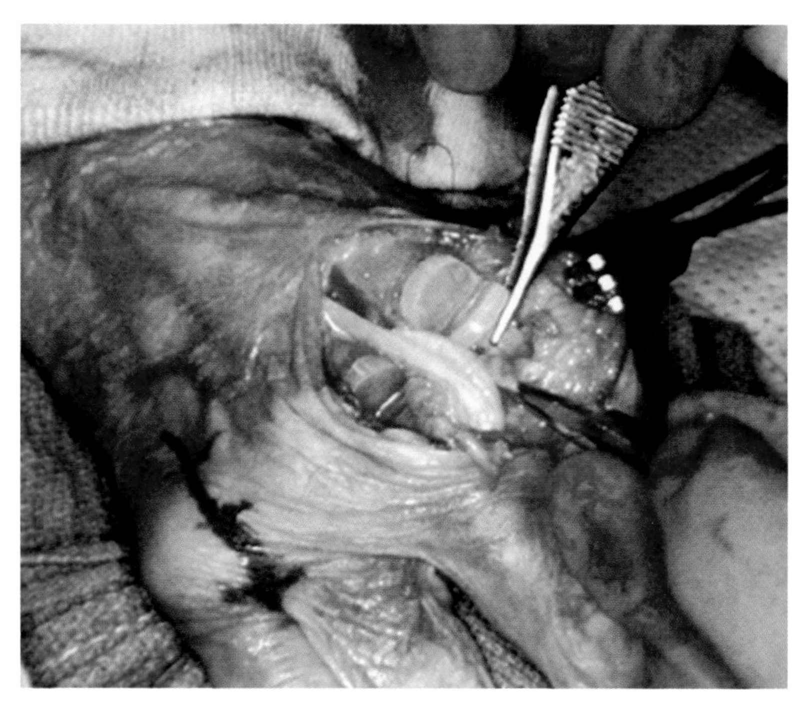

Figure 29.13. Implants are placed, and range of motion is checked.

In the index finger, make two radially based drill holes through the distal portion of the metacarpal shaft for later repair of the collateral ligament. Place a 4-0 nonabsorbable, braided suture into the radial collateral ligament that was detached from the metacarpal head prior to its resection. Thread each of the two suture ends into the drilled holes in the metacarpal shaft, going inside-out so that the two suture ends are left on the outside of the metacarpal shaft ready for tying. Insert the appropriate-size implant into each MCP space (Fig. 29.13). Again, perform a check of range of motion to ensure that the soft-tissue release and balance is appropriate (Fig. 29.14). In the index finger, the radial collateral

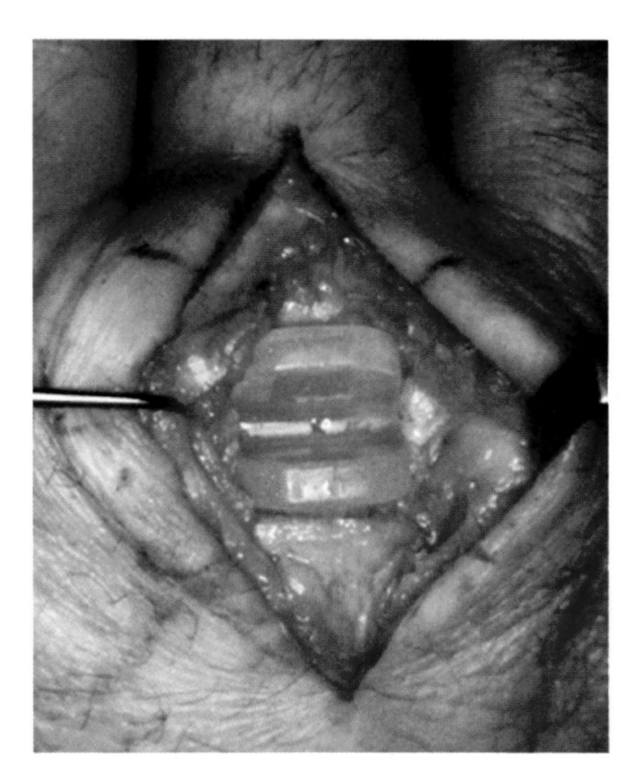

Figure 29.14. The implant should be well balanced in the joint resection area (as in this patient with osteoarthritis).

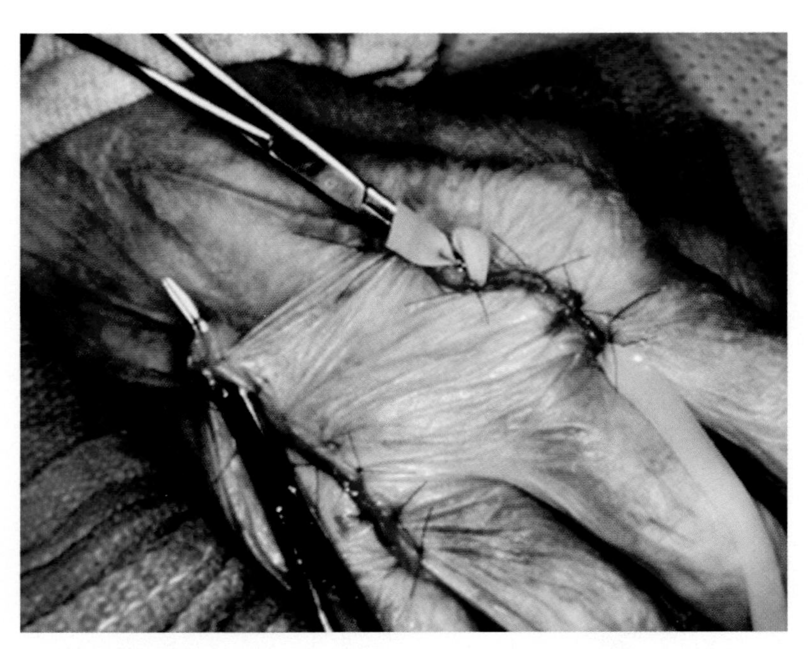

Figure 29.15. Drains are placed to prevent hematoma formation.

ligament is now repaired. Using the threaded sutures, repair the preserved radial collateral ligament under appropriate tension to the distal metacarpal by tying the passed sutures. If repair of the joint capsule is desired, this step is now performed to tighten the joint and improve stability, in hope of preventing ulnar drift in the future. The stretched radial aspect of the extensor hood is reefed and imbricated to relocate the extensor tendon to its dorsal midline position. It is important to ensure that the extensor tendon is not displaced into a radial position, which may create a pronation deformity. Again, take the joint through a trial range of motion to ensure that there is no soft-tissue or bone impingement and that the soft-tissue repair allows appropriate excursion.

Copiously irrigate the wounds. Using an electrocautery, achieve careful hemostasis. Place small drains into each wound to prevent hematoma formation (Fig. 29.15). Apply a large, bulky dressing and a volar plaster splint with the fingers in full extension.

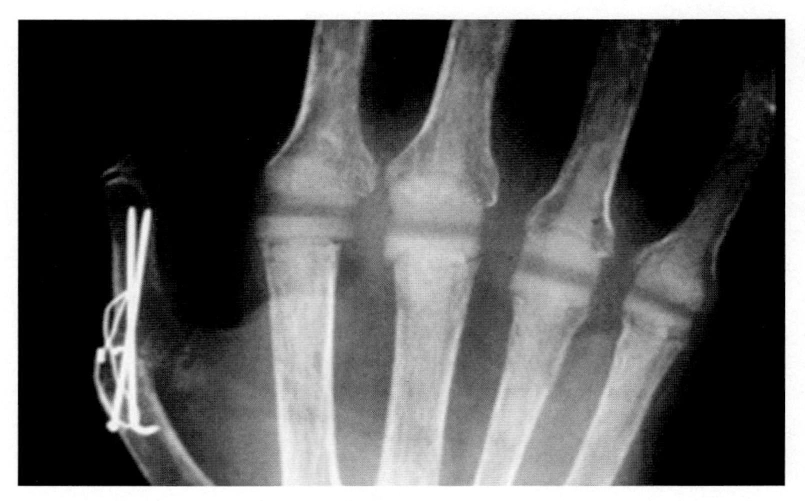

Figure 29.16. Postoperative radiographs are taken to check implant position.

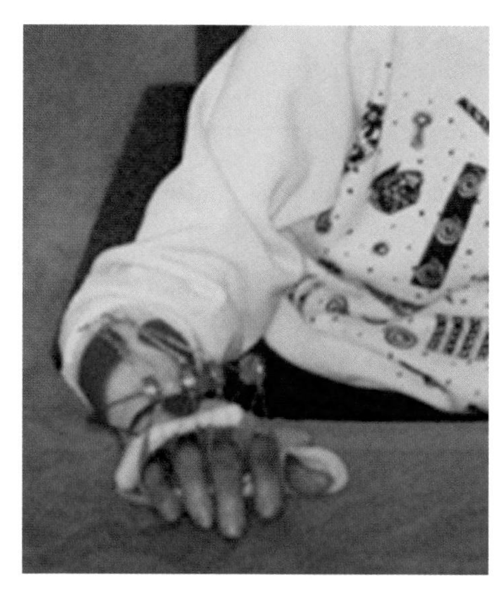

Figure 29.17. A dynamic extension splint is an important part of the patient's rehabilitation.

POSTOPERATIVE MANAGEMENT/REHABILITATION

Patients are usually admitted to the hospital for overnight observation, the drains removed the next morning, and the patient discharged with early follow-up to hand therapy. Radiographs of the hand are taken to confirm implant position (Fig. 29.16). The extension splint is maintained for approximately 5 to 10 days, after which a full extension pan splint is applied in conjunction with a dynamic extension splint allowing early motion of the digits (Fig. 29.17). Nighttime full extension splinting is maintained for at least 2 to 3 months postoperatively to prevent any recurrence of extensor lag.

An alternative splinting regimen was published by Burr in 2002. The fifteen patients in this study underwent a rehabilitation program of alternating MCP joint flexion and extension splints. Range-of-motion results in this study appear similar to the results obtained with dynamic splinting.

RESULTS

A study published by Gellman in 1997 examined the outcome of 901 Swanson silastic arthroplasties of the MCP joints in 294 patients. Average time to follow-up was 8 years. Active range of motion was 40° preoperatively and 50° postoperatively, an increase of 10°. Extensor lag improved from 50° preoperatively to 10° postoperatively, resulting in an arc of motion from 10° to 60°.

Similarly, Bieber published a study in 1986 that examined the results of 201 Swanson silicone MCP arthroplasty implants in 46 patients and found an average range of motion of 51° (10° to 61°).

In 2001, Weiss and Strickland conducted a study of 50 consecutive patients undergoing NeuFlex MCP joint arthroplasty. Forty-six patients had rheumatoid arthritis and four had osteoarthritis. A total of 168 implants were placed in these 50 patients. At a mean follow-up time of 28 months, all patients were satisfied with the appearance of their hands. No complications were related to the implant. No evidence of fracture of the implant was found on postoperative radiographs.

Active range of motion of respective fingers was: index finger 15°/75°, middle finger 14°/78°, ring finger 13°/73°, small finger 7°/65°. Average extensor lag was 12° and average flexion was 73°, or an average arc of motion of 61°. Of note, these findings demonstrate that a 30° prebend in the implant does not create a significantly greater extensor lag as compared to the Swanson implant. It is thought that this finding is likely secondary to the increased tendon excursion and moment arm, which allow the NeuFlex implant to be extended actively by the patient.

A recent prospective, random, and double-blind study (Wrightington Hospital, United Kingdom, 2003) of the clinical outcome comparing NeuFlex versus Swanson silicone MCP arthroplasty demonstrated a statistical significantly ($p < 0.05$) improved arc of motion (70 degrees vs. 42 degrees, respectively), greater flexion (77 degrees vs. 52 degrees, respectively), and less extensor lag (7 degrees vs. 11 degrees, respectively) for the patients receiving the NeuFlex implant at two-year follow-up examination.

COMPLICATIONS

Gellman's study of Swanson silastic MCP arthroplasty found that the most common complications were dehiscence and delayed wound healing (2%), superficial infection (0.5%), deep infection (3%), and prosthetic fracture (14%). In 1994, Olsen published results of 60 MCP arthroplasties in 16 patients and found an implant fracture in 13 joints (21%). The ability of the more recent implant designs to withstand implant fracture remains to be seen, although kinematic studies appear to demonstrate no significant fracture rate after 10 million motion cycles for the NeuFlex implant.

CONCLUSIONS

Since the 1960s, silicone implant arthroplasty has proven to be dependable and effective in the treatment of the pain and deformity of rheumatoid arthritis involving the MCP joints. The more recent designs have improved on the mechanical parameters of the implant and demonstrated superior clinical function. It appears that anatomically neutral (30°), designed implants, such as the NeuFlex, improve positioning of the center of rotation and tendon moment arm following arthroplasty. These improvements allow for a greater clinical arc of motion while preserving extension of the joint.

RECOMMENDED READING

1. Abernathy PJ, Dennyson WG. Decompression of the extensor tendons at the wrist in rheumatoid arthritis. *JBJS* 61(B):64–68, 1979.
2. Alsheik N, Bliss J, Moore DC, et al. Cyclic Loading of Silicone NeuFlex MCP Implants. Personal Communication.
3. Backhouse KM. The mechanics of normal digital control in the hand and an analysis of the ulnar drift of rheumatoid arthritis. *Ann R Coll Surg Engl* 43:154–173, 1968.
4. Bass RL, Stern PJ, Nairus JG. High implant fracture incidence with Sutter silicone metacarpophalangeal joint arthroplasty. *J Hand Surg* 21A:813–818, 1996.
5. Beckenbaugh RD. Implant arthroplasty in the rheumatoid hand and wrist: current state of the art in the United States. *J Hand Surg* 8: 675–678, 1983
6. Beckenbaugh RD, Dobyns JH, Linscheid RL, et al. Review and analysis of silicone-rubber metacarpophalangeal implants. *JBJS* 58(A):483–487, 1976.
7. Bieber EJ, Weiland AJ, Volenec-Dowling S. Silicone-rubber implant arthroplasty of the metacarpophalangeal joints for rheumatoid arthritis. *JBJS Am* 68(2):206–209, 1986.
8. Burr N, Pratt AL, Smith PJ. An alternative splinting and rehabilitation protocol for metacarpophalangeal arthtroplasty in patients with rheumatoid arthritis. *J Hand Ther* 15(1):41–47, 2002.
9. Delaney R, Trail IA, Nuttall D. A comparativestudy of outcome between the Neuflex and Swanson silastic metacarpophalangeal joint replacements. *J Hand Surg, In Press.*
10. Gellman H, Stetson W, Brumfield RH Jr, et al. Silastic metacarpophalangeal joint arthroplasty in patients with rheumatoid arthritis. *Clin Orthop* 342:16–21, 1997.
11. Loebl WY. Mobility of the metacarpophalangeal joints in rheumatoid arthritis. *Hand* 5:165–169, 1973.
12. Murray PM. Currrent status of metacarpophalangeal arthroplasty and basilar joint arthroplasty of the thumb. *Clin Plast Surg* 23:395–406, 1996.
13. Olsen I, Gebuhr P, Sonne-Holm S. Silastic arthroplasty in rheumatoid MCP joints. 60 joints followed for 7 years. *Acta Orthop Scand* 65(4):430–431, 1994.
14. Shapiro JS. The etiology of ulnar drive: A new factor. *JBJS* 50(A);634, 1968.

15. Swanson AB. Silicone rubber implants for replacement of arthritic or destroyed joints in the hand. *Surg Clinic North Am* 48:1113–1127, 1968
16. Weiss APC. NeuFlex Prosthesis. In: Simmen BR, Allieu Y, Lluch A, et al., eds. *Hand Arthroplasties*. London: Martin Dunitz, 2000:315–322.
17. Weiss APC, Moore DC, Crisco JJ. Metacarpophalangeal Mechanics After Silicone Joint Replacement. *Trans Amer Soc Surg Hand*, Boston, 1999.
18. Welsh RP, Hastings DE. Swan-neck deformity in rheumatoid arthritis of the hand. *Hand* 9:109–116, 1977.

30

Small Joint Fusions

Richard W. Barth and J. Robert Anderson

INDICATIONS/CONTRAINDICATIONS

The most common indications for proximal interphalangeal (PIP) and distal interphalangeal (DIP) joint arthrodesis are pain, instability, deformity, and ultimately functional loss. Common etiologies for these symptoms include osteoarthritis, inflammatory arthritis, and trauma. Less commonly, chronic tendon ruptures, burns, Dupuytren's disease, and postinfectious arthritis result in symptoms for which arthrodesis may be a recommended treatment. Arthritis mutilans, with progressive disintegration, is another indication for arthrodesis to prevent further shortening and bone loss.

Although not an indication for surgery, cosmetic appearance is clearly an issue for many patients. We have found patients to be as unhappy with the appearance of a deformed, "knobby" joint as they are with the pain and limited motion. Since this is a consideration in the patient's decision-making, the surgeon cannot ignore the cosmetic element.

Absolute contraindications to small joint arthrodesis include active infection. A lack of soft-tissue coverage may be a concern, yet shortening the bony column through fusion usually facilitates coverage because the osteoarticular column is effectively shortened. Relative contraindications include previous arthrodesis at adjacent joints in patients with specific jobs or hobbies that require the maintenance of some motion of the index digit.

PREOPERATIVE PLANNING

Patient evaluation begins with the history; pain, instability, and deformity are the most common complaints. An unstable index finger PIP joint or thumb interphalangeal joint can lead to weakness of pinch. A fixed boutonniere deformity can lead to difficulty with gripping and grasping. Severe degenerative arthritis can cause activity-limiting pain.

Richard W. Barth, M.D.: George Washington University School of Medicine, Georgetown University School of Medicine, Washington, DC

J. Robert Anderson, M.D.: Department of Orthopaedic Surgery, George Washington University School of Medicine, Washington, DC

The underlying cause of the arthritis or instability is important as it affects the treatment options. Relevant physical findings include the range of motion of the affected and surrounding joints, the stability of the joint, and the quality of the soft tissues and tendons. There will often be deformity of the joint, tenderness to palpation, and crepitus with passive motion.

A locked trigger finger can coexist with an arthritic PIP joint and result in a stiff, painful digit. A cortisone injection may be helpful to differentiate the relative contribution of the trigger finger from the arthritis. Routine radiographs of the affected digit are generally the only imaging study necessary. Rarely, computed tomography is necessary to evaluate the articular surface, the bone quality, or the extent of fracture healing.

Treatment alternatives must be considered. A patient with a stiff arthritic joint may elect nonoperative treatment if the major complaint is loss of motion. Volar plate arthroplasty may be a better option for a malunited PIP fracture-dislocation. Patients with a previous DIP arthrodesis may function better with a PIP arthroplasty than with an arthrodesis. The patient may "test drive" a particular small joint fusion by wearing a limited splint for a period of time or for a particular test of function. Sometimes a short dorsal splint for the DIP or PIP joint is best to model a fusion because it still permits tactile capability. If pain relief and functional improvement are realized through splinting, arthrodesis is a logical treatment option.

Once the choice is made to proceed with an arthrodesis, there are several technical considerations. The first consideration is choice of fixation, and there are a number of options. Kirschner wire (K-wire), tension band fixation, intraosseous wiring, variable-pitch headless bone screws (Herbert, Herbert-Whipple, Acutrak, EBI VPC), and plating have all been successfully used in small joint arthrodesis. Obviously, intramedullary implants have inherent benefits over relatively bulky plate-and-screw constructs in areas where coverage may be tenuous. Each surgeon has his or her own preference for a routine fusion.

However, there are situations in which fixation options may be limited. The distal phalanx may be too small for a screw. A plate may be the best choice if there is significant bone loss after a failed arthroplasty of the PIP joint. K-wires are quick and easy and may be the best choice when the fusion is a small part of a lengthy procedure.

The second consideration is the use of bone graft. Although bone grafting is rarely necessary, it may be indicated in managing bone defects. Significant bone defects may be encountered when converting a failed implant arthroplasty, in cases of post-traumatic bone loss, and in arthritis mutilans.

Finally, it is important that the digit be fused at the proper angle to allow maximum function. We generally fuse the DIP joint in full extension. The ideal PIP joint fusion angle depends on the digit and the portfolio of the patient's functional needs. Usually, the index and middle fingers are more important for pinch, and 15 to 30 degrees is optimal. The ring and small fingers are more important for grip, and these digits are arthrodesed in 30 to 45 degrees of flexion.

A preoperative splint trial can assist the surgeon and patient in choosing the optimal position for each individual. Preoperatively, we are careful to make it clear to the patient that the results of the surgery are permanent.

SURGERY

Interphalangeal joint arthrodesis is performed with the patient in the supine position. We generally perform DIP arthrodesis under digital block utilizing a Penrose drain as a tourniquet. In an anxious patient, intravenous sedation can be helpful. By performing the digital block with a mixture of marcaine and xylocaine, patients have 6 to 8 hours of pain relief. PIP arthrodesis is performed under regional anesthesia, generally a Bier block or an axillary block. The operating room should be equipped with power equipment for the placement of K-wires. Appropriate implants must be available. A mini-fluoroscopy unit vastly simplifies the procedure.

The PIP joint is approached most easily through a dorsal curvilinear incision, which should extend from the distal portion of the middle phalanx to the midportion of the prox-

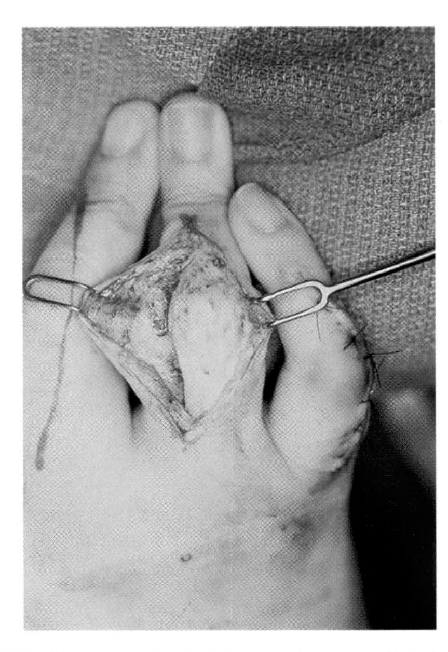

Figure 30.1. The proximal interphalangeal (PIP) joint is exposed through a curvilinear incision extending from the distal interphalangeal (DIP) to the metacarpophalangeal (MCP) joints, raising a large flap to the level of the extensor mechanism epitenon.

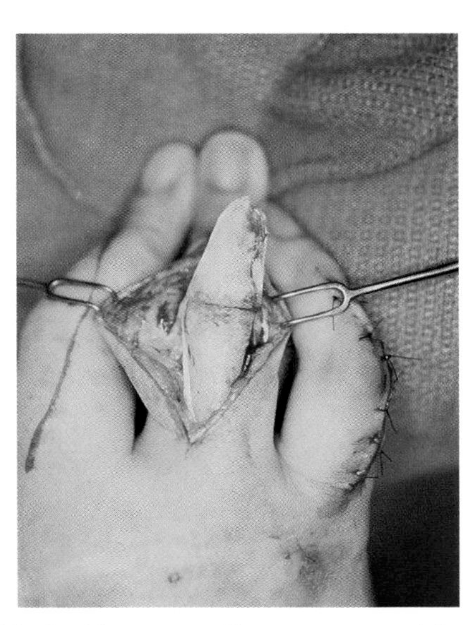

Figure 30.2. In this case, a Chamay approach is used to expose the PIP joint using a distally based flap of the extensor mechanism.

imal phalanx (Fig. 30.1). The skin and subcutaneous tissues are elevated in a flap, exposing the extensor mechanism. The extensor mechanism is usually split in a longitudinal fashion, exposing the PIP joint surface. Alternatively, a Chamay-type approach is used, elevating the extensor mechanism in a distally based flap (Fig. 30.2). The extensor hood is retracted distally, exposing the base of the middle phalanx as well as the proximal phalangeal head.

Regardless of exposure route, the collateral ligaments are then released from their origins, and the articular surface is easily visualized by hyperflexing the joint. In a minority of cases, a limited traction tenolysis of the flexors can be performed through the interval between the prepared bone ends.

Once the articular surface is exposed, we remove the remaining cartilage and subchondral bone. The joint can be prepared for fusion in one of two ways. The first is to prepare the joint surfaces in a cup-and-cone fashion by forming the proximal phalangeal head into a cone and the base of the middle phalanx into a cup. Although commercially available reamers may aid in the preparation of these surfaces, we have not found these to be necessary (Fig. 30.3).

The second option is to cut the articular surfaces flush. While some surgeons prefer this technique, we find in easier to fine-tune the fusion angle and rotation with the cup-and-cone method. The use of hand tools to prepare the fusion surfaces should be familiar to all surgeons. Alternatively, to prepare the base of the middle phalanx, we have found it useful to use a burr at low speed with continuous irrigation. It is important to avoid generating excessive heat when using power tools to prepare the joint surfaces; this can result in thermal necrosis and potentially an increased incidence of nonunion.

Many different fixation techniques have been described for the PIP joint. We prefer to use pins and a tension band technique. A transverse drill hole is made with a 0.035-inch K-wire approximately 9 to 10 mm from the joint surface (Fig. 30.4). Two parallel 0.045-inch K-wires are then placed across the PIP joint; the volar cortex of the middle phalanx is engaged but not penetrated (Fig. 30.5). This helps to prevent the pins from migrating volarly. The tensioning wire is then secured around the pin ends. Standard tensioning techniques are used, and wires are cut short and oriented to prevent interference with the extensor mechanism

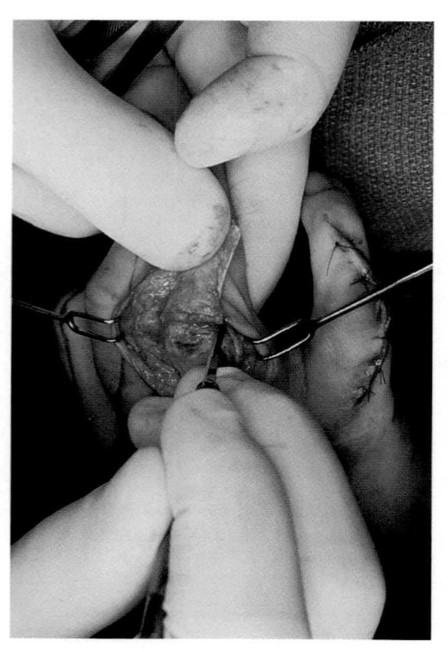

Figure 30.3. The collateral ligaments are released using a Beaver blade. The subchondral bone is removed from the distal portion of the proximal phalanx and the proximal portion of the middle phalanx.

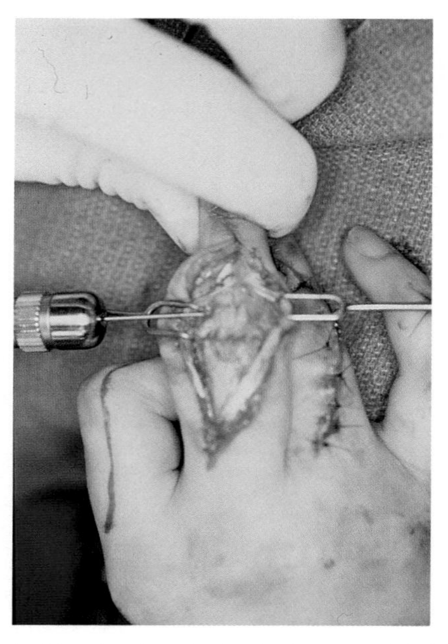

Figure 30.4. Tension band wire technique. A 0.035-inch K-wire is advanced across the proximal portion of the middle phalanx approximately 10 mm distal to the joint.

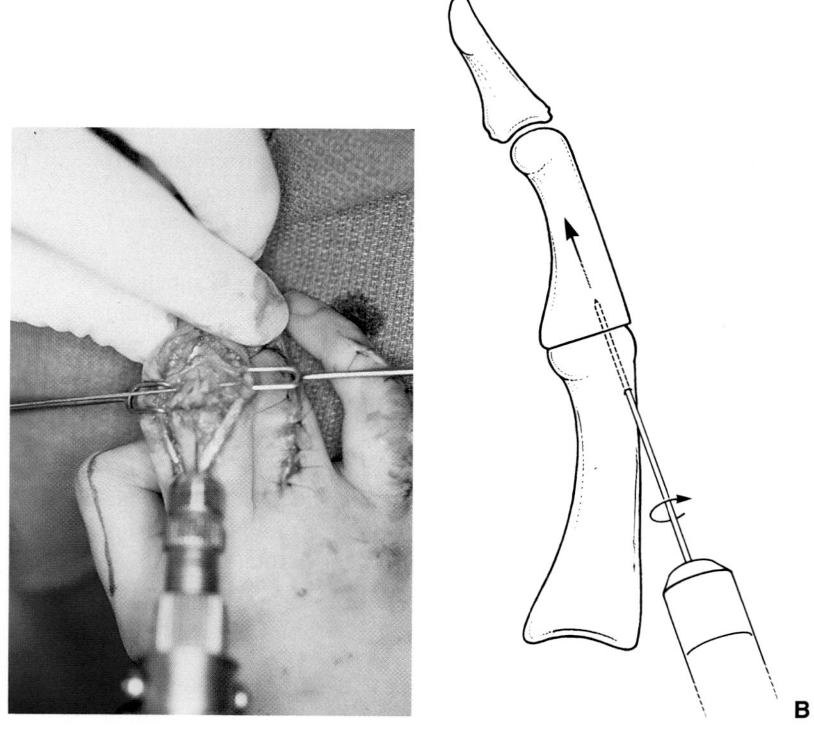

Figure 30.5. A: After resection of the articular surface and subchondral bone, a 24-gauge wire is advanced through the previously made drill hole. **B:** A 0.045-inch K-wire is advanced across the PIP joint from the proximal to the middle phalanx.

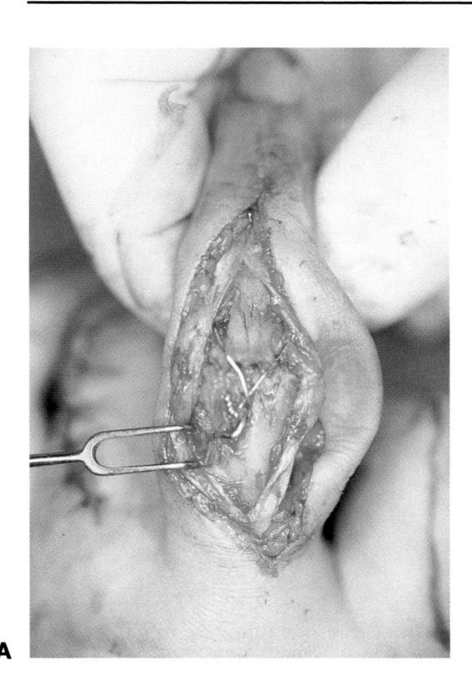

A

Figure 30.6. A: The 24-gauge wire and 0.045-inch K-wires are cut short. **B:** The wires are turned down to prevent interference with the extensor mechanism.

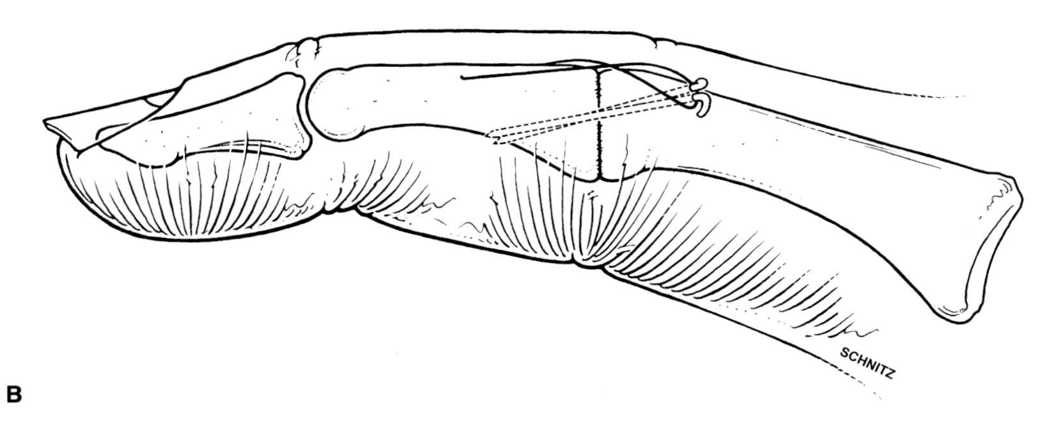

B

(Fig. 30.6). The wire knot can be placed in the fusion site to avoid hardware irritation. The extensor mechanism is repaired with nonabsorbable suture.

A number of alternative fixation methods have been described. K-wire fixation is quick, easy, and requires no special implants. One wire is driven obliquely and the second wire axially, or both wires are placed obliquely, in a crossed fashion.

The technique of 90/90 wiring provides excellent stability. In this technique, two loops of stainless steel wire, either 24 or 26 gauge, are placed at right angles to one another. It may be difficult to place the dorsal-to-palmar wire because of the flexor tendon mechanism. When this technique is used, it may be necessary to supplement the fixation with a transarticular K-wire. The use of plates and screws is an excellent technique to provide fixation in cases of segmental bone loss. This technique may necessitate hardware removal at a later date.

Finally, fixation with a variable-pitch, headless screw has been described for PIP joint fusion. In this technique, the headless screw drill must be placed proximal enough to prevent fracture of the dorsal cortex of the proximal phalanx (Fig. 30.7). This is most safely achieved by entering the proximal phalanx at 5 mm or more from the articular surface. In most cases, a 1.9-mm drill is all that is required to provide a path for the headless screw. In cases of hard bone, taps may be required. In cases of poor bone stock, such as in rheumatoid arthritis, a 0.062-inch K-wire may provide adequate entry into the bone, with the head-

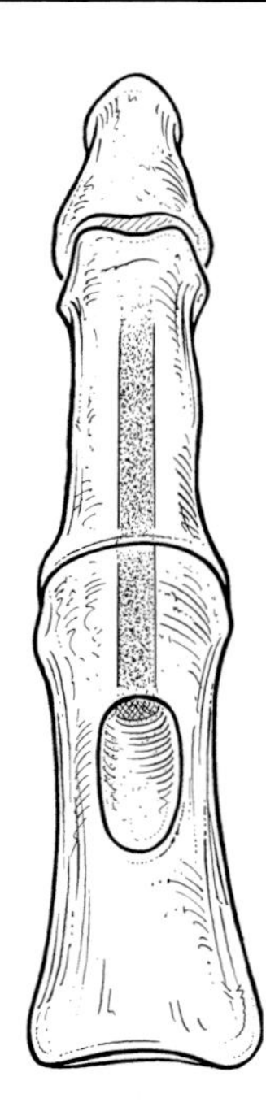

Figure 30.7. Bone preparation for Herbert screw placement includes the removal of a portion of the dorsal cortex.

less screw easily passing through the drill hole (Fig. 30.8). Whatever the status of the bone stock, a small portion of the cortical bone just distal to the drill hole should be removed using a curette or rongeur (Fig. 30.9) to allow full countersinking of the threads without cortical fracture of the proximal phalanx (Fig. 30.10). The extensor mechanism is repaired with nonabsorbable suture with the knots buried (Fig. 30.11). Other devices, such as a cannulated screw, may also be used for fixation using the same principles.

DIP Arthrodesis

We usually approach the DIP joint through a dorsal H incision. Transverse or Y-shaped incisions are also effective. The germinal matrix of the nail is protected. The extensor

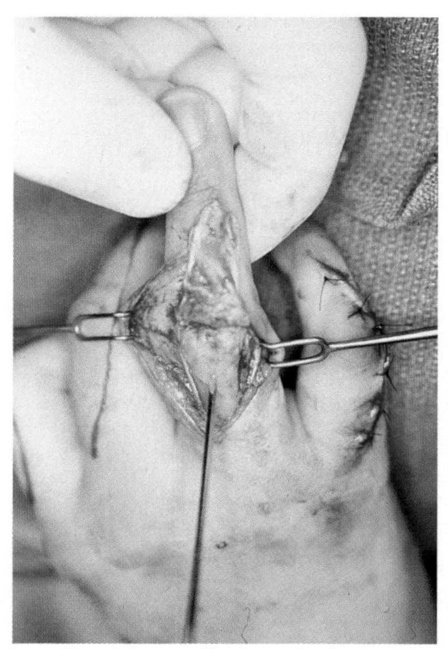

Figure 30.8. A 0.062-inch K-wire is advanced across the distal portion of the proximal phalanx into the middle phalanx with the joint held at the appropriate fusion angle.

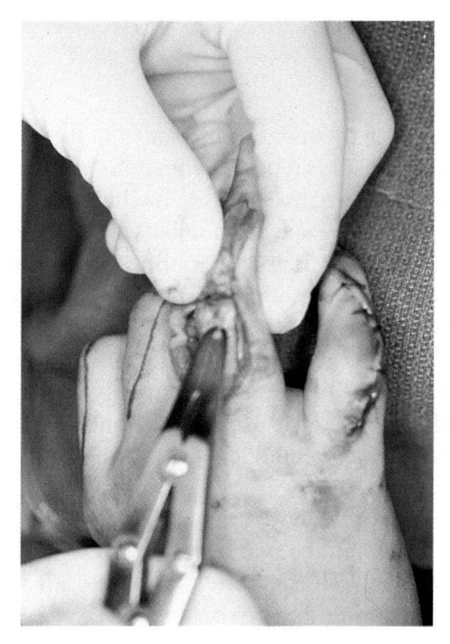

Figure 30.9. A small portion of the cortical bone at the distal portion of the drill hole is removed to allow full countersinking of the threads without cortical fracture.

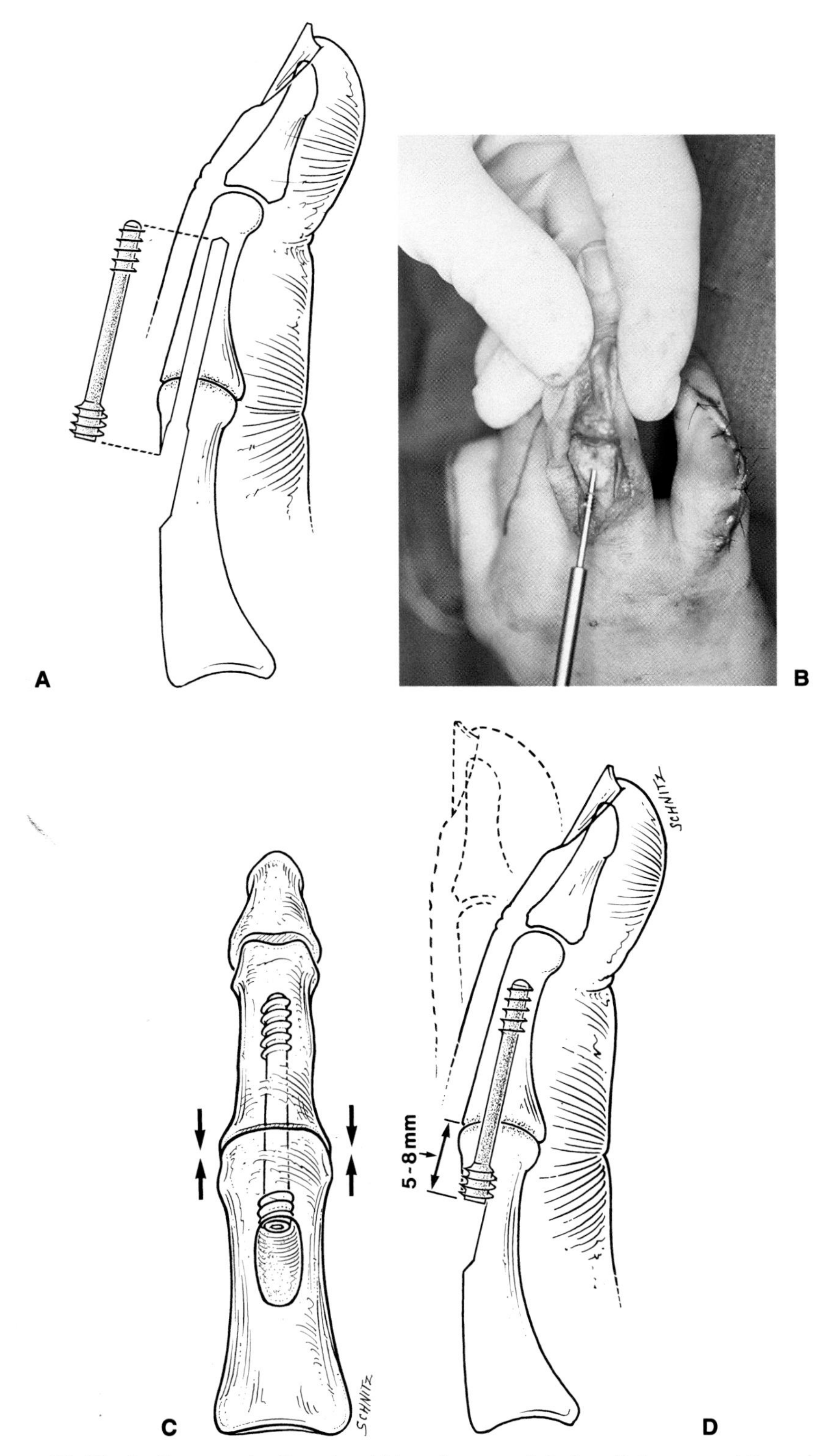

Figure 30.10. A: Screw selection should be of appropriate length to prevent thread protrusion proximally. **B, C:** A 24-mm Herbert screw is advanced across the PIP joint using the 0.062-inch drill hole. **D:** Screw placement must be made to avoid threads at the fusion site.

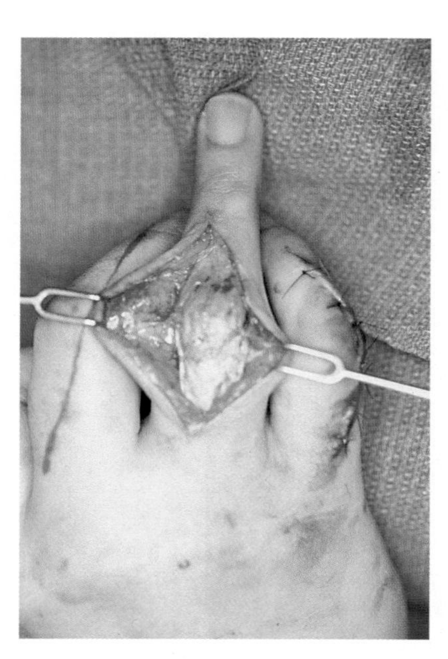

Figure 30.11. The extensor mechanism is reapproximated using buried nonabsorbable suture.

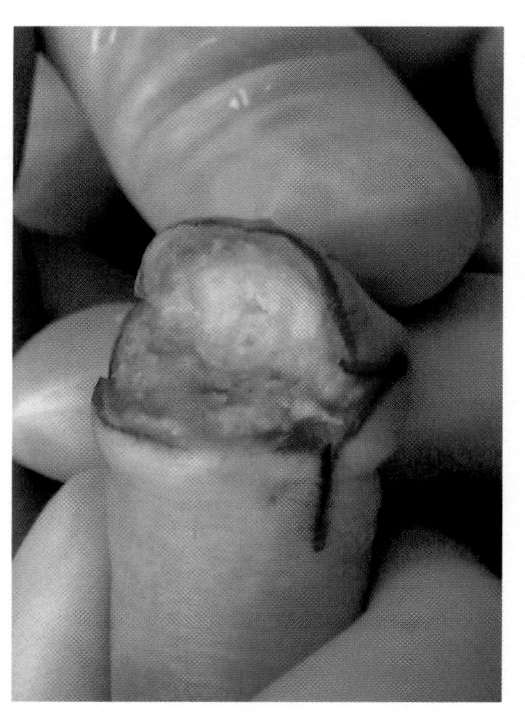

Figure 30.12. The DIP joint is exposed through a dorsal H-shaped incision. The collateral ligaments are released. The articular surface and subchondral bone are resected.

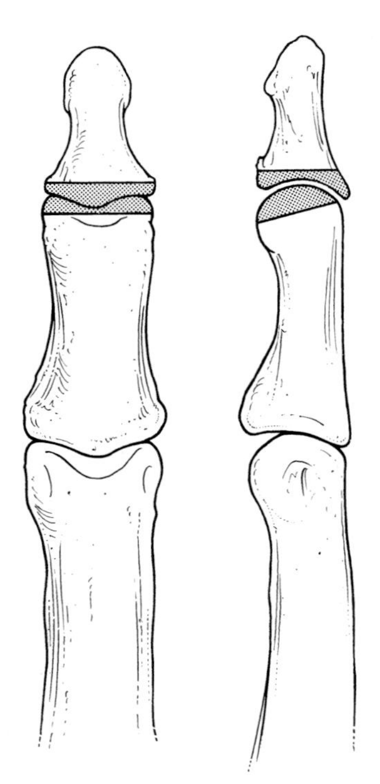

Figure 30.13. Bone resection illustrated for a DIP fusion. Bone preparation should allow fixation in full extension.

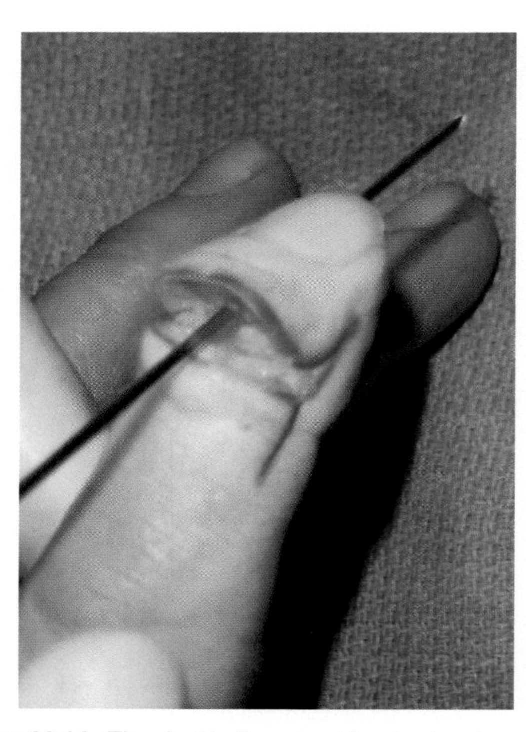

Figure 30.14. The double-tipped guide wire is advanced in an antegrade fashion into the distal phalanx. The guide wire exits centrally just below the nail plate.

mechanism is exposed and sectioned transversely. The collateral ligaments are released, the joint is hyperflexed, and the remaining articular cartilage and subchondral bone are removed. We create two opposing flat surfaces (Figs 30.12 and 30.13).

There are several fixation options for DIP arthrodesis. We prefer to use an Acutrak screw (Acumed, Hillsburg, OR). The fusion screw comes in several sizes. A standard screw and a mini-screw are also available, depending on the joint to be fused. Templates are used preoperatively to determine the most appropriately sized screw. The joint is prepared as described above. The middle phalanx is predrilled centrally with a K-wire. Under fluoroscopic guidance, a 0.062-inch double tipped K-wire is advanced proximal to distal in the distal phalanx (Fig. 30.14). The joint is then reduced and, under fluoroscopic guidance, the K-wire is driven retrograde centrally into the middle phalanx using the predrilled hole as a starting point. As we advance the screw into the middle phalanx, we find it helpful to use fluoroscopy to confirm central positioning in both planes. The appropriate size drills are then used. The joint is reduced and the screw is inserted. We visualize the fusion site during screw advancement to confirm that the surfaces are firmly opposed. Skin flaps are trimmed to remove redundant skin (Fig. 30.15).

Alternative fixation options include K-wires, a Herbert screw, an EBI VPC screw, or one of the newer locking screws. K-wires may be advanced through the distal phalanx with the

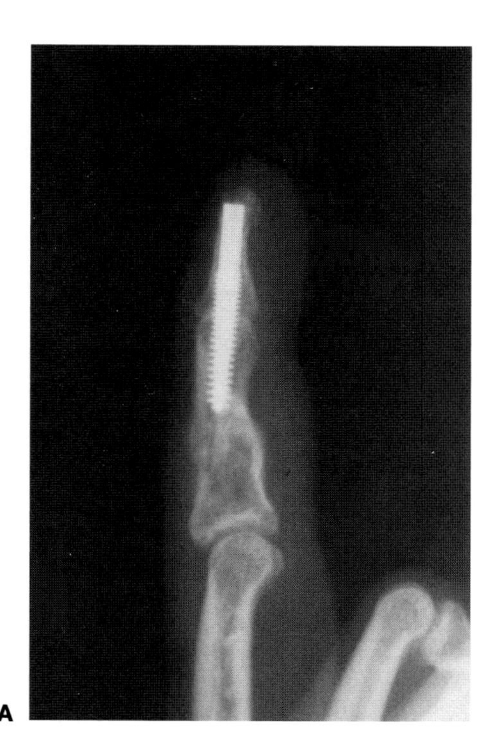

Figure 30.15. DIP fusion illustrated. **A:** Note that the trailing portion of the screw is not threaded and is well within the distal phalanx. **B:** The DIP joint is fixed in full extension.

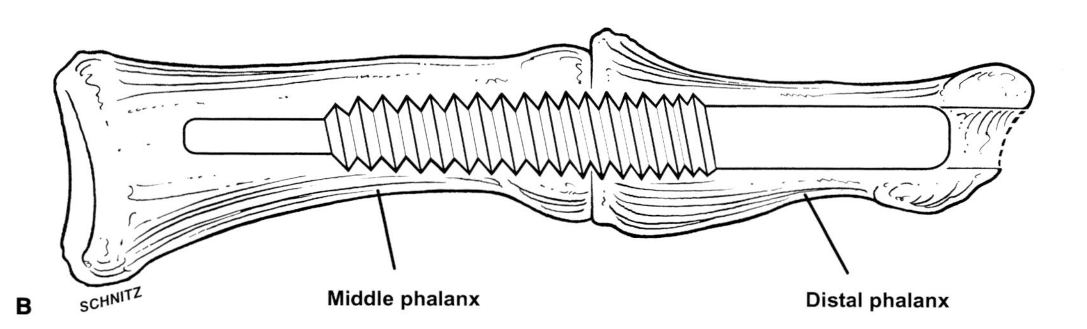

joint hyperflexed. They are then driven in a retrograde fashion into the middle phalanx. When using the Herbert or VPC screw, a 0.062-inch K-wire provides a satisfactory drill to create a path. The drill should exit the tip of the finger just volar to the nailbed. A 24- or 26-mm screw is most commonly used. Attention should be given to the size of the trailing screw threads, as these often are wider than the anterior-posterior (AP) diameter of the distal phalanx. In cases of poor bone quality, the distal phalanx may fracture with advancement of this screw.

Finally, there is a relatively new fusion screw (StayFuse; Zimmer, Warsaw, IN) that appears promising. The joint surfaces are prepared in a standard fashion, the implants are inserted into the proximal and distal phalanx, and the implants are then snap-locked together.

POSTOPERATIVE MANAGEMENT

The involved digit is placed in a bulky dressing and the hand is elevated above the heart for 72 hours. Postoperative pain is generally minimal and well controlled with oral narcotic medication. We generally see the patient at 7 to 10 days after surgery for a wound check and provision of digital splints.

REHABILITATION

For isolated DIP joint fusions, the patient is placed in a splint immobilizing only the DIP joint. Early active and passive range of motion of the PIP joint are initiated to prevent stiffness. The DIP joint is protected for 6 to 8 weeks, or until radiographs confirm bony union. For patients undergoing PIP joint fusion, a custom Orthoplast splint is applied. This splint should not restrict motion at the metacarpophalangeal or DIP joint to allow range of motion of these joints.

Radiographs are used to confirm fusion site healing, which usually occurs at 6 to 8 weeks. When percutaneous K-wires have been used, they are usually removed 6 to 8 weeks after surgery. After the wires are removed, we protect the digit for an additional 3 to 4 weeks using a removable splint. Once the fusion site has healed, no further protective splinting is required. Soft-tissue swelling may remain for several months. The patient must have realistic expectations regarding the ultimate appearance; the surgeon should not overpromise and then underdeliver on the ultimate cosmetic appearance of the fused digit.

RESULTS

In our experience, patients are generally pleased with the results of small joint arthrodesis. Successful fusion predictably relieves pain and improves strength. Most patients find that the benefits of a stable, painless joint far outweigh the loss of motion. Unsatisfactory results are secondary to complications or unrealistic patient expectations. We avoid the latter problem by a thorough preoperative discussion with the patient about the benefits and drawbacks of a motion-sacrificing procedure.

COMPLICATIONS

There are a number of complications of small joint arthrodesis. Superficial pin-tract infections are treated with antibiotics and generally resolve uneventfully. Persistent infection necessitates early pin removal. Deep infection and osteomyelitis require irrigation, incision, and debridement in addition to long-term antibiotic treatment.

Occasionally, symptomatic hardware may need to be removed after the fusion has healed. Malunion can be prevented by intraoperative attention to detail and nonunion by stable fixation. Nonunion of the PIP joint, although unusual, requires revision arthrodesis.

Nonunion at the DIP joint has been reported, but in our experience this has not been a problem with screw fixation. Cold intolerance has been noted by some patients. In rare instances, there may be vascular compromise when the severely contracted finger is extended to the eventual fusion position. This situation may require additional bone shortening.

RECOMMENDED READING

1. Allende BT, Engelem JC. Tension band arthrodesis in the finger joints. *J Hand Surg* 5:269–271, 1980.
2. Ayres JR, Goldstrohm GL, Miller GJ, et al. Proximal interphalangeal joint arthrodesis with the Herbert screw. *J Hand Surg* 13A:600–603, 1988.
3. Büchler U, Aiken MA. Arthrodesis of the proximal interphalangeal joint by solid bone grafting and plate fixation in extensive injuries to the dorsal aspect of the finger. *J Hand Surg* 13A:589–594, 1988.
4. Burton RJ, Margles SW, Lunseth PA. Small joint arthrodesis in the hand. *J Hand Surg* 11A:678–682, 1986.
5. Carroll RE, Hill NA. Small joint arthrodesis in hand reconstruction. *J Bone Joint Surg* 51A:1219–1221, 1969.
6. Leibovic SJ, Strickland JW. Arthrodesis of the proximal interphalangeal joint of the finger: comparison of the use of the Herbert screw with other fixation methods. *J Hand Surg* 19A:181–188, 1993.
7. Stahl S, Rozen N. Tension-band arthrodesis of the small joints of the hand. *Orthopedics* 10:981–983, 2001.
8. Peimer CA, Putnam MD. Proximal interphalangeal joint following traumatic arthritis. *Hand Clinics* 3:415–416, 1987.

31

Reconstruction for Boutonniere Deformity

James R. Doyle

INDICATIONS/CONTRAINDICATIONS

Boutonniere deformity may result from closed or open injuries, fractures or dislocations, infections, burns, and inflammatory arthropathies in and about the proximal interphalangeal (PIP) joint. Treatment of boutonniere deformity may be open or closed and is based on recognition of the etiology, stage, and pathomechanics of the deformity.

A system of classification is mandatory when discussing treatment indications and contraindications.

In general, in closed, nonflexible boutonniere deformity, conservative treatment is advised in the form of splinting and exercises. Surgery is not required in this type of deformity because conservative treatment is usually successful. Even in a fixed deformity, it is best to defer surgery until the PIP joint contracture is corrected by dynamic splinting and exercises.

In some cases, the fixed deformity cannot be corrected, and reconstruction must include surgical release or simultaneous joint release at the time of boutonniere reconstruction.

Because of the significant variations in the manifestations of boutonniere deformity, the indications/contraindications are presented in Table 31.1.

ETIOLOGY, ONSET, AND DIAGNOSTIC TESTS

Etiology

Disruption of the central slip of the extensor tendon at the PIP joint level, along with volar migration of the lateral bands, results in the so-called "boutonniere deformity," with subsequent loss of extension at the middle joint and compensatory hyperextension at the distal joint. This lesion may be secondary to closed blunt trauma with acute forceful flex-

James R. Doyle, M.D.: Department of Orthopaedic Surgery, John A. Burns School of Medicine, University of Hawaii, Honolulu, HI.

Table 31.1. *Indications/contraindications*

Type	Treatment method	Indications	Contraindications
IA	Dynamic splinting	Supple PIP, DIP joints	Fixed PIP, DIP joints
B	(1) Extensor tenotomy, PIP joint release	(1) Fixed PIP joint, failed splinting	(1–2) Irreparable PIP joint damage, loss of articular cartilage
	(2) PIP joint release, shorten central slip, dorsal transfer of lateral bands	(2) Fixed PIP joint, attenuated central slip	Absence or extreme attenuation of central slip
II	Reduction, fixation fracture	Large fracture fragment	Fixed PIP joint contracture, PIP joint subluxation
III	Reattach central slip	Supple, reduced PIP joint	Fixed PIP joint contracture, joint subluxation
IV	Free tendon graft to central slip	Loss of substance of central slip	Joint instability, chronic infection, loss of articular cartilage, inadequate skin coverage
V	PIP joint arthrodesis	Loss of articular cartilage	Uncontrolled infection, inadequate dorsal skin coverage
VIA	Extensor tenotomy and splinting	Mild deformity (10–15 degree extensor lag at PIP)	Moderate deformity or fixed joint, psoriatic arthritis
B	Extensor tendon shortening and dorsal transfer of lateral bands	Moderate deformity (30–40 degree extensor lag at PIP)	Fixed joint contracture, loss of articular cartilage, psoriatic arthritis
C	Arthrodesis PIP joint	Severe fixed deformity with loss of articular cartilage	Poor skin coverage or infection

PIP, proximal interphalangeal; DIP, distal interphalangeal

ion of the PIP joint, producing avulsion of the central slip from its insertion on the dorsal base of the middle phalanx, with or without fracture and laceration of the extensor tendon at or near its insertion. Volar dislocation of the PIP joint may also result in avulsion of the central slip and subsequent boutonniere deformity. With disruption of the central slip and volar migration of the lateral bands, flexion of the distal joint is markedly decreased. In fresh cadavers, Harris and Rutledge and Micks and Hager observed that section of the central slip alone did not result in the boutonniere deformity. However, the boutonniere deformity did develop if the PIP joint was repetitively flexed while tension was applied to the extrinsic extensor. The lateral bands tore away from the other fibers, producing a boutonniere deformity.

Onset. In closed injuries, the characteristic boutonniere deformity may not be present at the time of injury and usually develops over a 10- to 21-day period following injury. This condition is often missed even in an open wound.

Diagnostic Tests. A painful, tender, and swollen PIP joint that has been recently injured should arouse suspicion. Active motion of the PIP joint is decreased, and the finger is held semiflexed. Boyes noted that early diagnosis may be facilitated by holding the PIP joint in full extension and testing the amount of passive flexion of the distal joint. Rubin et al. said, in a study that used various published clinical tests to diagnose an early boutonniere lesion, that only the Elson test was said to be reliable. This test relies on abnormal tone between the PIP and distal interphalangeal (DIP) joints. Normally, with the PIP joint blocked in flexion, there is limited active extension of the DIP joint. Figure 31.1 demonstrates the clinical appearance and pathomechanics of the boutonniere deformity.

With disruption of the central slip and loss of the check-rein effect, extension of the DIP can occur by tightening the dorsal apparatus. In a boutonniere lesion, attempted active extension of the finger with the PIP joint held in flexion will increase the rigidity of the DIP joint. The Elson test is demonstrated in Fig 31.2.

Clinical Relevance of the Various Diagnostic Tests

Early diagnosis of boutonniere gives the best chance of a satisfactory outcome. Boyes' test becomes positive only at a late stage. The Elson test relies on abnormal tone between

A

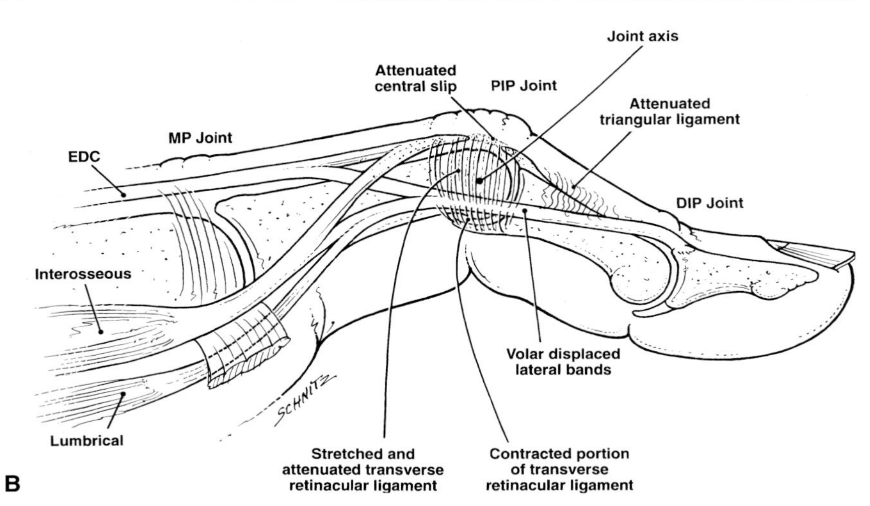

Figure 31.1. A: Chronic boutonniere deformity with extension of the metacarpophalangeal (MCP) joint, a fixed flexion contracture of the proximal interphalangeal (PIP) joint, and an extension contracture of the distal interphalangeal (DIP) joint. **B:** Pathomechanics of the chronic boutonniere deformity: The cascade of deformity begins with attenuation of the central slip of the extensor tendon and subsequent volar migration of the lateral bands below the axis of joint rotation, due to stretching of the dorsal aspect of the transverse retinacular ligaments and the triangular ligament between the central slip and the lateral bands. Subsequent contracture of the volar portion of the transverse retinacular ligaments keeps the lateral bands in this nonanatomic position. The end result is total absence of extension force at the PIP joint and secondary hyperextension at the DIP joint due to contracture of the lateral bands.

the PIP and DIP joints and may be the most reliable test for the early diagnosis of the boutonniere lesion. The diagnosis in these early cases in which the characteristic deformity is not evident is made by noting (a) a 15- to 20-degree or greater loss of active extension at the PIP joint when the wrist and metacarpophalangeal (MCP) joint are fully flexed, (b) weak extension of the middle phalanx against resistance, and (c) loss of passive flexion of the DIP joint when the PIP joint is held in extension. These findings will be present before the characteristic boutonniere deformity is present and always should be looked for in a suspected case of boutonniere deformity.

In the author's practice, the following classification has provided a useful basis for management of this difficult condition. It has helped the author to select the proper treatment and has provided a suitable rationale for closed versus open treatment. Treatment

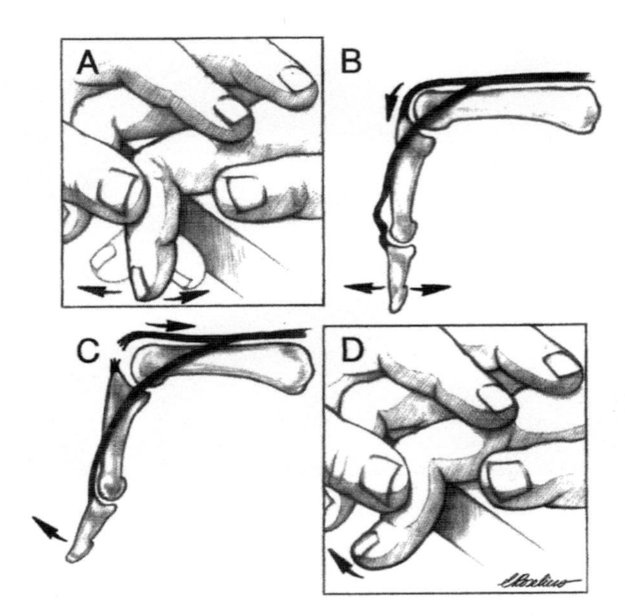

Figure 31.2. The Elson Test. **A, B**: The finger to be examined is flexed comfortably to a right angle at the PIP joint over the edge of a table and firmly held in place by the examiner. The patient is then asked to extend the PIP joint against resistance. Any pressure felt by the examiner over the middle phalanx can only be exerted by an intact central slip (CS). Further proof is that the DIP joint remains flail during the effort, since the competent central slip prevents the lateral bands from acting distally. **C, D**: In the presence of a complete rupture of the CS, any extension effort perceived by the examiner will be accompanied by rigidity at the DIP joint, with a tendency to extension. This is produced by the extensor action of the lateral bands. Note: This test will not demonstrate the presence of a partial rupture of the CS, and it may be impeded by pain or lack of patient cooperation. Consideration may be given to nerve block for pain relief, as indicated. (From: Doyle JR, Botte MJ. *Surgical Anatomy of the Hand and Upper Extremity*. Philadelphia: Lippincott, Williams, and Wilkins, 2002.)

recommendations are based on the following etiologic classification of the boutonniere deformity:

Type I Closed due to blunt trauma
- A: DIP, PIP joints not fixed
- B: DIP, PIP joints fixed

Type II Large avulsion fracture fragment from the dorsal base of the middle phalanx

Type III Palmar dislocation of the PIP joint

Type IV Loss of substance of the central slip due to old, untreated laceration, deep abrasion, or burn

Type V PIP joint infection

Type VI Inflammatory arthropathies
- A: Mild deformity (10–15 degree extension lag at PIP joint)
- B: Moderate deformity (30–40 degree extensor lag at PIP joint)
- C: Severe fixed deformity with loss of articular cartilage

PREOPERATIVE PLANNING

Anteroposterior and lateral radiographs of the entire finger to evaluate the MCP, PIP, and DIP joints are required to evaluate the status of the joints.

Most traumatic boutonniere lesions are due to closed blunt trauma without fracture or dislocation and are due to sudden, forceful flexion of the PIP joint, which avulses the central slip from its insertion on the dorsal base of the middle phalanx. In some closed cases, a small portion of bone is avulsed from the middle phalanx and can be ignored in the treatment plan. It must be noted, however, that this is not the same situation in which a large fragment is avulsed (see Type II).

In the author's experience, the boutonniere deformity seen after closed injuries may not be evident until 10 to 21 days after injury. This condition is often overlooked, but should be suspected in a patient with a painful, tender, and swollen PIP joint that has been recently injured and diagnosed as a "jammed" or "sprained" finger. Radiographs are most often normal. These acute cases secondary to closed blunt trauma, if diagnosed and treated early with splinting, can be successfully corrected in most instances by such splinting. The key to success is to diagnose and treat before the deformity becomes fixed.

NONSURGICAL TREATMENT

Type 1A: Closed Blunt Trauma Without Fixed Deformity

Correction of the deformity is dependent on restoration of the normal tendon balance and precise length relationships of the central slip and the lateral bands, and restoration of the lateral bands to their anatomic position above the axis of rotation of the PIP joint.

Surgical correction of this deformity is technically difficult and not always successful; therefore, it must be recognized that the best treatment of boutonniere deformity is early recognition of the problem and prevention of the natural progression of the lesion into an established and fixed deformity.

This correction may be achieved by progressive static or dynamic splinting of the PIP joint into full extension. Corrective methods include small serial casts or splints, dynamic splints, or an oblique transarticular K-wire inserted across the PIP joint (Fig. 31.3). Whatever method is used to obtain PIP joint extension, the DIP joint must be left free for active and passive flexion exercises, and the splint or cast must not block this DIP joint movement. The earlier the splinting and exercise program is begun, the quicker the correction is achieved.

Results. In my experience, static and/or dynamic splinting in Type IA deformity has usually resulted in nearly complete resolution of the deformity. Patient compliance in the use of the selected splint is mandatory for success, and splinting must be continued until rebalancing of the extensor components has been achieved.

Surgery. Surgery should not be considered a shortcut in these cases and cannot take the place of splinting and exercises. The results in cases that respond to conservative treatment equal or exceed the results of surgery.

Type I B: Closed Blunt Trauma with Fixed Deformity

Even in fixed deformities, a trial of dynamic splinting is worthwhile to see whether the PIP joint can be brought into full extension and the DIP joint actively flexed. Full extension may be achieved even in late cases with persistent splinting if secondary joint changes are not present. If correction cannot be achieved, operative intervention is required, with the understanding that there is damage to the central slip of the extensor and disruption of the transverse retinacular fibers that permit palmar subluxation of the lateral bands, which become fixed in this abnormal position. The lateral bands shorten, and the oblique retinacular ligaments shorten and thicken. All these structures, including the flexor digitorum supeficialis (FDS) and flexor digitorum profundus, produce unopposed PIP joint flexion. In late cases, secondary joint changes can occur, such as palmar plate scarring and contracture and intra-articular fibrosis. The surgical result is more likely to succeed in those patients who have full passive PIP joint extension. In Type I B(1) deformities, the central slip is intact, and in Type I B(2) deformities, the central slip is attenuated.

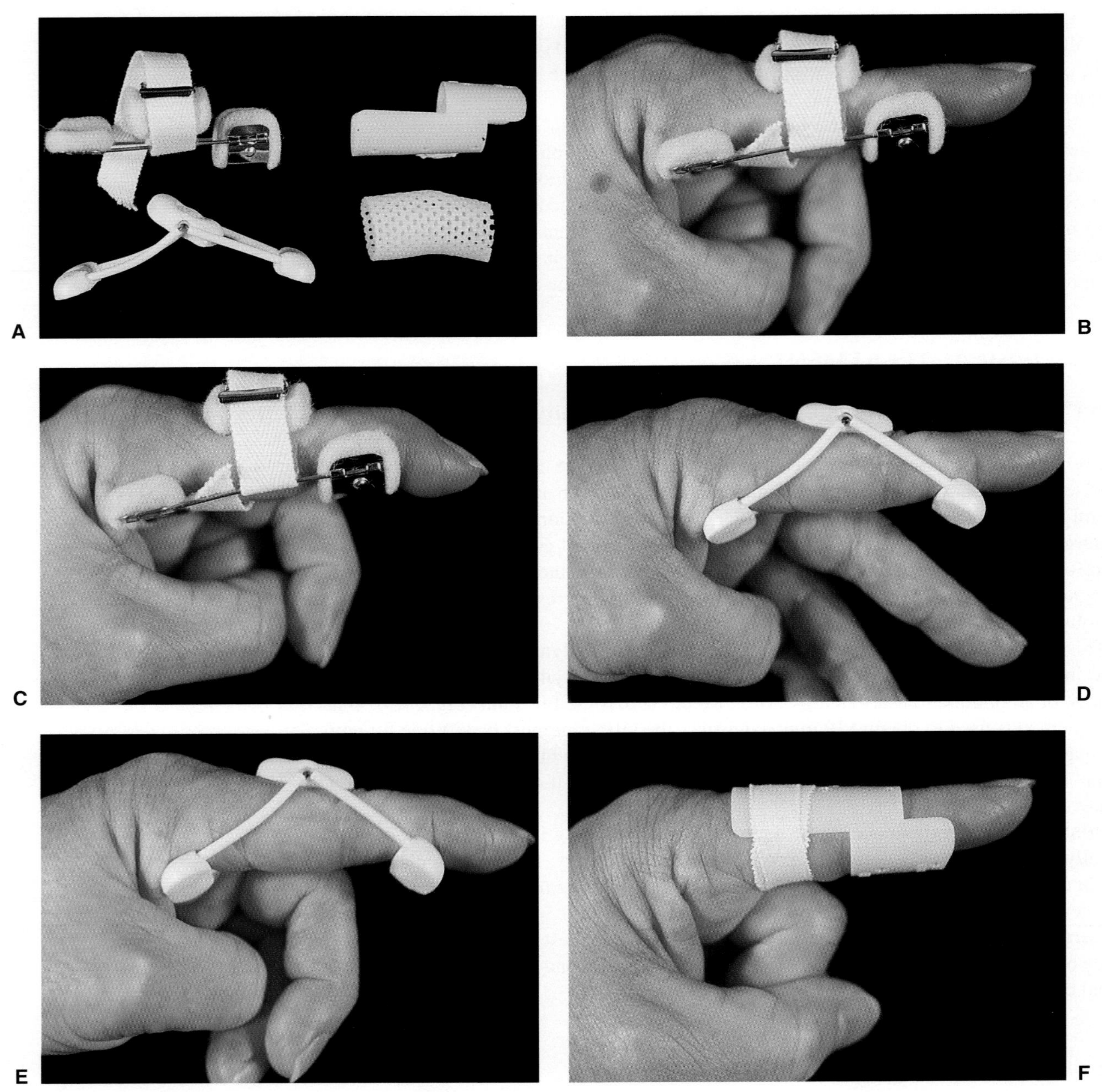

Figure 31.3. A: Various methods of splinting may be used for rebalancing the extensor mechanism. All the splints use the principle of three-point fixation, with the proximal and distal fixation points being palmar and the third point dorsal at or proximal to the proximal interphalangeal (PIP) joint. Useful splints in my practice are the safety-pin splint (*upper left*); the Link boutonniere splint (*upper right*); the LMB splint (*lower left*); custom-made perforated plastic splint (*lower right*). The first three splints are available in various sizes to fit each digit. Both static and dynamic methods require that the distal interphalangeal (DIP) joint be left free for active and passive flexion exercises. These methods, if applied appropriately before irreversible joint fibrosis, will correct the Type 1A boutonnière deformity by restoring the appropriate anatomic length of the central slip and the dorsal position of the lateral bands at the PIP joint. **B, C**: The safety-pin splint is held in place by a strap and buckle placed over or just proximal to the PIP joint. The strap is progressively tightened until full passive PIP joint extension is obtained. All splints are positioned so that active and passive DIP joint flexion can be performed. **D, E**: The LMB splint in place. The plastic-covered proximal and distal wire limbs may be bent to obtain the appropriate amount of extension force on the PIP joint. **F, G**: The Link boutonniere splint is a static splint and is most useful in boutonniere deformities that are passively correctable to full extension at the PIP joint.

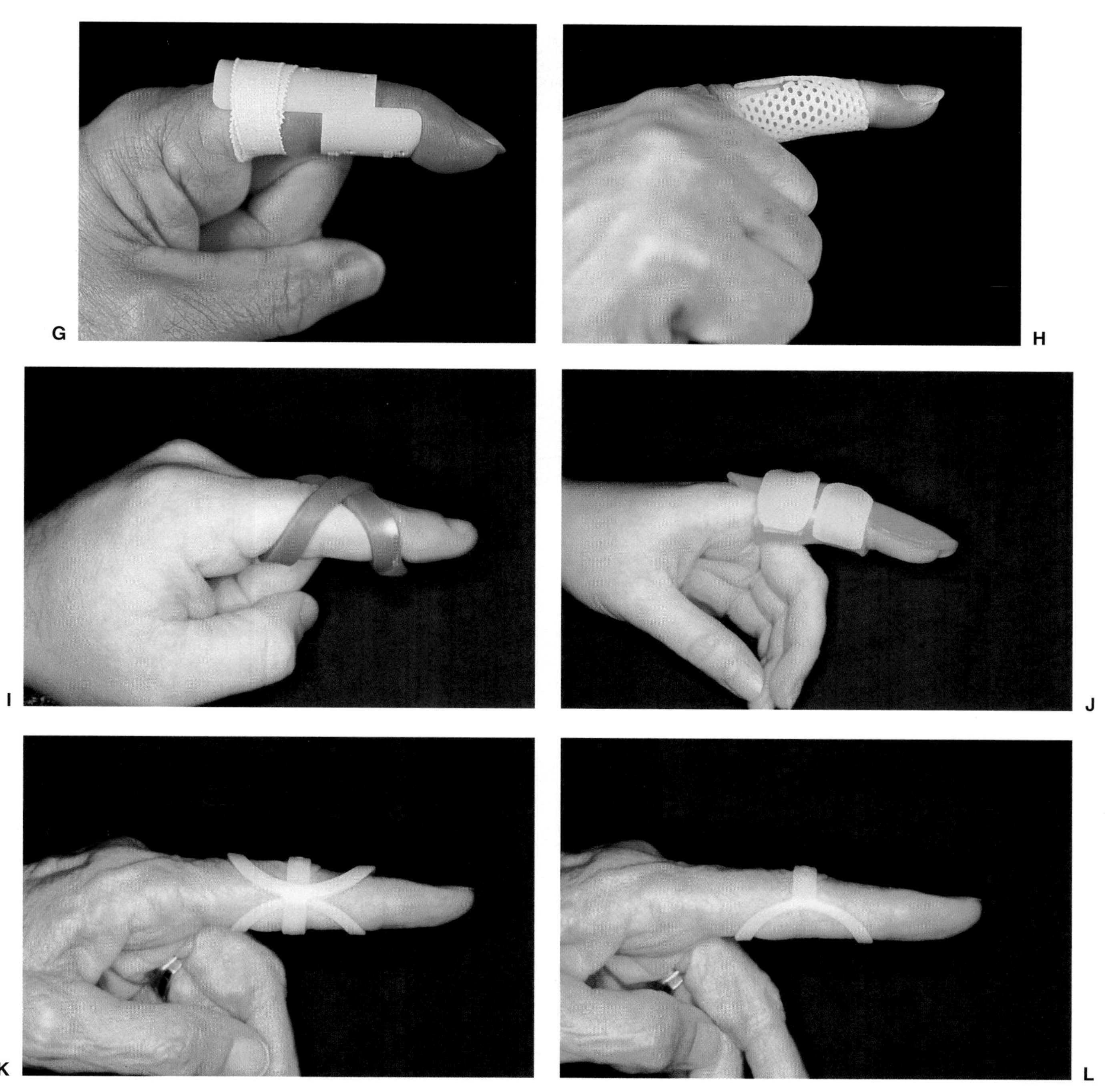

Figure 31.3. *Continued.* **H:** Serial custom-made splints of plastic or plaster of paris are useful in patients that, for one reason or another, might not be suitable candidates for any of the other splints. These custom-made splints are changed once or twice each week as the PIP joint is progressively brought into extension. **I, J**: Two other custom-made splints are demonstrated here. One is a plastic cylinder with Velcro straps, and the second is a figure-of- eight three-point fixation splint (both splints courtesy of Valley Hand Rehabilitation and Ergonomic Center, Napa, CA). **K, L**: This commercially available finger splint, called the Oval-8, is available from 3-Point Products, 1610 Pincay Court, Annapolis, MD 21401. These finger splints are available in multiple sizes and may be used in a single or double configuration.

Type 1B(1): Central Slip Intact

With the patient under appropriate anesthesia and tourniquet control, and the arm resting on a hand table, a 2.5-cm longitudinal incision is made at the midportion of the middle phalanx. The underlying extensor mechanism is identified and freed from the osseous phalanx by a small, curved elevator, along with sharp dissection as needed using a No. 64 Beaver blade. The entire mechanism must be freed for a distance of 1.5 cm over the middle phalanx, after which it is incised from ulnar to radial, with care taken to preserve the oblique retinacular ligament on the radial side. The incision of the extensor mechanism is at the middle third of the middle phalanx. The PIP joint is passively extended and the DIP joint passively flexed, which results in separation of the just-incised extensor (Fig. 31.4A). If the PIP joint cannot be fully extended at this time, the incision is extended proximally over the PIP joint to the midportion of the proximal phalanx. Flaps are reflected down to the flexor

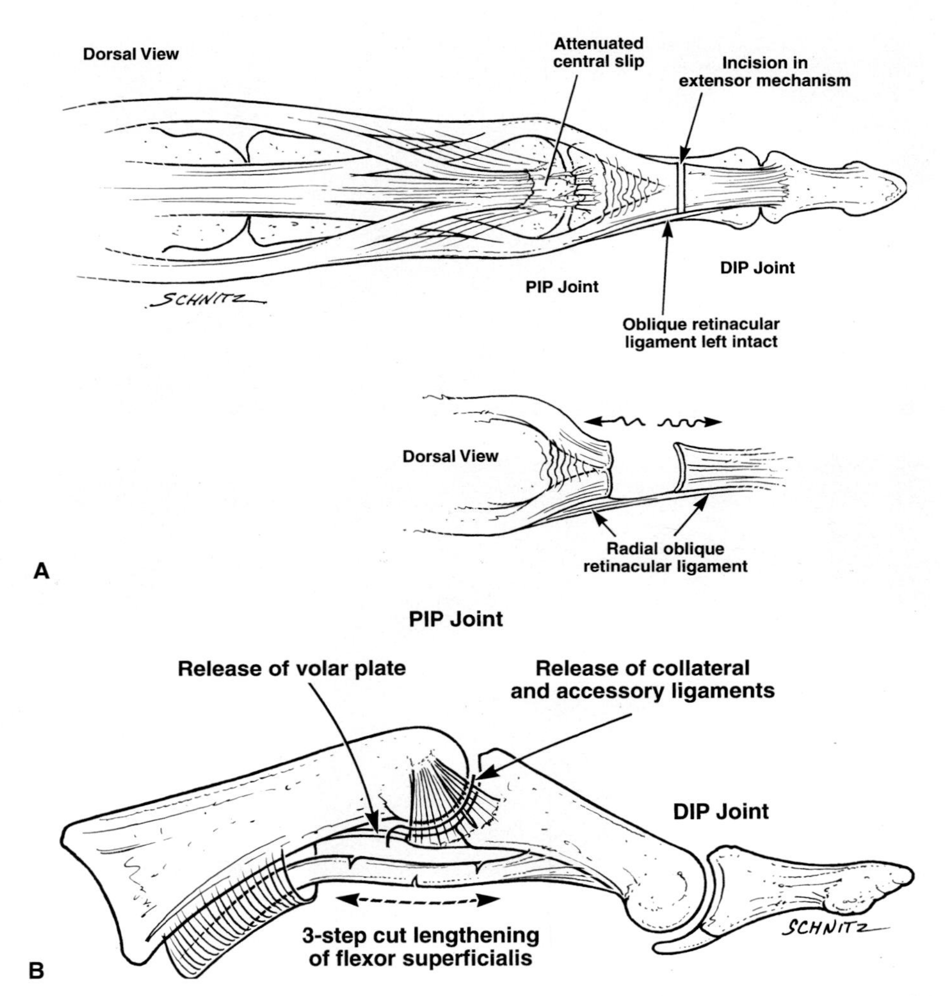

Figure 31.4. In type 1 B deformity, two surgical approaches are useful. **A:** Release of the extensor mechanism over the middle phalanx through a longitudinal approach, with release of the extensor mechanism in the middle third of the middle phalanx. The radial oblique retinacular ligament must be preserved to maintain extension of the DIP joint. **B:** If the PIP joint cannot be fully extended after these maneuvers, the incision is extended proximally to the midportion of the proximal phalanx, and flaps are reflected to each side to expose the flexor aspect of the PIP joint on each side. Through a small window between the C-1 and A-3 pulleys, the proximal edge of the volar plate is identified and the check-rein ligaments released with a No. 64 Beaver blade. If passive PIP joint extension is still incomplete, the collateral ligaments are lengthened on each side, along with step-cut release of each slip of the superficialis tendon.

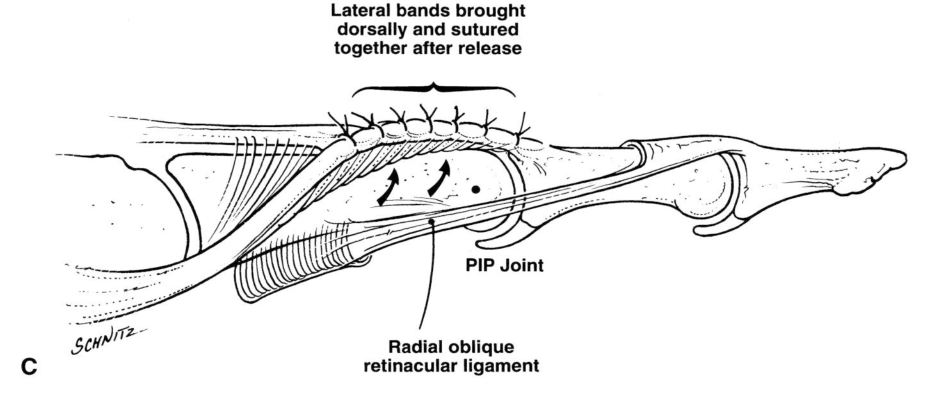

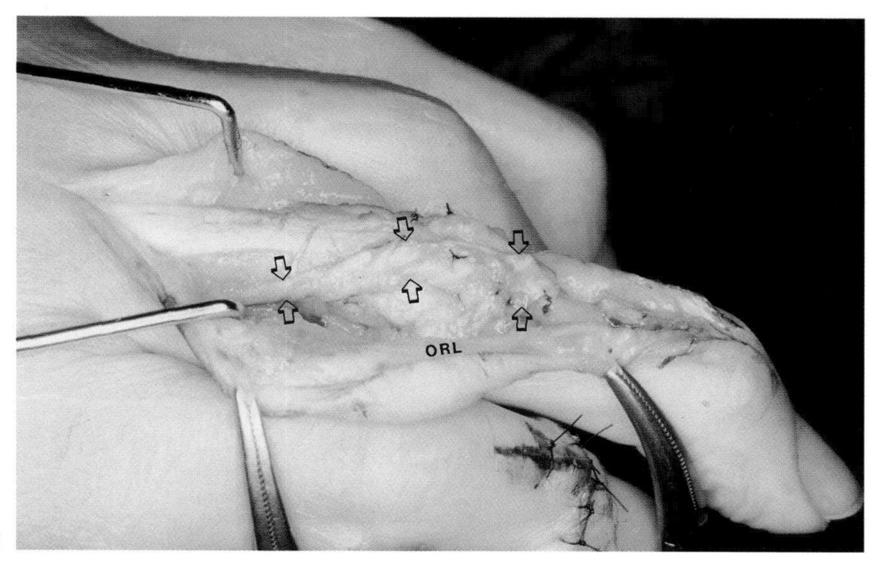

Figure 31.4. *Continued.* **C:** In cases with significant stretching or laxity of the central slip, the lateral bands, after division, are brought dorsally and sutured to the remnants of the central slip, which converts an abnormal flexion force into an extension force. **D:** The opposing arrows demonstrate the dorsally transposed radial lateral band, which is sutured to its ulnar counterpart over the PIP joint.

side of the digit on each side. A small window is made in the flexor sheath on each side of the PIP joint, the proximal edge of the palmar plate is identified, and the check-rein ligaments are released using a No. 64 Beaver blade. This window is usually between the C-l and A-3 pulleys, and the A-3 pulley should be preserved to avoid increasing the moment arm of the flexor tendons about the PIP joint and thus promote a recurrence of the flexion deformity. In addition to the volar plate release, it is often necessary to release the collateral ligaments, including the fan-like accessory collateral ligament and the cord-like proper collateral ligament. It also may be necessary to lengthen the two slips of the FDS (Fig. 31.4B). If the remaining oblique retinacular ligament is tight and is preventing full PIP joint extension, it can be lengthened in its proximal aspect by a similar step-cut incision, followed by passive manipulation of the PIP joint into full extension. The incised lateral bands and extensor mechanism are allowed to seek their own position.

Postoperative Management/Rehabilitation. The PIP joint is splinted in full extension, and the DIP joint is left free to flex actively. If a flexion posture is noted at the DIP joint, this joint is splinted in full extension between exercises. Splinting of the PIP joint is continued for 6 to 8 weeks, or until maximum extension has been obtained.

Results. In the author's experience, extensor tenotomy has been useful in the redistribution of the extensor mechanism forces about the PIP and DIP joints. It may result in a slight flexion posture at both the PIP and DIP joints that is functionally and cosmetically acceptable. Although full extension of the PIP and DIP joints is seldom obtained, most patients are happy to exchange the boutonniere deformity for a slight flexion posture at these joints.

Type I B(2): Central Slip Attenuated

In cases with significant stretching or attenuation of the central slip, the lateral bands, after division (as noted in Fig. 31.4A), are freed on each side and brought dorsally and sutured to the remnants of the central slip, thus converting the abnormal flexion force to an extension force (Fig. 31.4C and D). The radial oblique retinacular ligament is carefully separated from the adjacent radial lateral band by sharp dissection with a No. 64 Beaver blade and is left intact in its normal location to provide for extension of the DIP joint; PIP extension results in increased tension on the oblique retinacular ligament, which extends the DIP joint. After this repair, it is important to verify that passive flexion of the PIP joint to 60 degrees can be obtained; if not, some of the dorsal sutures used to maintain the lateral bands on the dorsum of the PIP joint must be removed. An oblique transarticular 0.045 K-wire is used to maintain the joint in extension to protect the repair. This procedure is contraindicated if the central slip is absent or too attenuated to accept sutures; if this is the case, a free tendon graft is required. (see Type V repair). In some cases, the attenuated central slip may be shortened by excising the pseudotendinous tissue interposed between the central slip and its normal site of attachment. The central slip is freed on each side, advanced to its normal insertion, and reattached (Fig. 31.5). Advancement of the central slip is facilitated by proximal tenolysis as needed. Passive flexion of the PIP joint to 60 degrees indicates that the reinsertion is not too tight. Shortening and reattachment of the central slip are performed before and in addition to the dorsal transposition of the lateral bands as described above.

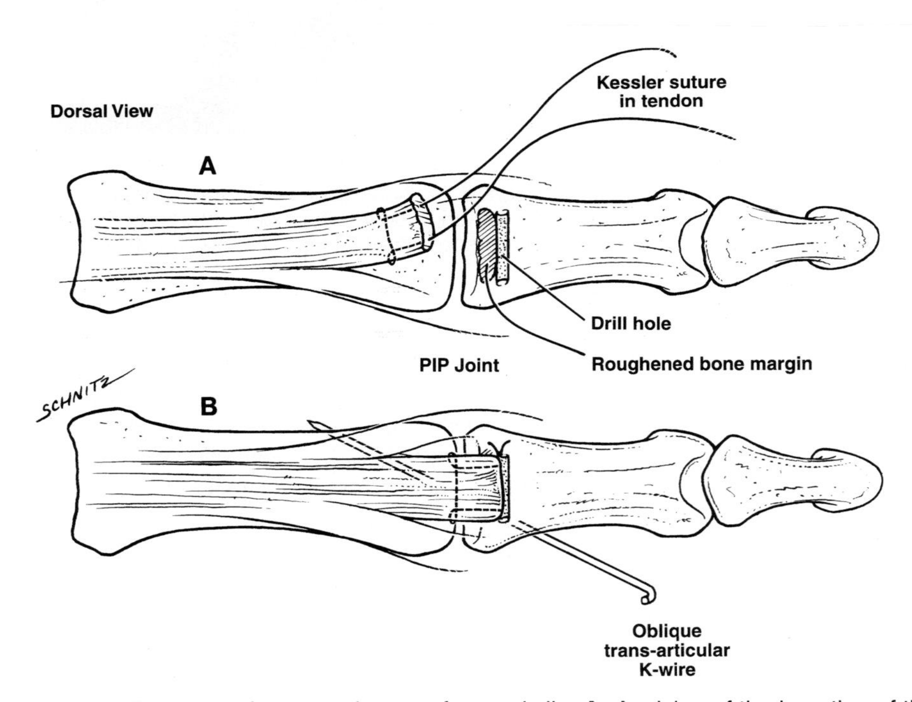

Figure 31.5. Technique for reattachment of central slip. **A:** Avulsion of the insertion of the central slip requires firm reattachment to bone and is best performed by a grasping-type suture in the central slip, which is tied through a small drill hole in the dorsal base of the middle phalanx. Reattachment is promoted by curetting the bone at the tendon-insertion site. **B:** Appropriate tension at the repair site may be determined in the operating room by noting the position of the PIP joint in comparison to adjacent digits and whether or not 60 degrees of passive flexion can be obtained after repair. The joint is immobilized in full extension by an oblique transarticular Kirschner wire.

Postoperative Management/Rehabilitation. Immediate postoperative care includes active flexion exercises at the DIP joint. The PIP joint K-wire is left in place for four weeks, after which it is removed and active range-of-motion exercises to the PIP joint begun. The PIP joint is splinted in extension between exercises for 2 to 4 months.

Results. Although expectations for this procedure may be slightly less than in those cases with an intact central slip, as noted above, the cosmetic and functional improvement is usually significant. Complete PIP joint extension is seldom obtained, but most patients appreciate the improved motion and function in both the PIP and DIP joints.

Type II: Boutonniere Deformity Due to Avulsion of the Central Slip with a Large Bone Fragment

The operative site is exposed through a 4.0-cm curved dorsal incision centered over the PIP joint. The bone fragment attached to the central slip is freed from the surrounding soft tissues, but care is taken to preserve its attachment to the central slip. It is then anatomically reduced and fixed with a nonabsorbable lasso suture or one or two 0.028 K-wires placed through the fracture fragment into the middle phalanx. The key factor for success is to restore accurately the normal length relationships between the central slip and lateral bands, and to reattach securely the tendon to bone. If the bone fragment is too small to reattach, I carefully excise the small fragment and use a Kessler-type grasping suture in the tendon of 4-0 nylon or similar suture, which is passed through a small transverse drill hole in the dorsal base of the middle phalanx and tied securely (Fig. 31.5). The repair is protected by maintaining the PIP joint in full extension with an oblique 0.045 transarticular K-wire or by splinting.

Postoperative Management/Rehabilitation. Immobilization in full extension is continued until the fracture has healed and/or the tendon has reattached to bone (usually three to four weeks). Protected range of motion should be started at that time.

Results. Because of the probability for earlier diagnosis and treatment, this type of boutonniere carries a more favorable prognosis than Type I B or other boutonniere deformities with significant disruption of the central slip. If seen and treated early, nearly full restoration of function can be anticipated.

Type III: Volar Dislocation of the PIP Joint

Although volar dislocations of the PIP joint are rare injuries, they may be associated with injury to the extensor mechanism and a subsequent boutonniere deformity. It is important to note that there are two types of volar dislocations: One type is most often associated with significant disruption of the central slip of the extensor tendon. The most common type of dislocation is due to a rotatory longitudinal compression force on a semiflexed middle phalanx, and results in unilateral disruption of a collateral ligament and partial avulsion of the volar plate. The proximal phalanx condyle on the affected side usually ruptures through the interval between the central slip and adjacent lateral band. Although this particular type of dislocation may result in some trapping of the surrounding soft tissues about the neck of the proximal phalanx, reduction can usually be achieved by traction with the MP and PIP joints in flexion, accompanied by reversal of the malrotation deformity in the middle phalanx. After reduction, active extension of the PIP joint is tested and, if intact, indicates that the central slip is probably intact and a boutonniere deformity probably will not occur. In contrast to the rotatory-type dislocation, if the dislocation is straight volar without a rotatory component, the central slip is more likely to rupture; if it is not recognized and treated within 2 weeks of the injury, a progressive boutonniere is inevitable.

Although an argument can be made for splinting the PIP in full extension without surgical repair of the central slip after reduction of the volar dislocation, it is my practice and recommendation in this type of dislocation to repair the central slip by reattaching it to the dorsal base of the middle phalanx. Through a 4-cm-long, slightly curved incision centered over the PIP joint, the central slip is identified and released from any abnormal soft-tissue attachments. Then it is brought distally and attached to the dorsal base of the middle phalanx using a Kessler-type suture through a small drill hole (Fig. 31.5). An oblique 0.045 transarticular K-wire is used to immobilize the PIP joint in full extension.

Postoperative Management/Rehabilitation. Active flexion of the DIP joint begins immediately after repair. The K-wire is removed after 3 to 4 weeks, and the PIP joint is gradually mobilized. The PIP joint is splinted in full extension when it is not being exercised, and splinting may be required for several months.

Results. Boutonniere deformities that result secondary to volar dislocations carry a poor prognosis, especially in volar dislocations that are neglected and require extensive soft-tissue release to reduce the joint. Full extension and flexion are seldom obtained, and the patient should be so advised.

Type IV: Boutonniere Due to Loss of Substance of the Central Slip

This type of deformity may be due to an old, untreated laceration, a deep abrasion, or a burn that destroys the continuity of the extensor mechanism over the PIP joint. Treatment is complicated by the fact that the joint may be open, with exposed bone and cartilage, a contaminated joint space, and absent or unstable skin and subcutaneous tissue coverage. Some form of central slip reconstruction must be done, either by release and dorsal transposition of the lateral bands to the dorsal base of the middle phalanx (Fig. 31.4C), or by complete reconstruction of the central slip by a free tendon graft inserted into the proximal portions of the extensor and inserted into the dorsal base of the middle phalanx (Fig. 31.6). If the lateral bands are attenuated, partially destroyed, or severely scarred, it may be best to perform a free tendon graft rather than to attempt dorsal transposition of the lateral bands. In cases with inadequate or unstable skin coverage, appropriate skin and subcutaneous tissue coverage must be obtained before tendon reconstruction. In late cases with chronic infection with joint destruction or in severe deformities after a burn, arthrodesis is the procedure of choice (Fig. 31.7). The resultant bone shortening with arthrodesis sometimes will permit excision of marginal skin coverage over the PIP joint at the same time. If the DIP joint remains in fixed extension after PIP arthrodesis, an extensor tenotomy is performed over the middle phalanx, as previously described for Type lB deformity (Fig. 31.4A).

Central Slip Reconstruction by Tendon Graft

Central slip reconstruction is performed through a dorsal incision beginning at the dorsal base of the proximal phalanx and continuing distally to the midportion of the middle phalanx. The distal end of the central slip is identified and freed from any adhesions in the proximal phalanx. If full PIP joint extension is not present, joint release must be performed as previously described (Fig. 31.4B). The radial and ulnar lateral bands are freed from any soft-tissue attachments that might keep them below the PIP joint axis. A free tendon graft, 8- to 10-cm long, is obtained either from the palmaris longus or an accessory slip of the extensor digiti minimi. An interweave technique is used to attach the graft to the proximal portion of the central slip (Fig. 31.6A). The distal aspect of the graft is split into two tails, which are passed through a transverse drill hole in the dorsal base of the middle phalanx. The two tails are brought back proximally and sutured together over the neck of the proximal phalanx. Tension of the graft is determined by noting nearly full extension of the PIP joint with the finger at rest and 60 degrees of passive flexion of the PIP joint. If the lateral bands do not lie above the axis of the PIP joint, they are loosely sutured to the margins of the central slip reconstruction. An oblique transarticular 0.045 K-wire is placed to immobilize the PIP joint in extension.

Postoperative Management/Rehabilitation. Active flexion exercises of the DIP joint are started in the immediate postoperative period. The PIP joint K-wire is removed after 3 to 4 weeks, and active PIP joint flexion and extension exercises are started. The pa-

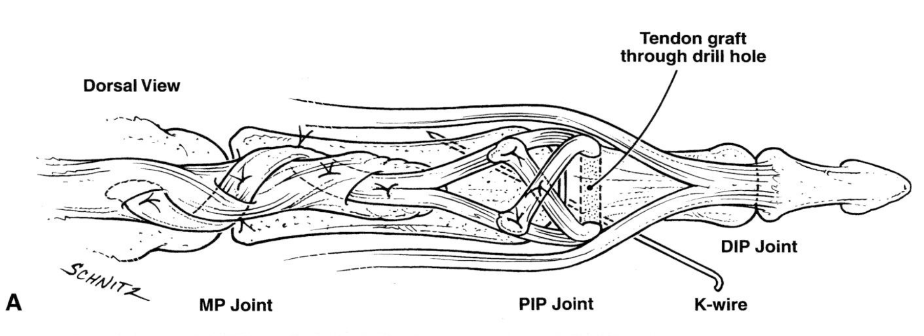

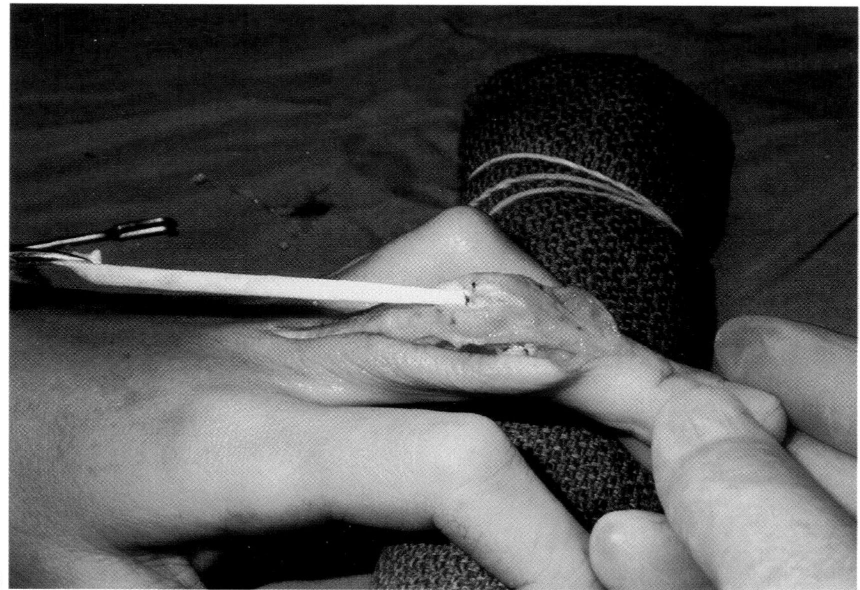

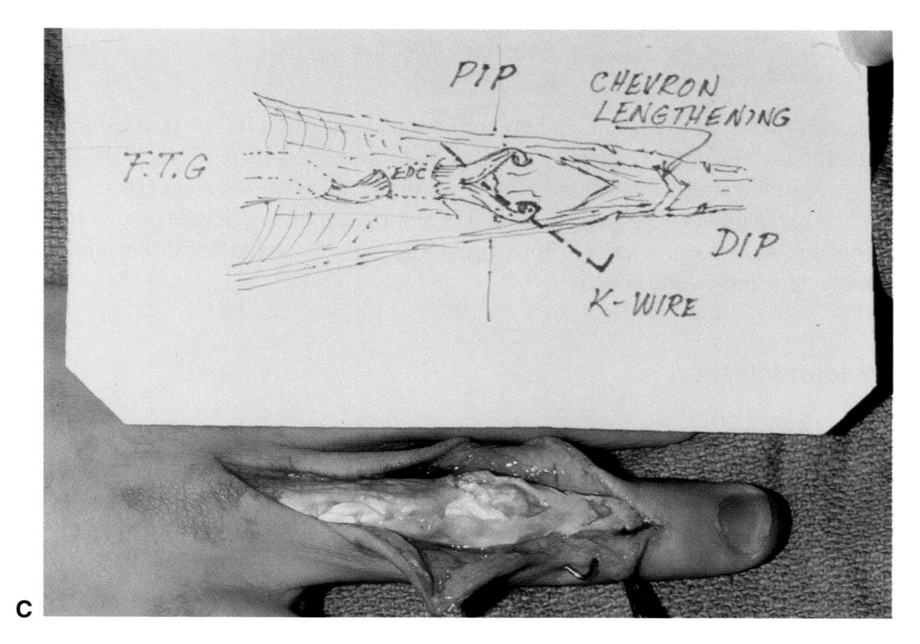

Figure 31.6. A: In digits with complete loss of substance of the central slip and in which the lateral bands are also absent or severely compromised, a free tendon graft is required for restoration of the central slip of the extensor tendon. **B:** The palmaris longus or similar-size tendon is split into two tails distally, which are passed in opposing directions through a transverse drill hole in the dorsal base of the middle phalanx and then sutured back to themselves in a crossover pattern. **C:** The graft then is woven into the proximal remnants of the central slip. An oblique transarticular Kirschner wire is used for 3 to 4 weeks, followed by active exercises and splinting. Lengthening of the extensor mechanism over the DIP joint is required for correction of the hyperextension deformity, but care is taken to preserve at least one oblique retinacular ligament, which may be done by chevron-shaped incisions or an incision as in Figure 31.3-A to lengthen the extensor mechanism over the middle phalanx.

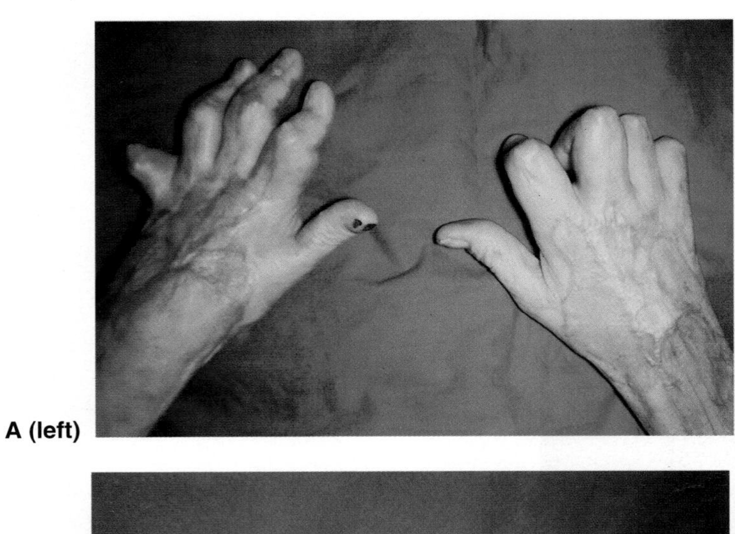

A (left)

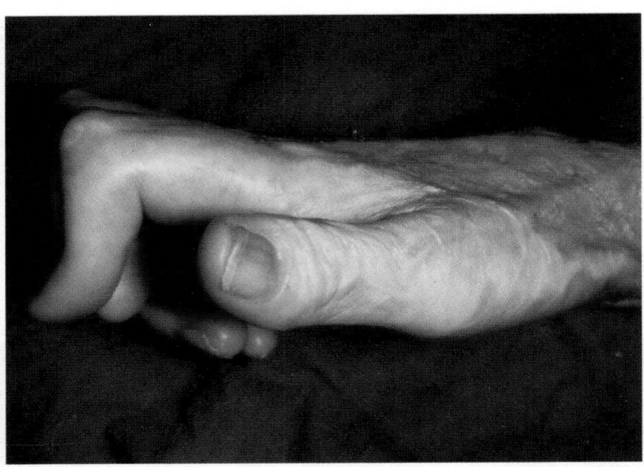

(right)

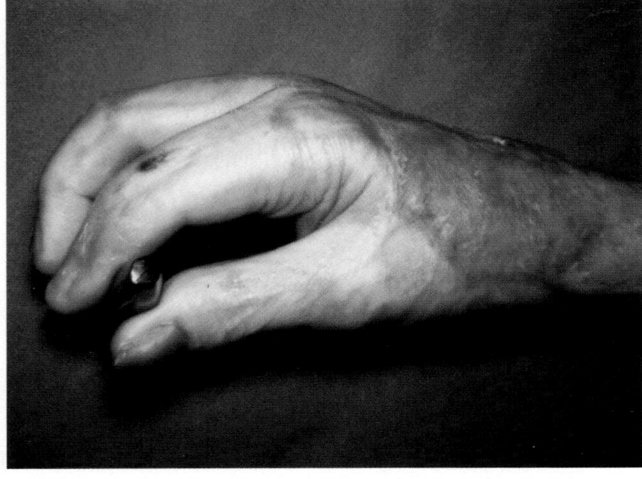

B

Figure 31.7. A: Severe irreparable boutonniere contractures following a thermal burn. **B:** Result following arthrodesis of the PIP joints of the right hand with improved position and function.

tient is instructed to hold the proximal phalanx in flexion as the PIP joint is extended to direct the force of the extensor more distally and thus to promote extension of the PIP joint. The PIP joint is splinted in full extension between these exercises for several weeks.

Results. Full extension or flexion is seldom, if ever, obtained in this severe type of boutonniere deformity and reconstruction. However, most patients are grateful for the improved cosmetic appearance and function.

Type V: PIP Joint Infection

Boutonniere deformity may be seen as a complication of pyogenic arthritis of the PIP joint and usually is seen as a late complication of untreated cases. Pus under pressure in the PIP joint escapes the dorsum of the joint, which is the path of least resistance. The extensor mechanism is attenuated and eventually destroyed. Early treatment is preventive and relates to management of the infection. In late cases, if the joint articular cartilage has not been destroyed and the joint is not fixed, it may be possible to achieve some correction by extensor tenotomy in the midportion of the middle phalanx, as described for Type lB.

If the joint is destroyed, it is best to fuse the PIP joints in a cascade of 5-degree increments, beginning with 25 to 30 degrees at the index and ending with 40 to 45 degrees in the little finger, along with extensor tenotomy as previously described over the middle phalanx if a DIP joint hyperextension deformity is present. These recommended arthrodesis angles should be tailored to the functional needs of the individual patient.

Results. The results of extensor tenotomy are as noted under Type IB. However, an arthritic joint due to the infection may be painful and ultimately require fusion. The results following arthrodesis are usually associated with improved cosmetic appearance and improved function due to improved and functional positioning of the joints and pain relief.

Type VI: Chronic Boutonniere Due to Inflammatory Arthropathies

The most common inflammatory arthropathy that causes boutonniere deformity is rheumatoid arthritis, although this deformity can also be associated with psoriatic arthritis and systemic lupus erythematosus. In my experience, soft-tissue procedures or arthroplasty in psoriatic arthritis for the correction of boutonniere deformity have not been successful, and arthrodesis or splinting and exercises are the procedures of choice for the management of boutonniere deformity in psoriatic arthritis. It must be appreciated that surgery for boutonnière deformity in rheumatoid arthritis is surgery performed in a chronic and progressive disease and, therefore, is less likely to produce a permanent result due to the progressive nature of the underlying disease. Boutonniere deformity due to rheumatoid arthritis may be mild, and there is only a slight PIP joint extension lag of 10 to 15 degrees and minimal to slight hyperextension of the DIP joint, in which the major functional loss is due to loss of flexion of the DIP joint (Type VI A). Moderate deformity is characterized by 30- to 40-degree extensor lag at the PIP joint (Type VI B), and severe deformity by a fixed boutonnière posture with loss of articular cartilage (Type VI C).

Type VI A: Mild Finger Deformity

Mild deformities can be treated with extensor tenotomy, as previously described for Type I B(1) deformities, followed by PIP joint splinting and active flexion of the DIP joint (Fig. 31.4).

Postoperative Management/Rehabilitation. Splinting and exercises are as described for Type I B(1) boutonniere.

Results. Similar to IB(1) deformity, but useful results may diminish due to progression of the disease.

Type VI B: Moderate Finger Deformity

If the PIP joint deformity is more significant (30–40 degrees), the central slip of the extensor tendon is shortened (4–6 mm), and the lateral bands are freed and brought dorsally (Fig. 31.4C).

Postoperative Management/Rehabilitation. Splinting and exercises are as described for type I B (2) boutonniere.

Results. Similar to IB (1). Success is most likely if there is good dorsal skin, good PIP joint surfaces, intact flexor tendons, and a nonfixed deformity at the PIP joint.

Type VI C: Severe Finger Deformity

In severe fixed deformities with articular surface damage and loss of joint space, arthrodesis or arthroplasty is indicated; arthrodesis is the more predictable of the two procedures. If arthroplasty is chosen, the central slip must be reconstructed and adjusted to its proper length. Reconstruction may be performed using the lateral bands brought dorsally or by a free tendon graft as previously described (Figs. 31.4C and 6A).

Postoperative Management/Rehabilitation. Splinting and exercise are as described for Type I B(2) if arthroplasty is chosen. In arthrodesis, the joint is immobilized until fusion has occurred.

Results. Function and cosmetic appearance may be improved, but progression of the disease may adversely affect long-term results.

BOUTONNIERE DEFORMITY OF THE THUMB

The preceding comments have applied specifically to the boutonniere deformity of the fingers that occurs at the PIP joint. Although thumb boutonniere deformity is quite common in inflammatory arthropathies, especially rheumatoid arthritis, a less-common traumatic form of boutonniere deformity may occur at the thumb MP joint secondary to dorsoradial capsular injury with a partial tear, attenuation, or avulsion of the attachment of the extensor pollicis brevis (EPB). This injury allows subluxation and retraction of the extensor pollicis longus (EPL) tendon that causes an extensor lag at the MP joint and hyperextension at the interphalangeal (IP) joint. In thumb boutonniere, the displaced EPL mimics the action of the displaced lateral bands in the finger boutonniere. Established traumatic boutonniere deformity of the thumb is best treated by advancement of the EPB tendon and realignment of the EPL by imbrication of the MP joint capsule. Isolated ulnar subluxation of the EPL may cause a form of "pseudoboutonniere" deformity of the thumb.

Results. In the author's limited experience with this rare type of boutonniere, the deformity may be improved, but not completely corrected, especially in long-standing cases.

COMPLICATIONS

Nonsurgical Treatment

The following complications may occur:

1. Failure to recognize and treat this injury before the PIP joint develops a fixed contracture that requires extensive surgery to correct. Most closed boutonniere-type injuries not associated with fracture or dislocation of the PIP joint, if recognized and treated within 3 to 4 weeks of injury with splinting and exercises, can be expected to recover nearly normal function.
2. Overzealous application of force instead of intermittent, progressive tension over the PIP joint with the splint, which may produce skin necrosis.
3. If transarticular K-wires are used for fixation of the PIP joint, the entry site must be kept clean and dry to avoid pin-tract and joint infections.
4. These K-wires also may break and should be protected by a splint to avoid this potential complication. Complications 3 and 4 also apply to surgical treatment.
5. Finally, the splint must be applied so that active and passive flexion of the DIP joint can be performed while the PIP joint is in extension. If the splint is placed too far distally and the DIP joint cannot flex, correction will not be achieved.

Surgical Treatment

Several complications of surgical treatment are worthy of mention and include the following:

1. A high failure and recurrence rate in the management of this disorder. This is especially true in advanced deformities, as most commonly seen in rheumatoid arthritis. The results in these cases are unpredictable and often disappointing. Patients with severe deformities, rigid deformities, or failed boutonniere reconstructions should be left alone or offered an arthrodesis.
2. Failure to leave at least one oblique retinacular ligament intact when performing a tenotomy of the extensor mechanism over the middle phalanx. Failure to do so will result in a mallet finger deformity at the DIP joint.

3. Central slip reconstructions that are too tight. When reconstructing the central slip over the PIP joint by dorsal transfer of the lateral bands or insertion of a free tendon graft, it is important to be sure that the reconstruction is not too tight. Passive flexion must be tested and tension of the repair adjusted so that at least 60 degrees of PIP joint flexion can be achieved with the wrist in neutral and the MCP joint in full extension.
4. Premature discontinuance of splinting and exercises. Both the patient and surgeon must realize that postoperative splinting and exercises must not be discontinued prematurely, because prolonged splinting may be required to achieve rebalancing of these critical joint linkages. Resumption of splinting and exercises may be required if there is recurrence of the deformity, especially in cases of free tendon graft or dorsal reconstruction by transposition of the lateral bands.

RECOMMENDED READING

1. Bowers WH, Wolf J, Bittinger S, et al. The proximal interphalangeal joint. I. An anatomic and biochemical study. *J Hand Surg* 5-A:79–88, 1980.
2. Boyes JH. *Bunnell's Surgery of the Hand*, 5th ed. Philadelphia: JB Lippincott 1970: 439–442, 616–618.
3. Carducci AT. Potential boutonniere deformity: its recognition and treatment. *Orthop Rev* 10:121–123, 1981.
4. Cardon LJ, Toh S, Tsubo K. Traumatic boutonniere deformity of the thumb. *J Hand Surg* 25B:505–508, 2000.
5. Churchill M, Citron N. Isolated subluxation of the extensor pollicis longus tendon-A cause of 'boutonniere' deformity of the thumb. *J Hand Surg* 22B:790–792, 1997.
6. Dray G J, Eaton RG. Dislocations and ligament injuries in the digit. In: Green DP, ed. *Operative Hand Surgery*, 3rd ed. New York: Churchill Livingstone, 1993:767–798.
7. Eaton RG. *Joint Injuries of the Hand*. Springfield, IL: Charles C. Thomas, 1971.
8. Elson RA. Rupture of the central slip of the extensor hood. *J Bone Joint Surg* 68B:229–231, 1986.
9. Evans RB. Therapeutic management of extensor-tendon injuries. *Hand Clinics* 2:157–169, 1986.
10. Feldon P, Terrono AL, Nalebuff, EA, et al. Rheumatoid arthritis and other connective tissue diseases. In: Green DP, ed. *Operative Hand Surgery*, 4th ed. New York: Churchill Livingstone, 1999:1717– 1723.
11. Fowler SB. The management of tendon injuries. *J Bone Joint Surg* 41A:579–580, 1959.
12. Garroway RY, Hurst LC, Leppard J, et al. Complex dislocation of the proximal interphalangeal joint. *Orthop Rev* 8:21–28, 1984.
13. Grant IR. Irreducible rotational anterior dislocation of the proximal interphalangeal joint. A spin-drier injury. *J Hand Surg* 18B:648–651, 1993.
14. Green DP, Butler TE Jr. Fractures and dislocations in the hand. In: Rockwood and Green's *Fractures in Adults*. Philadelphia: Lippincott-Raven, 1996.
15. Groenevelt F, Schoori R. Reconstructive surgery of the post-burn boutonniere deformity. *J Hand Surg* 1IB:23–30, 1986.
16. Harris C, Rutledge GL Jr. The functional anatomy of the extensor mechanism of the finger. *J Bone Joint Surg* 54A:713–726, 1972.
17. Imatami J, Hashizume H, Wake H, et al. The central slip attachment fracture. *J Hand Surg* 22B:107–109, 1997.
18. Kiefhaber TR, Strickland JW. Soft tissue reconstruction for rheumatoid swan neck and boutonniere deformities: long term results. *J Hand Surg* 18A:984–989, 1993.
19. Littler JW. Extensor tendon injuries. In: Converse JM, ed. *Reconstructive Plastic Surgery*, vol. 6. Philadelphia: WB Saunders, 1977:3166–3214.
20. Lovett WL, McCalla MA. Management and rehabi1itation extensor tendon injuries. *Orthop Clin North Am* 14:811–826, 1983.
21. McCue FC, Honner R, Johnson MD et al. Athletic injuries of the proximal interphalangeal joint requiring surgery. *J Bone Joint Surg* 52-A:937–955, 1970.
22. Micks JE, Hager D. Role of the controversial parts of the extensor of the finger. *J Bone Joint Surg* 55A:884, 1955.
23. Peimer CA, Sullivan DJ, Wild WR. Palmar dislocation of the proximal interphalangeal joint. *J Hand Surg* 9A:39–48, 1984.
24. Rubin J, Bozentha DJ, Bora FW. Diagnosis of closed central-slip injuries. *J Hand Surg* 21B: 614–616, 1996.
25. Spinner M, Choi BY. Anterior dislocation of the proximal interphalangeal joint, a cause of rupture of the central slip of the extensor mechanism. *J Bone Joint Surg* 52A:1329–1336, 1970.
26. Stewart IM. Boutonniere finger. *Clin Orthop* 23:220–226, 1962.
27. Zancolli E. *Structural and Dynamic Basis of Hand Surgery*. Philadelphia: JB Lippincott, 1966:105–106.

32

Reconstruction for Flexible and Fixed Swan-Neck Deformities

Drew Engles, Konstantinos Ditsios, and Martin I. Boyer

The swan-neck deformity is typified by proximal interphalangeal (PIP) joint hyperextension and distal interphalangeal (DIP) joint flexion. A concomitant flexion posture at the metacarpophalangeal (MCP) joint may be part of the deformity and an integral component of the digital imbalance (Fig. 32.1). The swan neck, with its hyperextension posture at the PIP joint and its shortcomings in extension distally, is typically the result of a compromise of the restraints to overexuberant PIP joint extension and failure of the DIP joint to summon the requisite extension via the lateral bands tensioning the terminal tendon. These individual deficiencies may result initially from trauma or disease to either site in the linkage system, but ultimately the finger decompensates due to the insidious imbalance, which leads to concomitant failure at both sites.

There are a number of etiologies that may ultimately result in a swan-neck deformity. It may originate from untreated or undertreated injuries of the PIP joint volar plate. The multiply dorsally dislocated digit is the prime example.

It may occur after injury or attenuation to the terminal tendon at the DIP joint. This is especially true in the patient with a pre-existing tendency for hyperextension at the PIP joint. Apex volar angulated fractures of the middle phalanx may alter the tension of the lateral bands and, thus, ultimately lead to the swan neck. Muscle imbalance, such as that seen in patients with spastic hemiplegia from cerebral palsy, may produce the deformity as well. Rheumatoid arthritis and its ubiquitous synovitis may devitalize the volar plate proximally or distend the capsule and attenuate the terminal tendon distally. Either initially, or both in combination, may surreptitiously lead to the swan-neck posture.

Drew Engles, M.D.: Summit Hand Center, The Crystal Clinic, Akron, OH
Konstantinos Ditsios, M.D.: Department of Orthopaedic Surgery, Washington University School of Medicine, St. Louis, MO
Martin I. Boyer, M.D.: Department of Orthopaedic Surgery, Washington University School of Medicine, St. Louis, MO

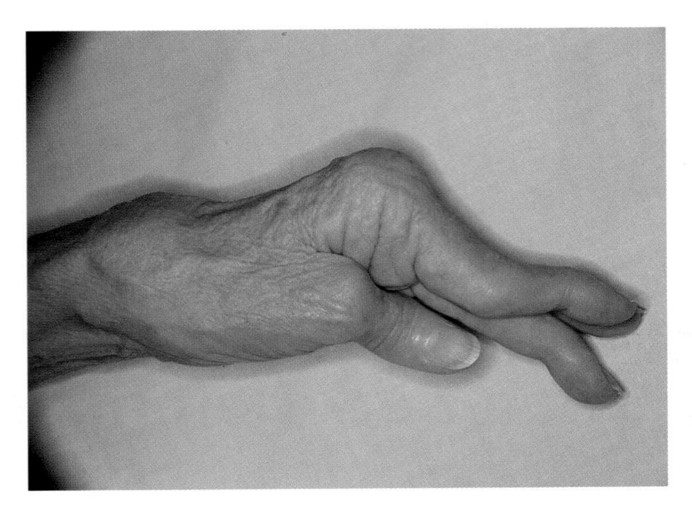

Figure 32.1. Swan-neck deformity of the index finger in a patient with rheumatoid arthritis. Hyperextension of the proximal interphalangeal (PIP) joint and flexion deformities of the metacarpophalangeal (MCP) and distal interphalangeal (DIP) joints.

The pathological processes are perhaps best illustrated in the rheumatoid patient, in whom PIP joint synovitis results in attenuation of the palmar restraints to the joint and resultant hyperextension. This is further exacerbated by the flexed posture of either the wrist or the MCP joint proximally, the limited flexion force of synovitic and adherent flexor tendons, and intrinsic myotendinous tightness associated with chronic MCP joint volar subluxation (Fig. 32.2). Although the swan-neck configuration may be limited to the PIP and DIP joints, the MCP joint is frequently involved, and a three-joint sequence often is present (Fig 32.3).

Mallet deformities also can contribute to a hyperextension deformity of the PIP joint. The forces of digital extension concentrate at the PIP joint, as their action on the distal joint is lost as a result of attenuation or rupture of the terminal tendon. Unopposed flexor digitorum profundus action at the DIP joint exacerbates the deformity.

A

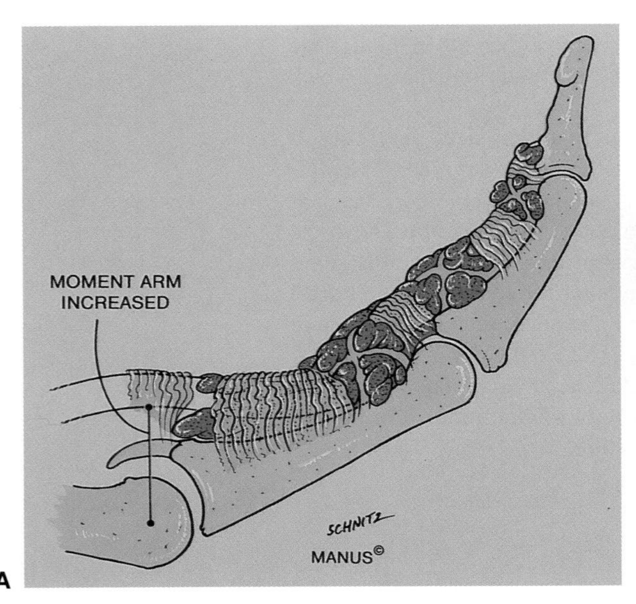

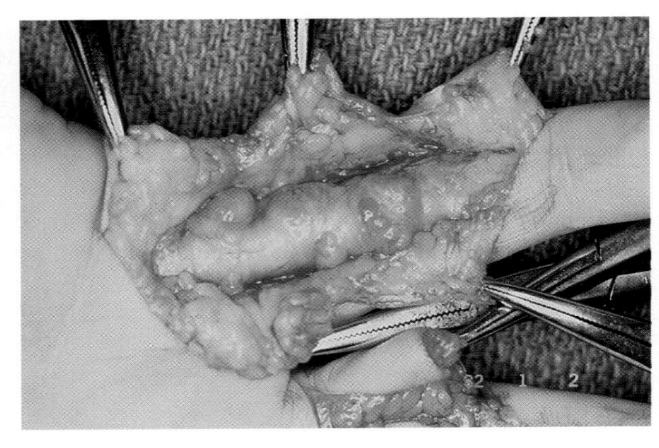

B

Figure 32.2. A: A drawing depicting flexor tenosynovitis of a rheumatoid digit. **B:** Photograph of the flexor tendon sheath in a rheumatoid patient with severe flexor tenosynovitis. Note the synovial bulging of cruciate components of the sheath and attenuation of the annular pulleys. Flexor tenosynovitis results in a decreased excursion of the flexor tendons within the digit, increasing their pull at the MCP joint and decreasing their efficiency at the proximal PIP joint.

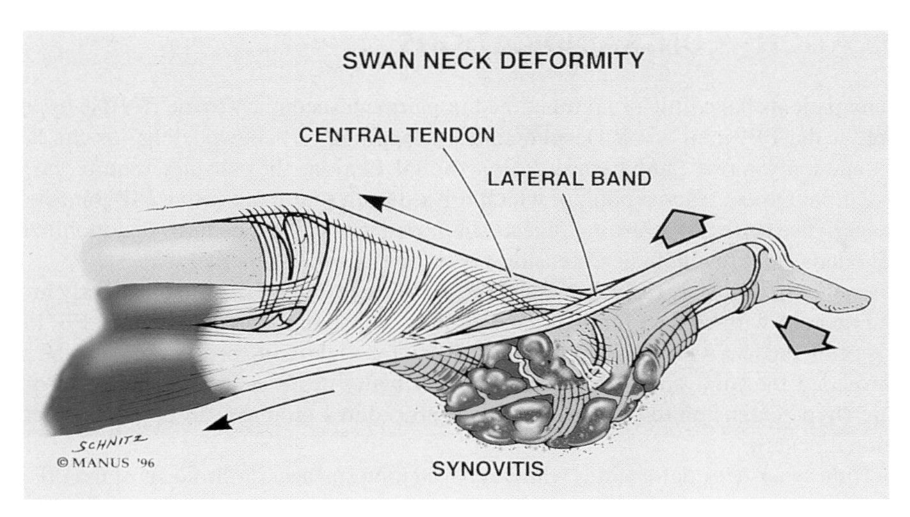

Figure 32.3. A drawing of the pathoetiology of a swan-neck deformity: synovitis of the palmar side of the PIP joint, dorsal migration of the lateral bands, and increased extension pull of the central extensor and intrinsic tendons.

Unlike the care for other common disorders of the digital extensor apparatus (e.g., the claw deformity, the boutonniere deformity, and the soft-tissue mallet finger), there is no effective, let alone provisional, nonoperative course of treatment of the swan-neck deformity. At best, there is the palliative figure-of-eight splint. Therefore, the care of this deformity is almost always surgical.

EVALUATION OF THE SWAN-NECK DEFORMITY

Swan-neck deformities are either flexible (passively correctable) or fixed. In the flexible swan neck, the PIP joint can be flexed either actively or passively. In some instances, there may be an associated snapping phenomenon if the intrinsic mechanism is required to initiate flexion preferential to the flexor tendons themselves. In the fixed swan neck, PIP flexion is not possible either actively or passively. Fixed deformities are divided into those with preservation of some joint space and those with destroyed articular surfaces. This classification has direct implications in the choice of surgical procedure for the deformity.

Over time, dorsal subluxation of the lateral bands becomes fixed and the central slip tendon and the triangular ligament shorten. The lateral retinacular ligaments become attenuated and the dorsal skin and subcutaneous tissue also may contract with long-standing PIP joint hyperextension.

In rheumatoid arthritis, the PIP joint may deteriorate and become fixed. Thus, the flexible deformity becomes a rigid one. Long extensor tendon subluxation, loss of the MCP joint cartilage, and volar subluxation and dislocation of the proximal phalanx on the metacarpal head may decrease this effect of relative shortening of the long digital extensors as the disease advances. These effects, which would decrease the tendency of the finger to assume a swan-neck configuration, may mitigate some of the deforming force. Once the PIP joint has collapsed into hyperextension and the lateral bands subluxate dorsally, it is rare to see any significant reversal of the condition. The multifactorial nature of the deformity must be appreciated for a rational approach to restoration to be developed.

In the previous edition of this monograph, the authors focused on treating the deformity as it related to rheumatoid arthritis. These recommendations have stood the test of time and thus remain unchanged. In this edition, the discussion is expanded to include not only patients with swan-neck deformity as a result of rheumatoid arthritis but also those patients who exhibit symptomatic swan neck as a result of chronic mallet finger and cerebral palsy as well. Thus, four surgical procedures are discussed.

INDICATIONS/CONTRAINDICATIONS

Many patients have little or no functional impairment secondary to the flexible hyperextension at the PIP joint level. Despite some "snapping" or "cogwheeling" as the lateral bands suddenly move palmarward during digital flexion, they do not require surgical intervention. Others reach a point at which it is difficult to initiate active PIP joint flexion and experience difficulty grasping objects. In those instances, procedures that mobilize the lateral bands and prevent hyperextension via tenodesis are of benefit.

When the deformity is fixed, patients lack the ability to wrap their hands tightly around curved objects, with contact limited to the palmar surface of the hyperextended PIP joints. Pain is often present with rigid contractures; PIP joint-mobilizing procedures may be helpful, provided the joint articular surfaces are not badly destroyed. The change in digital posture (hyperextension to flexion) that these procedures produce can be of considerable functional benefit.

For rigid swan-neck deformities with destroyed joint surfaces, arthrodesis of the PIP joint is usually the most practical option. Although there may be instances in which a flexible implant arthroplasty can be used to address the cartilage deficiencies, we have found those procedures to be generally unreliable in the rheumatoid patient, mainly because of the complex rebalancing of deforming forces that must be employed during such reconstructive efforts.

PREOPERATIVE PLANNING

A detailed history must be taken and a physical examination performed. Additional concerns in the rheumatoid patient include the status of the cervical spine, corticosteroid suppression of the pituitary-hypothalamic axis, and proximal joint disease. In cerebral palsy, proximal contractures are often addressed concomitantly. A complete evaluation of all coexistent deformities is required. To ignore the contributions of the long extensor tendon, the MCP joint, the wrist joint, the intrinsic musculature, or the skin and subcutaneous tissue in the creation of the digital swan-neck deformity is to invite the failure of surgical correction. The PIP joint deformity cannot be addressed in isolation.

Flexor tenosynovitis, which restricts tendon excursion, may be a significant factor in the development of swan-neck deformities. In these instances, tenosynovectomy or a palmar traction tenolysis of the flexor tendons may be an important addition to corrective procedures.

Long extensor tendon subluxation or dislocation must be recognized in the preoperative evaluation so that it can be corrected by an extensor tendon realignment procedure. A fixed flexion deformity of the MCP joint will relatively tighten the extrinsic digital extensors. In these instances, consideration should be given to either an MCP joint synovectomy or, in the presence of gross joint destruction or dislocation, a flexible implant arthroplasty.

The presence of ulnar subluxation or dislocation of the MCP joint also serves to tighten the intrinsic digital extensors. If a flexible MCP arthroplasty is performed, the surgeon should plan on resection of sufficient bone at the level of the metacarpal head and the base of the proximal phalanx to relatively lengthen both the intrinsic and the extrinsic digital extensors. Although these procedures at the MCP joint alone may improve mild flexible swan-neck deformity, it is frequently necessary to carry out additional surgery at the PIP joint level to rebalance or reposition that joint.

Incisions should be planned so that they are not in the plane of PIP joint motion and thus the dorsal tension created by joint flexion does not compromise healing. In the long-standing fixed deformity, contraction of the dorsal skin and subcutaneous tissue over the PIP joint may make wound closure difficult after the joint is corrected into a flexed position. In those instances, it is preferable to leave the distal portion of the wounds open. These small open wounds can be expected to heal quickly and will not compromise postoperative therapy.

In patients with spastic hemiplegia, there must be a satisfactory modicum of volitional control to warrant surgery. As these patients often are undergoing multiple simultaneous proximal procedures, the simplicity of a central slip tenotomy is quite appealing.

SURGERY

Overview

For flexible deformities, we prefer a lateral band tenodesis of the PIP joint using a lateral band rerouting procedure as advocated by Zancolli and by Tonkin et al. This procedure can be used even in the presence of modest joint-space narrowing.

For fixed PIP hyperextension deformities without gross joint destruction, we perform an extensor tenolysis, dorsal capsulotomy, partial collateral ligament release, and lateral band mobilization after the techniques described by Nalebuff and Millender and Gainor and Hummel. In this procedure, soft-tissue releases are sequentially carried out until the PIP joint can be brought into full unrestricted flexion with the lateral bands displaced palmar to the axis of rotation of the PIP joint. For a fixed deformity with gross joint destruction and pain, we recommend arthrodesis or, on rare occasions, arthroplasty with flexible implants.

In patients with compensatory hyperextension of the PIP joint following a mallet injury, we use the technique espoused by Kleinman. Although it utilizes some of the biomechanical principles first described by Thompson et al., it is performed without bony anchorage and thus is a completely soft-tissue reconstruction.

Patients with swan-neck deformity secondary to spastic hemiplegia are treated with a simple central slip tenotomy. This procedure has been previously described and critically examined by Gerwin Carlson.

Flexible Deformity

The patient is positioned supine on the operating table. A digital block, wrist block, or axillary block is administered. In most instances, an axillary block is favored. A well-padded pneumatic tourniquet is placed around the upper arm. A standard sterile prep and draping is performed. The pressure of the tourniquet is set at systolic blood pressure plus 100 mm Hg. The limb is elevated and exsanguinated, and the tourniquet is inflated. A brachial tourniquet is preferred to a Penrose drain placed on the digit, as the mobilization of the lateral band is more difficult when proximal exposure is hampered by the presence of the digital tourniquet.

A dorsal curvilinear incision around the PIP joint is made 1 to 2 mm dorsal to the midlateral line of the finger, from the midpoint of the proximal phalanx to the DIP joint. This approach permits easy access to the dorsally subluxated lateral bands, which are to be mobilized. Dissection is carried across the dorsum of the digit so that the reflected flap provides exposure of the extensor apparatus, the retaining ligaments, and the flexor tendon sheath. Punctate bleeding is controlled using bipolar cautery. Cleland's ligament is divided to allow access to the palmar aspect of the finger. The fibrous flexor sheath is approached directly, as the neurovascular structures are usually safely palmar to the surgical field. However, care must be taken to identify the digital artery and nerve when there is severe PIP joint hyperextension.

The subluxated lateral band is now identified, passing dorsal to the axis of rotation of the PIP joint. Using a scalpel, the lateral band is dissected free of its dorsal attachment to the extensor apparatus and is allowed to displace volar to the axis of rotation of the PIP joint as the joint is passively flexed. Sufficient proximal and distal release of the lateral band should be carried out so that it may be displaced down to the level of the flexor sheath at the level of the PIP joint. The mobilized lateral band should not be detached either proximally or distally, and excessive mobilization should be avoided to preserve sufficient tension for the tenodesis effect.

The location of the PIP joint is now determined. The collateral ligament, volar plate, and fibrous flexor sheath (the A3 pulley at this level) are identified and exposed. The digital artery and nerve are retracted in a volar direction. A scalpel is used to create a 1-cm-wide, dorsally based flap of flexor sheath at the level of the joint. The sheath flap is incised as far palmarward as possible and left attached to the volar plate and adjacent PIP joint structures.

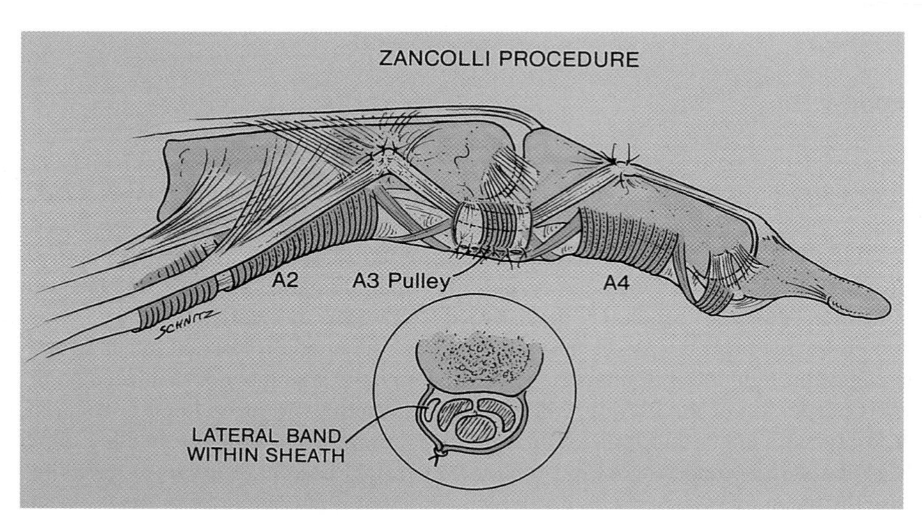

Figure 32.4. Lateral band rerouting procedure for flexible swan-neck deformities. Artist's depiction of the position of the palmarly displaced lateral band within the flat created in the flexor tendon sheath.

The incision in the flexor sheath is made as close to the midline of the digit in the anteroposterior plane as the exposure will afford.

The mobilized lateral band is displaced in a palmar direction and brought to lie under the sheath flap. With the PIP joint held in flexion, the flap of flexor sheath is now replaced in its anatomic position, trapping the lateral band inside. The band now lies within the fibrous flexor sheath, adjacent to the flexor tendons. The base of the flap prevents subluxation of the lateral band in a dorsal direction and ensures that it will remain palmar to the axis of rotation of the PIP joint. The flap of flexor sheath is now repaired anatomically using two or three 3-0 or 4-0 braided nonabsorbable sutures (Fig. 32.4).

The PIP joint is passively flexed, and the excursion of the mobilized lateral band within its new tunnel is confirmed. The lateral band is gently grasped proximal to the repaired flexor sheath "sling" using nontoothed forceps, and mild proximally directed traction is exerted on it to demonstrate that the band glides freely. Before wound closure, the resistance to the PIP joint extension is gently evaluated. The joint is first allowed to return to its new resting posture, with the finger supported by the surgeon's grasp of the proximal phalanx. Dorsally directed pressure is exerted on the tip of the digital pulp, and the tendency of the PIP to extend past neutral is evaluated. The PIP should extend no farther than 10 to 15 degrees of flexion and, on release of dorsally directed pressure, should return to its new resting posture of approximately 30 to 35 degrees of PIP flexion. If the tension on the displaced lateral band is not sufficient to prevent hyperextension, proximal and distal sutures can be used to tighten it back to the central tendon or the triangular ligament.

Wound closure then is carried out after a thorough irrigation of the surgical wound. Nonadherent 5-0 monofilament sutures are used in an interrupted fashion. Both simple and mattress-type sutures are used. The surgical assistant prevents any extension of the PIP joint from its flexed resting posture during wound closure. Protective flexion of the PIP joint to 45 degrees or greater is encouraged.

A sterile nonadherent dressing is applied. Gauze padding is applied over the dressing, and a circumferential wrap is applied to the finger. A dorsal static extension block splint is applied to the finger, holding the PIP joint in 45 degrees of flexion with the DIP joint fully extended. The tourniquet is then deflated.

Fixed Deformity

In the absence of PIP joint pain and gross destruction of the articular cartilage, an extensor tenolysis, dorsal capsulectomy combined with partial collateral ligament release, and lateral band mobilization constitute our preferred procedure. The components related to the selection of anesthesia, draping, and tourniquet use described previously apply to this description.

A curvilinear dorsal incision is made beginning at the midline of the proximal aspect of the proximal phalanx. The incision gently curves radially or ulnarly toward the middle of the incision at the PIP joint. It then curves back toward the midline until the dorsal DIP joint crease is reached. A radial- or ulnar-based flap of skin, subcutaneous tissue, and fat then is raised across the entire dorsum of the PIP joint and distal aspect of the proximal phalanx. The dorsal draining veins are included in the flap. Epitenon is left overlying the extensor apparatus and is not included in the flap. Punctate bleeding is controlled using bipolar cautery.

Dissection is continued in a volar direction, dividing or retracting the transverse retinacular ligaments to gain exposure of the cord component of the collateral ligaments. The dorsally subluxated lateral bands, central slip, contracted triangular ligament, and collateral ligaments of the PIP joint are all well visualized.

A longitudinal incision is made between each lateral band and the central slip (Fig. 32.5A). Proximally, the incision is made between the lateral band and the central extensor tendon. Distal to the insertion of the central tendon at the base of the middle phalanx, the incision is then brought through the contracted triangular ligament. Gentle sharp dissection is used to free the undersurface of the lateral bands from the underlying bone and joint capsule.

Tenolysis of the central extensor tendon is performed. A round-edged elevator is passed underneath the central tendon at the level of the joint and is passed proximally against the undersurface of the central tendon, freeing it from any adhesions and scar (Fig. 32.5B). After completion of the tenolysis, an incision is made in the PIP joint on both sides of and beneath the central tendon. A small scalpel blade is passed from dorsal to palmar directly into the point parallel to the opposing articular surfaces of the proximal and middle phalanges and adjacent to the central slip. The dorsal capsulotomy is now complete. This can be converted to capsulectomy by using a small rongeur to remove the dorsal capsular tissue.

With the finger held in the surgeon's hand, flexion pressure is applied to the PIP joint (Fig. 32.5C). The scalpel blade then is placed inside the collateral ligaments, parallel to the long axis of the finger. In this manner, it can be used to release the dorsal-most ligament fibers from their bone origin on the proximal phalanx. Small incremental cuts are placed alternately underneath the radial and ulnar ligaments until the joint moves easily into full flexion. If there is any "rebound" tendency for the joint to spring back into extension, additional collateral division should be carried out. Occasionally, in severe fixed deformities, transarticular pinning of the PIP joint for 7 to 10 days may be required to overcome the residual tendency for extension contracture.

As the PIP joint is delivered into full flexion, palmar subluxation of the mobilized lateral bands occurs. The lateral bands now lie volar to the axis of rotation of the PIP joint. No fixation of the lateral bands in this position is required. If the bands appear attenuated and incapable of fully extending the DIP joint, imbricating sutures may be used to shorten and tighten them distal to the PIP joint.

Wound closure then is carried out after a thorough irrigation of the surgical wound. Monofilament sutures (5-0) are used in an interrupted fashion. Both simple and mattress-type sutures are used. If the wound closure is difficult or appears to be excessively tight with the PIP joint in flexion, the distal part of the wound over the middle phalanx should be left open and uncomplicated healing can be expected (Fig. 32.6).

A sterile nonadherent dressing is applied. Gauze padding is applied over the dressing, and a circumferential wrap is applied to the finger. The tourniquet is then deflated. A dorsal static-extension block plaster splint is applied to the finger, holding the PIP joint in 45 degrees of flexion and the DIP joint fully extended.

Swan-Neck Deformity Secondary to Chronic Mallet Finger

Regional anesthetic is used. A brachial tourniquet is applied, and after prepping, draping, and exsanguination, the tourniquet is inflated. The incision is carried from the ulnar

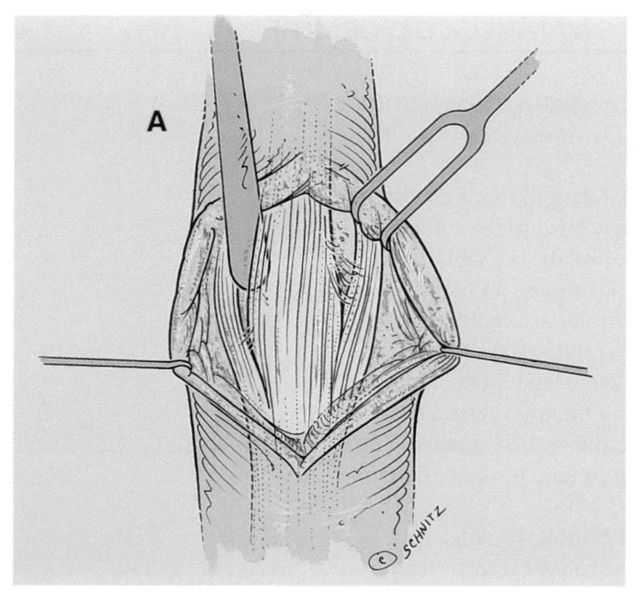

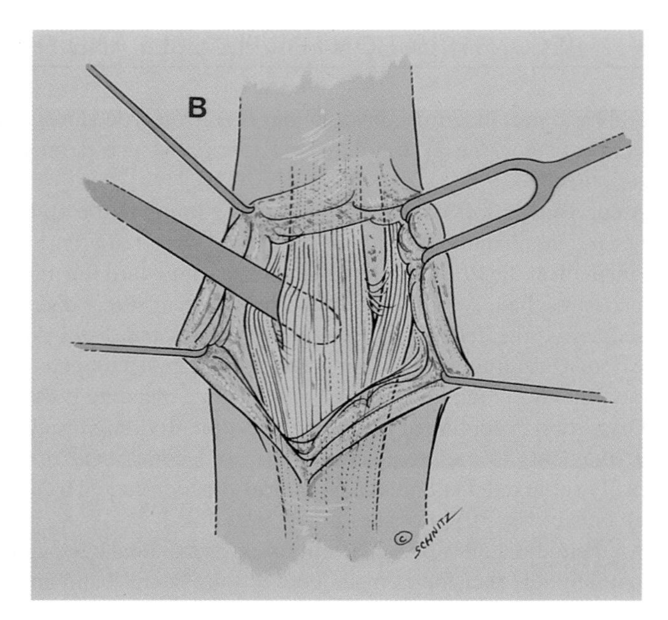

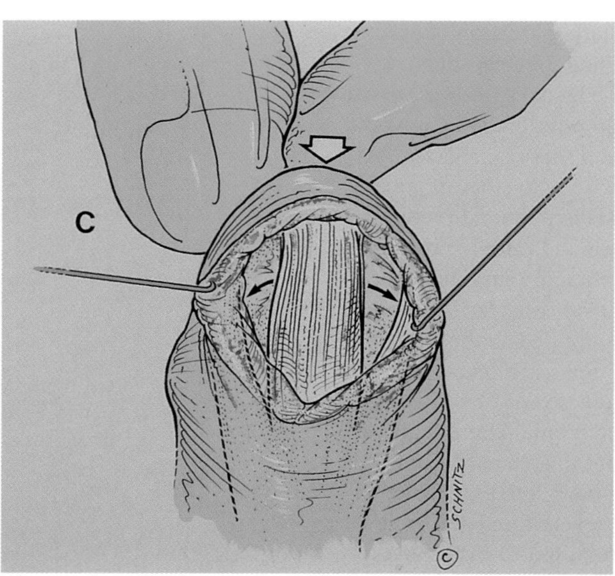

Figure 32.5. A: Correction of fixed swan-neck deformity by lateral band mobilization, extensor tenolysis, and capsulotomy. **B:** Exposure of the extensor mechanism over the PIP joint and mobilization of the lateral bands and extensor tenolysis. **C:** The surgeon's finger applies gentle flexion force to the PIP joint while capsulectomy is performed. Note the lateral and palmar displacement of lateral bands.

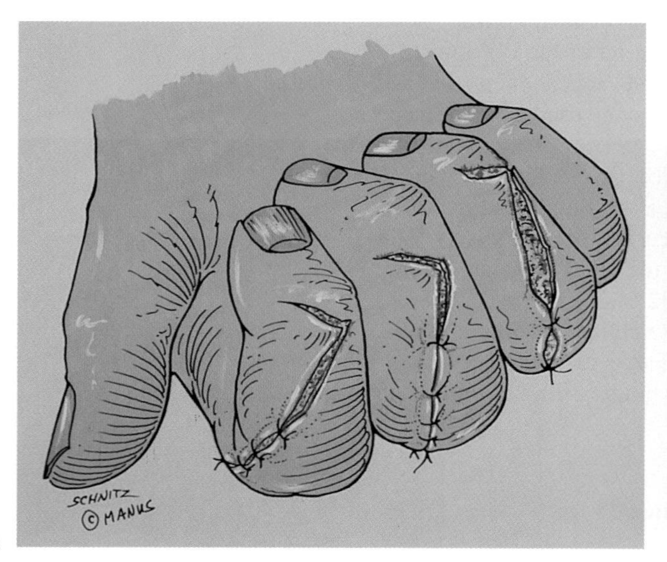

A

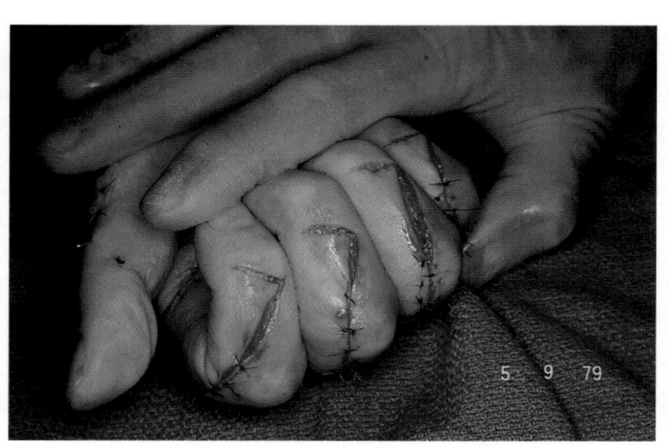

B

Figure 32.6. A: Completed restoration of PIP joint flexion on three rheumatoid swan-neck deformities. Note that distal wounds have been left open to avoid excessive tension. **B:** Photographs at the conclusion of the lateral band mobilization, extensor tenolysis, and capsulectomy sequence for four rheumatoid fingers with fixed swan-neck deformities.

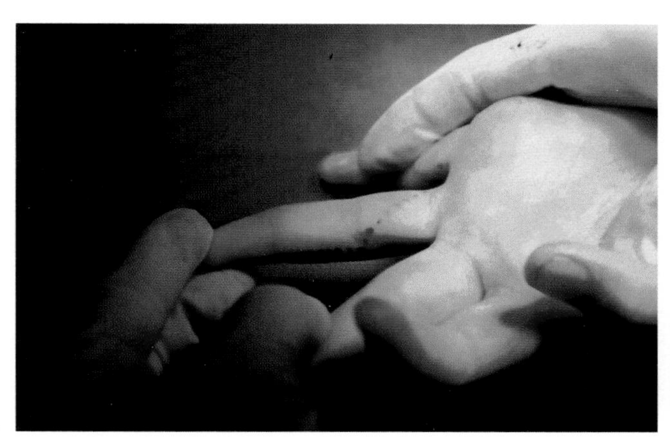

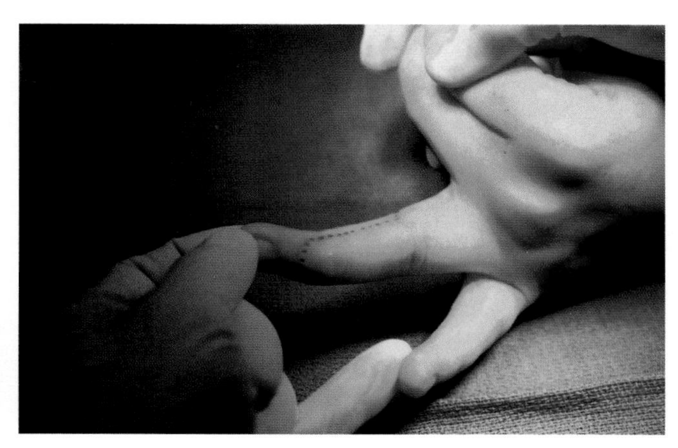

Figure 32.7. A: The incision is carried from the ulnar aspect of the MCP flexion crease to the midlateral line in the ulnar aspect of the digit at the PIP joint. **B:** The incision travels distally along the midlateral line of the middle phalanx and curves dorsally to end over the DIP joint.

aspect of the proximal phalanx distally to the radial aspect of the PIP joint flexion crease in the midlateral line. The incision is then continued distally in the midlateral line over the middle phalanx, to the level of the DIP joint. The incision is completed transversely over the dorsal aspect of the DIP joint (Fig. 32.7). Full-thickness skin flaps are raised, and the neurovascular bundle on the radial side of the digit is isolated and dissected free of soft-tissue attachments. The insertion of the conjoined terminal extensor tendon at the dorsal base of the distal phalanx is identified. The distal edge of the A2 pulley is identified proximally.

A transverse incision 1 cm in length is made over the palmaris longus tendon in the distal forearm. The palmaris longus tendon is identified and removed using a tendon stripper. The tendon is kept moist and is divided longitudinally so as to decrease its caliber by half.

A 0.035-inch Kirschner wire transfixes the DIP joint in 0 degrees of flexion. One end of the palmaris longus tendon graft is sewn to the terminal tendon insertion using multiple 6-0 braided nonabsorbable sutures. The tendon graft is then passed deep to the neurovascular bundle, against the fibrous flexor sheath (Fig. 32.8). An additional 0.035-inch Kirschner wire transfixes the PIP joint in 25 degrees of flexion. The tendon graft is then sewn under slight tension to the distal edge of the A2 pulley using 6-0 braided nonabsorbable sutures (Fig. 32.9). The wound is irrigated and closed using 4-0 nonabsorbable nylon suture. A hand-based compressive dressing with plaster slab augmentation is applied. The authors do not routinely deflate the tourniquet before closure.

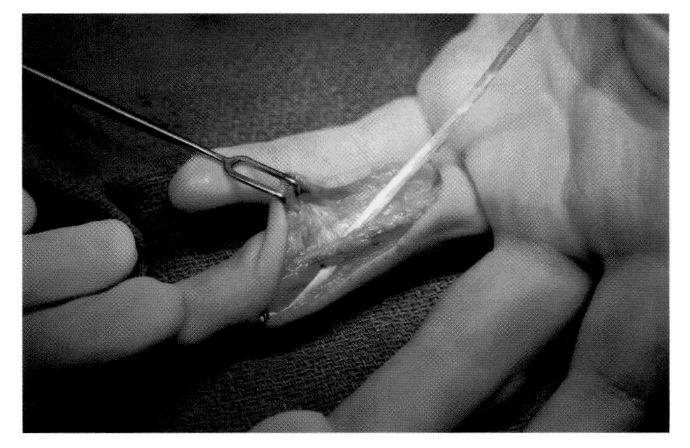

Figure 32.8. After harvest, the palmaris longus tendon graft is divided longitudinally. An axial transfixation pin is placed across the DIP joint, and the tendon graft is sewn to the terminal tendon insertion. The graft is passed deep to the neurovascular bundle as shown.

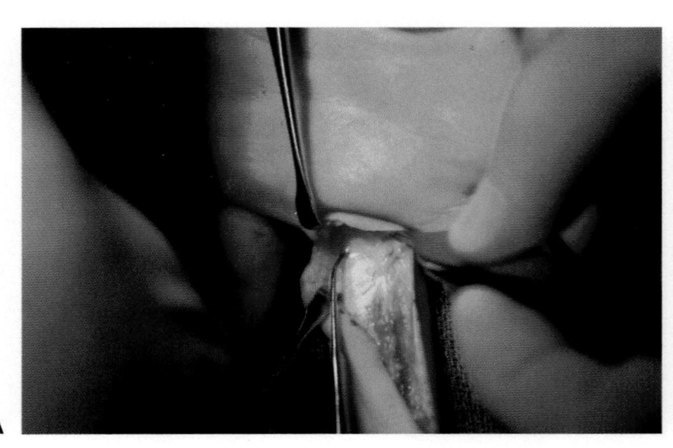

A

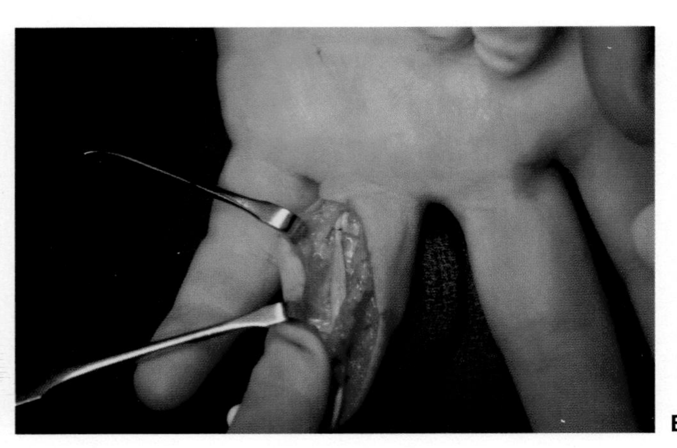

B

Figure 32-9. A: The transfixation pin is placed across the PIP joint to hold it at 25 degrees of flexion. **B:** The free end of the graft is sewn to the distal aspect of the A2 pulley.

Swan-Neck Deformity Secondary to Spastic Hemiplegia

Regional anesthetic is used. A brachial tourniquet is applied, and after prepping, draping, and exsanguination, the tourniquet is inflated. A transverse incision approximately 1 cm proximal to the PIP joint is utilized. The interface between the central slip and the lateral bands is identified. Grasping the central slip and lifting it dorsally facilitates this. The central slip in transected proximal to the joint over the proximal phalanx. As the central slip fibers are divided, the lateral bands fall away laterally. After fully tenotomizing the central slip, a 0.035-inch Kirschner wire is placed obliquely across the articulation with the joint in 10 degrees of flexion. Hemostasis is obtained via bipolar cautery. The wound is then irrigated and closed. Monofilament sutures (5-0) are utilized in horizontal mattress fashion. A nonadherent dressing is applied and covered with additional gauze in a compressive, nonconstricting fashion. If surgery on one digit is performed, a single-digital splint is used. If multiple digits are treated, then a hand or forearm-based splint is utilized.

POSTOPERATIVE MANAGEMENT

Lateral Band Tenodesis

The surgical dressing is removed 10 to 14 days postoperatively. If earlier removal is mandated because of pain or risk of infection, a dorsal digit-based extension block splint is constructed to keep the PIP joint in at least 30 degrees of flexion and the DIP joint fully extended. At the time of suture removal (10–14 days), a molded dorsal extension block splint is applied, maintaining the PIP joint at 30 degrees of flexion and permitting full composite digital flexion. The splint is discontinued 4 weeks postoperatively, and active flexion and extension exercises are begun. Passive extension of the PIP joint is discouraged until about 6 weeks. Any flexion deformities that persist usually can be corrected with dynamic splinting designed to stop at neutral extension.

Lateral Band Mobilization and Capsular/Collateral Ligament Release

Hyperextension deformity of the PIP joint rarely recurs after this procedure. In fact, some modest amount of extension lag usually results and is quite acceptable to patients who are accustomed to rigid recurvatum of their digits. For that reason, active flexion and extension exercises may begin as soon as pain subsides, usually 1 to 2 weeks postoperatively. If the PIP joints are pinned in flexion after mobilization of the lateral bands, the pins are removed 7 to 10 days postoperatively and active range of motion is then begun.

Static palmar gutter finger splints are to be used between exercises. A dorsal block splint is helpful in those rare instances in which the joint has a tendency to return to hyperextension. Dynamic PIP flexion or extension splinting may be used after 3 weeks to improve the arc of motion of the PIP joint.

Oblique Retinacular Ligament Reconstruction

At 2.5 weeks postoperatively, sutures are removed and the proximal transfixation pin is pulled. A splint is worn to immobilize the DIP joint only, and active and active assisted range of motion of the PIP joint from zero to maximal flexion is begun. At 5 weeks postoperatively, the distal Kirschner wire is removed and active range of motion of the DIP joint along with grip strengthening begins.

Postoperatively, if a PIP joint flexion deformity coupled with a DIP joint hyperextension deformity occurs during attempted digital extension, the graft has been sewn in under too much tension and a step-cut lengthening is required.

Central Slip Tenotomy

At 2 weeks postoperatively, the patient's sutures are removed and the pins are cleaned and redressed. Gutter splints are applied. At 4 weeks postoperatively, the transarticular pins are removed and the digits are placed in figure-of-eight splints. These are continued for 4 weeks full time and then for 4 weeks at night only (Fig. 32.10).

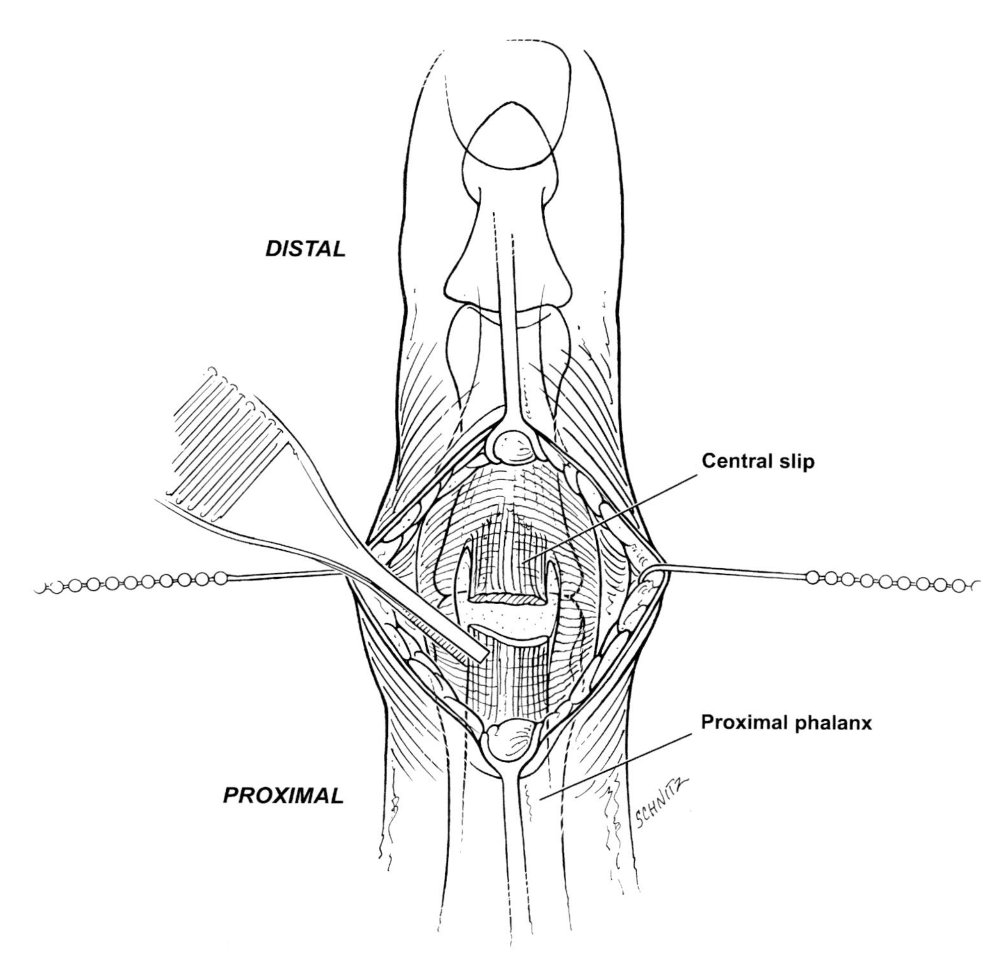

Figure 32.10. A drawing of the central slip tenotomy. Gentle dorsal traction of the central slip fibers aids in delineating the central slip boundaries from the lateral bands.

REHABILITATION

In all of the aforementioned procedures, rehabilitation is directed at maximizing flexion and preventing recurrence of the hyperextension at the PIP joint while simultaneously optimizing DIP joint extension. If dynamic splinting is utilized for excessive PIP joint flexion posturing, it must be carefully modulated to prevent any extension beyond neutral. Custom splint fabrication and close supervision by a certified hand therapist is the optimal scenario.

RESULTS

It would be difficult and counterproductive to list the compendium of procedures and their subsequent variations for the four aforementioned swan-neck deformities. The techniques chosen and highlighted in this monograph are those that have proven effective for the authors. In most instances, our experience has paralleled that which has been described in the literature.

Tonkin et al. reported their results of a procedure similar to that described herein for flexion deformity. They reported successful correction of PIP joint hyperextension deformity (on average, 16 degrees preoperatively) to 11 degrees of PIP joint flexion postoperatively. Their patients either regained or improved their range of preoperative flexion. Our results are in agreement with those reported.

Kiefhaber and Strickland reported their results with lateral band release and dorsal capsulotomy for fixed deformity. Although patients initially gained an average of 55 degrees of flexion in the immediate postoperative period, gradual postoperative loss of some of the arc of flexion was the rule. A mean loss of almost one-third (17 degrees) was seen postoperatively over 3 to 12 months. The authors recognize that "the long term loss of flexion may be unavoidable" because of the progression of the underlying rheumatoid disease. The key benefit, however, was that the entire arc of PIP joint motion shifted into flexion, allowing improved use of the fingers in prehensile and grasping activities.

The experience reported by Kleinman and Petersen is that the soft-tissue retinacular ligament reconstruction predictably restored DIP joint extension and corrected secondary PIP joint hyperextension. Two of 12 patients required additional surgery. One required a tenolysis, the other a lengthening of the palmaris graft to achieve full extension at the PIP joint. This procedure has been predictably successful for the authors as well.

Gerwin Carlson reported 88% good or excellent results in 26 fingers. She found that the preoperative degree of the swan-neck angle correlated with the ultimate degree of correction. The authors have likewise found this procedure simple and effective. No patients have developed a subsequent boutonniere deformity despite the release of the central slip.

COMPLICATIONS

Infections or hematomas are managed in the standard fashion. When dorsal skin tension prohibits closure, distal wounds on the digits may safely be left open. They are dressed in a sterile fashion with routine moist to dry dressing changes until they are healed.

Recurrent deformity should be addressed in a manner similar to the initial deformity; that is, an assessment of contributing abnormalities should be undertaken, followed by evaluation of the flexibility of the deformity. When the disease continues to affect the joint, radiographs will help determine the extent of articular destruction and whether there is any hope of preserving joint motion. In the event of severe joint destruction or refractory pain, arthroplasty or, more commonly, arthrodesis is performed.

RECOMMENDED READING

1. Ferlic DC, Clayton ML. Flexor tenosynovectomy in the rheumatoid finger. *J Hand Surg* 3:364–367, 1978.
2. Gainor BJ, Hummel GL. Correction of rheumatoid swan-neck deformity by lateral band mobilization. *J Hand Surg* 10A:370–376, 1985.
3. Gerwin Carlson M, Wolff A, Brooks C. Easy surgical treatment of dynamic digital swan neck deformity in cerebral palsy. Presented at: 56th Annual Meeting, American Society for Surgery of the Hand, Baltimore, MD, October 4–6, 2001.
4. Kiefhaber TR, Strickland JW. Soft tissue reconstruction for rheumatoid swan-neck and boutonniere deformities: long-term results. *J Hand Surg* 18A:984–989, 1993.
5. Kleinman WB, Petersen DP. Oblique retinacular ligament for chronic mallet finger deformity. *J Hand Surg* 9A:399–404, 1984.
6. Nalebuff EA. The rheumatoid swan-neck deformity. *Hand Clinics* 5:203–214, 1989.
7. Nalebuff EA, Millender LH. Surgical treatment of the swan-neck deformity in rheumatoid arthritis. *Orthop Clin North Am* 6:733–752, 1975.
8. Nalebuff EA, Feldon PG, Millender LH. Rheumatoid arthritis in the hand and wrist. In: Green DP, ed. *Operative Hand Surgery*. 2nd ed. New York: Churchill Livingstone, 1988:1724–2736.
9. Thompson JS, Littler JW, Upton J. The spiral oblique retinacular ligament (SORL). *J Hand Surg* 3:482–487, 1978.
10. Tonkin MA, Hughes J, Smith KL. Lateral band translocation for swan-neck deformity. *J Hand Surg* 17A:260–267, 1992.
11. Zancolli EA, Zancolli E Jr. Surgical rehabilitation of the spastic upper limb in cerebral palsy. In: Lamb DW, ed. *The Paralyzed Hand*. New York: Churchill Livingstone, 1987:163–165.

33

The Rheumatoid Thumb: Evaluation and Surgical Reconstruction of the Swan Neck Deformity

Andrew L. Terrono

INDICATIONS/CONTRAINDICATIONS

Rheumatoid thumb deformities are seen commonly in patients with advanced hand involvement as a result of inflammatory arthropathy and can cause significant functional disability. Surgery can improve thumb function and remains one of the most effective reconstructive procedures for patients with rheumatoid arthritis.

The second most common pathologic thumb posture, and one that frequently requires surgical intervention, is the swan neck (type III) rheumatoid thumb deformity. In the development of thumb swan neck deformity, the carpometacarpal (CMC) joint is initially involved, with subsequent development of flexion and adduction of the first metacarpal, leading to hyperextension of the metacarpophalangeal (MCP) joint and loss of extension of the interphalangeal (IP) joint (Fig. 33.1). The degree of involvement varies from minimal deterioration and instability of the CMC joint to severe fixed deformities of both the CMC and MCP joints.

Treatment of these deformities depends upon the degree of pain and functional disability. Surgery is usually not the primary recommendation for inflammatory CMC arthritis in an effort to prevent the development of the deformity because patients often have remarkably good function in the early stages of the condition. Surgery can be delayed or avoided if nonoperative measures are effective in alleviating pain and preserving function.

A carefully fabricated CMC splint may be effective in stabilizing the joint and relieving pain. Aspirin or nonsteroidal agents can be used during light activities requiring modest thumb participation. Hand therapists also can help the patient with adaptive devices. The

Andrew L. Terrono, M.D.: Department of Orthopaedics, Tufts University School of Medicine, Boston, MA, and Hand Surgery, New England Baptist Bone and Joint Institute, Boston, MA

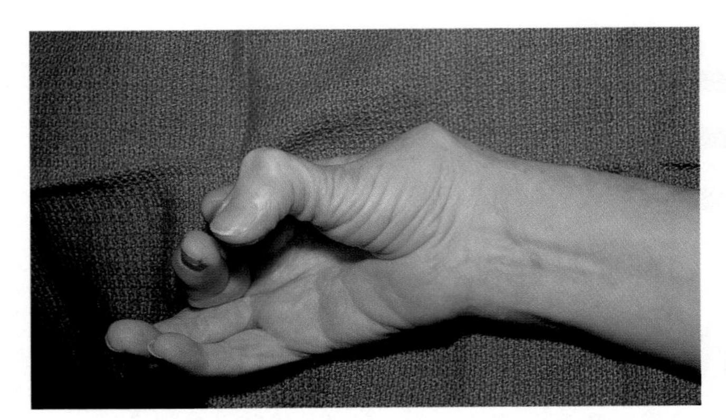

Figure 33.1. Classic type III deformity with carpometacarpal (CMC) joint dislocation and metaphalangeal (MP) joint hyperextension.

judicious use of steroid injections can provide transient benefit, particularly in the acute stage with active synovitis. In general, the indications for surgery are persistent pain not responsive to conservative treatment and instability and deformity that impair the use of the thumb for pinch and grasp activities.

PREOPERATIVE PLANNING

To adequately evaluate the patient with rheumatoid involvement of the thumb, the surgeon must understand the pathophysiology and functional disability that this collapse deformity produces. In the type III deformity, synovitis initially attacks the CMC joint, resulting in varying degrees of cartilage and bone destruction and joint instability.

Early in the type III deformity, there is primarily cartilage erosion without significant bony destruction or capsular attenuation. The clinical presentation is that of stiffness of the CMC joint, mild to moderate discomfort, and minimal deformity. The patient has pain and/or instability associated with activities that require axial loading of the thumb ray, including key pinch and cylindrical grasp activities, such as opening jar lids. Complaints also may include the inability to write, sew, or do other manipulative activities without considerable discomfort. Weakness, often resulting in a tendency to drop objects, also may be reported.

The initial examination usually will reveal tenderness at the level of the CMC joint. Pain, crepitus, or instability may be elicited when carrying out the "grind" test, which is performed by longitudinal loading of the first metacarpal, and thus the CMC joint, while rotating and translating the ray (Fig. 33.2). Pinch strength assessment will give the examiner an objective appreciation of the degree of disability. Comparing the pinch strength of the two hands is recommended, but many patients have bilateral movement.

As the joint manifestations of the underlying inflammatory disease progress, dorsal and radial subluxation of the joint develops secondary to soft-tissue disruption with or without bony erosion. Radial subluxation results from attenuation of the CMC joint supporting structures, including the anterior oblique ligament, the CMC capsule, and the dorsal radial ligament. The subluxation is augmented by the pull of the abductor pollicis longus, which inserts on the radial base of the first metacarpal (Fig. 33.3).

As the deformity progresses, a complete dislocation of the CMC joint may develop, resulting in adduction of the first metacarpal (promoted by the intrinsic adductor), which creates forces that will produce hyperextension of the MCP joint (dorsal translation of the extensor tendons, attenuation of the volar plate and capsule) followed by accentuated flexion of the IP joint. The degree of deformity depends on the amount of ligamentous laxity, the extent of joint destruction, and the pathologic tendon forces resulting from the altered anatomy.

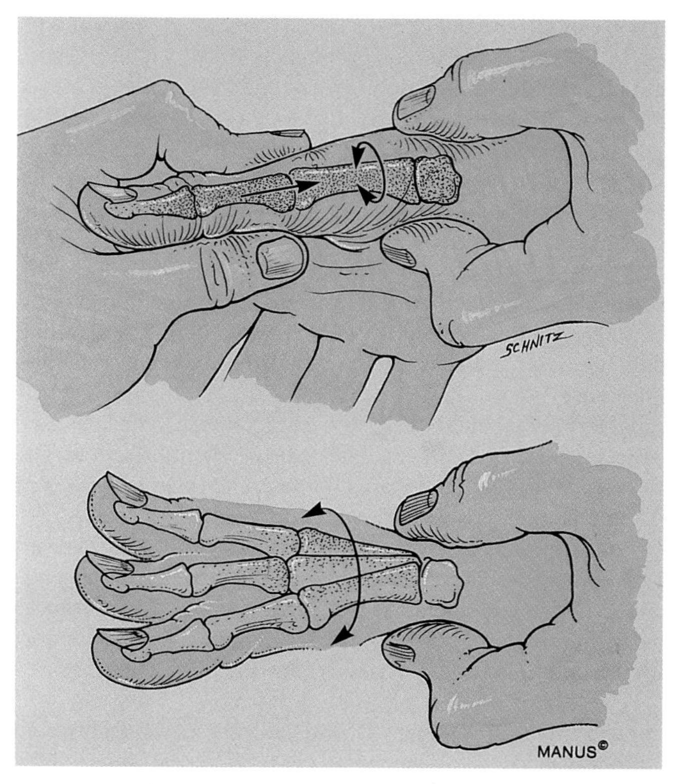

Figure 33.2. Grind test demonstrated.

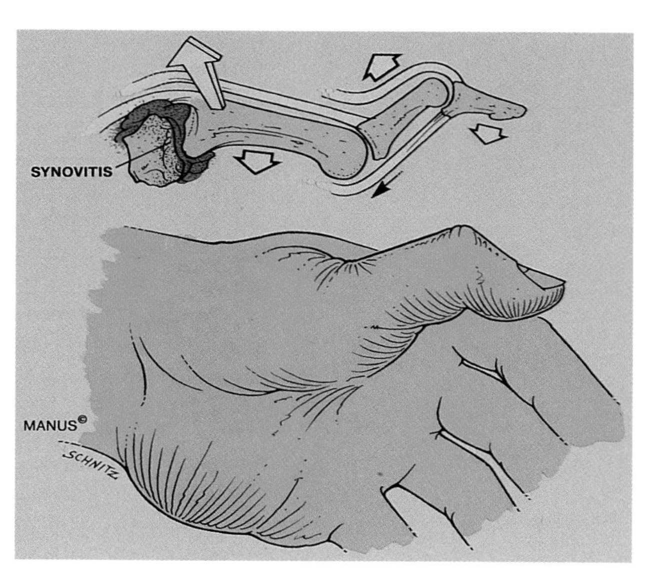

Figure 33.3. Pathophysiology of the type III deformity. Synovitis causing cartilage and bone destruction and capsular insufficiency. Subluxation develops. The abductor pollicis longus accentuates this deformity. Secondary metacarpophalangeal (MCP) hyperextension and interphalangeal (IP) flexion develop.

In its advanced stages of collapse, the thumb develops a recognizable "zigzag" configuration, which severely restricts both pinch and grasp activities. At this stage, the thumb index web space is markedly diminished and, when the patient attempts to grasp large objects, the thumb MCP joint extends, thus increasing the deformity. Secondary contracture of the adductor pollicis and first dorsal interosseous fascia will contribute to a fixed deformity. The loss of pinch and grasp capability will lead the patient to seek treatment. At this stage, pain is usually a secondary factor, as functional loss is significant.

In planning a reconstructive procedure for the type III collapse deformity, a thorough study of posterior-anterior (PA), lateral, and hyperpronated (anteroposterior) views of the thumb CMC joint is essential. The status of the articular cartilage of the CMC, metaphalangeal (MP), and IP joints are all important in determining the appropriate procedure at each level. Complete dislocation of the CMC joint will result in significant shortening of the thumb, necessitating complete trapezium excision for correction. Physical examination will also give important information to be used in the preoperative planning.

If the first metacarpal can be passively abducted, first web space release or deepening procedures may not be necessary. In addition, if repositioning of the first metacarpal results in balancing of the MCP joint and/or the patient can actively stabilize the MCP joint, preventing hypertension, stabilization or arthrodesis of the MCP joint may not be necessary. If MCP motion is less than 30 degrees even if the joint surfaces are intact, I prefer an MP joint fusion.

SURGERY

The typical surgical treatment "package" of the type III deformity includes trapeziumectomy and soft-tissue arthroplasty of the CMC joint, correcting any adduction deformity of the metacarpal, any web space procedure, and/or deep release and stabilizing of the MCP joint by one of a variety of acceptable methods (capsulodesis, sesamoid-to-phalanx fusion, tenodesis, or MCP arthrodesis).

A notable exception in the family of inflammatory arthritides would be the patient with systemic lupus erythematosus. In this case, the major problem is joint instability with preservation of the cartilage and bone: CMC joint fusion is recommended in these cases.

With the patient in the supine position and the arm extended on the hand surgical table, a pneumatic tourniquet is placed on the upper arm. Axillary block and general anesthesia are both appropriate choices. After routine preparation and draping, the tourniquet is inflated to approximately 100 mm Hg greater than the systolic blood pressure. A zigzag incision is used that extends from the proximal third to the thumb metacarpal to the first dorsal compartment.

The sensory branch of the radial nerve is identified and protected. The first dorsal compartment is usually released with the tendons retracted with Penrose drains. The radial artery is identified, freed from the underlying fascia, and retracted. The artery may be displaced if the CMC joint is dislocated.

The periosteum on the proximal third of the metacarpal and CMC joint capsule is incised longitudinally. The capsule is preserved, if possible, for later closure by imbrication. The thumb metacarpal base is exposed by releasing the capsule on the volar and ulnar sides of the metacarpal. This facilitates CMC joint exposure and reduction (Fig. 33.4).

The amount of trapezial resection is determined by the deformity of the trapezium as well as the space needed to correct the first web space contracture and the presence or absence of scaphoid-trapezium-trapezoid (STT) involvement. At least the distal half of the trapezium is resected in most patients. Preserving as much trapezium as possible is not as important in this day as it was when silicone implant arthroplasty was the "gold standard" of CMC reconstruction.

A majority of the time, complete trapezial resection is selected; this is especially true when the STT joint presents with advanced involvement. In cases of partial trapezial resection, the base of the thumb metacarpal is also resected to form a flat surface that will eventually accommodate the soft-tissue interposition.

Because the CMC deformity is typically advanced and the quality of cartilage and bone are poor, complete trapezial resection is the rule rather than the exception. This allows reduction of the subluxation and correction of the adduction deformity and provides an adequate space. The metacarpal then can be easily delivered into the joint and resected. Occasionally, it may be necessary to release a tight fascial band between the thumb metacarpal and the index metacarpal (Fig. 33.5). Rarely is any formal adductor release necessary to correct an adduction deformity.

A standard ligament reconstruction tendon interposition arthroplasty as described by Burton and Pellegrini using one-half of the flexor carpi radialis is performed. The flexor carpi radialis or a slip of the abductor pollicis tendon can be used to reinforce the capsule.

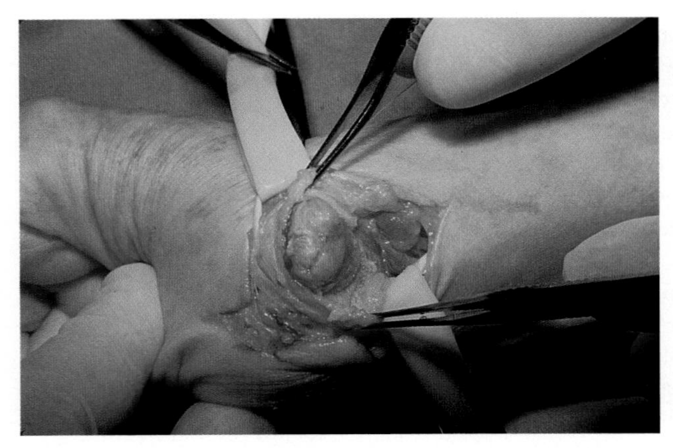

Figure 33.4. The first compartment tendons are retracted with Penrose drains. The metacarpal base is exposed after soft-tissue dissection.

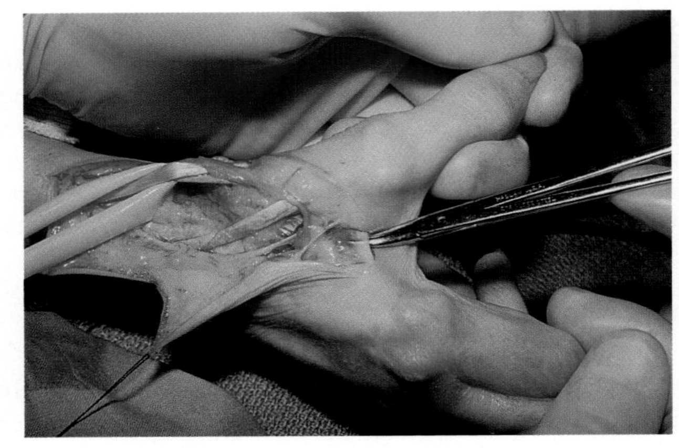

Figure 33.5. A tight fascial band that occasionally may have to be released.

Temporary Kirschner wire (K-wire) fixation of the first to the second metacarpal or carpus is usually not necessary.

In most cases, when the MCP joint is involved, arthrodesis of the MCP joint in approximately 10 to 20 degrees of flexion is carried out; this procedure is thought by most hand surgeons to be one of the most predictably successful alternatives in the repertoire of rheumatoid hand reconstruction. In the rare patient who has MCP hyperextension, minimal MCP joint destruction and good active MP flexion, a "sesamoidesis" (sesamoid-to-phalanx fusion) is performed.

To perform a joint fusion, the MCP joint is exposed through a dorsal longitudinal incision. This usually is a distal extension of the previous zigzag incision. The capsule and collateral ligaments are released, exposing the joint. With the metacarpal joint flexed to expose the articular surface of the metacarpal head and the base of the proximal phalanx, a rongeur is used to remove the remaining cartilage, creating a proximal concave and distal convex "cup-and-cone" relationship between the two bones. If necessary, bone from the resected trapezium can be used as a graft.

Fixation of the arthrodesis may be achieved using the tension band technique (Fig. 33.6), screw fixation, or crossed K-wires. I find the tension band technique to be reliable and straightforward in the soft bone usually encountered in the patient with rheumatoid arthritis.

The thumb is splinted in opposition-abduction with the wrist in slight extension, and a bulky hand dressing is applied. This may be modified depending on the procedures that might have been performed in combination with thumb reconstruction. If the thumb MP joint has not been fused, care should be taken not to inadvertently hyperextend the MP joint during the effort to immobilize the first metacarpal in abduction. The fingers are left free, and postoperative motion is encouraged.

In a subset of patients, the interphalangeal (IP) joint presents with angular deformity and either stiffness or instability. In some of these patients, there is tremendous deformity, yet

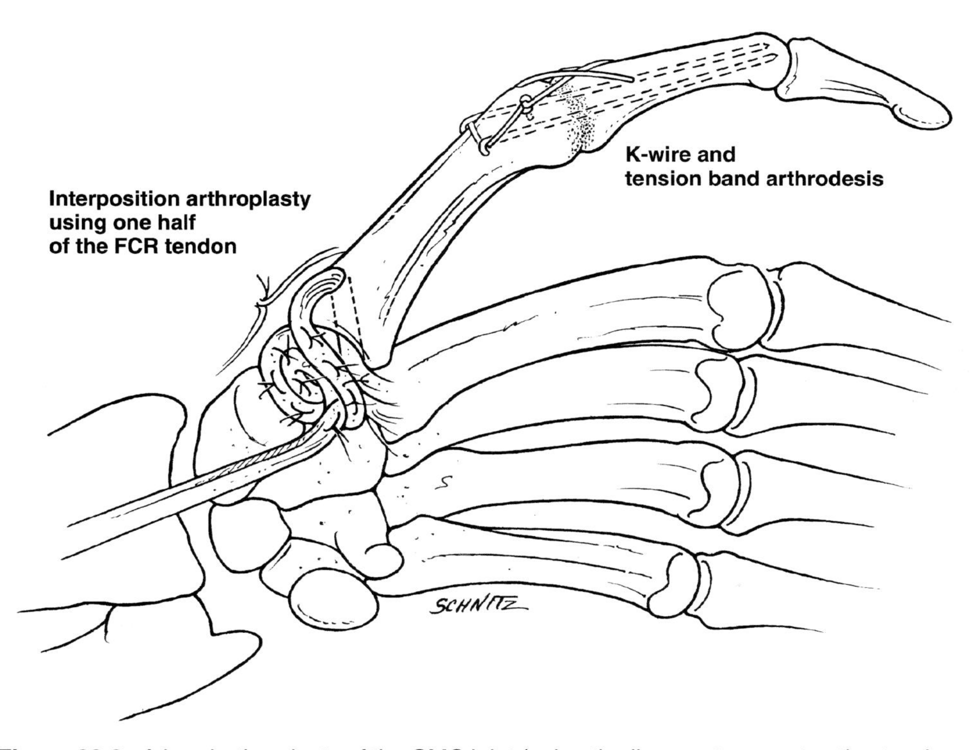

Figure 33.6. A hemiarthroplasty of the CMC joint (using the ligament reconstruction tendon interposition technique) is performed, and the MCP joint is stabilized by arthrodesis using a tension band technique.

it appears well tolerated. Consideration of IP reconstruction, the only logical choice for which is arthrodesis, is made based on comfort and function. Unlike surgery for the other two joints of the thumb's osteoarticular column, IP joint surgery can "stand alone" and be performed as an isolated procedure at a remote time from CMC and MCP reconstruction. Some surgeons will want to fuse the IP joint in slight flexion with K-wires, whereas others may decide that the bone quality and dimension can accommodate a variable-pitch screw and fuse the joint in neutral with this implant.

In a minority of cases, web space deepening (a combination of skin flap creation and deep soft-tissue release) is needed to complete the rheumatoid thumb reconstruction. Incision planning is important, as the coverage needs for the newly deepened web space must often be considered simultaneously with exposure needs for multiple joint levels. The conventional two-flap Z-plasty gives the maximum depth, although the contour can be more acute than some patients prefer. More elaborate flaps that may serve to improve the contour can lead to necrosis and are not recommended. Aside from the necessary capsular contractures that may need release along with the CMC and MCP reconstructions, the fascia over the first dorsal interosseous muscle sometimes requires release. Rarely, myotomy is needed to maximize the web space recovery.

POSTOPERATIVE MANAGEMENT

A cast is applied after the sutures are removed at approximately 10 to 14 days. The thumb is immobilized for a total of 4 or 5 weeks in an appropriate anteposed posture to allow for adequate soft-tissue healing. Protected CMC joint exercises then are initiated, with splinting continued between exercises. Light dorsal splinting for the MCP joint is continued until bony union has occurred, but the splint should not impede CMC or IP joint motion. If the tension band technique was used and the bone quality was reasonable, the arthrodesis construct is extremely stable and the wires rarely require removal. At 6 to 8 weeks, if the arthrodesis has healed, strengthening exercises can be commenced and include pinching and grasping activities.

This procedure usually results in a gratifying improvement of appearance and function of these badly deformed thumbs with excellent relief of pain. Patients rarely complain of postoperative discomfort, and restoration of the first web space significantly improves grasping capabilities (Fig. 33.7). The patient will be better able to hold larger objects, although weakness often persists for many months. Postoperative pinch strength averages 4.6 pounds. The involvement of other joints of the upper extremity hampers the ability to improve strength.

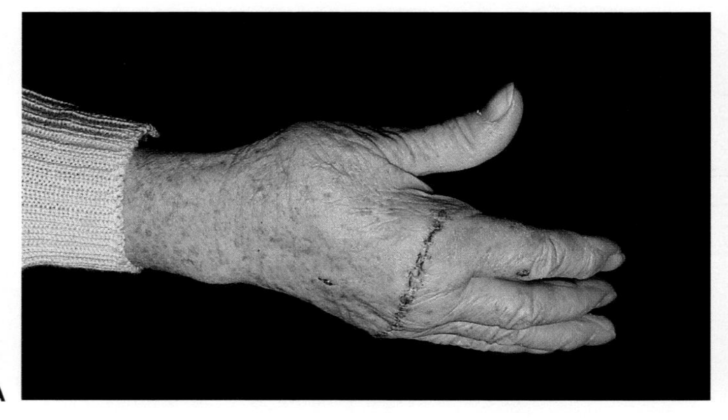
A

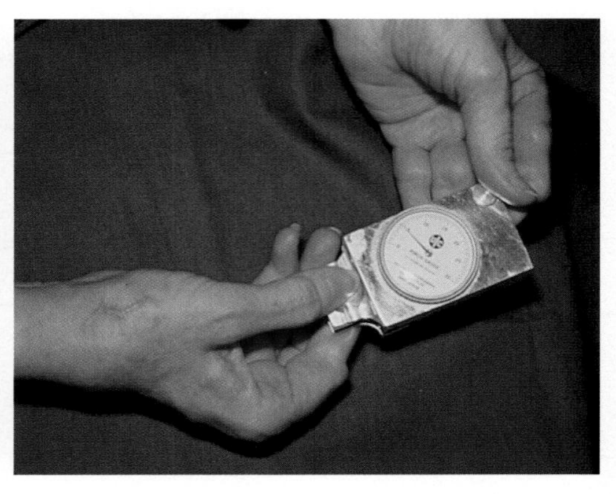
B

Figure 33.7. A: A 55-year-old female with a type III deformity secondary to rheumatoid arthritis. **B:** Postoperative appearance with functional pinch and a good web space at 6 months after surgery.

COMPLICATIONS

Complications of the procedures used to correct the type III collapse deformity of the rheumatoid thumb are uncommon. Failure to provide adequate soft-tissue stabilization at surgery, or initiation of CMC joint motion before adequate soft-tissue healing, can lead to recurrent deformity. If partial trapezial resection was performed, pain may recur or persist at the STT joint. If needed, excision of the remaining trapezium and/or the proximal portion of the trapezoid may be necessary. Impingement of the thumb and index metacarpal or thumb metacarpal and trapezoid is rarely seen. Nonunion of the MCP fusion is extremely rare in the rheumatoid patient. Hardware may have to be removed occasionally.

RECOMMENDED READING

1. Burton RI, Pellegrini VD. Surgical management of basal joint arthritis of the thumb. Part II. Ligament reconstruction with tendon interposition arthroplasty. *J Hand Surg* 11A:324–332, 1986.
2. Feldon P, Terrono AL, Nalebluff EA, et al. Rheumatoid Arthritis and Other Connective Tissue Diseases. In: Green DP, Hotchkiss RN, Pedersen WC, eds. *Green's Operative Hand Surgery*. Philadelphia: Churchill Livingstone, 1999:1651–1739.
3. Ijsselstein CB, van Egmond DB, Hovius SER, et al. Results of small-joint arthrodesis: comparison of Kirschner wire fixation with tension band wire technique. *J Hand Surg* 17A:952–956, 1992.
4. Kessler I. Aetiology and management of the adductor contracture of the thumb in rheumatoid arthritis. *Hand* 5:170–174, 1973.
5. Millender LH, Nalebuff EA, Amadio P, et al. Interpositional arthroplasty for the rheumatoid carpometacarpal joint disease. *J Hand Surg* 3:533–541, 1978.
6. Nalebuff EA. Diagnosis, classification and management of rheumatoid deformities. *Bull Hosp Joint Dis* 29:119–137, 1968.
7. Terrono AL. The rheumatoid thumb. *J Am Soc Surg Hand* 1(2):81–92, 2001.
8. Terrono AL, Nalebluff EA, Philips CA. The Rheumatoid Thumb. In: Mackin EJ, Callahan AD, Skirven TM, et al., eds. *Rehabilitation of the Hand: Surgery and Upper Extremity*. St. Louis: Mosby, 2002:1555–1568.

34

Repair of Ruptured Finger Extensors in Rheumatoid Arthritis

Donald C. Ferlic

INDICATIONS/CONTRAINDICATIONS

Rupture of the extensor tendons at the wrist is most often due to the erosive effect of the distal ulna. Other factors that may be involved are bone irregularity of the radius or carpal bones, compressive effects of the dorsal retinaculum, direct rheumatoid invasion of the tendons, local steroid injections, and infarcts of the tendons by hypertrophic rheumatoid tissue.

The diagnosis of rupture of the extensor tendons at the wrist usually poses no problem, but in the rheumatoid patient other conditions must be considered in the differential diagnosis. The first condition is the result of metacarpophalangeal (MCP) synovitis, where the extensor tendons have slipped off the metacarpal heads into the intermetacarpal areas so that the extensor tendons are below the axis of rotation, impeding their mechanical advantage. The second condition is that of posterior interosseous nerve palsy secondary to rheumatoid involvement at the elbow. Last, extensor tendons can rupture over the metacarpal heads as a result of bone spurs at this level.

The most frequently ruptured tendon is the common extensor to the little finger, followed by the ring finger. Next, in order of frequency of rupture, are the extensor pollicis longus (EPL), extensor digiti minimi, long-finger extensor, index extensor, extensor indicis proprius (EIP), and extensor carpi ulnaris. Ideal management is to perform surgery consisting of tenosynovectomy, dorsal retinacular ligament reposition, and treatment of the distal ulna and other bony prominences before the tendons rupture. The tendon that is prevented from rupturing will work better than the one that must be reconstructed. Many patients with dorsal tenosynovitis will suffer ruptured tendons, and rarely can they be repaired, primarily because it would be necessary to resect a considerable amount of frayed tendon, leaving it too short for end-to-end suture, which, if done, will result in an extension deformity of the digit.

Donald C. Ferlic, M.D.: P/SL Professional Plaza West, Denver, CO

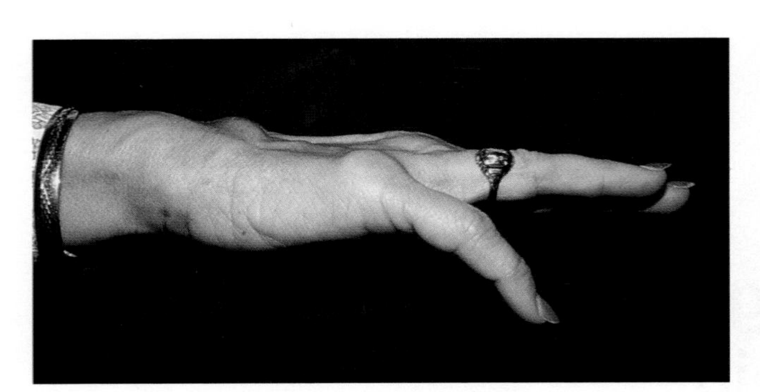

Figure 34.1. Rupture of the extensor digiti minimi and extensor digitorum communis to the little finger.

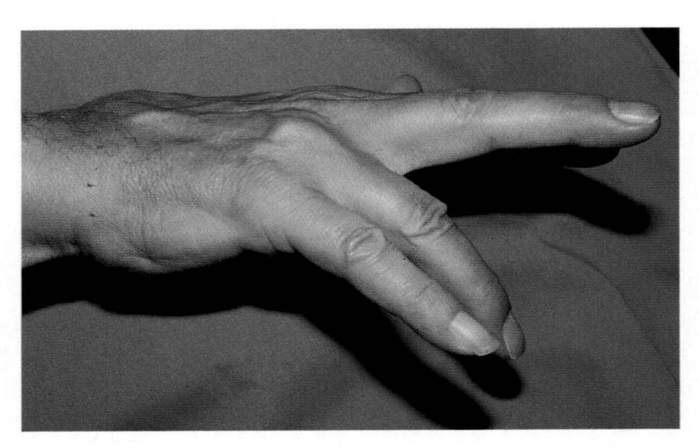

Figure 34.2. Rupture of common extensor to the ring and little fingers as well as the extensor digiti minimi.

Rupture of the EPL is common, but often is overlooked because of minimal functional deficit, and the extensor pollicis brevis often provides adequate extension of the MCP and interphalangeal joints. If the rupture is an isolated one, a number of alternatives are available. Arthrodesis of the interphalangeal joint of the thumb may be all that is warranted if the joint is already destroyed or if it does not have satisfactory passive motion. As far as tendon reconstruction is concerned, transfer of the brachioradialis, extensor carpi radialis longus (ECRL), extensor pollicis brevis, or the EIP, which is my preferred transfer, have been used.

For treatment of the rupture of the finger extensors, individual transfers will work better than mass transferral of one tendon into all that are ruptured. If the extensor tendons to the little finger are gone (Fig. 34.1), transfer of the communis into the adjacent intact ring-finger extensor works well. The same principle applies when any single extensor tendon is ruptured. If the extensor to the little and ring fingers has ruptured (Fig. 34.2), the ring-finger extensor is sutured into the long-finger tendon, and the EIP is used to motor the little finger. It is not necessary to suture the proximal muscles of the ruptured tendon into the transferred tendon motor. If the adjacent tendon is frayed, it may not be suitable for transfer. In such a case, a free tendon graft is taken to reinforce the weakened area.

In the case of a triple rupture (Fig. 34.3) (communis to the long, ring, little, and extensor digiti minimi) where both the extensors to the index finger are intact, the EIP is transferred to the ring and little fingers, and the ruptured long-finger tendon is sutured to the communis of the index. A ring-finger superficialis may also be used, but I have not had as good results with this transfer. If the index communis and EIP are not intact, the ECRL can be transferred into all three ruptured tendons, but goals will be limited. Normal finger motion

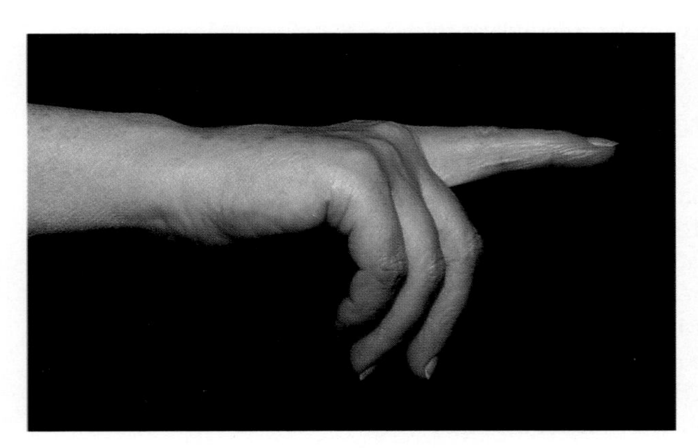

Figure 34.3. Triple rupture.

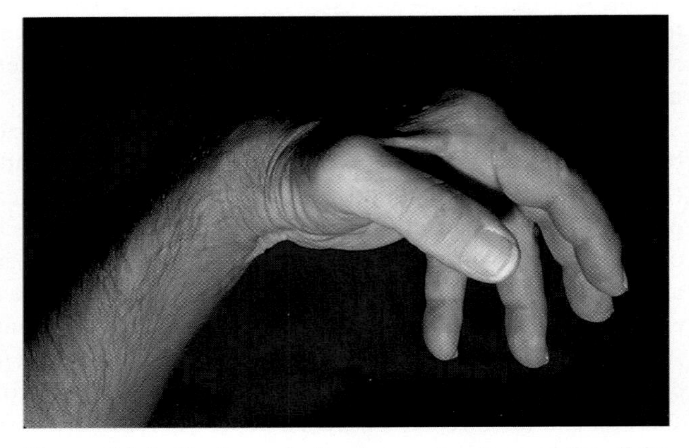

Figure 34.4. Rupture of all extensor tendons of the digits and wrist. A wrist fusion is necessary to reconstruct this wrist.

cannot be expected because of the limited excursion of this muscle, but if the wrist is supple, a tenodesis effect will aid the excursion but will not be enough for full finger motion. Other transfers that may be used are brachioradialis, extensor carpi ulnaris, or flexor carpi ulnaris if none of the above is available.

In cases where the wrist as well as the finger extensor is ruptured (Fig. 34.4), reconstruction is not possible unless the wrist is fused. The wrist tendons then can be used for transfers. If the wrist is to be fused, the extensor carpi ulnaris makes an excellent transfer, even in triple ruptures. Surgery to these hands certainly has limited goals, and the patient needs to be aware of the limitations before reconstructive attempts are made.

PREOPERATIVE PLANNING

The wrist with an acute rupture should be treated with some urgency, because a single rupture is often followed by a second rupture, and prompt surgery may prevent this occurrence. The result of surgery for ruptured tendons is related to the number of tendons involved. A hand with a triple rupture (extensor tendons to the little, ring, and long fingers) cannot be expected to turn out as well as the hand where only the tendons to the little finger are separated.

Some of the other general principles of tendon surgery applicable to the traumatically divided tendons may not rigidly apply to the rheumatoid patient. The usual period of immobilization may need to be shortened, arthrodesis of the affected joint may be the procedure of choice instead of tendon reconstruction, and free grafts are less likely to be useful, especially in a wrist that has marked involvement of the soft tissues. In these wrists, the chances of these devascularized structures gliding will be minimal. Other principles of tendon transfer need to be appreciated, such as excursion, direction, and power of the transferred muscle, although some bending of these rules may be necessary.

SURGERY

A straight-line dorsal longitudinal incision is made (Fig. 34.5); it may be diagonal or placed more to the radial or ulnar side, depending on where the tenosynovitis is most promi-

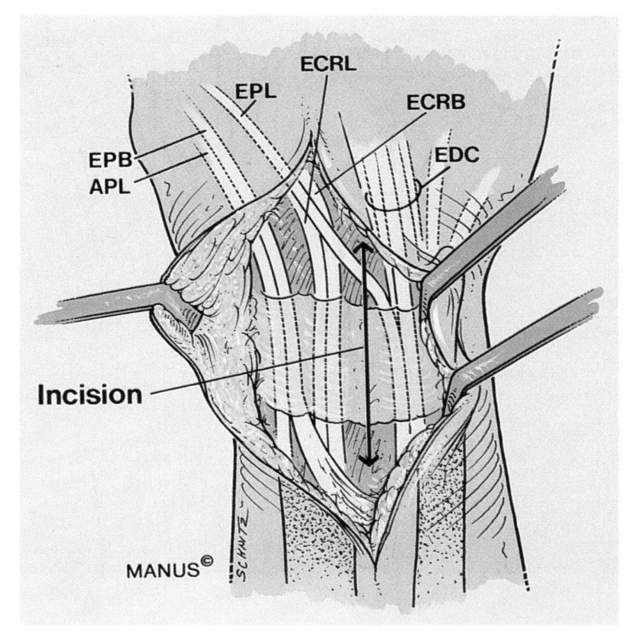

Figure 34.5. A straight dorsal incision is made.

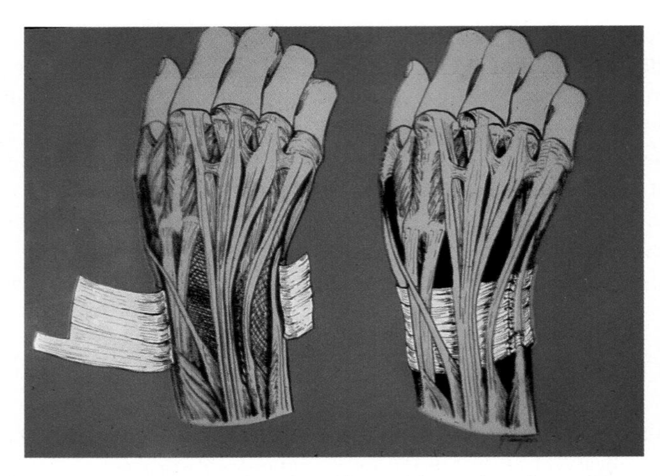

Figure 34.6. A: The dorsal retinaculum is reflected from the ulnar side, exposing the extensor tendons. **B:** The dorsal retinaculum is passed beneath the extensor tendons.

nent. The incision is long enough so that retraction is gentle. The skin is not dissected from the subcutaneous fat. Dorsal veins should be preserved as much as possible, and dorsal sensory nerves are protected. The dorsal retinaculum is reflected from the ulnar side, leaving it attached radially (Fig. 34.6A). All extensor compartments are opened. A tenosynovectomy is performed. The ruptured extensor tendons are identified (Fig. 34.7A). Appropriate surgery to the radiocarpal joint (synovectomy), distal ulna (Darrah, hemiresection arthroplasty, Sauve-Kapandji procedure), and dorsal capsule (dorsal ulnar capsule reconstruction) is carried out if indicated. The dorsal retinaculum is passed beneath the extensor retinaculum (Fig. 34.6B). The tendons for transfer then are chosen. If the EIP is selected, it is harvested with a narrow strip of hood expansion by detaching it from the ulnar side of the

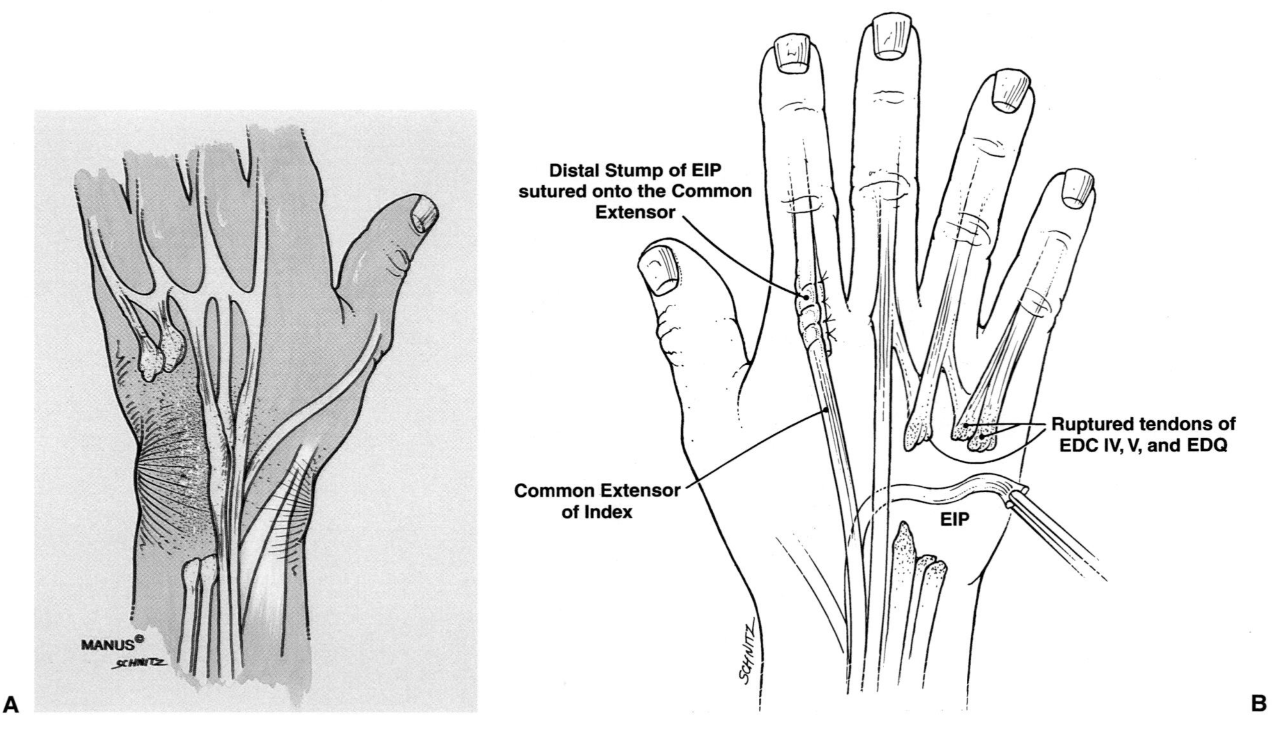

Figure 34.7. A: The ruptured extensor tendons are identified. **B:** The extensor indicis proprius (EIP) is taken for transfer, and the extensor hood is closed to prevent an extensor lag.

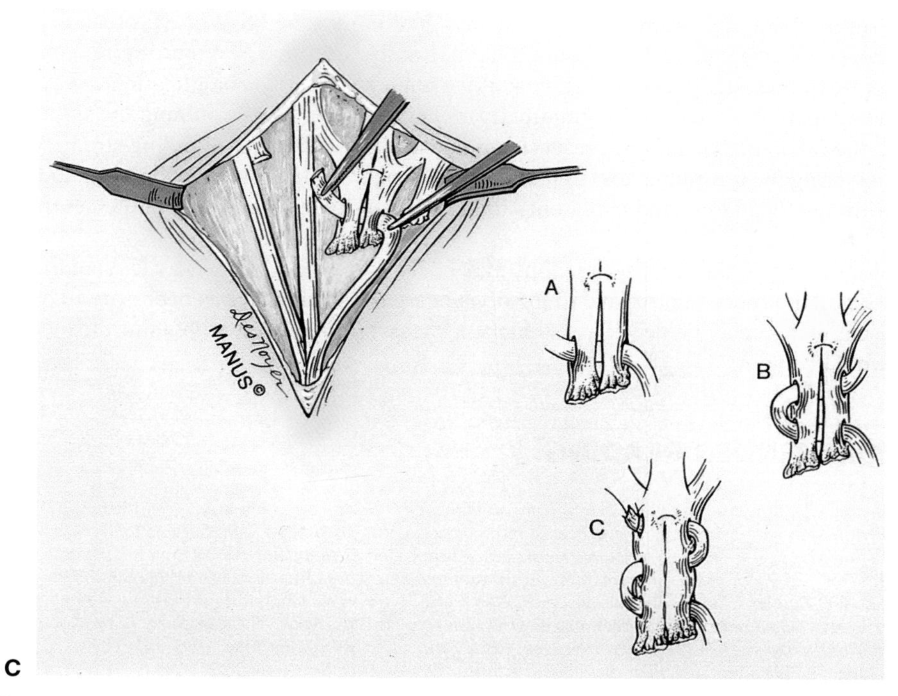

C

Figure 34.7. *Continued.* **C:** The tendon is transferred using a rigid interweave technique.

extensor mechanism just proximal to the MCP joints. A deficit is created in the extensor mechanism, which must be closed with sutures; an extensor lag at the proximal interphalangeal joint may develop if this is not done (Fig. 34.7B). Transfers are carried out by interweaving the distal end of the ruptured tendon into the intact tendon (Fig. 34.7C).

Suturing is done with 3-0 nonabsorbable undyed suture. This technique will provide adequate fixation so that early motion is possible using dynamic extension splints. If sufficient length to obtain this type of suture is not possible, a longer immobilization period may be necessary, but should be avoided if at all possible. In setting tension, one should err on the side of increased tension. The tendon should be sutured with the MCP joints slightly flexed, the wrist in slight extension, and maximal passive excursion of the transferred tendon. The tourniquet is lowered, hemostasis obtained, a suction drain inserted, and the wound closed. A bulky dressing is applied with the wrist splinted in neutral and the affected digits extended to neutral.

POSTOPERATIVE MANAGEMENT

The postoperative dressings are changed in 3 to 5 days, and hand therapy is started. Dynamic extension splints are made by the hand therapist, and gentle protected range-of-motion exercises are started. A static splint may be used during sleep. The transferred tendons are protected for 4 weeks, longer if an extensor lag develops.

The outcome is variable. If a single rupture is present and the hand is otherwise minimally involved, near-normal function may be anticipated. If there are multiple ruptures and the wrist and finger joints are involved, the goals and expectations are limited.

COMPLICATIONS

Rerupture of extensor tendons is not common after this procedure, but has occurred with an unstable distal ulna after resection. Wound breakdown may be encountered with dorsal wrist surgery; we have seen it in fewer than 5% of our cases. Most often, breakdown involves a small area and heals without problem. Rarely will there be a more significant area of the wound that necessitates debridement or even grafting. This complication can be minimized by making a straight, longitudinal, ample incision; not undermining the skin; leaving all the fat on the skin flaps; preserving all possible dorsal veins, avoiding strong retraction; lowering the tourniquet and obtaining hemostasis; wound drainage; dressing to finger tips with much padding, and using only light compression and splinting in the neutral position.

Bowstringing of the extensor tendons may occur but can be avoided by leaving the dorsal fascia in the forearm proximal to the dorsal carpal ligament. If it is necessary to release the fascia, it also may be necessary to make a check-rein ligament with a thin strip of dorsal carpal ligament.

RECOMMENDED READING

1. Clayton MD. Surgery of the thumb in rheumatoid arthritis. *J Bone Joint Surg* 44A:1376–1385, 1962.
2. Clayton ML. Surgical treatment at the wrist in rheumatoid arthritis. *J Bone Joint Surg* 47A:741, 1965.
3. Clayton ML, Ferlic DC. The wrist in rheumatoid arthritis. *Clin Orthop* 106:182, 1975.
4. Ferlic DC. Extensor indicis proprius transfer for ruptured extensor pollicis longus in rheumatoid arthritis. In: Blair WF, Stevers CM, eds. *Techniques in Hand Surgery.* New York: Churchill Livingstone, 1996:649–653.
5. Ferlic DC. Management of the rheumatoid wrist. In: Clayton ML, Smyth CJ, eds. *Surgery for Rheumatoid Arthritis: A Comprehensive Team Approach.* New York: Churchill Livingstone, 1992:155–187.
6. Goldner JL. Tendon transfers in rheumatoid arthritis. *Orthop Clin North Am* 5:425, 1974.
7. Harrison RD, Swannell AJ, Ansell BM. Repair of extensor pollicis longus using extensor pollicis brevis in rheumatoid arthritis. *Ann Rheum Dis* 31:490–492, 1972.
8. Marmot L, Lawrence JF, Dubois EL. Posterior interosseous nerve palsy due to rheumatoid arthritis. *J Bone Joint Surg* 49A:381, 1967.
9. Midgley RD. In: Creuss RL, Mitchell NS, eds. *Surgery of Rheumatoid Arthritis.* Philadelphia: JB Lippincott, 1971:159–163.
10. Millender LH, Nalebuff EA, Albin R, et al. Dorsal Tenosynovectomy and tendon transfer in the Rheumatoid Hand. *J Bone Joint Surg* 56A:601–609, 1974.
11. Millender LH, Nalebuff EA, Holdsworth DE. Posterior interosseous nerve syndrome secondary to rheumatoid arthritis. *J Bone Joint Surg* 55A:753, 1973.
12. Moore JR, Weiland AJ, Valdata L. Tendon ruptures in the rheumatoid hand; analysis of treatment and functional results in 60 patients. *J Hand Surg* 12A:9–14, 1987.
13. Pressley JA, Goldner JL. Extensor pollicis longus rupture due to old fracture, collagen degeneration, or rheumatoid arthritis; analysis and treatment by transfer of the extensor carpi radialis longus. *J Bone Joint Surg* 56A:1093, 1974.
14. Schnieder LH, Rosenstein RG. Restoration of extensor pollicis longus function by tendon transfer. *Plast Reconstr Surg* 71:533–537, 1983.
15. Sharman FT, Barton NJ. Surgery for rupture of extensor tendons in rheumatoid arthritis. *The Hand* 8:279–286, 1976.
16. Straub LR, Wilson EH. Spontaneous rupture of extensor tendons in the hand associated with rheumatoid arthritis. *J Bone Joint Surg* 38A:1208, 1956.
17. Trimpathi R, Ferlic DC, Clayton ML, et al. Rupture of the extensor tendons over the metacarpal heads. *The Hand* 15:149–150, 1983.

35

Subtotal Palmar Fasciectomy for Dupuytren's Contracture

James W. Strickland

INDICATIONS/CONTRAINDICATIONS

Limited (subtotal) palmar fasciectomy is indicated for patients with advanced contracture of one or more digits. The procedure is designed to remove only the pathologic fascia responsible for joint contracture. Hueston applied the term *regional fasciectomy* to this procedure and defined it as the removal of diseased fascia within the area. Howard perhaps said it best when he wrote that surgery was indicated for the release of "bothersome contractures."

A painful or annoying palmar nodule is rarely an indication for surgery, because the potential complications of the procedure outweigh the nuisance value of the lesion. Because metacarpophalangeal (MCP) joint deformities almost always can be corrected, surgery at this level is less urgent than that undertaken to correct developing contractures at the proximal interphalangeal (PIP) joint. At about 30 degrees of flexion, an isolated MCP joint contracture begins to become annoying to many patients, and surgery may be appropriate. It is much more difficult to correct PIP joint contractures secondary to Dupuytren's disease than MCP joint deformities, and the greater the magnitude of the presenting contracture, the less likely it is that significant, long-term improvement can be achieved by surgery. The author concurs with McFarlane that PIP surgery should be considered before joint contractures exceed 30 degrees.

Patients undergoing surgery for Dupuytren's disease should be counseled carefully about the nature of the disease process and the prognosis for the additional contracture and functional impairment should they elect not to proceed with surgery. The intricacies of the operation also should be reviewed, including the possibility of complications and the need to commence early postoperative digital motion to minimize stiffness or recurrent contracture. Make every effort to identify patients who develop a postoperative sympathetic "flare," and often the author more reluctant to proceed with surgery in these patients. It has been said that a moist, sweaty hand is a bad prognostic sign, as is the thickened hand of a laborer. Alcoholics, epileptics, and patients with Dupuytren's diaphysis (strong family history, early onset of the disease, multiple areas of fibromatosis, ectopic fibromatosis, Pey-

James W. Strickland, M.D.: Reconstructive Hand Surgery of Indiana, Carmel, IN, and Indiana University School of Medicine, Indianapolis, IN

ronie's disease, knuckle pads, or foot involvement) can be expected to do less well than patients who do not have these characteristics. In addition, there is a strong feeling that female patients are more likely to develop a postoperative sympathetic "flare" than male patients. Although the indications for surgery are generally the same in these patients, it may be appropriate to follow them longer to ensure that their disease is progressive and to consider alternative methods designed to lessen the magnitude of the operative procedure, such as subcutaneous fasciotomy or a more limited open fasciectomy.

PREOPERATIVE PLANNING

In preparation for subtotal palmar fasciectomy, drawings are made of the position and the extent of the fascial involvement, and accurate measurements of digital motion, including the extent of the MCP or PIP joint flexion contractures, should be made. In some instances, radiographs may be important to rule out any arthritic involvement of the joints one expects to mobilize during the operative procedure.

SURGERY

The author carries out all subtotal palmar fasciectomies for Dupuytren's contracture on an outpatient basis, with the patient under axillary block anesthetic. The advantages of regional anesthesia are considerable and include the fact that the procedure produces a sympathetic blockade, which may be of value in diminishing the incidence of postoperative sympathetic "flare." Most of our axillary blocks are done using bupivacaine so that patients will have prolonged postoperative anesthesia, which will permit them to return comfortably to their homes before experiencing any postoperative discomfort.

The axillary block is administered in a remote anesthetic area, with the provision of additional sedation depending on the patient's desires. The patient then is brought into the regular operating room, where preparation and draping are carried out in the exact manner described in Chapter 12, Subcutaneous Fasciotomy for Dupuytren's Contracture.

Incisional decisions are made according to the exact location of the offending fascia. If the digital cord is midline, the incisions will be centered over the midportion of the palmar digit. If the fascia is located more to the radial or ulnar side of the involved digit, incisions should be centered over the fascia rather than over the digit to lessen the amount of dissection necessary to expose the offending fascia and to decrease the often-precarious length of the digital flaps.

Limited fasciectomy requires wide surgical exposure of the offending fascia. My goal is to release contractures of the MCP and PIP joints fully, even if that requires concomitant capsulectomy. Incisional options include the use of a continuous Z-plasty; multiple, long zigzag incisions as described by Brunner, or shorter, Y-shaped incisions that are converted to V-shaped incisions to bring additional skin to the midline (Fig. 35.1). The zigzag incision with the Y-V closure, advocated by King and associates, has the advantage of allowing mobilization of considerable skin into the longitudinal axis of the palm and digit, and is the author's preference. There is rarely a need for skin grafting following correction of the deformity, and parallel incisions may be made if the disease involves adjacent digits.

Subtotal palmar fasciectomy is a meticulous, technique-intensive surgical procedure (Fig. 35.2A). Incisions are centered directly over the involved fascia, beginning at the proximal palm and extending to a level distal to the terminal fibers of the diseased cord. If several digits are involved, carefully planned, parallel incisions may be made continuously in the palm and digit. All incisions are drawn on the finger at the onset of the procedure using a skin-marking pen, following which the hand and arm are exsanguinated with an Esmarch bandage, and the tourniquet is elevated to the appropriate pressure (100 to 150 mg greater than systolic blood pressure, not to exceed 300 mm Hg). Although many surgeons prefer to use a magnifying loupe, magnification of greater than ×2 may hinder dissection by limiting the surgeon's field of vision. Magnification for Dupuytren's fasciectomy is rarely used. Throughout the dissection, small bleeding vessels should be cauterized immediately to minimize bleeding at the time of tourniquet release. Skin flaps are dissected carefully off the un-

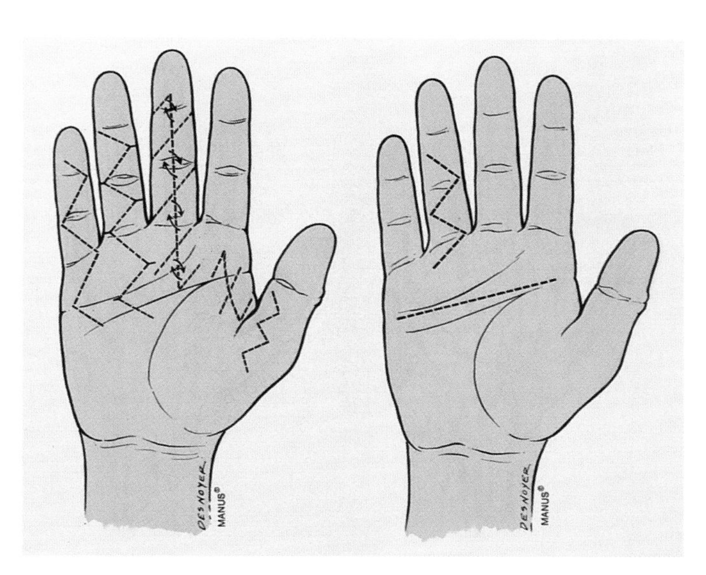

Figure 35.1. Incision options for subtotal palmar fasciectomy. The author prefers the short (two incisions per phalangeal segment) right-angle zigzag incisions shown on the ring fingers of both drawings. They may be easily converted to Y-V closures.

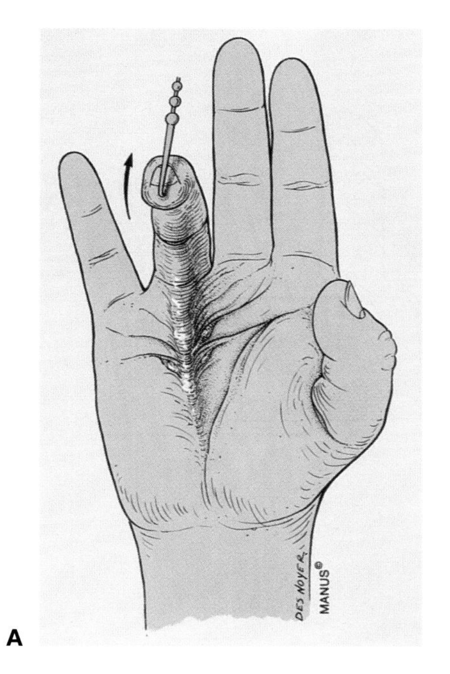

A

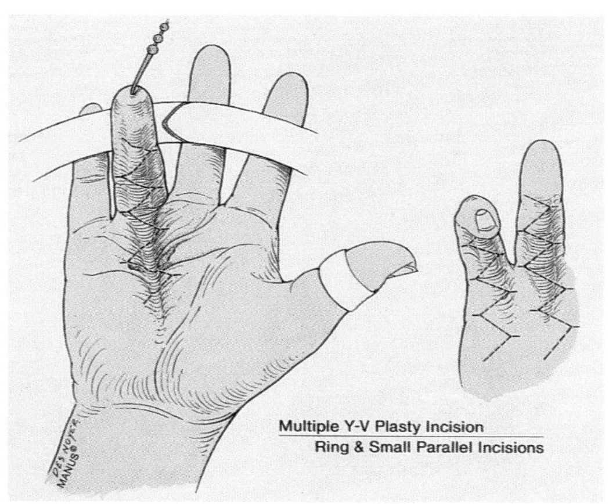

B

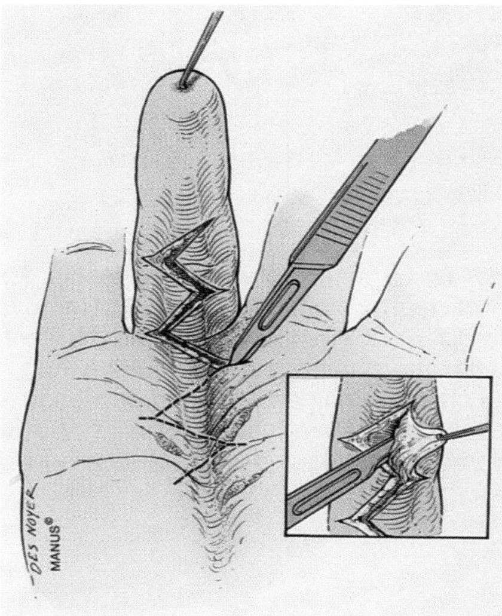

C

Figure 35.2. Illustrations of surgical technique for subtotal palmar fasciectomy. **A:** Palmar-digital cord of the ring finger with contracture. **B:** Hand positioned on table and planned incisions are shown. **C:** Skin incisions and subcutaneous dissection.

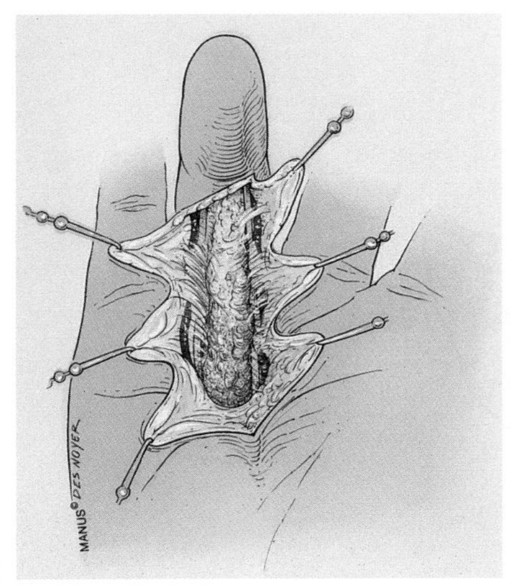

D,E

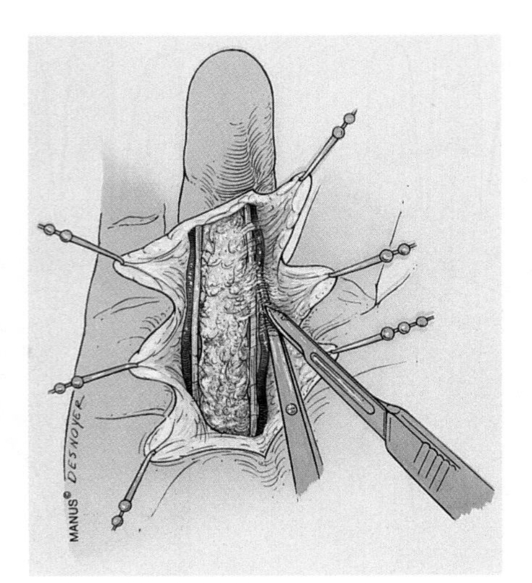

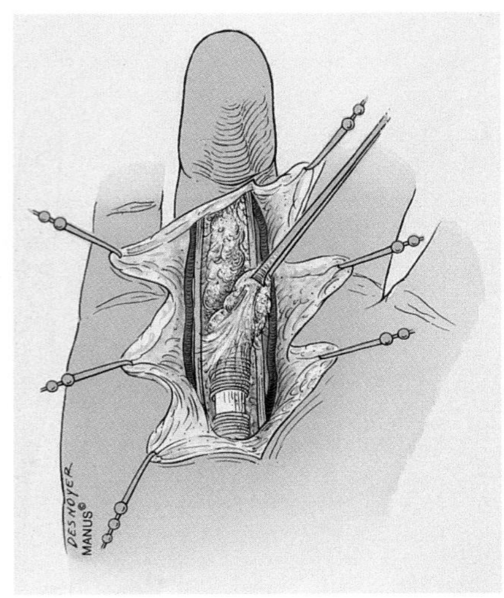

F

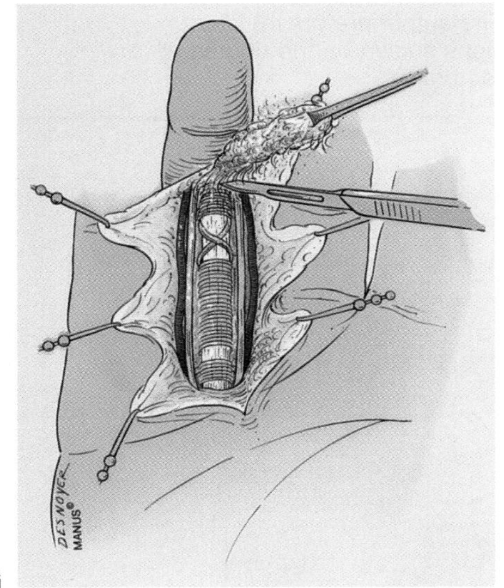

G

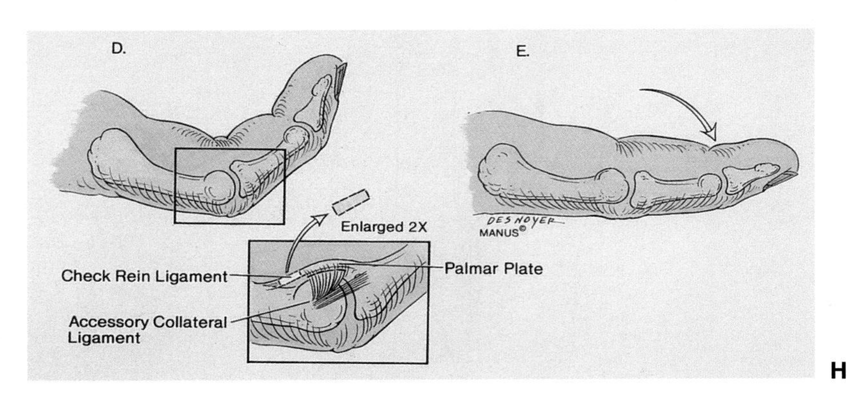

H

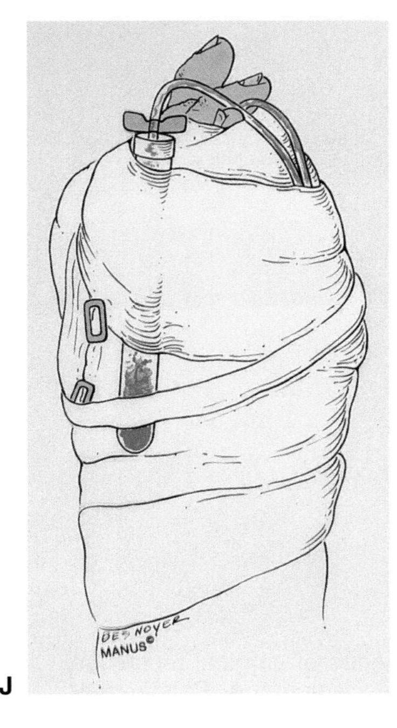

J

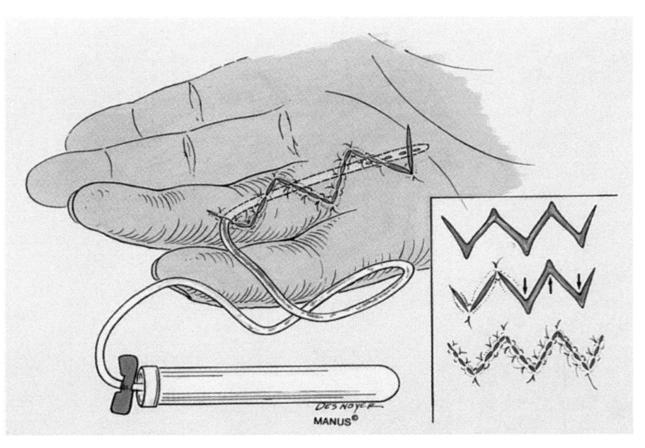

I

Figure 35.2 *Continued.* **D:** Exposure of diseased fascia. **E:** Identification and careful dissection of neurovascular bundles. **F:** Removal of diseased fascia from proximal to distal. **G:** Removal complete. **H:** Technique of capsulectomy of the proximal interphalangeal (PIP) joint (when necessary) release or removal of the check-rein ligaments and accessory collateral ligaments. **I:** Wound closure by flap advancement (Y-V). Small catheter drainage. **J:** Bulky compression dressing with catheter and suction collecting tube incorporated.

derlying diseased area, and, despite the intimate relationship between the fascia and its overlying skin, a satisfactory plane always can be identified. Sharp dissection with a No. 15 blade is used, and flaps are mobilized until the entire diseased cord has been exposed.

At this point, neurovascular bundles from the distal palm to the distal digital level on both the radial and ulnar sides of the cord are exposed, and one must take particular care to identify spiral cords and to protect the vulnerable neurovascular bundles that are delivered in a superficial and medial direction by these fascial projections. The spiral cords arise from either the pretendinous cords or the intrinsic muscle tendons and extend deep via the spiral band to the neurovascular bundle, displacing it both superficially and medially, and rendering it vulnerable to surgical dissection. The presence of a spiral cord often can be identified before surgery by the observation and palpation of a large nodular, fascial accumulation eccentrically located at the base of an involved digit. Flaps are dissected carefully off the spiral cord area, and the vulnerable nerves and vessels should be identified early and protected thereafter.

It is usually preferable to remove the fascia en bloc in a proximal to distal fashion once the neurovascular bundles are well exposed; however, when a spiral cord exists, or the nerve and artery are intricately involved with the digital disease, it is preferable to remove the fascia in a piecemeal fashion to protect these structures. It is also important to preserve as much fatty tissue as possible to provide a well-padded bed for the neurovascular bundles at the conclusion of the procedure. Vertical septa are divided deep to the plane of the fascia, but the author usually makes no effort to remove them at the deeper level, as they are not a cause of contracture.

When necessary, similar dissection in the adjacent palmar digital areas is carried out, and, when all diseased fascia has been excised, determine whether full joint extension has been achieved. In almost every instance, the MCP joints are fully extensible following removal of the offending fascia, but persisting PIP joint contractures may require capsulectomy. When capsulectomy is required at the PIP level, the technique of Watson and colleagues is recommended. For this procedure, open the flexor tendon sheath just proximal to the A-3 pulley and, with the flexor tendons alternately retracted into the radial and ulnar sides of the digits, excise the check-rein proximal extensions of the palmar plate. It is also possible to release the palmarmost fibers of the collateral ligament (accessory collateral ligaments) and gently manipulate the digit to achieve full or near-full extension. Failure to achieve full extension may require additional exploration and release of portions of the lateral digital sheet or further V-Y skin extension incisions.

In the little finger, expose the ulnar aspect of the digit to determine whether a hypothenar cord is present. If so, it should be excised, as it may represent the most likely cause of recurrence of deformity in that digit. Similar isolated digital cords may be present in other digits and should be identified before surgery by the palpable presence of a PIP joint contracture without an associated palmar fascial communication. Again, the use of zigzag incisions centered directly over the cord will usually provide adequate exposure for cord excision, with the realization that the neurovascular bundle is displaced medially in the proximal digit and passes underneath the cord distally.

At the conclusion of the fascial excision and any necessary capsulectomies, the tourniquet should be released and compression applied to the hand for 10 minutes to control the resulting wound hyperemia. At this point, cauterize all brisk bleeders; while the tourniquet is released, carefully inspect all skin flaps to be sure that they return adequate vascularity. If the entire flap remains white, it may be necessary to excise it and use skin-graft coverage, as that flap almost surely will be necrotic at the time of the initial dressing change. If only the distal 2 or 3 mm of the flap remain white, that segment of the flap may be excised and the flap advanced further at the time of the wound closure. At the time of closure, do not hesitate to reinflate the tourniquet if there is a vascular ooze.

It is preferred to close the wound somewhat loosely using 5-0 nonabsorbable sutures with about two-thirds the normal number of skin sutures that might normally be used for a tight wound closure. As the wound is being closed, introduce the tubing of a pediatric scalp vein set into each wound in a distal to proximal fashion after several small holes have been placed along the length of the tube. After wound closure is complete, it has been the author's habit to instill 3 to 5 ml of triamcinolone into each digital wound with a small flexible catheter. This local steroid eliminates postoperative pain and reduces the amount of postoperative wound reaction that these patients so commonly experience.

A bulky compressive dressing is applied in such a manner as to produce anterior/posterior compression of the hand. The fingers are splinted into nearly full extension using a palmar plaster slab. If the tourniquet has been reinflated, it is then deflated, and the scalp vein needle, which exits from the distal part of the dressing, is placed in the rubber stopper of a suction collection tube. The drainage tube then can be incorporated in the outer layer of the dressing, and an additional tube can be placed adjacent to it in case the first tube should fill. Clinical photographs of the surgical steps of subtotal palmar fasciectomy are illustrated in Figure 35.3.

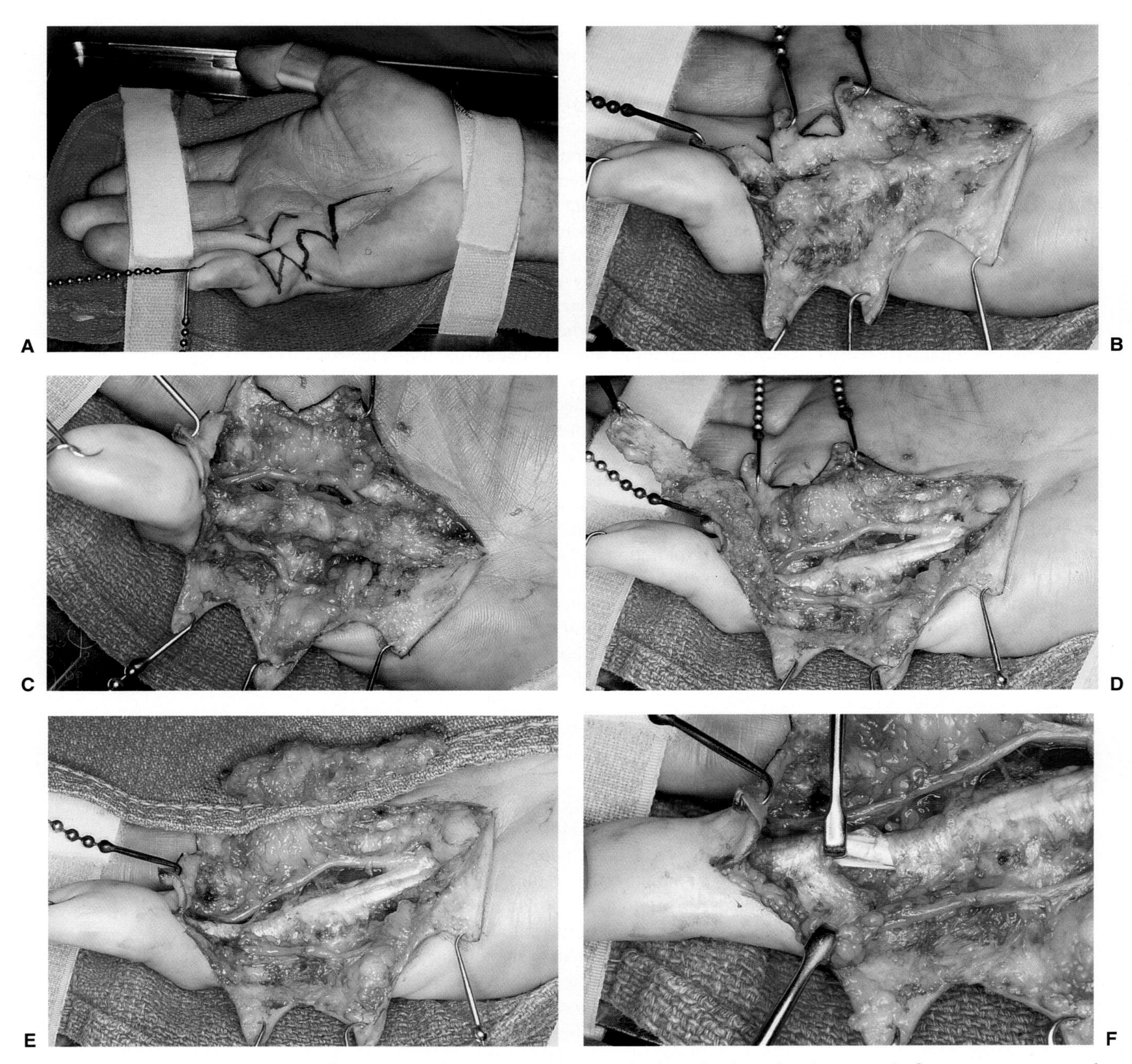

Figure 35.3. Clinical photographs of subtotal palmar fasciectomy. **A:** Severe contracture of the fifth finger with associated distal palmar disease proximal to ring finger. Incisions have been marked. **B:** Appearance of diseased fascia with all flaps elevated. **C:** Identification and dissection of neurovascular bundles. **D:** Fascia removed from proximal to distal. **E:** Appearance of digit with fascia removed (*shown above digit*). **F:** Sheath opened over proximal interphalangeal (PIP) joint, and flexor tendons retracted in preparation for capsulectomy.

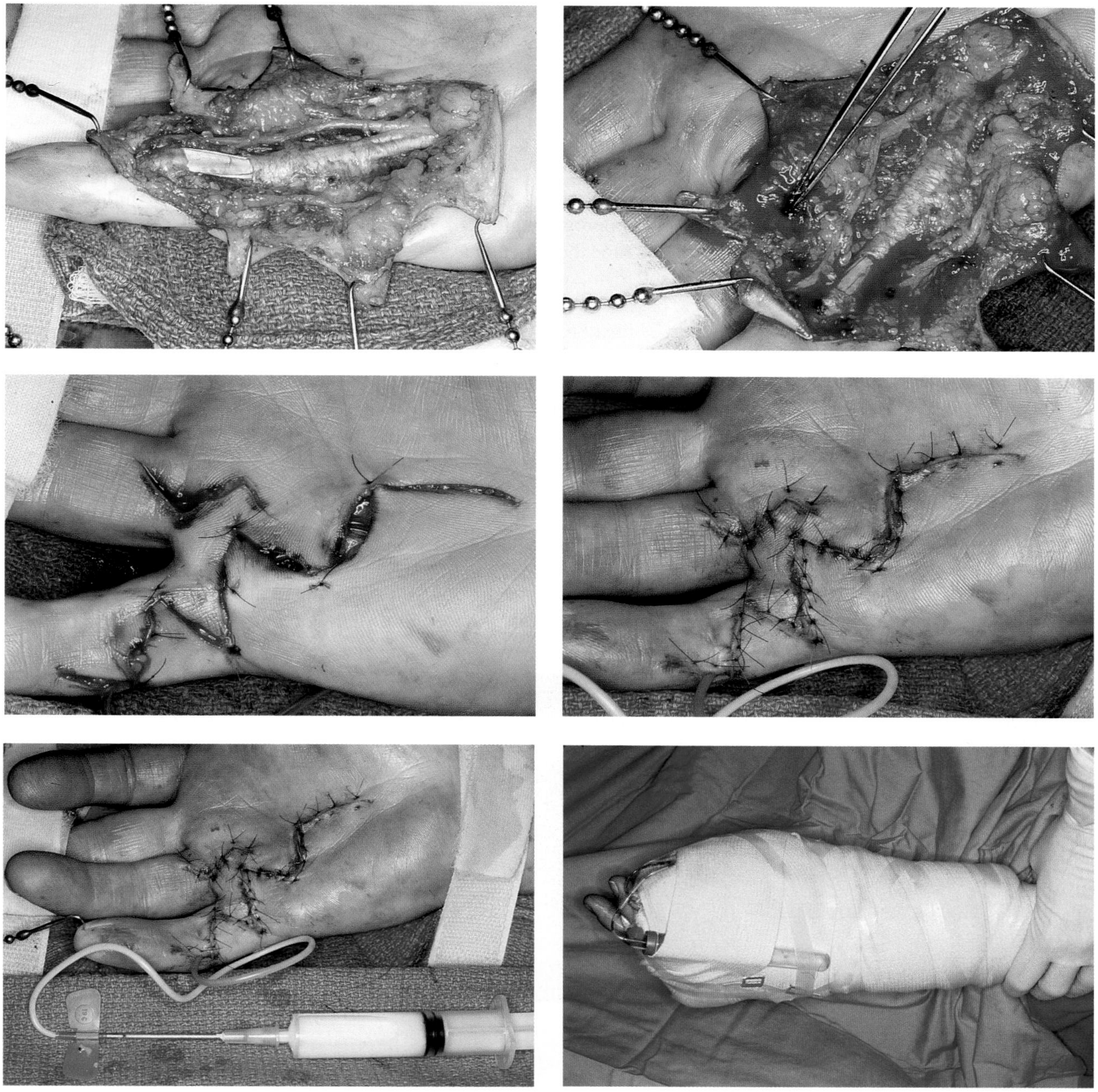

G H I J K L

Figure 35.3 *Continued.* **G:** Digit fully extended following capsulectomy. **H:** Small bleeding vessels cauterized with tourniquet deflated. **I:** Skin flaps advanced before closure. **J:** Wound closure with drainage catheter in place. **K:** Instillation of several milliliters of triamcinolone before applying dressing. **L:** Compression dressing with collecting tube incorporated.

POSTOPERATIVE MANAGEMENT

At the time of discharge, instruct both the patients and their families about the method of removing the drain from the dressing on the following day. Any problems are to be reported to the doctor's office, and, for patients who have traveled a long distance for their surgery, they may be asked to spend the night in an adjacent lodge so the drain can be removed on the following day before the trip home. All patients are scheduled for follow-up appointments within 3 to 5 days of surgery, at which time the bulky dressing is removed and a vigorous digital-motion program initiated. Every effort is made to achieve a full range of digital motion by the time the patient leaves the facility. Continuous extension splinting of the involved digits is maintained for several weeks, although the splint is removed frequently for active and passive range-of-motion exercises. Skin sutures are removed at 2 weeks, and formal therapy is instituted for patients who have difficulty with active flexion and extension. Night extension splinting for the involved digits is currently continued for 6 to 12 months in an effort to minimize the possibility of recurrent contractures.

The author has been impressed that patients have little or no discomfort in the immediate postoperative period, and this may be attributable to the use of steroids in the operative wound. Some discomfort is associated with the initial therapy, and it is not unusual for the digits to be somewhat swollen for several weeks. A complete composite fist is sometimes quite difficult because of this digital swelling, but most patients can bring their digits to or close to their palms at the conclusion of the initial therapy. The surgical wounds from Dupuytren's contracture are often hypertrophic and angry-looking for 4 to 8 weeks. When the patient is struggling with postoperative exercises and the wounds are firm and hypertrophic, initiate a short course of oral steroids (Methylprednisone Dose-Pak) for 6 days and,

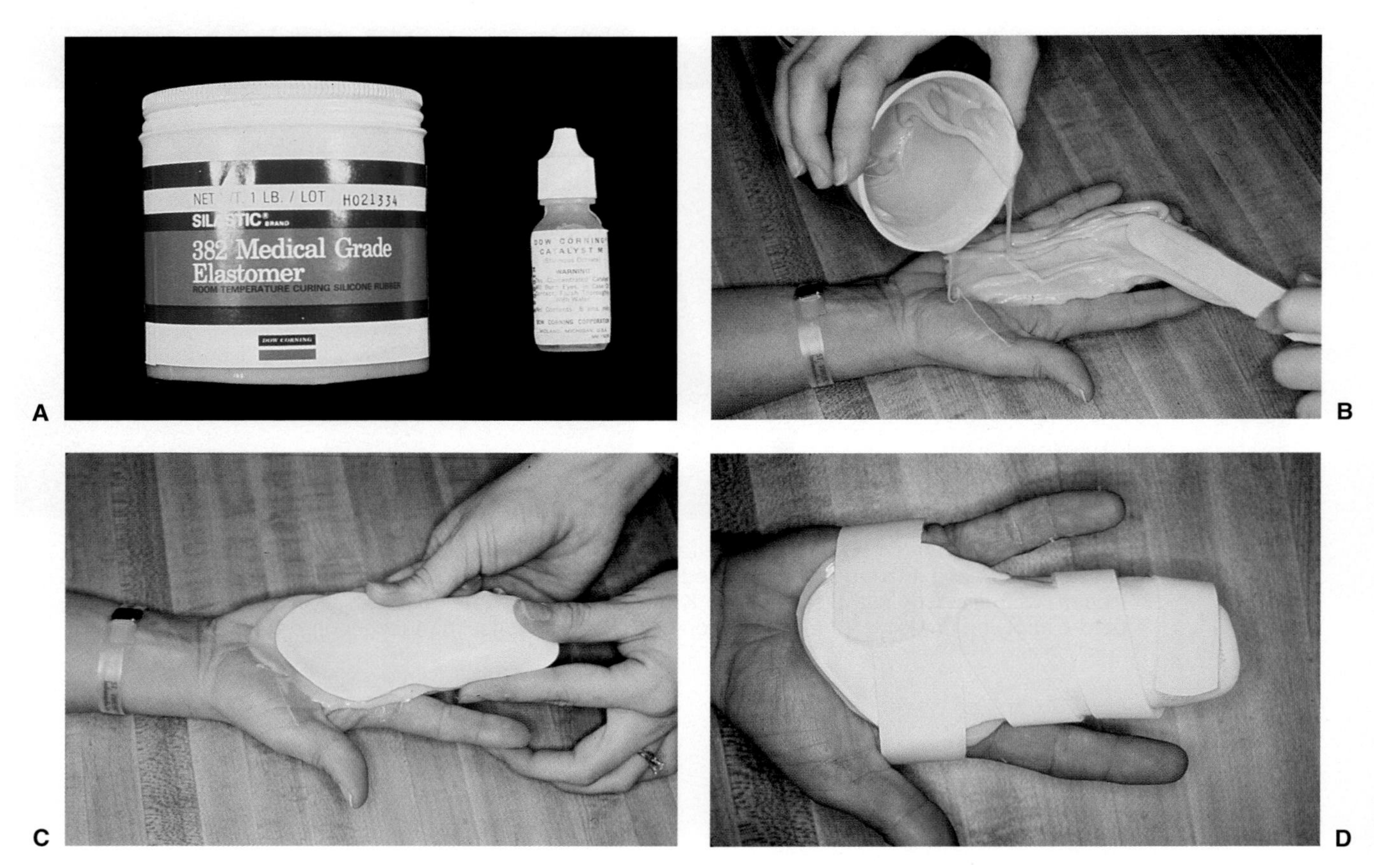

Figure 35.4. Preparation of customized digital splint inlaid with molded Medical Grade Elastomer (Dow Corning). **A:** Commercial components of Elastomer. **B:** Material is prepared and conformed to the patient's middle and ring fingers. **C:** Supporting rigid splint is bonded to Elastomer. **D:** Appearance of splint when strapped in position.

in some patients, extend the use of steroids for an additional two to three weeks in a low dosage, not to exceed 8 mg a day. The use of steroids for these somewhat reactive wounds is beneficial.

For patients who experience some difficulty maintaining a satisfactory range of digital motion on their own, formal hand therapy may be appropriate. In addition to active and passive range-of-motion exercises and the use of static or dynamic splints, therapists also may employ massage techniques in an attempt to soften the surgical scar, and we find that the use of Coban elastic wrapping or small elastic digital "socks" have been helpful in reducing edema. The inclusion of soft, custom-molded materials, such as Medical Grade Elastomer, in the contact areas of postoperative Dupuytren's splints also has been helpful in reducing swelling and softening the surgical scar (Fig. 35.4). Most important, therapists can recognize deteriorating function by serial digital measurements and wound observations. The therapy program may be altered as a result of these changes, and frequent dialogue with the surgeon is important so that appropriate measures can be carried out to minimize functional loss.

COMPLICATIONS

The immediate potential complications of surgery for Dupuytren's contracture include palmar hematoma and skin necrosis. The use of low-suction drainage should minimize the likelihood of hematoma, but, when it occurs, prompt evacuation is recommended. Skin necrosis may be managed by careful observation if the diameter of the area is no greater than 1 cm; however, larger areas must be excised as soon as possible. The defect that results from excision of the necrotic skin may be left open or closed by the use of a free graft.

A postoperative sympathetic disturbance or "flare" is probably the most severe complication after surgery for Dupuytren's contracture. The condition is thought to be secondary to an overresponse of the sympathetic nervous system and may be quite difficult to manage. Pain, swelling, and stiffness may involve not only the operated digits but also the unoperated fingers, the hand, and to some extent the entire extremity. Wounds may be inordinately reddened and firm, and the hand may sweat excessively. Onset of this unfortunate complication may be suspected when the degree of pain, edema, and stiffness experienced by the patient exceeds that normally seen during the early stages of surgical recovery.

Treatment of severe "flare" usually consists of a gentle but vigorous therapeutic program that includes active and passive range-of-motion exercises, dynamic splinting, continuous passive-motion devices, transcutaneous nerve stimulation, and the administration of anti-inflammatory medications or steroids. Oral steroids may be of considerable value in patients with particularly severe dystrophy characterized by marked inflammation and stiffness. Carpal tunnel decompression is of value when the median nerve is compromised. Occasionally, one or more stellate ganglion blocks may help to reverse this phenomenon.

When postoperative flare or dystrophy occurs, patients should be advised that their recovery will be considerably slower than originally expected and that a great deal of patience and effort will be required to maximize the eventual recovery. Failure to comply with the vigorous therapeutic program may result in permanent stiffness of the involved digital joints and sometimes even of the uninvolved digits of the operated hand.

The author concurs with the statement made many years ago by Howard that surgery for Dupuytren's contracture is palliative rather than curative. Recurrence of diseased fascia and flexion contractures are, unfortunately, fairly common following this procedure. Our results suggest that complete correction of the MCP joint deformities are almost always achieved, and recurrent deformity at that level is rare. The redevelopment of PIP joint flexion contractures is much more frequent, and these deformities often recur fairly rapidly following surgical correction. We found that the degree of PIP joint contracture at the time of surgery could be used to predict the likelihood of recurrence. If the presenting contracture was less than 30 degrees, long-term postoperative follow-up indicated that recurring contractures almost never exceeded 30 degrees. If the preoperative deformity was between 30 and 60 degrees, 20% of patients redeveloped deformity that was as great as or greater than the original contracture. If the initial contracture was greater than 60 degrees, 50% went on to recurrent severe deformity. Without question, the PIP joint of the small finger is the most troublesome, and trying to correct and prevent the recurrence of deformity at that joint is an enigma for all hand surgeons.

Recurrent Dupuytren's disease is common and almost always involves the PIP joint. Because of the added difficulty in correcting recurrent contractures, the indications for additional surgery are somewhat different from those governing the original procedure. If the degree of contracture is not great and the condition appears to be reasonably stable, the surgeon and the patient may elect to accept the results of the initial operation rather than to attempt surgical correction again. If, however, the contracture is severe and progressive, additional efforts at ablation of the offending disease may be indicated. Reoperation is more difficult, because the diseased fascia is intertwined with scar secondary to the previous surgery. As with the original fasciectomy, complete exposure of the neurovascular bundles is required. Defining and protecting those structures may be considerably more difficult than with the initial procedure, and digital capsulectomy is almost always required when dealing with recurrent disease. If the skin is of good quality, it may be retained and closed, but poor-quality skin should be excised and replaced by full-thickness skin grafts, as advocated by Hueston. Local rotational flaps or cross-finger flaps may be employed on some occasions when vascularized tissue is required to cover complex defects resulting from skin and fascial excision for recurrent contracture.

When an irreparable contracture exists at the PIP joint, several salvage operations are available. The most rational salvage procedure is arthrodesis of the PIP joint. A sufficient wedge of dorsal bone is removed to allow the digit to be brought into about 40 degrees of extension, and a tension band technique or Herbert screw may be used to secure fixation. Given the fact that the MCP joint function is usually normal, a good grasping digit can be preserved in this manner. When severe deformities (greater than 90 degrees) are present, or for patients who request amputation because of occupational concerns or disdain for the digit, amputation either through the proximal phalanx or by ray excision may provide a satisfactory final solution.

RECOMMENDED READING

1. Bruner JM. Incisions for plastic and reconstructive (non-septic) surgery of the hand. *Br J Plast Surg* 4:48, 1951.
2. Howard LD. *Dupuytren's Contracture: A Challenge, Not a Blessing.* AAOS Instructional Course Lecture. Presented at the 32nd annual meeting of the American Academy of Orthopaedic Surgeons (self-published), 1965.
3. Hueston JT. Dupuytren's contracture: the trend to conservatism. *Ann R Coll Surg Engl* 36:134, 1965.
4. Hueston JT. In: Flynn JL. *Hand Surgery.* Baltimore, MD: Williams and Wilkins, 1982:797–822.
5. King EW, Exeter NH, Bass DM, et al. The treatment of Dupuytren's contracture by extensive fasciectomy through multiple Y-V plasty incisions. *J Hand Surg* 4:234, 1979.
6. McFarlane RM. The current status of Dupuytren's disease. *J Hand Surg* 8:703, 1983.
7. McFarlane RM. In: Green DP, ed. *Operative Hand Surgery.* Churchill-Livingstone, New York, 1983.
8. McFarlane RM. Patterns of the diseased fascia in the fingers in Dupuytren's contracture: displacement of the neurovascular bundle. *Plast Reconstr Surg* 54:31, 1974.
9. McFarlane RM, Jamieson WB. Dupuytren's contracture: the management of 100 patients. *J Bone Joint Surg Am* 48-A:1095, 1966.
10. McGrouther DA. In: Watson N, Smith RJ, eds. *Methods and Concepts in Hand Surgery.* Boston: Butterworth and Company, 1986:75–96.
11. McGrouther DA. In: Hueston JT, Tubiana R, eds. *Dupuytren's Disease.* Churchill-Livingstone, London, 1985.
12. McGrouther DA. The microanatomy of Dupuytren's contracture. *Hand* 14:215, 1982.
13. Michon J. In: Hueston JT, Tubiana R, eds. *Dupuytren's Disease.* Churchill-Livingstone, London, 1985: 177–183.
14. Stein AMH, Jr. The relation of median nerve compression to Sudeck's syndrome. *Surg Gynecol Obstet* 115:713, 1962.
15. Strickland JW, Bassett RL. The isolated digital cord in Dupuytren's contracture: anatomy and clinical significance. *J Hand Surg* 10-A:118, 1985.
16. Torstrick RF, Hartwig RH, Strickland JHW. Long-term results of regional fasciectomy of Dupuytren's contracture of the proximal interphalangeal joint. *J Hand Surg* 6:297, 1981.
17. Watson HK, Light TR, Johnson TR. Check-rein resection for flexion contracture of the middle joint. *J Hand Surg* 4:67, 1970.

36

Decompression and Lavage for Suppurative Flexor Tenosynovitis

John A. McAuliffe

INDICATIONS/CONTRAINDICATIONS

The digital flexor tendon sheaths lie within millimeters of the palmar skin on the working surface of our hands. It is logical that most cases of suppurative flexor tenosynovitis result from direct penetrating trauma. Even the most innocent-looking wounds can be problematic. An almost imperceptible puncture wound that inoculates the tendon sheath but does not allow for drainage can result in fulminant infection within the confines of this closed space within 12 to 36 hours.

A small percentage of flexor tendon sheath infections occur in the absence of penetrating injury, presumably resulting from hematogenous seeding of the offending organism, usually from another focus of infection. Such "spontaneous" infections are encountered more frequently in immunocompromised hosts, including diabetics and patients with acquired immunodeficiency syndrome. Gonococcal flexor tenosynovitis also presents in this fashion.

Whatever the source of infection, edema of the tendon and surrounding soft tissues increases the drag on the flexor system, and pain due to inflammation and swelling further inhibits motion. Purulent exudate within the sheath compromises synovial nutrition of the tendon, while increased pressure caused by the accumulation of fluid may impair vincular and intratendinous blood flow. All of these factors conspire to disrupt the normal gliding mechanisms that are critical to finger function and may ultimately result in tendon necrosis.

The slightest suspicion of suppurative flexor tenosynovitis should prompt urgent evaluation and treatment. Although some authors suggest that patients with early signs and symptoms of tendon sheath infection can be treated with antibiotics, immobilization, and elevation, it is imperative that these patients be reassessed frequently. If obvious clinical

John A. McAuliffe, M.D.: Department of Orthopaedic Surgery, Cleveland Clinic Florida, Weston, FL

improvement is not appreciated within 12 to 24 hours, surgical drainage should be performed without further delay.

The sequelae of delayed or inadequate treatment of suppurative flexor tenosynovitis include functional loss due to stiffness and adhesions, tendon necrosis, spread of infection to adjacent areas of the hand, and possible need for amputation. These consequences are potentially so severe that it is far safer to err on the side of draining a finger that proves to be culture-negative than to defer surgical treatment. This is one of those clinical situations in which if one even considers the need for surgical care, it is probably wisest to proceed, particularly when caring for immunocompromised patients, for whom delay could prove catastrophic. The risks of inadequate treatment far exceed those of a carefully performed decompression and lavage.

PREOPERATIVE PLANNING

Given an appropriate history, the diagnosis of suppurative flexor tenosynovitis is made on clinical grounds, taking note of the four cardinal signs of flexor sheath infection described by Kanavel in 1943:

- flexed posture of the finger,
- fusiform swelling of the finger,
- tenderness over the entire course of the flexor tendon sheath, and
- pain on passive extension of the finger.

I find tenderness over the tendon sheath at a distance from the zone of injury to be the most helpful finding, although pain with passive extension may be the first sign to become apparent in patients seen very early in the disease process. Although Kanavel noted the flexed posture of these infected fingers, and they are certainly never fully extended, it is worth noting that because of the increased hydrostatic pressure within the flexor sheath, these digits are usually slightly more extended at rest than the normal flexion cascade of the adjacent digits (Fig. 36.1).

The synovial flexor tendon sheaths of the index, long, and ring fingers run from the proximal extent of the A1 pulley to the flexor digitorum profundus insertion. Typically, the synovial sheaths of the thumb and small fingers are prolonged proximally through the carpal tunnel to the distal forearm as the radial and ulnar bursae, respectively. Rarely, the sheaths of the index, long, and ring fingers may communicate with the ulnar bursa. Neglected in-

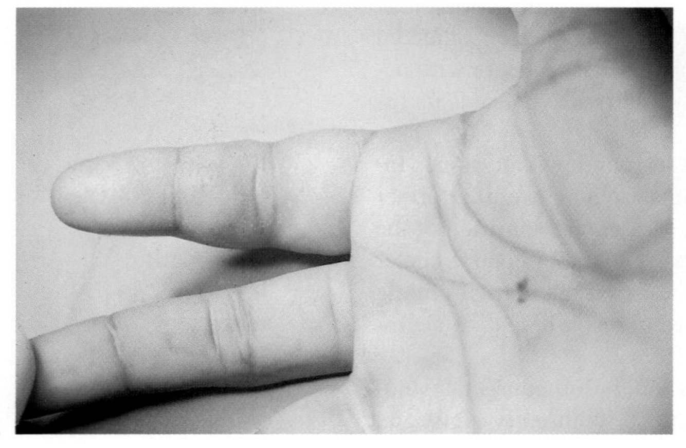

A

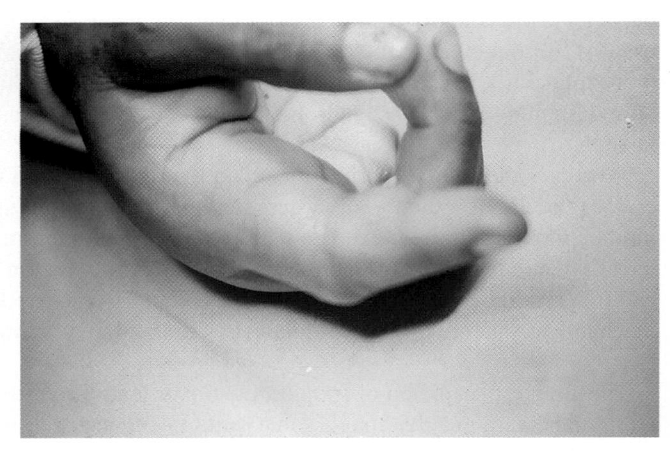

B

Figure 36.1. A: Note the fusiform swelling of this index finger with suppurative flexor tenosynovitis. **B:** Although the involved index finger is "semi-flexed," as described by Kanavel, note that the increased pressure within the tendon sheath causes this finger to be relatively more extended than the flexion cascade of the adjacent fingers at rest.

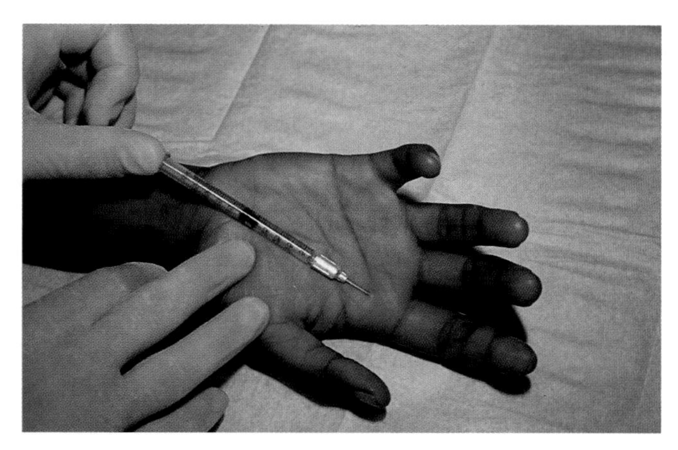

Figure 36.2. The flexor tendon sheath may be aspirated at the level of the A1 pulley in the palm.

fection may rupture the sheath at any point along its course, resulting in the spread of infection to contiguous spaces. Distal rupture may result in a felon, more proximal rupture may involve the thenar or midpalmar spaces, and communication between the radial and ulnar bursae deep to the contents of the carpal tunnel in the distal forearm (Parona's space) may cause a so-called "horseshoe abscess" in which infection beginning in the thumb comes to involve the small finger, or vice versa.

Animal bites often involve both the dorsal and palmar surfaces of the hand, potentially penetrating the flexor tendon sheath palmarly and the metacarpophalangeal or interphalangeal joints dorsally. The possibility of each of these additional sites of infection must be carefully considered.

Plain radiographs may be helpful to exclude the possibility of retained foreign bodies in the case of penetrating injury or to search for early signs of osteomyelitis in neglected cases. Acute calcific tendonitis can also be diagnosed on plain radiographs, but this does not rule out the possibility of a concomitant or superimposed infectious process.

Additional imaging is seldom indicated in acute cases. Although edema of the tendons and fluid within the tendon sheath have been demonstrated on ultrasound, I think these findings should be clinically obvious and would not help to differentiate suppuration from inflammation. In the rare instance in which gout or some other metabolic or inflammatory process is strongly suspected, aspiration of the sheath to search for crystals or other microscopic findings may be helpful (Fig. 36.2). Never delay lavage and decompression for days while awaiting culture results.

Baseline white blood cell count and erythrocyte sedimentation rate may be helpful if the response to treatment does not follow the anticipated course over the ensuing days or weeks. Additional laboratory evaluation may be necessary depending upon the patient's general health or the choice of antibiotics to be administered. If the patient is being taken to the operating room urgently and has no signs or symptoms of systemic toxicity, I prefer to withhold antibiotic therapy until deep specimens for culture are obtained during surgery.

SURGERY

The patient is placed supine on the operating table with the upper extremity on a hand table. A well-padded pneumatic tourniquet is placed proximal to the elbow. General anesthesia is usually preferred. Infiltration anesthesia at the level of the hand or wrist is likely to be ineffective in the presence of local infection and runs the risk of potentially contaminating uninvolved tissues. Many anesthesiologists prefer not to perform axillary block

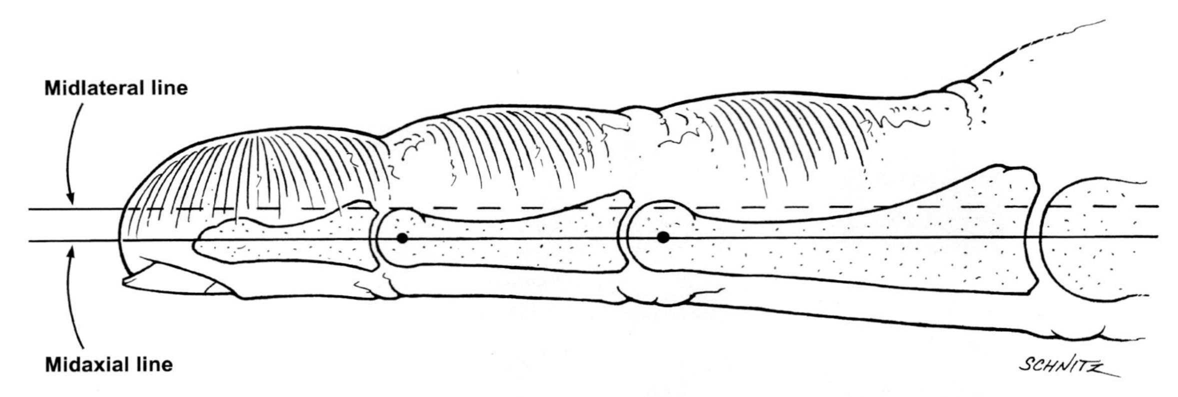

Figure 36.3. The midaxial line passes through the centers of rotation of the PIP and DIP joints, approximately 2 to 3 mm dorsal to the midlateral line.

anesthesia to avoid the possibility of violating lymphatics that drain the affected area, although I am not aware of any documented complications of regional anesthesia when infection is confined to the hand and there is no clinical evidence of proximal lymphangitis or adenopathy.

Adequate lighting and magnification are mandatory. The extremity is exsanguinated by gravity and the tourniquet inflated to 100 mm Hg above systolic blood pressure. The use of an Esmarch bandage or other compression wrap is avoided so as not to spread infection.

Ignore the traumatic wound and make a midaxial incision on the side of the digit that is least likely to have tactile contact (the ulnar side of the index, long, and ring fingers and the radial side of the small finger and thumb). The midaxial line is approximately 2 or 3 mm dorsal to the midlateral line and passes through the center of rotation of the heads of the proximal and distal phalanges (Fig. 36.3). This incision in the line of minimal skin tension facilitates early active motion and healing of the wound by secondary intention.

Depending upon the severity of infection, this incision can involve only a small portion of the digit at the level of the distal interphalangeal (DIP) joint to allow the flexor sheath to be entered distal to the A4 pulley, or it may encompass the entire length of the finger. In most cases, the incision will proceed from just proximal to the proximal interphalangeal (PIP) joint to just distal to the DIP joint, allowing entry into the sheath both distal to the A4 pulley and between the A2 and A4 pulleys. In all but the very mildest cases of flexor tendon sheath infection, this incision has the added benefit of relieving the significantly elevated subcutaneous pressures that have been measured in these edematous digits.

The incision is carried through the transverse retinacular ligament at the level of the PIP joint and Cleland's ligament along the length of the digit, reflecting the palmar skin and the neurovascular bundle from the flexor tendon sheath (Fig. 36.4). The dorsal branch of the digital nerve courses obliquely across the incision proximal to the PIP joint and should be protected if possible, but in cases of severe infection, it may not be identifiable due to swelling, scarring, and distortion of the soft tissues.

The tendon sheath can be opened at the level of the PIP and DIP joints, taking care not to violate the critical A2 and A4 pulleys (Fig. 36.5). As the sheath is opened, specimens of the fluid are obtained for Gram's stain and aerobic and anaerobic cultures. If present, hypertrophic synovial tissue should be debrided thoroughly and collected for histologic examination. It is necessary to visualize the flexor digitorum superficialis insertion to be certain that the separate synovial sheath that sometimes encircles this tendon has also been opened and drained. The interphalangeal joints can be opened and irrigated if necessary by excising the accessory collateral ligament to gain access to the joint (Fig. 36.6).

I now prefer to orient the palmar incision slightly obliquely so that it can more easily be extended if necessary. This incision is made at the proximal extent of the A1 pulley,

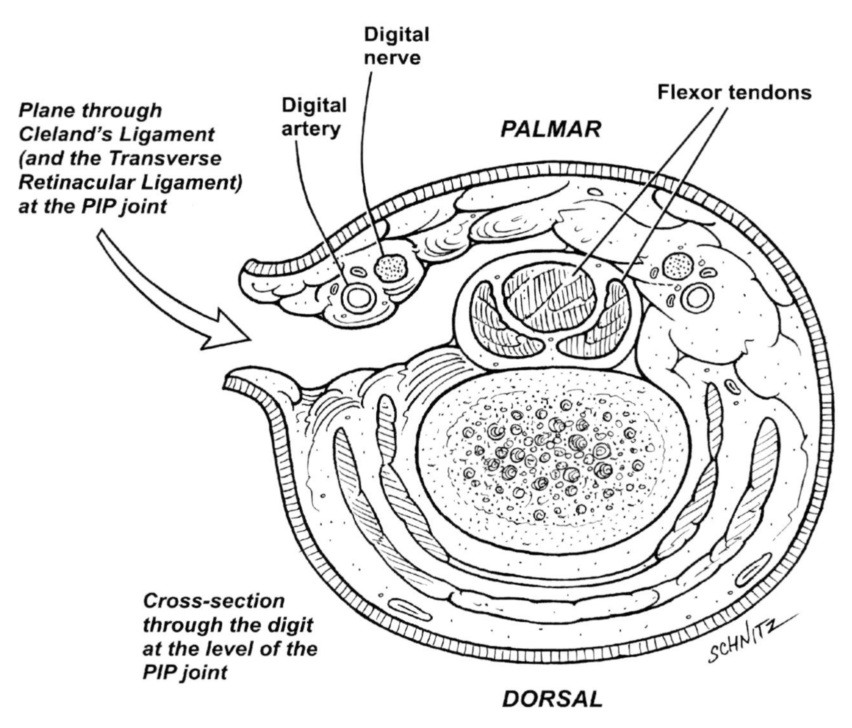

Figure 36.4. The plane of dissection in the digit reflects the neurovascular bundle with the palmar skin flap.

and I attempt to dissect directly down to the flexor sheath without exposing the neurovascular bundles to either side, but if there is any doubt about their location, they should be visualized. I make two parallel incisions along the radial and ulnar borders of the pulley so that it can be hinged distally to open the sheath. Hypertrophic synovium is again debrided.

In cases of more severe infection, it can be helpful to excise a portion of palmar fascia overlying the A1 pulley, and to fix the proximal edge of the pulley to the distal skin flap with an absorbable suture to promote drainage and prevent the wound from sealing rapidly

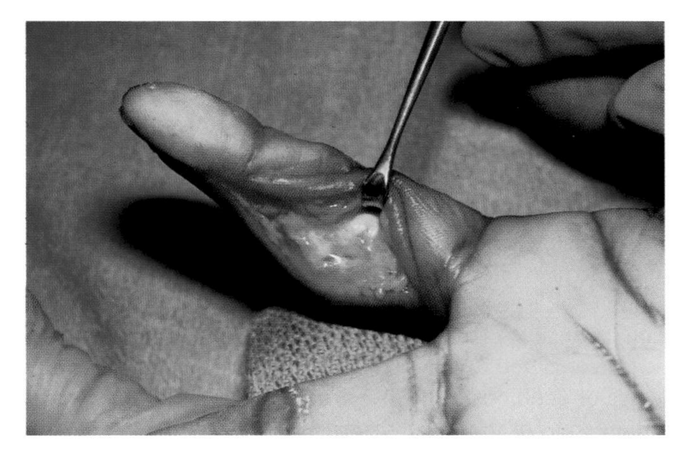

Figure 36.5. The flexor tendon sheath has been opened between the A2 and A4 pulleys. Note the purulent exudate.

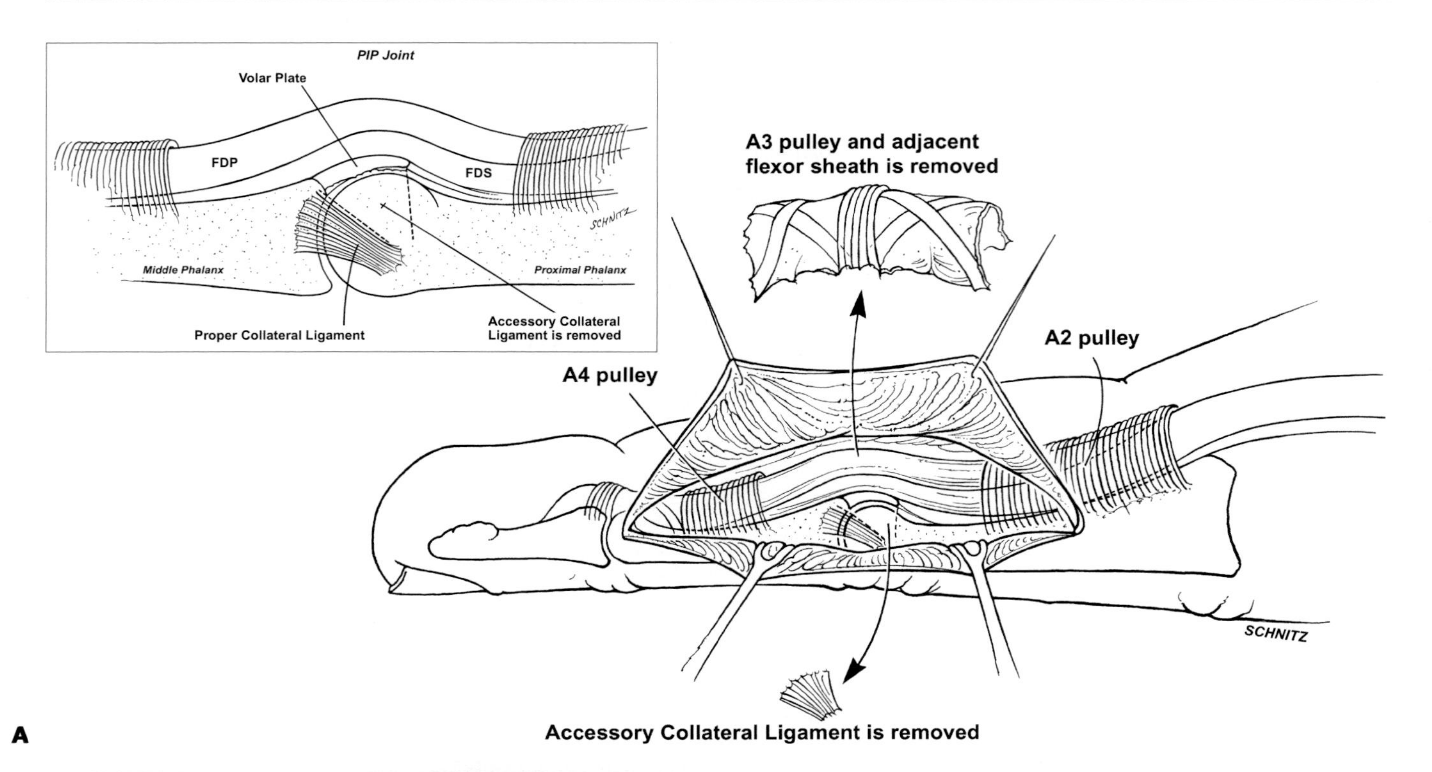

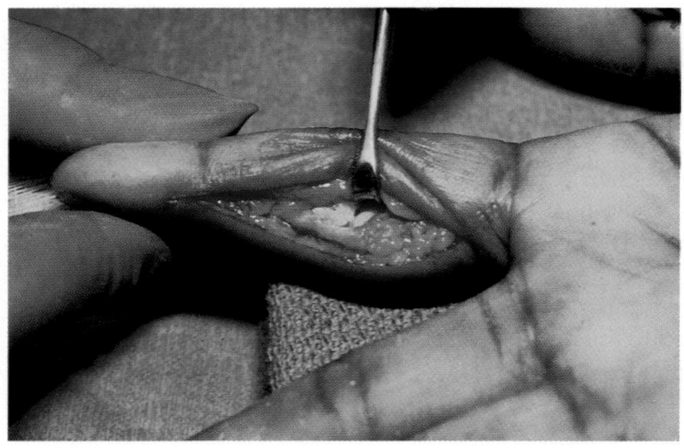

Figure 36.6. A: The flexor digitorum profundus and superficialis tendons can be visualized between the A2 and A4 pulleys. The inset demonstrates how excision of the accessory collateral ligament can be used to gain exposure to the PIP joint. **B:** The articular surface of the PIP joint can be seen after excision of the accessory collateral ligament in this clinical photograph.

(Fig. 36.7). Digital pressure over the course of the involved tendons from the distal forearm, across the carpal tunnel, and into the palm will help to demonstrate any proximal spread of infection that may require further exploration and drainage.

The tendon sheath can now be irrigated from proximal to distal using a 16-gauge intravenous catheter, irrigating first beneath the A2 pulley and then beneath A4 (Fig. 36.8). It is often easiest to first pass the catheter on the dorsal side of the tendon sheath; however, efforts should be made to also introduce it between the tendons and on the palmar surface as well. A blunt tendon hook is used to atraumatically apply traction to the tendons and glide them from beneath the intact A2 and A4 pulleys to be sure that any loculated pockets have been drained and irrigated and to excise as much hypertrophic synovium as possible. No advantage to the use of antibiotic-containing irrigation has ever been demonstrated. Once one is certain that all areas of the sheath have been drained, the pneumatic tourniquet can be deflated during the final phases of irrigation. Intravenous antibiotics can now be administered if this has not already been done. Hemostasis is achieved using a bipolar electrocautery device.

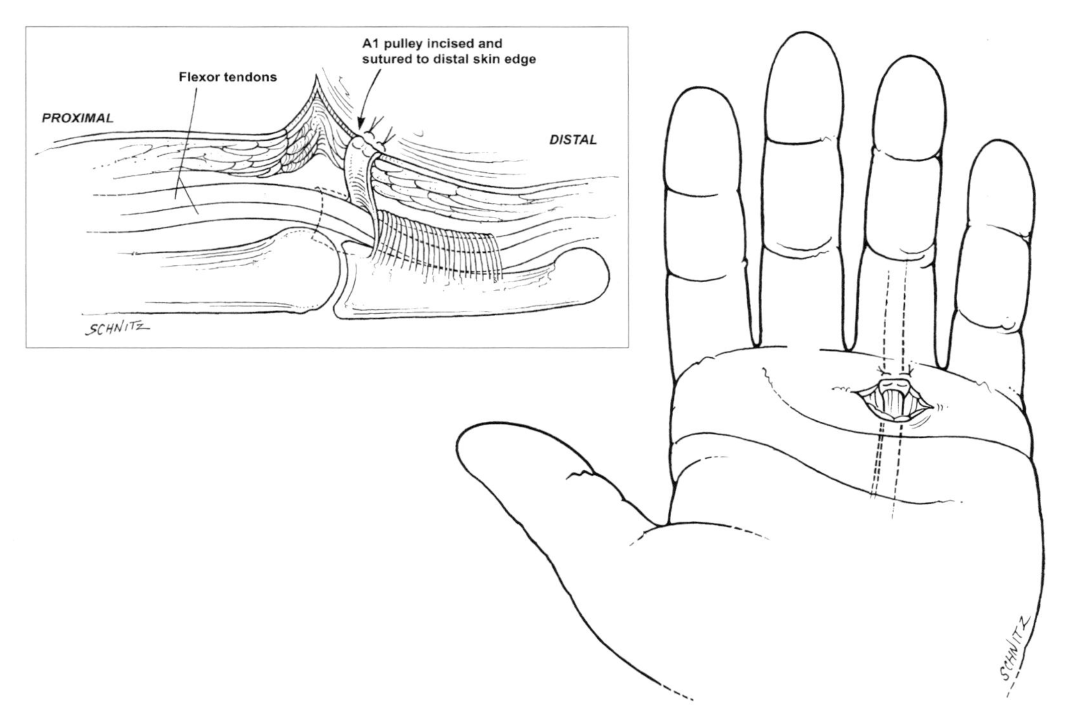

Figure 36.7. The proximal portion of the tendon sheath is exposed at the level of the A1 pulley in the palm. The inset shows how a distally based flap of the pulley can be sutured to the distal skin edge to promote proximal drainage of the sheath.

Although many authors have recommended the use of an indwelling catheter (Fig. 36.9) for continuous or intermittent irrigation for 24 to 48 hours postoperatively, I have never found this necessary or advantageous. In my limited experience with indwelling catheters, they are painful for the patient, messy for the patient and staff, and difficult to manage for the patient, staff, and physician. In my opinion, the severe or neglected flexor tendon sheath infection is best managed with repeat debridement and irrigation in the operating room as necessary.

The wounds are left open and a bulky dressing is applied. Nonadherent dressings are not used on the wounds so that drainage is not inhibited. Palmar and dorsal plaster slabs main-

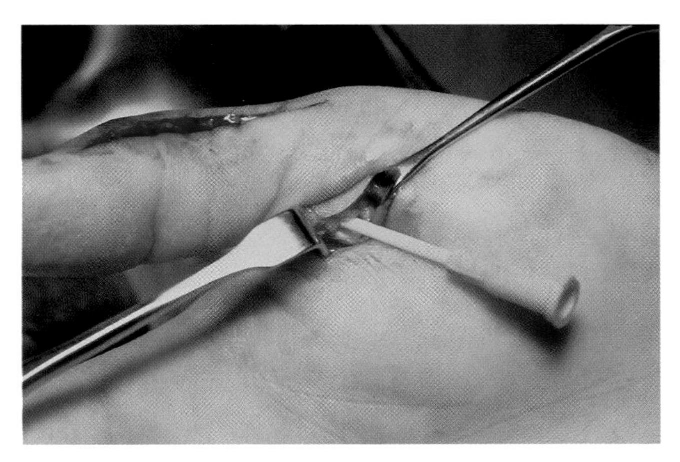

Figure 36.8. A 16-gauge intravenous catheter has been placed in the flexor tendon sheath of this infected thumb after opening the A1 pulley. Irrigation beneath the oblique pulley can be performed, allowing the fluid to exit through the distal wound.

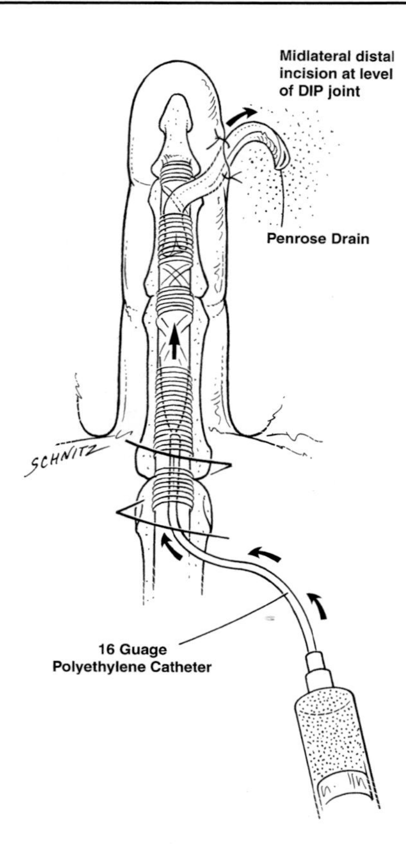

Figure 36.9. Diagram of an indwelling catheter in the proximal tendon sheath and a small drain placed distally through a limited incision, as advocated by Neviaser.

tain the wrist in slight extension and the digits in the intrinsic plus position. An arm-elevating device is applied before the patient leaves the operating room.

POSTOPERATIVE MANAGEMENT

Strict elevation of the hand is maintained postoperatively, and frequent neurocirculatory checks are ordered for the first 24 hours. Adequate pain management is essential and is facilitated by the use of nonsteroidal anti-inflammatory agents in addition to narcotics.

The operative dressing is removed on the first postoperative day when wound care and supervised therapy are initiated.

Prolonged intravenous antibiotic therapy is not necessary if the patient progresses as anticipated. Hospital discharge on oral antibiotics can often be accomplished by 48 to 72 hours postoperatively, at which time culture and sensitivity results can be used to guide therapy. Hospital stays may be prolonged in cases of severe or neglected infection or when caring for immunocompromised or untrustworthy patients.

REHABILITATION

The patient washes the affected hand under clean running water in the sink or shower using a mild soap three times daily. The lightest possible dry dressing that does not interfere with digital motion is applied.

The instruction and supervision of a knowledgeable hand therapist are essential. Daily therapy may be necessary for the first week or two. It is especially helpful if the same therapist sees the patient regularly so that subtle changes in the clinical course that may indicate recrudescence of infection are appreciated early.

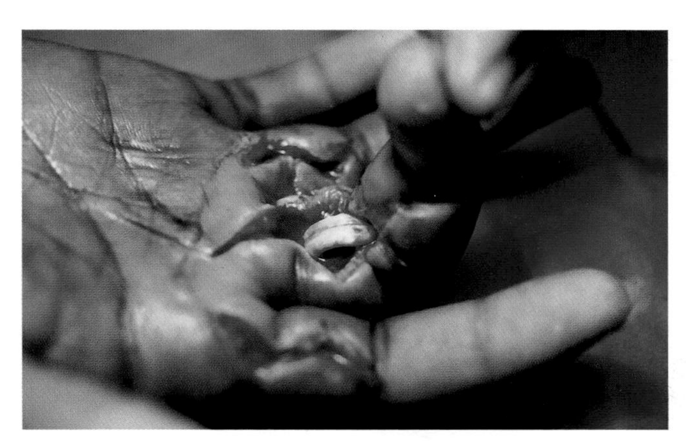

Figure 36.10. Note that passive flexion of this edematous infected finger causes the flexor tendon to bunch up in the wound and produces no gliding beneath the proximal pulleys. The tendon cannot be pushed through the sheath; it must be pulled. Active motion is necessary to produce tendon gliding in these circumstances.

The mainstay of therapy after flexor tendon sheath infection is active assisted digital range of motion. Passive motion may help to avoid joint contracture, but only active motion can move edematous tendons through the digital pulleys and help to restore and maintain the gliding surfaces that are crucial to hand function (Fig. 36.10). Active motion is also essential to promote wound drainage. A wrist support is often helpful to allow the patient to concentrate his efforts at active flexion of the fingers. Without proximal splinting, a good deal of such effort is often wasted on dysfunctional flexion posturing of the wrist that limits the flexion power applied to the digits. In rare instances, a metacarpophalangeal joint flexion block splint may help the patient to maximize critical PIP joint motion. Impending digital joint contractures will usually respond to static night splinting.

Following wound healing, scar management and desensitization can be performed if necessary, but well-placed incisions seldom require such long-term care. The most important role of the therapist often proves to be in educating patients to assume increasing responsibility for their own care and enabling them to move early and actively despite the natural reluctance to do so based on pain and the appearance of the hand.

RESULTS

Outcomes following the treatment of flexor tendon sheath infections are as variable as the infections themselves and the patients who present with them. An otherwise healthy patient with suppurative tenosynovitis caused by *Staphylococcus aureus,* who presents for treatment within 24 hours of sustaining a penetrating wound and has slightly cloudy fluid in the tendon sheath at the time of surgery, will have nearly normal range of motion within 1 week and healed wounds in about twice that time (Fig. 36.11). A diabetic patient with a polymicrobial infection who presents after 96 hours of progressive digital pain and swelling, who is noted to have thick purulence within the sheath and softening of the tendons, may ultimately require digital amputation to control infection.

Most large series of hand infections in the literature emanate from urban centers that treat large numbers of uninsured and indigent patients who have limited access to health care, present late for treatment, and often do not return for follow-up. The findings of these studies are remarkably consistent, with 3% to 10% of patients requiring more than one operation to control their infection, and nearly the same rate of amputation. These numbers probably do not reflect expectations in a community hospital setting, where the great majority of patients would be anticipated to recover nearly normal range of motion and a small number would sustain modest limitations of motion. Of greatest concern is the severity of

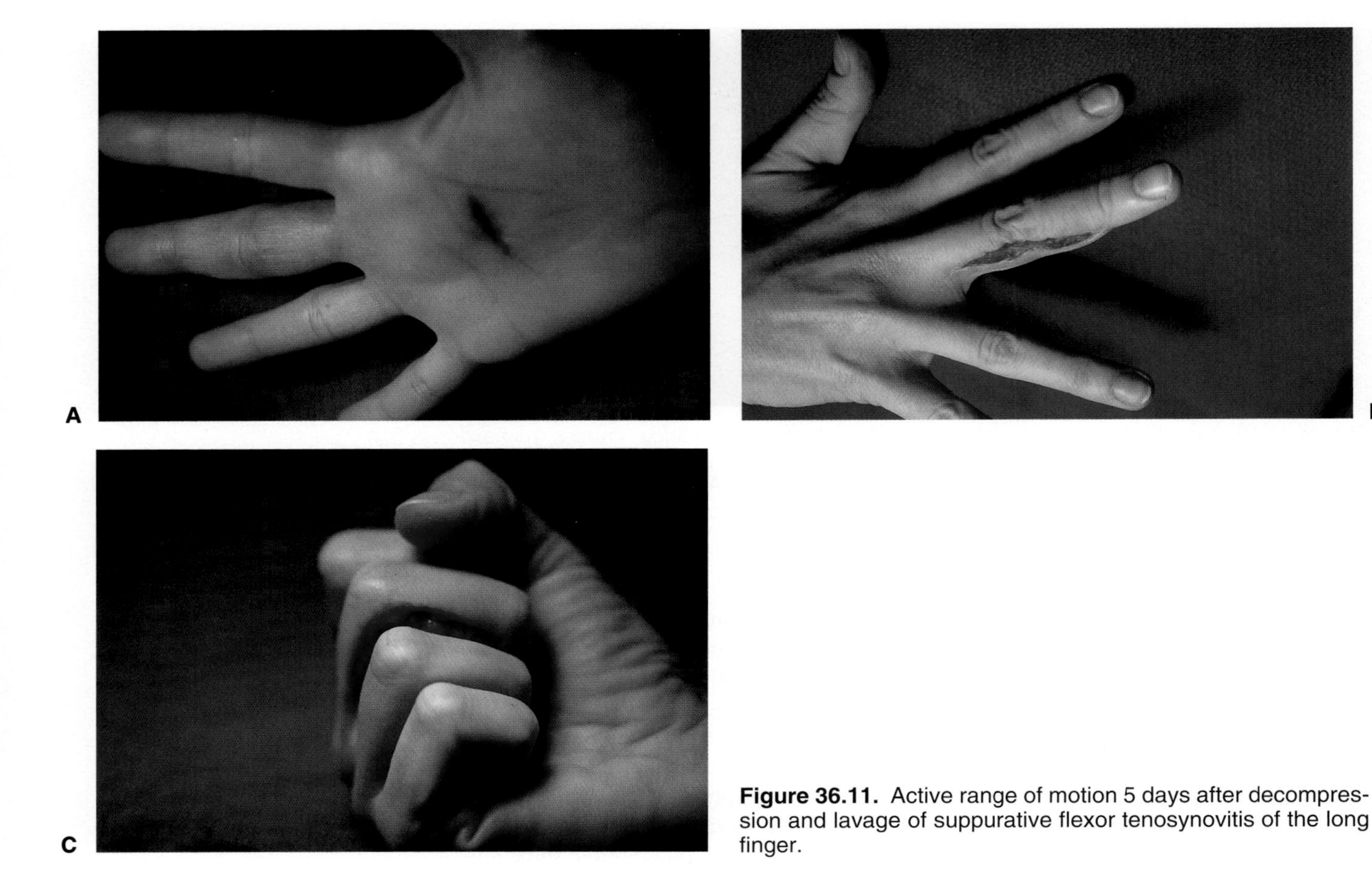

Figure 36.11. Active range of motion 5 days after decompression and lavage of suppurative flexor tenosynovitis of the long finger.

infection in the diabetic or immunocompromised host who may be encountered in any health care venue. Amputation rates of 40% to 60% are frequently reported in diabetic patients, and one study demonstrated a 100% amputation rate in 10 diabetic renal transplant patients.

The commonly reported risk factors for poor outcome include the following:

- infection in an immunocompromised host,
- presentation for treatment delayed by more than 48 hours,
- Gram-negative or anaerobic infection,
- infection involving the tendon sheath, joint, or bone, and
- spread of infection to adjacent closed spaces in the hand.

Unfortunately, the treating physician can control none of these factors.

COMPLICATIONS

The generally reported complications that follow the treatment of flexor tendon sheath infections include those enumerated above: loss of motion, the need for repeated operations to control infection, and amputation. These often reflect the severity of infection rather than the result of the treatment.

Of more concern are complications that result from avoidable errors in treatment. The foremost of these is a delay in surgical treatment while antibiotics are administered. One study noted that delay in treatment beyond the 48 hours that frequently distinguishes good

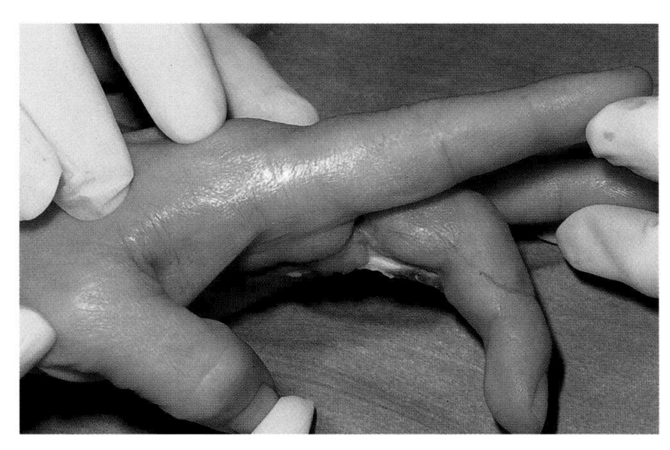

Figure 36.12. A Bruner incision was used to drain this infected flexor tendon sheath. The infection has resolved, but partial necrosis of the palmar skin flaps has left the tendon exposed and desiccated. Ray amputation was performed to salvage the function of this hand.

from bad results was most often attributable to the doctor. Only the very earliest of suspected tendon sheath infections should be considered for treatment with antibiotics alone, and this course of action should be re-evaluated and altered if dramatic improvement is not seen in 12 to 24 hours. In cases of hand infection, errors of commission (operating on a finger that may not have required surgical decompression and lavage) are far less costly than errors of omission (delaying surgery in the presence of closed space infection).

Other avoidable complications include skin loss and tendon necrosis resulting from the use of palmar digital incisions. Although the underlying infection is adequately controlled, the use of palmar incisions may result in partial flap loss, tendon desiccation, and necrosis, ultimately necessitating amputation (Fig. 36.12). Bruner incisions should never be used when infection is suspected to avoid this potential complication.

RECOMMENDED READING

1. Boles SD, Schmidt CC. Pyogenic flexor tenosynovitis. *Hand Clinics* 14:567–587, 1998.
2. Francel TJ, Marshall KA, Savage RC. Hand infections in the diabetic and the diabetic renal transplant recipient. *Ann Plast Surg* 24:304–309, 1990.
3. Glass KD. Factors related to the resolution of treated hand infections. *J Hand Surg* 7A:388–394, 1982.
4. Juliano PJ, Eglseder WA. Limited open-tendon-sheath irrigation in the treatment of pyogenic flexor tenosynovitis. *Orthop Rev* 20:1065–1069, 1991.
5. Kanavel AB. *Infections of the Hand.* 7th ed. Philadelphia: Lea and Febiger, 1943.
6. Lille S, Hayakawa T, Neumeister MW, et al. Continuous postoperative catheter irrigation is not necessary for the treatment of suppurative flexor tenosynovitis. *J Hand Surg* 25B:304–307, 2000.
7. Monstrey SJM, Van Der Werken C, Kauer JMG, et al. Tendon sheath infections of the hand. *Neth J Surg* 37:174–178, 1985.
8. Neviaser RJ. Closed tendon sheath irrigation for pyogenic flexor tenosynovitis. *J Hand Surg* 3A:462–466, 1978.
9. Schnall SB, Vu-Rose T, Holtom PD, et al. Tissue pressures in pyogenic flexor tenosynovitis of the finger: compartment syndrome and its management. *J Bone Joint Surg* 78B:793–795, 1996.
10. Stern PJ, Staneck JL, McDonough JJ. Established hand infections: a controlled, prospective study. *J Hand Surg* 8A:553–559, 1983.

Index

R